Methods in Molecular Biology

Series Editor
John M. Walker
School of Life and Medical Sciences
University of Hertfordshire
Hatfield, Hertfordshire, AL10 9AB, UK

For further volumes:
http://www.springer.com/series/7651

Rational Drug Design

Methods and Protocols

Edited by

Thomas Mavromoustakos and Tahsin F. Kellici

Division of Organic Chemistry, Department of Chemistry, National and Kapodistrian University of Athens, Panepistimiopolis, Zografou, Athens, Greece

Humana Press

Editors
Thomas Mavromoustakos
Division of Organic Chemistry
Department of Chemistry
National and Kapodistrian
University of Athens
Panepistimiopolis, Zografou
Athens, Greece

Tahsin F. Kellici
Division of Organic Chemistry
Department of Chemistry
National and Kapodistrian
University of Athens
Panepistimiopolis, Zografou
Athens, Greece

ISSN 1064-3745 ISSN 1940-6029 (electronic)
Methods in Molecular Biology
ISBN 978-1-4939-8629-3 ISBN 978-1-4939-8630-9 (eBook)
https://doi.org/10.1007/978-1-4939-8630-9

Library of Congress Control Number: 2018948185

Printed on acid-free paper

This Humana Press imprint is published by the registered company Springer Science+Business Media, LLC part of Springer Nature.
The registered company address is: 233 Spring Street, New York, NY 10013, U.S.A.

Preface

As you set out on the way to Ithaca
hope that the road is a long one,
filled with adventures, filled with discoveries.
The Laestrygonians and the Cyclopes,
Poseidon in his anger: do not fear them, . . .
And if you find her poor, Ithaca didn't deceive you.
As wise as you will have become, with so much experience,
you will understand, by then, these Ithacas; what they mean.

C. P. Cavafy
Translated by Daniel Mendelsohn

What excites us as guest editors in the rational drug design is the decision of beginning a trip toward Ithaca that can lead to the liberation from the thefts that steal our health. This trip that involves Laestrygonians and Cyclops is exciting and adventure. We do not mind if our Ithaca did not fill our expectations. We become mature and happy as we discover new avenues for reaching a new Ithaca. The rational drug design is an Odyssey that never ends and this is the essence of life.

This volume of Methods in Molecular Biology covers several aspects of rational drug design. Such aspects include (a) synthesis of novel bioactive drugs; (b) development and application of new methodologies to tackle problems related to discovery of potent molecules; (c) comprehend on concepts strictly related to the bioactivity, i.e., lipophilicity; (d) development and application of computational methods valuable toward the establishment of new approaches in the Ithaca trip of drug discovery; and (e) the effects of physicochemical and ADMET properties of the designed potential drugs.

Hereby is given an outline of the chapters covered in the volume. The first three chapters are dedicated to the design of peptides and peptidomimetics targeting the amyloid deposits and multiple sclerosis. Chapter 4 offers applications and comprehends on saturation transfer difference (STD) NMR in the mapping of the protein-ligand interface. In the fifth chapter the performance of docking tools is assessed. The use of structural biology in drug design is reviewed in the sixth chapter. Chapter 7 introduces new essential cheminformatic tools in ligand-based drug design. In Chapter 8 a thorough method of bioguided design of trypanosomicidal compounds is explained. The use of hybrid screening protocols is given in Chapter 9. Chapter 10 explains a novel method for the determination of unlabeled compound kinetics using the technique of time-resolved fluorescence resonance energy transfer. The new computational method of dynamic undocking is introduced in Chapter 11. The importance of lipophilicity in drug discovery is explained in Chapter 12. Chapters 13 and 14 explore the polypharmacology and the development of nuclear receptor modulators. An extensible orthogonal protocol that combines structure-based and ligand-based screening tools is introduced in Chapter 15. In Chapter 16 the synthesis of various adamantane derivatives with σ-receptor affinity is described. Examples of supervised molecular dynamics approaches are reviewed in Chapter 17. In Chapter 18 the synergistic action of biomolecular NMR methodologies is explained. Chapter 19 introduces the use of the dynamic and in silico pharmacophore approach in drug discovery. Chapters 20 and 21 deal with the rational design of inhibitors targeting MAGL and methyllysine reader protein spindlin1. The design of natural product hybrids bearing triple antiplatelet profile is described in Chapter 22. Pharmacophore generation using phase is explained in Chapter 23. The design of inhibitors targeting histone deacetylases by filtering through ADMET, physicochemical and ligand-target flexibility properties is provided in Chapter 24. The occurrence of reactions in NMR tubes that may lead to new drug leads is explored in Chapter 25. The two last chapters deal with the angiotensin II type 1 receptor (AT1R). Chapter 26 provides the application of structure-based methods to develop new antagonists of the receptor, while Chapter 27 explores the importance homology modeling played in the case of AT1R.

This book, as can be understood from the analysis of its contents, was made possible through the generous contributions of many scientists, who shared their knowledge, for which we are very grateful. We are also sincerely grateful to the series editor, Professor John Walker, for his help, advice, and patient guidance in preparing this volume.

Athens, Greece

Thomas Mavromoustakos
Tahsin F. Kellici

Contents

Contributors

Antreas Afantitis • *NovaMechanics Ltd., Nicosia, Cyprus*
Busecan Aksoydan • *Department of Biophysics, Computational Biology and Molecular Simulations Laboratory, School of Medicine, Bahcesehir University, Istanbul, Turkey*
Guzmán Ignacio Álvarez Touron • *Laboratorio de Moléculas Bioactivas, CENUR Litoral Norte, Universidad de la República, Paysandú, CP, Uruguay*
Andrew Anighoro • *Department of Life Science Informatics, B-IT, LIMES Program Unit Chemical Biology and Medicinal Chemistry, Rheinische Friedrich-Wilhelms-Universität, Bonn, Germany*
Jürgen Bajorath • *Department of Life Science Informatics, B-IT, LIMES Program Unit Chemical Biology and Medicinal Chemistry, Rheinische Friedrich-Wilhelms-Universität, Bonn, Germany*
Flavio Ballante • *Department of Biochemistry and Molecular Biophysics, Washington University School of Medicine, Saint Louis, MO, USA; Department of Cell and Molecular Biology, Uppsala Biomedicinska Centrum BMC, Uppsala University, Uppsala, Sweden*
Xavier Barril • *Institut de Biomedicina de la Universitat de Barcelona (IBUB) and Facultat de Farmàcia, Universitat de Barcelona, Barcelona, Spain; Catalan Institution for Research and Advanced Studies (ICREA), Passeig Lluís Companys 23, Barcelona, Spain*
Martiniano Bello • *Laboratorio de Modelado Molecular, Bioinformática y Diseño de Fármacos, de la Escuela Superior de Medicina, Instituto Politécnico Nacional, Plan de San Luis y Díaz Mirón s/n, Col. Casco de Santo Tomas, Delegación Miguel Hidalgo, C.P., Ciudad de México, Mexico*
Anirban Bhunia • *Department of Biophysics, Bose Institute, Kolkata, India*
Maria Birkou • *Department of Pharmacy, University of Patras, Patras, Greece*
Jeffrey R. Brender • *Radiation Biology Branch, National Cancer Institute, National Institutes of Health, Bethesda, MD, USA*
Isabella Caligiuri • *Division of Experimental and Clinical Pharmacology, Department of Molecular Biology and Translational Research, National Cancer Institute and Center for Molecular Biomedicine, IRCCS, Pordenone, Italy*
Steven J. Charlton • *School of Life Science, Queen's Medical Centre, University of Nottingham, Nottingham, UK*
Maria V. Chatziathanasiadou • *Section of Organic Chemistry and Biochemistry, Department of Chemistry, University of Ioannina, Ioannina, Greece*
Magda S. Chegkazi • *Institute of Biology, Medicinal Chemistry and Biotechnology, National Hellenic Research Foundation, Athens, Greece; Faculty of Life Sciences and Medicine, Randall Centre for Cell and Molecular Biophysics, King's College London, London, UK*
Evangelia D. Chrysina • *Institute of Biology, Medicinal Chemistry and Biotechnology, National Hellenic Research Foundation, Athens, Greece*
Jose Correa-Basurto • *Laboratorio de Modelado Molecular, Bioinformática y Diseño de Fármacos, de la Escuela Superior de Medicina, Instituto Politécnico Nacional, Plan de San Luis y Díaz Mirón s/n, Col. Casco de Santo Tomas, Delegación Miguel Hidalgo, C.P., Ciudad de México, Mexico*

RUEL Z. B. DESAMERO • *Department of Chemistry, York College and The Institute for Macromolecular Assemblies, Jamaica, NY, USA; Ph.D. Programs in Chemistry and Biochemistry, The Graduate Center of the City University of New York, New York, NY, USA*

SERDAR DURDAGI • *Department of Biophysics, Computational Biology and Molecular Simulations Laboratory, School of Medicine, Bahcesehir University, Istanbul, Turkey*

YOUNESS ELKHOU • *Department of Chemistry, York College and The Institute for Macromolecular Assemblies, Jamaica, NY, USA; Ph.D. Programs in Chemistry and Biochemistry, The Graduate Center of the City University of New York, New York, NY, USA*

LEIF A. ERIKSSON • *Department of Chemistry and Molecular Biology, University of Gothenburg, Gothenburg, Sweden*

ISMAIL EROL • *Department of Biophysics, Computational Biology and Molecular Simulations Laboratory, School of Medicine, Bahcesehir University, Istanbul, Turkey*

ANIRBAN GHOSH • *Department of Biophysics, Bose Institute, Kolkata, India*

CONSTANTINOS GIAGINIS • *Department of Food Science and Nutrition, School of Environment, University of the Aegean, Myrina, Lemnos, Greece*

CARLOTTA GRANCHI • *Department of Pharmacy, University of Pisa, Pisa, Italy*

ISIK KANTARCIOGLU • *Department of Biophysics, Computational Biology and Molecular Simulations Laboratory, School of Medicine, Bahcesehir University, Istanbul, Turkey*

TAHSIN F. KELLICI • *Division of Organic Chemistry, Department of Chemistry, National and Kapodistrian University of Athens, Panepistimiopolis, Zografou, Athens, Greece*

ANTONIOS KOLOCOURIS • *Department of Pharmacy, National and Kapodistrian University of Athens, Panepistimiopolis, Zografou, Athens, Greece*

ATHINA KONSTANTINIDI • *Department of Pharmacy, National and Kapodistrian University of Athens, Panepistimiopolis, Zografou, Athens, Greece*

JANARTHANAN KRISHNAMOORTHY • *Department of Biosciences, Jimma University, Jimma, ET, USA*

PANAGIOTIS LAGARIAS • *Department of Pharmacy, National and Kapodistrian University of Athens, Panepistimiopolis, Zografou, Athens, Greece*

GEORGE LAMBRINIDIS • *Department of Pharmacy, National and Kapodistrian University of Athens, Panepistimiopolis, Zografou, Athens, Greece*

THIERRY LANGER • *Faculty of Life Sciences, Department of Pharmaceutical Chemistry, University of Vienna, Vienna, Austria*

CHIARA LUISE • *Department of Pharmaceutical Chemistry, Martin-Luther University of Halle-Wittenberg, Halle/Saale, Germany*

MARCO MACCHIA • *Department of Pharmacy, University of Pisa, Pisa, Italy*

MACIEJ MAJEWSKI • *Institut de Biomedicina de la Universitat de Barcelona (IBUB) and Facultat de Farmàcia, Universitat de Barcelona, Barcelona, Spain*

MICHAEL MAMAIS • *Institute of Biology, Medicinal Chemistry and Biotechnology, National Hellenic Research Foundation, Athens, Greece*

KONSTANTINOS D. MAROUSIS • *Department of Pharmacy, University of Patras, Patras, Greece*

ADRIANO MARTINELLI • *Department of Pharmacy, University of Pisa, Pisa, Italy*

MARLET MARTÍNEZ-ARCHUNDIA • *Laboratorio de Modelado Molecular, Bioinformática y Diseño de Fármacos, de la Escuela Superior de Medicina, Instituto Politécnico Nacional, Plan de San Luis y Díaz Mirón s/n, Col. Casco de Santo Tomas, Delegación Miguel Hidalgo, C.P., Ciudad de México, Mexico*

MINOS-TIMOTHEOS MATSOUKAS • *Department of Pharmacy, University of Patras, Patras, Greece*
THOMAS MAVROMOUSTAKOS • *Division of Organic Chemistry, Department of Chemistry, National and Kapodistrian University of Athens, Panepistimiopolis, Zografou, Athens, Greece*
GEORGIA MELAGRAKI • *NovaMechanics Ltd., Nicosia, Cyprus*
DANIEL MERK • *Institute of Pharmaceutical Chemistry, Goethe University Frankfurt, Frankfurt, Germany*
EMMANUEL MIKROS • *Department of Pharmacy, National and Kapodistrian University of Athens, Panepistimiopolis Zografou, Athens, Greece; "Athena" Research and Innovation Center, Athens, Greece*
FILIPPO MINUTOLO • *Department of Pharmacy, University of Pisa, Pisa, Italy*
STEFANO MORO • *Molecular Modeling Section (MMS), Department of Pharmaceutical and Pharmacological Sciences, University of Padova, Padova, Italy*
VASSILIOS MYRIANTHOPOULOS • *Department of Pharmacy, National and Kapodistrian University of Athens, Panepistimiopolis Zografou, Athens, Greece; "Athena" Research and Innovation Center, Athens, Greece*
SPYRIDON NIKOLAKOPOULOS • *NovaMechanics Ltd., Nicosia, Cyprus*
DIMITRIOS NTOUNTANIOTIS • *Department of Chemistry, Laboratory of Organic Chemistry, National and Kapodistrian University of Athens, Athens, Greece*
ALESSANDRO PADOVA • *Computer-Aided Drug Design Group, Fondazione Ri.MED, Palermo, Italy*
IOANNIS PAPANASTASIOU • *School of Health Sciences, Department of Pharmacy, Division of Pharmaceutical Chemistry, National and Kapodistrian University of Athens, Panepistimiopolis—Zografou, Athens, Greece*
UGO PERRICONE • *Computer-Aided Drug Design Group, Fondazione Ri.MED, Palermo, Italy*
ADAM A. PROFIT • *Department of Chemistry, York College and The Institute for Macromolecular Assemblies, Jamaica, NY, USA; Ph.D. Programs in Chemistry and Biochemistry, The Graduate Center of the City University of New York, New York, NY, USA*
FLAVIO RIZZOLIO • *Division of Experimental and Clinical Pharmacology, Department of Molecular Biology and Translational Research, National Cancer Institute and Center for Molecular Biomedicine, IRCCS, Pordenone, Italy; Department of Molecular Science and Nanosystems, Ca' Foscari Università di Venezia, Venezia-Mestre, Italy*
DINA ROBAA • *Department of Pharmaceutical Chemistry, Martin-Luther University of Halle-Wittenberg, Halle/Saale, Germany*
SERGIO RUIZ-CARMONA • *Institut de Biomedicina de la Universitat de Barcelona (IBUB) and Facultat de Farmàcia, Universitat de Barcelona, Barcelona, Spain*
DAVIDE SABBADIN • *Syngenta Crop Protection AG, Stein, Switzerland*
PATRICIA SAENZ-MÉNDEZ • *Department of Chemistry and Molecular Biology, University of Gothenburg, Gothenburg, Sweden; Computational Chemistry and Biology Group, Facultad de Química, UdelaR, Montevideo, Uruguay*
VERONICA SALMASO • *Molecular Modeling Section (MMS), Department of Pharmaceutical and Pharmacological Sciences, University of Padova, Padova, Italy*
SIMONE SCHIERLE • *Institute of Pharmaceutical Chemistry, Goethe University Frankfurt, Frankfurt, Germany*

THOMAS SEIDEL • *Faculty of Life Sciences, Department of Pharmaceutical Chemistry, University of Vienna, Vienna, Austria*
ANASTASIA I. SOTIROPOULOU • *Institute of Biology, Medicinal Chemistry and Biotechnology, National Hellenic Research Foundation, Athens, Greece*
GEORGIOS A. SPYROULIAS • *Department of Pharmacy, University of Patras, Patras, Greece*
MATTIA STURLESE • *Molecular Modeling Section (MMS), Department of Pharmaceutical and Pharmacological Sciences, University of Padova, Padova, Italy*
EVGENIOS K. STYLOS • *Section of Organic Chemistry and Biochemistry, Department of Chemistry, University of Ioannina, Ioannina, Greece; Biotechnology Laboratory, Department of Biological Applications and Technology, University of Ioannina, Ioannina, Greece*
DAVID A. SYKES • *School of Life Science, Queen's Medical Centre, University of Nottingham, Nottingham, UK*
ANNA TSANTILI-KAKOULIDOU • *Department of Pharmaceutical Chemistry, Faculty of Pharmacy, National and Kapodistrian University of Athens, Panepistimiopolis, Zografou, Athens, Greece*
ALEXANDROS D. TSELEPIS • *Atherothrombosis Research Centre/Laboratory of Biochemistry, Department of Chemistry, University of Ioannina, Ioannina, Greece*
THEODORE TSELIOS • *Department of Chemistry, University of Patras, Patras, Greece*
ANTONIS TSIAILANIS • *Section of Organic Chemistry and Biochemistry, Department of Chemistry, University of Ioannina, Ioannina, Greece*
AIKATERINI C. TSIKA • *Department of Pharmacy, University of Patras, Patras, Greece*
FOTIOS TSOPELAS • *Laboratory of Inorganic and Analytical Chemistry, School of Chemical Engineering, National Technical University of Athens, Athens, Greece*
MARIA TSOUMANI • *Atherothrombosis Research Centre/Laboratory of Biochemistry, Department of Chemistry, University of Ioannina, Ioannina, Greece*
ANDREAS TSOUMANIS • *NovaMechanics Ltd., Nicosia, Cyprus*
TIZIANO TUCCINARDI • *Department of Pharmacy, University of Pisa, Pisa, Italy*
ANDREAS G. TZAKOS • *Section of Organic Chemistry and Biochemistry, Department of Chemistry, University of Ioannina, Ioannina, Greece*
HARALAMBOS TZOUPIS • *Department of Chemistry, University of Patras, Patras, Greece*
DIMITRA-DANAI VARSOU • *NovaMechanics Ltd., Nicosia, Cyprus*
JAYSON VEDAD • *Department of Chemistry, York College and The Institute for Macromolecular Assemblies, Jamaica, NY, USA; Ph.D. Programs in Chemistry and Biochemistry, The Graduate Center of the City University of New York, New York, NY, USA*
ELENI VRONTAKI • *Department of Pharmacy, National and Kapodistrian University of Athens, Panepistimiopolis Zografou, Athens, Greece*
MARCUS WIEDER • *Faculty of Life Sciences, Department of Pharmaceutical Chemistry, University of Vienna, Vienna, Austria; Faculty of Chemistry, Department of Computational Biological Chemistry, University of Vienna, Vienna, Austria*

Chapter 1

Molecular Dynamics Simulations on the Bioactive Molecule of hIAPP22–29 (NFGAILSS) and Rational Drug Design

Panagiotis Lagarias, Youness Elkhou, Jayson Vedad, Athina Konstantinidi, Adam A. Profit, Tahsin F. Kellici, Antonios Kolocouris, Ruel Z. B. Desamero, and Thomas Mavromoustakos

Abstract

This chapter includes information about the structure in equilibrium of the bioactive molecule hIAPP22–29 (NFGAILSS). The experimental structure was derived using X-ray and its 2D NOESY NMR experiments in d_6-DMSO and d-HFIP solvents. This molecule contains eight of the ten amino acids of the 20–29 region of the human islet amyloid polypeptide (hIAPP) often referred as the "amyloidogenic core." Amyloid deposits are well-known to cause as many as 20 pathological neurodegenerative disorders such as Alzheimer, Parkinson, Huntington, and Creutzfeldt-Jakob. The experimental structure was relaxed using molecular dynamics (MD) in simulation boxes consisting in DMSO and HFIP; the latter not provided by the applied software. The calculations were performed in GPUs and supercomputers, and some basic scripting is described for reference. The simulations confirmed the inter- and intramolecular forces that led to an "amyloidogenic core" observed from NOE experiments. The results showed that in DMSO and HFIP environment, Phe is not in spatial proximity with Leu or Ile, and this is consistent with an amyloidogenic core. However, in an amphipathic environment such as the model lipid bilayers, this communication is possible and may influence peptide amyloidogenic properties. The knowledge gained through this study may contribute to the rational drug design of novel peptides or organic molecules acting by modifying preventing amyloidogenic properties of the hIAPP peptide.

Key words hIAPP22–29, Aggregation of proteins, Molecular dynamics, NMR, Amyloids

1 Introduction

The aggregation of proteins into structures known as amyloids is observed in many neurodegenerative diseases, including Alzheimer disease. Amyloids are composed of pairs of tightly interacting, stranded, and repetitive intermolecular β-sheets, which form the cross-β-sheet structure. This structure enables amyloids to grow by recruitment of the same protein, and its repetition can transform a weak biological activity into a potent one through cooperativity and avidity. Amyloids therefore have the potential to self-replicate and

Thomas Mavromoustakos and Tahsin F. Kellici (eds.), *Rational Drug Design: Methods and Protocols*, Methods in Molecular Biology, vol. 1824, https://doi.org/10.1007/978-1-4939-8630-9_1, © Springer Science+Business Media, LLC, part of Springer Nature 2018

can adapt to the environment, yielding cell-to-cell transmissibility, prion infectivity, and toxicity [1].

Due to the enormous conformational space of the full-length protein and the limitations of computational algorithms and capacity, the aggregation as an example of protein folding has not been understood yet. Therefore, the folding and aggregation mechanism of full-length proteins is studied using short fragments as models with key amino acid sequences which have been reported to form fibrils and cause toxicity in vitro. For this reason, the 20–29 region of the human islet amyloid polypeptide (hIAPP) is often referred as the amyloidogenic core. Amyloid deposits are well known to cause as many as 20 pathological neurodegenerative disorders such as Alzheimer, Parkinson, Huntington, and Creutzfeldt-Jakob [2–4]. The shorter peptide hIAPP22–29 (NFGAILSS) is still capable of aggregating into amyloid fibrils [5, 6] (Fig. 1a).

Several studies reported a β-strand formation of key amino acid sequences that may play an important role in the aggregation process. For example, Chakraborty et al. studied the amyloidogenic structure of hIAPP peptide (19–27) [7]. They illustrated a four-residue turn spanning (22–25) adopting preferentially helix-coil and extended β-hairpin. Residues 17, 22, and 23 are found to play an important role in amyloid formation. Mo et al. investigated the structural diversity of the soluble peptide trimmer of hIAPP20–29 by MD simulations. The amorphous trimmer in room temperature contains a central structural amino acid residue part FGAIL (23–27) capable of forming interpeptide β-sheets and antiparallel β-strands with higher propensity than parallel β-strands [8].

Cao et al. performed MD simulations for the NFGAILSS motif of hIAPP associated with the type 2 diabetes. They found that the stability of an IAPP22–28 oligomer was not only related with its size but also with its morphology. The driving forces to form and stabilize the oligomers are the hydrophobic effects and backbone H-bond interactions. The simulations indicate that IAPP22–28 peptides tend to form an antiparallel strand orientation within the sheet [9]. Crystal structures of IAPP amyloidogenic segments revealed a novel packing of out-of-register β-sheets [9, 10]. Comprehensive studies have been performed to examine the effect of electron donating and withdrawing groups along with heteroaromatic surrogates at position 23 (F) of the hIAPP22–29 to interrogate how π-electron distribution affects amyloid formation [11–13].

In an attempt to understand the first principles underlying the possibility of this peptide to form closed structures, NFGAILSS was synthesized, and its conformational properties are studied in the well-dissolved d_6-DMSO and *d*-HFIP using NMR spectroscopy and in silico using molecular dynamics (MD) in the former environments and 1-palmitoyl-2-oleoyl-*sn*-glycero-3-phosphocholine (POPC) bilayers. These bilayers simulate the cellular membranes involved in the formation of amyloids. This is a contribution to the

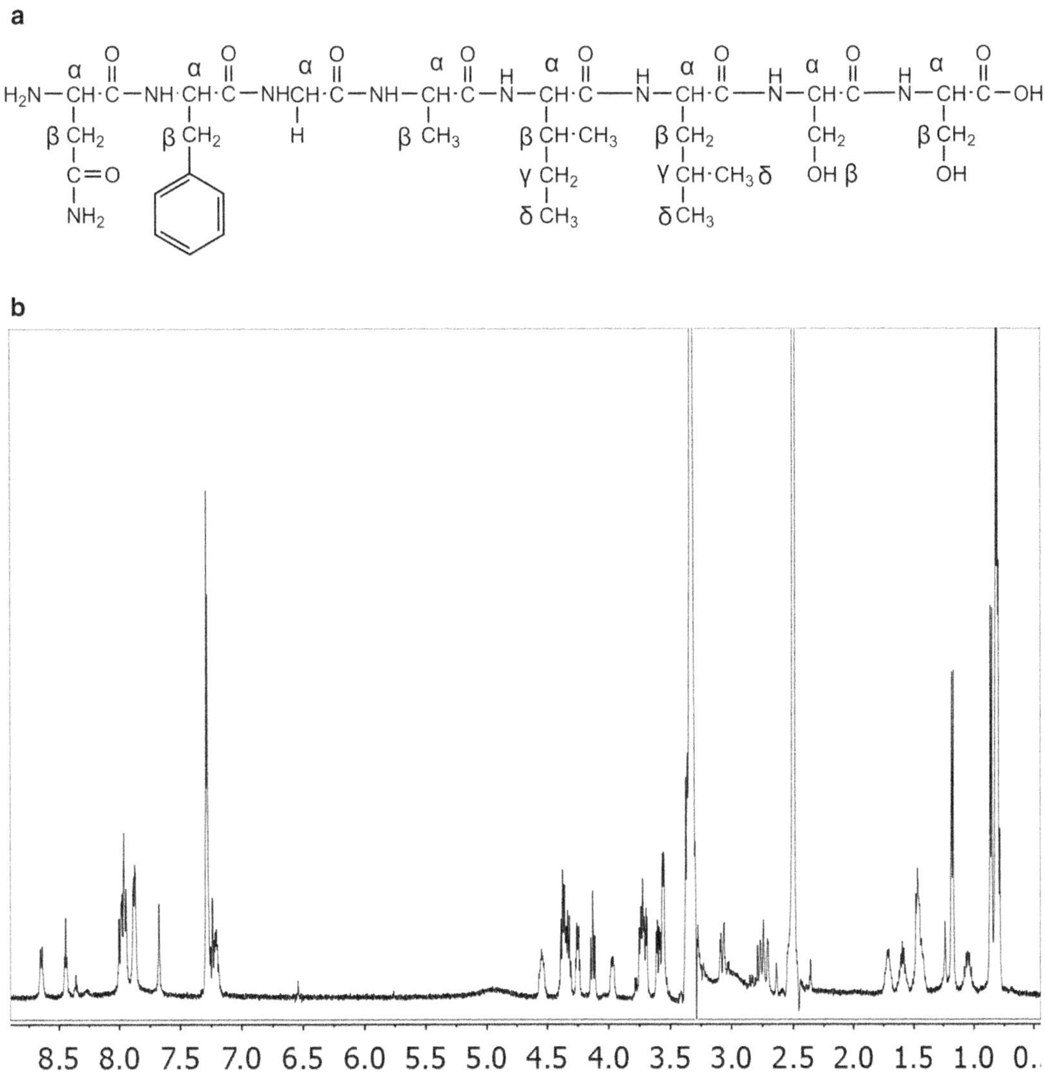

Fig. 1 (**a**) Structure of NFGAILSS; (**b**) 1H NMR spectrum of NFGAILSS run at DMSO-d_6 and using 500 MHz Agilent spectrometer at 25 °C. Through the combination of 2D TOCSY experiment (not shown), all the observed peaks are identified, and the peptide was structurally elucidated. This is an important step before proceeding to conformational studies using 2D NOESY experiments and in silico MD calculations [1]

understanding of intra- and intermolecular forces that govern the peptide NGFAILSS. NMR experiments cannot be directly utilized in lipid bilayers for hIAPP due to the rapid aggregation of the peptide, and studies are restrained in SDS micelles or solid state [14–16].

The understanding of these intra- and intermolecular forces is the driving force for our laboratories to design and synthesize novel peptide derivatives that might lack the ability of aggregation. In this chapter, the in silico MD methodologies will be described giving details for the procedure in ascending complexity systems.

In particular information of the MD simulation on the systems are as follows: (a) NFGAILSS simulated in implicit environment; (b) NFGAILSS simulated in DMSO a solvent existing in Desmond; (c) NFGAILSS simulated in the not common HFIP and not existing in Desmond; and (d) NFGAILSS in POPC bilayers.

2 Materials

For the current tutorial, we have chosen a variety of different versions in order to show that even the older versions seem quite exceptional for several specific purposes. More specifically:

Desmond Maestro, version 2011 or later (for building of the NFGAILSS oligopeptide).

Desmond Maestro, version 2013-1 or later (for energy minimization, system setup, equilibration, molecular dynamics production, and trajectory analysis and visualization).

Access at a high-performance computer cluster (HPC) is needed (for the Subheading 3.2.2 part of the tutorial).

3 Methods

The major emphasis in the chapter is given in the computational analysis using MD simulations. NMR spectroscopy was used as a complementary experimental technique to provide an initial low energy structure to start the in silico MD simulation.

3.1 NMR Spectroscopy

1. 2 mM peptide is dissolved in d_6-DMSO or *d*-HFIP (0.002 g peptide in 1 mL DMSO-d_6 or HFIP-*d*).
2. Tetramethylsilane (TMS) is added as a reference, and the sample is pipetted into a high-precision NMR tube.
3. Spectra are obtained using a 500 MHz Agilent NMR spectrometer using pulse sequence regular parameters stored in the library of the NMR spectrometer.
4. ROESY experiments are run at different mixing times (0.2–2 s) in order to ensure NOE buildups.
5. 2D TOCSY is also run at various spin locks in order to assure the best experimental conditions for observing all the expected correlations.

2D TOCSY experiment was sufficient to assign unequivocally all proton resonances appeared in the ^{1}H NMR spectrum (Fig. 1b). 2D NOESY and ROESY spectra did not provide any additional information in respect to the conformational properties of the molecule. Special care was given in the clustering of the phenyl ring of phenylalanine with the alkyl chains of leucine and isoleucine. No medium- or long-range ROEs are observed between phenylalanine ring and isoleucine or leucine amino acids. As no ROEs have been observed between the other amino acids, it is evident that the peptide adopts an opened conformation.

3.2 MD Simulations

The following steps are applied for the conformational analysis:

1. Building the 3D structure of NFGAILSS. The building of NFGAILSS peptide is achieved using the Maestro program. A table opens, and "grow" is selected and "from fragments" the small rectangle box, named "aminoacids." (Note: The procedure, for more recent Desmond releases, is identical, *see* **Notes 1** and **2**.
2. The various amino acids are presented under the fragments small rectangle box. The amino acid (NFGAILSS) consisting the peptide is chosen for building the peptide. Once all the amino acids have been selected and checked that the fragment matches with the (NFGAILSS), hydrogen atoms are added to complete the structure.
3. Then, the selected application tab located on top of the screen is chosen and scrolled down to macromodel and apply minimization. The "Minimization" tab opens and the parameters are used (Table 1, *see* **Notes 3** and **4**).
4. In the (Potential) tab, the parameters are used (Table 2).

Table 1
Minimization parameters used to obtain low energy structure of NFGAILSS peptide

Method	Optimal
Maximum iterations	10,000
Converge on	Gradient
Convergence threshold	0.05

Table 2
Applied parameters using the potential tab for NFGAILSS peptide

Force field	OPLS_2005
Solvent	None
Changes from	Force field
Cutoff	Extended
Electrostatic treatment	Dielectric constant
Dielectric constant	46

Table 3
MD parameters used for NFGAILSS peptide

Method	Molecular dynamics
Shake	Bond to hydrogen
Simulation temperature (K)	500.0 (used different temperatures)
Time steps (fs)	1.2
Equilibrium time (ps)	1000
Simulation time (ps)	1000

Table 4
MD parameters used in the (mini) tab for NFGAILSS peptide

Method	Optimal
Maximum iterations	10,000
Convergence on	Energy
Convergence threshold	0.05

5. The following MD parameters are used (Table 3).
6. In the (mini) tab, the following parameters are used (Table 4).
7. In the application tab located on top of the screen, scroll down to macromodel, and then click on dynamics. The dynamic window should pop up.
8. In the monitor tab, the number of desirable conformations to be produced by the dynamics experiment is selected, click on minimize sampled structure, and use the already described parameters. The conformations on the project table are processed to generate the desirable conformers. The clustering is performed at the script tab and scrolled down to cheminformatics and selected conformers for cluster, *see* **Notes 5–7**.
9. In the case of using explicit DMSO or HFIP or POPC, the following parameters are used (Table 5).

3.2.1 Desmond-Available Solvents to Run Molecular Dynamics Simulations, Using Either Workstation or High-Performance Computing (HPC)

The most common solvent systems, DMSO, TIP3P, and TIP3P-POPC membrane, are used in this study. The procedure is explained in details.

1. After opening Maestro (Desmond 2013-1 till Desmond 2016-3 Classic Edition GUI), the .mae structure is imported in the structure/directory/path/*.mae. The following utilities are consequentially selected: Protein Preparation Wizard, Assign bond order, Add hydrogens, Remove original hydrogens, Cap termini, and Preprocess button.

Table 5
MD parameters used for NFGAILSS peptide treated with explicit solvents of DMSO or HFIP or POPC

Method	Molecular dynamics
Force field	OPLS_2005
Simulation temperature	300
Time steps (fs)	1.2
Equilibration time (ps)	1200
Simulation time (ps)	50,200
Production class ensemble	NPT
Simulation cutoff	9.0 Angstrom
Recording interval (ps)	1.2
Number of frames	41,833
Thermostat	Nose-Hoover
Barostat	Martyna-Tobias-Klein
Restraints	None
Randomized velocities	None
Equilibration stages	8
Equilibration class ensemble	NVT

2. On the left side of GUI, "also display" → "all hydrogens" is selected, and the structure is checked.
3. The hybridization is selected by clicking on "label all" → atom type (macromodel).
4. Labels are deleted. The preferred tasks are selected as follows: molecular dynamics → system setup → predefined, DMSO; distances, 15.0; force field, OPLS_2005 (or OPLS3 if possible. OPLS3 is not freely available).
5. The box-shape orthorhombic (or cubic) and box size calculation method are used: buffer and press are run. DMSO solvent is detected after some seconds in the Workspace.

3.2.2 System Setup, Using TIP3P

1. Using the same protocol above on stage 5, TIP3P instead of DMSO is pressed.
2. "Setup Membrane" → POPC → (the POPC membrane appears red) and then "adjust membrane" are chosen. The middle mouse button to turn the red membrane barriers to be parallel to our system peptide is used.
3. The "adjust membrane position" and save membrane position → OK. → Run is selected.

As soon as the membrane is presented and the peptide is embedded within the lipid bilayer, the following steps are used:

1. Tasks → molecular dynamics.
2. "Load" is pressed (otherwise, Maestro will not allow you to continue with the next steps).
3. Simulation time used is 50 ns (or 250 ns) or the simulation time you wish.
4. Ensemble class, NPT; temperature, 300 K.
5. Advanced options → output → record velocities.
6. Advanced options → miscellaneous → and "Randomize Velocities" is unclicked, and then "apply" or "OK" is pressed.
7. The reversed triangle next to the cogwheel is chosen, and to run GPU simulation, job settings → host: localhost-gpu → run. To run CPU simulation, the following are chosen:

Job settings → host: localhost, Total: enter number on the "processors" box and "run."

To run the system on a computer cluster (high-performance computer, HPC), **steps 1–7** of the above protocol are applied. At the reversed triangle (next to the cogwheel) → write. The "write" command produces a .cfg, a .cms, and an .msj file. These files should be transferred to your HPC account, using scp command of Linux. To continue, Desmond Maestro should be already installed on your HPC cluster account.

1. A pbs script using a preferred editor is created (vi, emacs, nano, etc.) that needs to include the commands below, depending on the case.
2. CPU MD job is launched:

```
$SCHRODINGER/desmond -LOCAL -WAIT -HOST localhost:number-of-
cpu-cores -JOBNAME <jobname> -c <your>.cfg -in <your>.cms
```

(Files had been produced before, by pressing the "Write" button).

3. CPU MD job is restarted as follows:

```
$SCHRODINGER/desmond -LOCAL -WAIT -JOBNAME <job-continue>
-HOST localhost:<number-of-cores> -restore <jobname>.cpt
```

CPU MD job can be extended as follows:

```
$SCHRODINGER/desmond -LOCAL -WAIT -JOBNAME <job-extension>
-HOST localhost:<number-of-cores> -restore .cpt -cfg mdsim.
last_time=<till-xyz-ns>
```

4. GPU MD job is launched:

```
env SCHRODINGER_CUDA_VISIBLE_DEVICES="0" $SCHRODINGER/utili-
ties/multisim -WAIT -LOCAL -JOBNAME $JOBNAME1 -HOST localhost
-maxjob 1 -cpu 1 -m <your-job>.msj -c <your-job>.cfg <your-
job>.cms -mode umbrella -set 'stage[1].set_family.md.
jlaunch_opt=["-gpu"] -o $JOBNAME1-out.cms &
```

and

```
env SCHRODINGER_CUDA_VISIBLE_DEVICES="1" $SCHRODINGER/utili-
ties/multisim -WAIT -LOCAL -JOBNAME $JOBNAME2 -HOST localhost
-maxjob 1 -cpu 1 -m <your-job>.msj -c <your-job>.cfg <your-
job>.cms -mode umbrella -set 'stage[1].set_family.md.
jlaunch_opt=["-gpu"]' -o $JOBNAME2-out.cms.
```

5. GPU MD job is restarted:

```
env SCHRODINGER_CUDA_VISIBLE_DEVICES="0" $SCHRODINGER/desmond
-JOBNAME job_continue -HOST localhost:1 -gpu -restore jobname.
cpt -in job_continue-in.cms &
```

and

```
env SCHRODINGER_CUDA_VISIBLE_DEVICES="1" $SCHRODINGER/desmond
-JOBNAME job_continue -HOST localhost:1 -gpu -restore jobname.
cpt -in job_continue-in.cms.
```

6. GPU MD job is restarted:

```
env SCHRODINGER_CUDA_VISIBLE_DEVICES="0" $SCHRODINGER/desmond
-JOBNAME job_extend -HOST localhost:1 -gpu -restore job_ex-
tend.cpt -in <your_md_job>.cms -cfg mdsim.last_time=<till-
xyz-ns> &
```

and

```
env SCHRODINGER_CUDA_VISIBLE_DEVICES="0" $SCHRODINGER/desmond
-JOBNAME job_extend -HOST localhost:1 -gpu -restore jobname.cpt
-in job_continue-in.cms -cfg mdsim.last_time=<till-xyz-ns>
```

The following protocol using Desmond Maestro (2013-1 or later version) for the non-common solvent hexafluoroisopropanol -HFIP is applied.

1. A cubic array is created for the solvent.
2. The molecule is imported and the title for the entry is given hexafluoroisopropanol.
3. The "project table" is opened and the entry is selected.
4. The entry is duplicated till 16 entries were created by typing Ctrl+A Ctrl+D (i.e., four times).
5. All entries are selected (Ctrl+A) and included in the Workspace (Ctrl+N).
6. "Tile" is typed in the command line box of Desmond Maestro (i.e., the command input area) in the main window. The entries are placed in a grid in the plane of the Workspace, with new coordinates. (Warning: Do not use the Tile toolbar button, as this button does not change the coordinates but only the display.)
7. In the "project table" panel, all entries are selected, and then right click on "merge." A new entry is created with the molecules from the Workspace. This must be the only selected entry.
8. All entries are deleted, apart from the new one created on stage 7.
9. The "new entry" in the Workspace is chosen and then "view" and "align."
10. The "YZ" plane is selected to align three or more atoms in a plane. "Pick for alignment" is then selected to a plane and then the same atom in three of the molecules. Do *not* pick the same atom in three molecules of the same row/column. For instance, pick two from the first row and one from the second one.
11. "Align" and then "Update Coordinates" are selected. The plane of the "square-slices" of molecules will be rotated, and the coordinates will be updated.
12. The entry is duplicated once with Ctrl+A and Ctrl+D.
13. Stages 5–7 are repeated. One entry with two "square-slices" of molecules is formed.
14. The entry is duplicated with Ctrl+A Ctrl+D, and stages 5–7 are repeated again. Now a single entry with four "square-slices" of HFIP solvent molecules that make up a $4 \times 4 \times 4$ box was created. If not, please delete what you have done so far, and restart the procedure from the beginning, i.e., from stage 1.

For smaller molecules, you should probably double the size of the box, to produce a box with dimensions approximately 30 Å. To achieve this, follow the procedure above from stage 4, using the current entry as the original "molecule." In **step 4**, duplicate the molecule with Ctrl+A Ctrl+D a couple of times in order to create 4 entries only (rather than 16), and stop after stage 13—stage 14 can be omitted (17).

3.2.3 Molecular Dynamics of the HFIP System

Now that the box is created, Desmond can be used to create the solvent model box, as follows:

1. A model system without solvent, ions, or membrane in the system builder panel is created. The "cubic," buffer method for the box dimensions, and a distance of 1.0 (or more if you wish) are used. If the disordered system builder is used, this step is skipped, as the model system is already created.
2. The .cms file is edited and solute is changed to solvent.
3. The "molecular dynamics" option from "tasks" menu is opened.
4. In the "model system," the "import from file" from the option menu was chosen, and the .cms file is imported.
5. Ensemble class "NPT" is used.
6. Relax model system before simulation is selected (click on the "default relaxation" box. If not, the MD will probably fail during stage 4 of relaxation).
7. Simulation time used: 1 ns (but you can use the defaults if you want).
8. The simulation was started by clicking on "Run" button.

When the simulation results are incorporated, a property is added as follows:

1. "Property" and then "Add" are chosen.
2. It was named in the "num_component" and "integer" is typed.
3. "1" within the "Initial value" was added and the "add" was clicked. The internal name of the property must be edited to change the "family."

From Suite 2013-1 on the internal name in Maestro, it can be edited as follows (though editing the file is probably quicker):

1. "Property," "Columns," "Edit Name/Type," and then the property "Num_component" are selected.
2. "Num_component" in the visible name text box is entered, and "edit internal data" is selected.
3. In the "Family option" menu, "other" is selected. Enter "ffio" within the box. Finally, click on "Save Changes."
4. The HFIP solvent entry is exported to a .mae file "... and this .mae file will be used as a custom solvent file."

3.3 Results Summary

As the NMR spectroscopy did not provide any constraints, the molecule is built and minimized using the available minimization algorithms of Schrodinger Maestro until the energy convergence threshold of 0.05 Kcal mol^{-1} was achieved. The minimized structure was subjected to MD simulations using dielectric constant $\varepsilon = 46$ that simulates DMSO environment. The conformers obtained with equal propensity for both the "opened" and the "closed" structure (*see* Fig. 2).

Molecular dynamics experiments in explicit solvent DMSO showed the open structure of the molecule in accordance with NMR data. In 80% of the trajectory, isoleucine and leucine were far away (Fig. 3a) and only 20% were in proximity (Fig. 3b). Phenylalanine was far away from all amino acids and did not have any spatial correlations with isoleucine and leucine in accordance with NMR results.

Details of the clusters generated in the explicit HFIP solvent (not shown for simplicity) are depicted in Fig. 4b. Similar trends are found as with DMSO, and again all these clusters are in accordance with NMR results. The above clusters in the two solvents and NMR results clearly show the following: (a) in a polar environment Leu, Ile, and Phe are not in spatial proximity; (b) the peptide is most of the time in a linear form and when it adopts turns the key three amino acids Leu, Ile, and Phe not in a spatial proximity; and (c) Leu and Ile have a freedom to be far away or in spatial proximity.

MD simulations were applied in a more biologically relevant environment of POPC bilayers. In Fig. 5 are shown four clusters of the peptide (POPC bilayer is not shown for simplicity), and in Fig. 6 a snapshot of the whole system is observed.

NFGAILSS is clearly shown that in vacuum or in a membrane simulating environment can adopt hydrophobic interactions between Phe and Ile or Leu that enhance its ability to aggregate. These interactions are not observed when a polar environment is used as it is shown both experimentally by NMR spectroscopy using the two solvents DMSO or HFIP or MD simulations using the same explicit solvents. This information is valuable for drug design and discovery as it points out that (a) the environment may be decisive to aggregation for the peptide NFGAILSS, (b) the hydrophobic interactions between the key amino acids Phe and Ile or Leu may play a pivotal role in this aggregation, and (c) it provides means of using structural modifications to avoid the undesired aggregation.

4 Notes

1. The chirality of the structure was checked, and it was confirmed that all amino acids bear S configuration.

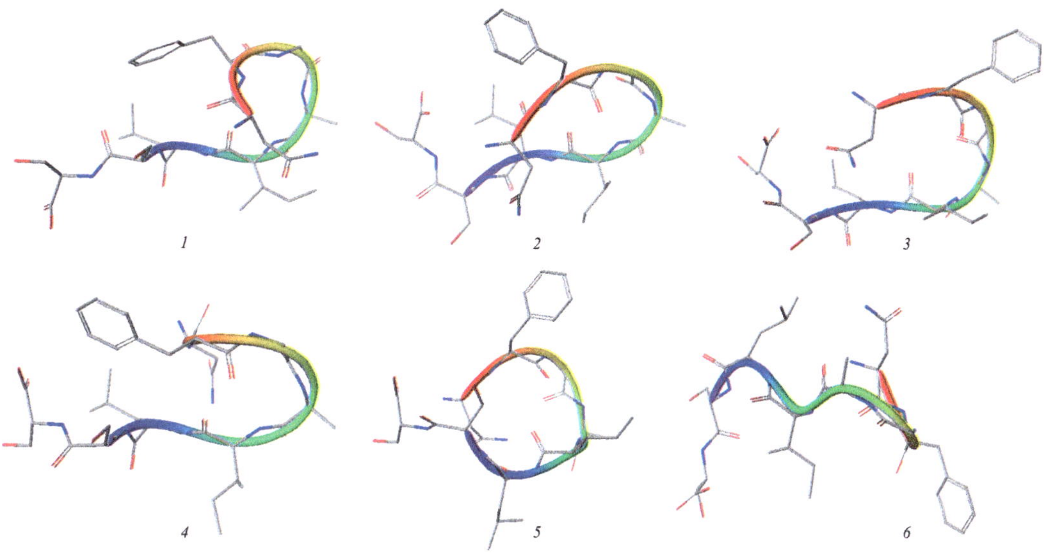

Fig. 2 Six culsters were generated in the implicit DMSO-simulating environments using stochastic MD. In the first cluster (top, left), phenylalanine is clustering with leucine which is on the opposite side. The characteristic of the second cluster (top, middle) is that asparagine and isoleucine are on the same side and leucine is in close proximity with phenylalanine. In the third cluster (top, right), asparagines are in a vicinal proximity with serine. Phenylalanine, isoleucine, and leucine are far away from each other. In the fourth cluster (left from the bottom), asparagine and serine are in proximity with isoleucine. Leucine and phenylalanine are far away from each other. The fifth cluster contains almost cyclic structures with serine and leucine being in close proximity, while leucine is far away from isoleucine and phenylalanine. The last cluster 6 is mostly linear. Serine and isoleucine are in close proximity and are on the same side as phenylalanines

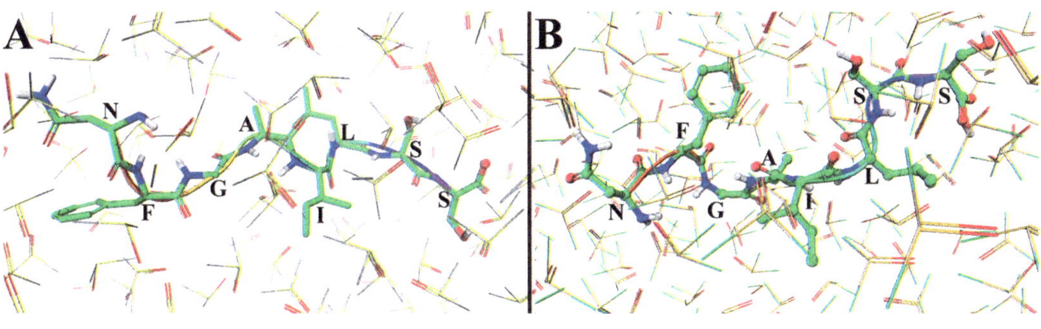

Fig. 3 MD simulation of the peptide NFGAILSS using explicit DMSO. Leucine and isoleucine (**a**) on opposite sides and (**b**) on the same side. As it can be seen, the peptide is linear, and phenylalanine does not form any cluster with leucine and isoleucine. Details of the clusters generated in the explicit DMSO solvent (not shown for simplicity) are shown in Fig. 4a

2. This was achieved with the "edit" tab; scroll down to adjust, and then click on chirality. After a window is opened, chiral centers label was clicked. If some of them have no desirable configuration, i.e., R chirality, switch to proper S configuration by clicking on the chiral center of the molecule, and select invert chirality or flip ring substituent located to the right toolbar of the Maestro 9.3 program.

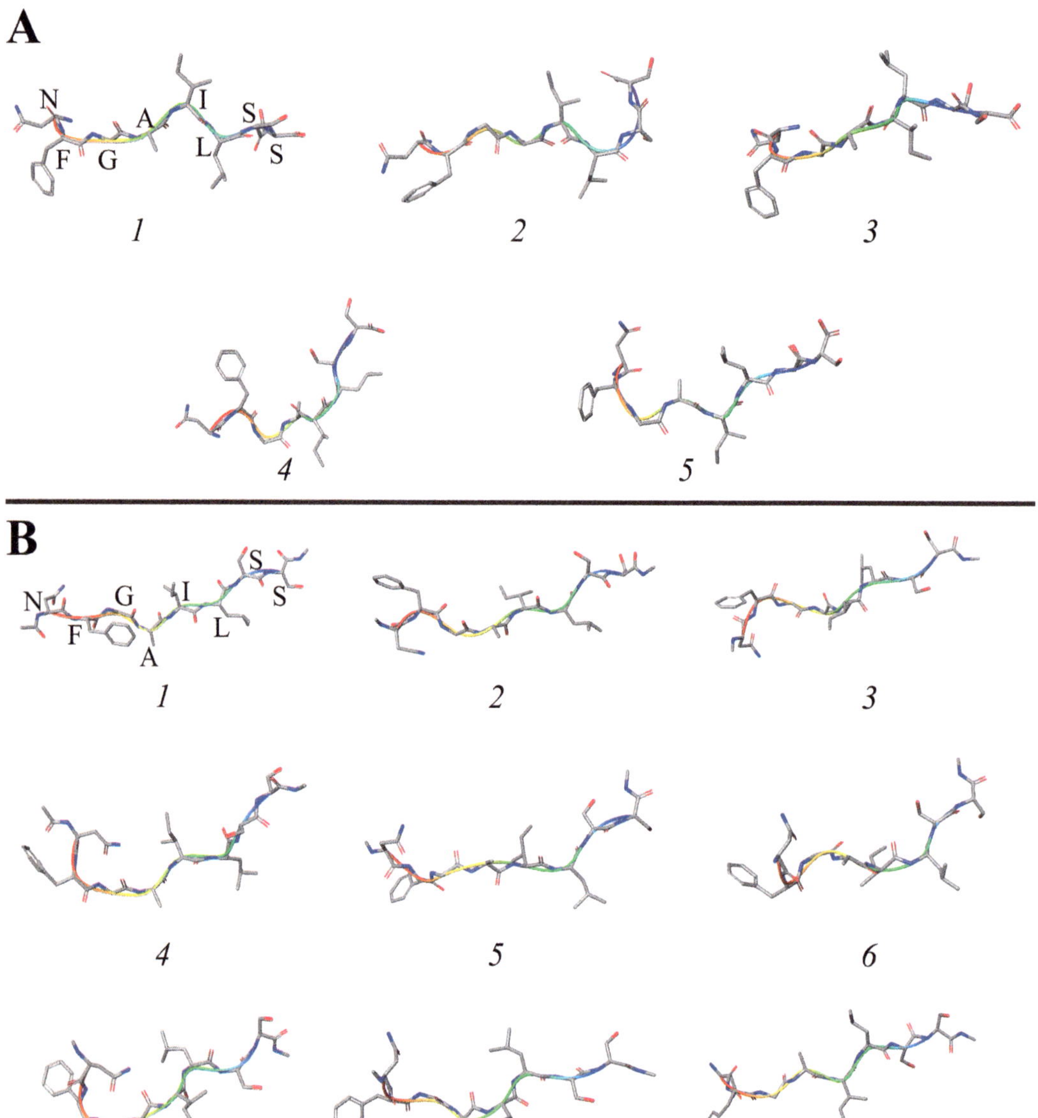

Fig. 4 (**a**) Five clusters generated in the explicit DMSO simulating environments using stochastic MD; (**b**) Nine clusters generated in the explicit HFIP-simulating environments using stochastic MD. The absence of vicinal proximity between Phe and Leu or Ile is evident in all clusters. In the first two top structures spatial vicinity of Leu and Ile is observed and a turn in AILSS region. The first cluster from the left (bottom) is characterized by a turn on the NFGA region. Again this turn orients Phe far away from Leu and Ile amino acids. The last two clusters (middle and right bottom) are almost open structures in an agreement with NMR absence of medium or long ROEs

3. The experiment was checked if it was run properly at the lower left side of the screen where it is written jobs 1/1. When it is completed, it changes to jobs 0/0.

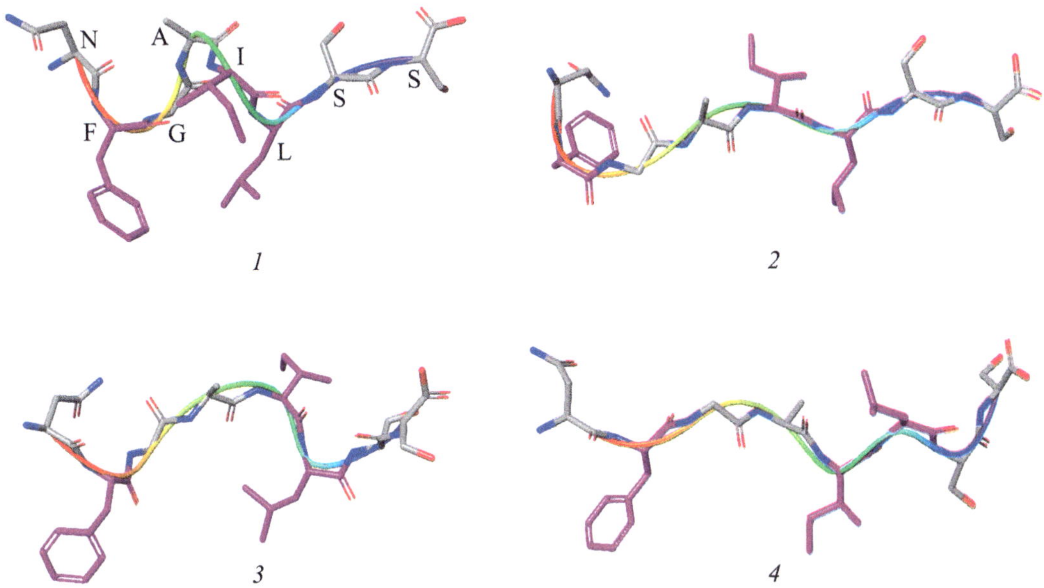

Fig. 5 Four clusters generated in the explicit TIP3P-POPC simulating environment, using stochastic MD, with the NFGAILSS peptide to be located within the POPC membrane. In this environment, it is evident that Phe, Leu, and Ile can form a cluster by coming to a spatial vicinity (*see* cluster 1). This clustering leads to a stable hydrophobic nucleus within the POPC lipid bilayer. This hydrophobic nucleus is absent in cluster 2 and is only consisting of phenylalanine with isoleucine in clusters 3 and 4

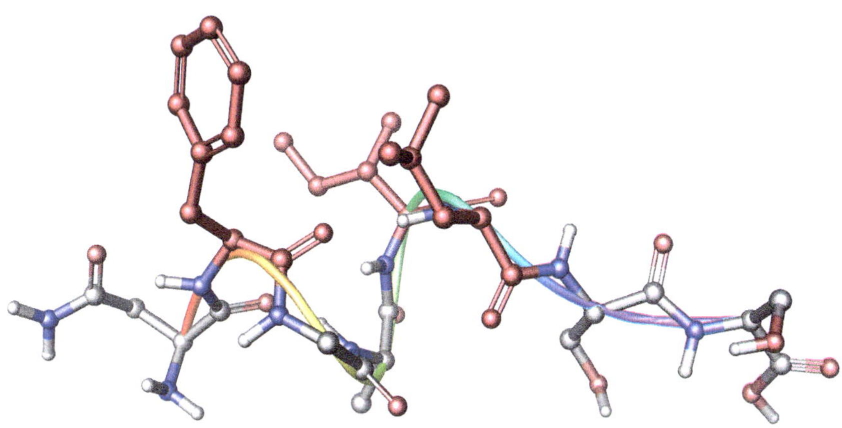

Fig. 6 Snapshot of the peptide NFGAILSS in POPC-TIP3P system. Leucine and isoleucine are on the same site. As it can be seen, the peptide is linear, and phenylalanine does come quite close to isoleucine and leucine creating a hydrophobic nucleus with leucine and isoleucine

4. Check if the convergence threshold has been reached; otherwise continue minimization to achieve it.
5. After choosing the conformations, Atoms RMSD is selected, and then click on pick and select all heavy atoms and retain a mirror image conformation. Then, the RMSD matrix is calculated.

6. Once the RMSD was calculated, it was able to calculate the clusters. If the linkage method has been chosen, various options appear, and then average was selected. Then, it was clicked on calculate clusters.
7. There are many other options, such as follow the hydrogen bonds, apply experimental NOE constraints, follow critical distances, etc.

References

1. Seuring C, Verasdonck J, Ringler P, Cadalbert R, Stahlberg H, Bockmann A, Meier BH, Riek R (2017) Amyloid fibril polymorphism: almost identical on the atomic level, mesoscopically very different. J Phys Chem B 121(8):1783–1792. https://doi.org/10.1021/acs.jpcb.6b10624
2. Westermark P, Wernstedt C, Wilander E et al (1987) Amyloid fibrils in human insulinoma and islets of Langerhans of the diabetic cat are derived from a neuropeptide-like protein also present in normal islet cells. Proc Natl Acad Sci U S A 84:3881–3885
3. Cooper G, Willis A, Clark A, Turner R, Sim R, Reid K (1987) Purification and characterization of a peptide from amyloid-rich pancreases of type II diabetic patients. Proc Natl Acad Sci U S A 84:8628–8632
4. Clark A, Cooper GJ, Lewis CE et al (1987) Islet amyloid formed from diabetes-associated peptide may be pathogenic in type-2 diabetes. Lancet 2:231–234. https://doi.org/10.1016/S0140-6736(87)90825-7
5. Tracz SM, Abedini A, Driscoll M, Raleigh DP (2004) Role of aromatic interactions in amyloid formation by peptides derived from human amylin. Biochemistry 43(50):15901–15908. https://doi.org/10.1021/bi048812l
6. Milardi D, Sciacca MF, Pappalardo M et al (2011) The role of aromatic side-chains in amyloid growth and membrane interaction of the islet amyloid polypeptide fragment LANFLVH. Eur Biophys J 40(1):1–12. https://doi.org/10.1007/s00249-010-0623-x
7. Chakraborty S, Chatterjee B, Basu S (2012) Mechanistic insight into the amyloidogenic structure of hiapp peptide revealed from sequence analysis and molecular dynamics simulation. Biophys Chem 168–169:1–9. https://doi.org/10.1016/j.bpc.2012.05.003
8. Mo Y, Lu Y, Wei G, Derrumaux P (2009) Structural diversity of the soluble trimers of the human amylin (20–29) peptide revealed by molecular dynamics simulations. J Chem Phys 130(12):125101. https://doi.org/10.1063/1.3097982
9. Soriaga A, Smriti S, Macdonald R, Sawaya M (2016) Crystal structures of IAPP amyloidogenic segments reveal a novel packing motif of out-of-register beta studies. J Phys Chem 120(26):5810–5816. https://doi.org/10.1021/acs.jpcb.5b09981
10. Wiltzius J, Sievers S, Sawaya M et al (2008) Atomic structure of the cross-β spine of islet amyloid polypeptide (amylin). Protein Sci 17(9):1467–1474. https://doi.org/10.1110/ps.036509.108
11. Guo J, Zhang Y, Ning L et al (2014) Stabilities and structures of islet amyloid polypeptide (IAPP22-28) oligomers: from dimer to 16 mer. Biochim Biophys Acta 1840(1):357–366. https://doi.org/10.1016/j.bbagen.2013.09.012
12. Profit A, Vedad J, Saleh M, Desamero R (2015) Aromaticity and amyloid formation: effect of π-electron distribution and aryl substituent geometry on the self-assembly of peptides derived from hIAPP22-29. Arch Biochem Biophys 567:46–58
13. Profit A, Felsen V, Chinwong J et al (2012) Evidence of π-stacking interactions in the self-assembly of hIAPP22-29. Proteins 81(4):690–703. https://doi.org/10.1002/prot.24229
14. Prakash R, Nanga R, Brender J, Vivekanandan S, Ramamoorthy A (2011) Structure and membrane orientation of IAPP in its natively amidated form at physiological pH in a membrane environment. Biochim Biophys Acta 1808:2337–2342. https://doi.org/10.1016/j.bbamem.2011.06.012
15. Mascioni A, Porcelli A, Ilangovan U et al (2003) Conformational preferences of the amylin nucleation site in SDS micelles: an nmr study. Biopolymers 69(1):29–41. https://doi.org/10.1002/bip.10305
16. Weirich F, Gremer L, Mirecka E et al (2016) Structural characterization of fibrils from recombinant human islet amyloid polypeptide by solid-state NMR: the central fgails segment is part of the β-sheet core. PLoS One 11(9):e0161243. https://doi.org/10.1371/journal.pone.0161243

Chapter 2

Development of Peptide-Based Inhibitors of Amylin Aggregation Employing Aromatic and Electrostatic Repulsion

Adam A. Profit and Ruel Z. B. Desamero

Abstract

Human islet amyloid polypeptide (hIAPP) is a 37-residue hormone that is co-stored and co-secreted with insulin. In type 2 diabetes, the polypeptide misfolds to form amyloid plaques in the pancreas. The self-assembly of hIAPP has been linked to the loss of insulin production and β-cell death. Recent investigations have revealed that soluble oligomers of hIAPP are the cytotoxic species responsible for β-cell death and not insoluble amyloid fibrils. Compounds that prevent the self-assembly of hIAPP or drive self-assembly to the state of innocuous insoluble amyloid may be of potential therapeutic value. In this report we summarize key methods employed in our efforts to identify peptide-based modulators of amylin self-assembly that utilize π-electronic effects or electrostatic charge repulsion. These peptide-based modulators may serve as lead compounds for the development of more drug-like molecules and demonstrate that tuning π-electron density and employing charged amyloid disrupting elements are viable approaches toward the design of potential amyloid inhibitors.

Key words Amylin, amyloid, type 2 diabetes, Raman, Peptide, Thioflavin-T assays

1 Introduction

Abnormal protein aggregation and the formation of amyloid deposits are the hallmark of over 20 human diseases including pathological neurodegenerative disorders such as Alzheimer's, Parkinson's, Huntington's, and Creutzfeldt-Jakob [1–3]. Amyloid formation has also been found to play a significant role in adult-onset diabetes or type 2 diabetes (T2D) [4–7].

Human islet amyloid polypeptide (hIAPP), also known as amylin, is a 37-residue hormone that is co-stored and co-secreted with insulin in pancreatic β-cells [8–10]. Normal functions of hIAPP include glucose homeostasis as well as regulating appetite suppression [11, 12]. However, in T2D, hIAPP misfolds to form insoluble amyloid deposits in the islets of Langerhans. Postmortem inspection has revealed amyloid deposits in up to 90% of all T2D patients

Thomas Mavromoustakos and Tahsin F. Kellici (eds.), *Rational Drug Design: Methods and Protocols*, Methods in Molecular Biology, vol. 1824, https://doi.org/10.1007/978-1-4939-8630-9_2, © Springer Science+Business Media, LLC, part of Springer Nature 2018

[10, 13]. In addition, the formation of amyloid is also believed to be a major contributor to the failure of islet grafts [14].

Initial theories postulated that insoluble amyloid fibrils of hIAPP were responsible for β-cell death and the associated loss of insulin production. However, more recent investigations suggest that it is actually soluble oligomers that are the causative agents of cellular toxicity [15–17].

Soluble oligomers of hIAPP are believed to exert their cytotoxic effects by rupturing the phospholipid membranes of β-cells. Other mechanisms of hIAPP cytotoxicity are also believed to include the activation of various stress-related signaling pathways ultimately leading to apoptosis [4].

The inhibition of abnormal protein aggregation may represent an effective strategy for potential therapeutic intervention in amyloid diseases. Current strategies employed to prevent amyloid formation include, but are not limited to, the development of novel compounds that block or disrupt the self-assembly process as well as the discovery and application of compounds that stabilize the native conformation of the amyloidogenic protein. Small molecule protease inhibitors directed at the enzymes that process polypeptide precursors of the amyloid protein are also a viable approach. Alternatively, novel chemical entities that hasten amyloid formation may also prove to be of therapeutic value. Compounds which rapidly drive the self-assembly process to the state of innocuous amyloid fibrils minimize cellular exposure to the toxic, membrane-disrupting effects of soluble oligomers.

In an effort to identify potential amyloid inhibitors, our laboratory systematically interrogated how the electronic nature of the π system affects the self-assembly process [18]. This was accomplished through the synthesis and biophysical characterization of $hIAPP_{22-29}$ peptide fragments containing phenylalanine derivatives with electron withdrawing groups (EWGs) or electron donating groups (EDGs) at the *para*-position of the aromatic ring. The phenylalanine derivatives with electron donating substituents used in these studies were 4-aminophenylalanine [(NH_2)Phe], tyrosine (Tyr), *O*-methyltyrosine [(CH_3O)Tyr], 4-methylphenylalanine [(CH_3)Phe], and 4-formamido phenylalanine [(HCONH)Phe]. The phenylalanine derivatives containing electron withdrawing groups utilized were 4-nitrophenylalanine [(NO_2)Phe], 4-cyanophenylalanine [(CN)Phe], 4-carboxyphenylalanine [(COOH)Phe], 4-fluorophenylalanine [(F) Phe], and pentaflurophenylalanine [(F5)Phe].

An alternative approach to fine-tuning aromaticity to develop potential amyloid inhibitors is to utilize electrostatic charge repulsion. Small peptide sequences carrying charged groups should prevent the self-assembly of amyloidogenic proteins by binding to the corresponding recognition sequence in the full-length protein to form a charged peptide/protein complex. Electrostatic repulsion between charged complexes should in theory prevent self-assembly and amyloid formation. To accomplish this we conjugated several benzene carboxylic acids to the N-terminal of the $hIAPP_{22-29}$ sequence [19]. The benzene carboxylic acids varied in the number and position of carboxyl substituents on the aromatic ring. By varying the degree of carboxyl group substitution, we were able to vary the net charge on the N-terminal.

In this report we summarize key methods employed in our efforts to identify peptide-based modulators of amylin self-assembly that employ π-electronic effects or electrostatic charge repulsion [18, 19]. These peptides may serve as lead compounds for the development of small molecule or peptide mimetic amylin aggregation inhibitors.

2 Materials

1. Reagents for peptide synthesis.
2. Acetonitrile (ACN), dimethylformamide (DMF), and dichloromethane (DCM).
3. Supelco solid-phase extraction (SPE) tubes for peptide synthesis.
4. Peptides are synthesized in 6 or 12 mL fritted polyethylene solid-phase SPE tubes equipped with a cap plug and stopper using a wrist action shaker for mechanical agitation.
5. Peptides are purified on a Varian ProStar, Palo Alto, CA, using a Vydac C_{18} column (2.2 × 25 cm).
6. Turbidity measurements were made using a Jasco V-570 spectrophotometer (Easton, MD).
7. Raman spectra were obtained on a Jasco NRS-3100 confocal dispersive Raman spectrometer equipped with a macro-Raman measurement accessory (Easton, MD).
8. Spectroscopic analysis was conducted with concentrated solutions or samples fixed on special Teflon-covered stainless steel slides. FTIR spectra were collected on a Nexus 8700 (Thermo Fisher Scientific, Waltham, MA), while ThT fluorescence was measured using a FluoroMax-4 spectrofluorometer (Horiba Jobin Yvon Inc., Edison, NJ).
9. All solutions were prepared with distilled water.

3 Methods

3.1 Manual Solid-Phase Peptide Synthesis

Peptides and peptide conjugates are synthesized using a standard Fmoc solid-phase synthesis protocol [18, 19]. The synthetic procedure is provided below:

1. 250–500 mg of Rink amide resin (substitution level between 0.22 and 0.53 mmol/g) is placed in an SPE tube and swelled in DMF for 10–30 min. Then the solvent was drained.

2. The resin-bound amine is then deprotected by the addition of 20% piperidine in DMF (v/v) for 20 min. Drain the solvent at the end of this time.
3. Wash the resin with DMF (3×) followed by DCM (3×) (*see* **Note 1**).
4. Remove a few beads of resin, and perform a Kaiser ninhydrin test to confirm the presence of free amine [20].
5. Amino acid coupling is then carried out using three equivalents each of Fmoc-protected amino acid, *N,N,N′,N′*-Tetramethyl-*O*-(1 *H*-benzotriazol-1-yl)uranium hexafluorophosphate (HBTU), 1-Hydroxy-benzotriazole (HOBT), and nine equivalents of *N*-methylmorpholine (NMM) relative to the resin-bound amine. The protected amino acid, HBTU, and HOBT are dissolved in DMF and NMM added. The solution is allowed to stand for a few minutes for activation to occur. The solution is then added to the resin and the mixture is shaken for 1 h (*see* **Notes 2** and **3**).
6. Drain the solution and wash the resin with DMF (3×) followed by DCM (3×) (*see* **Note 1**).
7. Confirm coupling is complete by Kaiser test.
8. Repeat **steps 2** through **7** using the appropriate Fmoc-protected amino acids in the coupling step.
9. Remove the terminal Fmoc group as described in **step 2**.
10. Wash the resin well with DCM and dry in a vacuum desiccator.
11. Cleave the peptide from the resin by the addition of a cocktail of trifluoroacetic acid (TFA), triisopropylsilane (TIS), and water (95:2.5:2.5). Shake the mixture for 2.5 h.
12. Drain and collect the cleavage cocktail into a round bottom flask. Wash the resin two or three times with 1 mL of TFA. Add washings to the round bottom flask.
13. Concentrate the mixture to approximately 20% of its original volume.
14. Precipitate the peptide by flooding with cold diethyl ether, and place mixture on ice for 5–10 min.
15. Isolate the crude peptide by vacuum filtration using a sintered glass funnel (fine to medium porosity) (*see* **Note 4**).
16. Dry and store the crude peptide in a vacuum desiccator until ready for purification.

3.2 Peptide Purification and Characterization

1. Dissolve the crude peptide in water or acetonitrile/water (1:1) containing 0.1% TFA. Remove any insoluble material by passing the solution through a syringe filter (≤0.45 μM). Peptides are then purified by preparative HPLC on a C_{18} column using a linear gradient of acetonitrile/water. Column effluent is monitored at 218 nm.

2. Combine and lyophilize appropriate HPLC fractions to provide the peptides as white solids/powders.
3. Peptide identity and structure are confirmed by matrix-assisted laser desorption ionization time of flight (MALDI-TOF) mass spectrometry.
4. Peptide purity is confirmed by analytical HPLC using a Vydac C_{18} column (4.6 × 250 mm) and a linear gradient of ACN/H_2O.

3.3 Spectroscopic Analysis of Peptide Samples

3.3.1 Turbidity Measurements

Turbidity measurements at 405 nm are employed to monitor the aggregation of peptides and peptide conjugates based the $hIAPP_{22-29}$ sequence [18, 19, 21]. Concentrated peptide stock solutions are prepared in either HFIP or DMSO to prevent aggregate formation. The final concentration of peptide in the turbidity assay is typically 1 mM, while the final concentration of DMSO or HFIP should be less than 5% (v/v). The assay is conducted by placing an appropriate aliquot of peptide stock solution in 10 mM Tris-HCl buffer (pH 7.5) to produce a 1 mM peptide solution and light scattering measured at 405 nm as a function of time. A generalized procedure is given below:

1. Prior to use, sonicate peptide stock solutions for a minimum of 30 min to disrupt any aggregates (*see* **Note 5**).
2. Mix an appropriate aliquot of peptide stock with Tris-HCl buffer (pH 7.5) in a semi-micro cuvette inside the sample compartment of a UV-vis spectrometer equipped with a stirring accessory to produce a 1 mM peptide solution.
3. Measure light scattering at 405 nm for 60 min or until aggregation is complete.
4. Monitor turbidity for 14 days if no aggregates are observed after the first few hours. If there is no signal change detected after 14 days, the sample is considered non-aggregating.

Data from turbidity studies on the EDG and EWG peptides are summarized in Table 1. The data clearly demonstrates that when electron donating substituents on Phe-23 are incorporated into the $hIAPP_{22-29}$ sequence, the peptides fail to self-assemble. Peptides **2**, **3**, **4**, **5**, and **10** are all incapable of undergoing fibrillization. The inability of the EDG peptides to form amyloid was corroborated by TEM analysis of the samples used for turbidity and confirmed the absence of amyloid fibrils. In contrast, electron withdrawing substituents on Phe-23 facilitate peptide aggregation (Table 1) [18, 21]. The NFGAILSS control [1] along with **6**, **7**, **8**, **9**, and **11** all readily form amyloid. TEM analysis verified the presence of amyloid fibrils in samples derived from the EWG peptides.

Our observations on the self-assembly properties of the various $hIAPP_{22-29}$ mutants were found to be highly consistent with the

Table 1
EDG and EWG peptides synthesized and their ability to undergo self-assembly to form amyloid as determined by turbidity assays and confirmed by transmission electron microscopy [18]

Peptide	Sequence	Self-assembly
1	NFGAILSS	Yes
2	NTyrGAILSS	No
3	N(CH_3O)PheGAILSS	No
4	N(NH_2)PheGAILSS	No
5	N(CH_3)PheGAILSS	No
6	N(NO_2)PheGAILSS	Yes
7	N(F_5)PheGAILSS	Yes
8	N(CN)PheGAILSS	Yes
9	N(F)PheGAILSS	Yes
10	N(HCONH)PheGAILSS	No
11	N(COOH)PheGAILSS	Yes

Hunter-Sanders rules of aromatic-aromatic interactions [22, 23]. Peptides containing electron-rich ring systems repelled each other and failed to aggregate, whereas electron-deficient peptides attracted each other and readily formed amyloid.

The structure of peptide conjugates employed to study the effects of charge repulsion are illustrated in Fig. 1. The NFGAILSS sequence is known to adopt a parallel β-sheet-like structure. Hence, parallel β-sheet formation would be prevented by repulsion of adjacent strands due the charged benzene carboxylic acids at the N-termini of each peptide. Conjugates were also designed to a have a free carboxyl terminal as to prevent the possible antiparallel association of peptide strands via repulsion of the negatively charged C-terminal of one strand and the benzene carboxylic acids ligated to the N-terminal of another.

Conjugates were evaluated for their ability to self-assemble using turbidity. Conjugates **C2**–**C7** were found not to form aggregates (Fig. 1) [19]. This is assumed to be due to charge repulsion. However, conjugate **C1** with a single carboxyl group on the N-terminal was capable of undergoing self-assembly, indicating that a charge greater than −1 is likely necessary to inhibit aggregation. In contrast to **C1**, conjugate **C7** which also carries a −1 charge did not aggregate. **C7** also contains sulfonic acid and hydroxyl functionalities as substituents on the benzene carboxylic acid. These polar groups likely provide enhanced water solubility that prevents the aggregation of the conjugate.

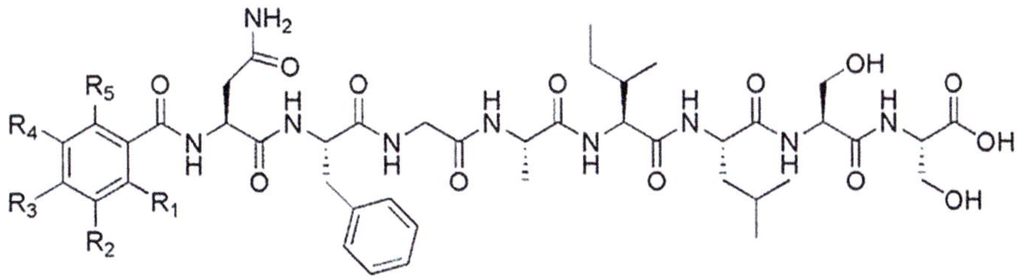

Conjugate	R_1	R_2	R_3	R_4	R_5	N-terminal charge	Self-Assembly
C1	H	H	$-CO_2H$	H	H	-1	Yes
C2	H	$-CO_2H$	H	$-CO_2H$	H	-2	No
C3	H	H	$-CO_2H$	$-CO_2H$	H	-2	No
C4	$-CO_2H$	H	$-CO_2H$	H	H	-2	No
C5	$-CO_2H$	H	$-CO_2H$	$-CO_2H$	H	-3	No
C6	$-CO_2H$	$-CO_2H$	$-CO_2H$	$-CO_2H$	$-CO_2H$	-5	No
C7	-OH	H	H	$-SO_3H$	H	-1	No

Fig. 1 General structure of peptide conjugates derived from benzene carboxylic acids and their ability to undergo self-assembly as determined from turbidity measurements and TEM [19]

3.3.2 Raman Measurements

Raman spectroscopy was used to probe the secondary structure of peptides and to ascertain the structural configuration of the aromatic rings of the aggregated samples.

Raman Measurements of Liquid Samples

1. Prepare 1 mM or higher concentration peptide sample solutions in appropriate buffer.
2. Transfer 30 μL of sample into a quartz cuvette and take its spectrum. Adjust spectrometer slit width, exposure time, number of repetitions, and spectral window accordingly.

Raman Measurement Using Drop Coat Deposition Technique

1. Prepare peptide sample solutions in appropriate buffer; often we will use the resulting samples from the turbidity and ThT fluorescence assay.
2. A 5–10 μL aliquot of the peptide sample is spotted on the special Teflon-covered stainless steel slides.
3. Evaporate the excess solvent until a solvated gel sample remains in the surface (do not dry until a precipitate is formed). A good

solvated gel sample will look superimposed concentric circles and not lumps of precipitated crystal or power.

4. Take the spectrum of the sample. Adjust spectrometer parameters accordingly (*see* **Note 6**).

Raman and FTIR spectroscopy, which measures the vibrational frequency of a group of bonded atoms, was employed to investigate the nature of the aromatic ring interactions during aggregation. The masses of the atoms and the force constant of the various bonds between the atoms determine this frequency, from which bond order, bond length, and bond energy can be derived [24]. The interactions that take place between molecular groups, such as hydrogen bonding or hydrophobic interaction, affect the force constant of certain bonds and hence their vibrational frequencies. Raman spectroscopy is so sensitive that minute changes in the environment of the bond of interest can be detected. Both vibrational techniques are very high-resolution tools (better than 0.01 Å) for determining bond lengths, bond orders, geometries, and ionization states. Crystallographic studies and multidimensional NMR spectroscopy do not characterize the electronic distributions between atoms and in bonds very well, and these distributions are keys to understanding mechanistic aspects. For example, a distortion of less than 0.01 Å was shown to be equivalent to six orders of magnitude of catalytic rate enhancement [25]. This distortion showed up in the vibrational spectrum as a change of 35 cm^{-1} shift of a key coordinate [25].

Raman spectra of aggregates not only provided direct evidence of β-sheet formation but also offer details into the nature of the interactions resulting from fibrillization. Perturbation in the aromatic ring modes and the Raman modes associated with the substituent helps ascertain the hydrophobicity and rigidity of the aromatic ring region and other peptide-specific substituents. The extent and direction of the observed peak shifts of the ring and substituent specific Raman modes are a direct measure of hydrophobicity. Spectral red shifts indicate a change to a more hydrophobic environment, while blue shifts indicate increased hydrogen bonding interactions [21, 26–29]. The full width at half height (fwht) of the same Raman modes indicates the heterogeneity of the sampled conformations; peak narrowing, indicated by low fwht, proves that the sample is fairly structured and uniform during the time frame of the Raman measurement [21, 29].

Raman spectroscopy was also employed to examine the conformational properties of aggregates derived from peptides **1**, **6**, 7, **8**, **9**, and **11** (Table 2) [18, 21]. The amide I vibrational mode ca. 1674 cm^{-1} in the Raman spectra of these aggregates indicates the presence of a parallel β-sheet secondary structure. Parallel ring stacking is evident from its effect on the observed ring modes exhibiting single peaks at ca. 1037 and 1610 cm^{-1} and split

Table 2
Summary of selected Raman modes for aggregated peptides from the kinetic turbidity assay taken from samples prepared using drop coat deposition technique and run using a 488 nm laser

	Raman modes			
Peptide	Ring –CH in plane bending mode 1 (cm^{-1})	Ring –CH in plane bending mode 2 (cm^{-1})	Ring –C=C– stretching (cm^{-1})	Amide I mode (cm^{-1})
1	1036	1204, 1211	1611	1676
6		1119, 1214	1607	1676
7	1037	1197, 1217	1616	1676
8	1032	1200, 1216	1618	1675
9	1039	1200, 1212	1608	1676
11	1034	1189, 1216	1617	1676

Parallel β-sheets were observed for peptides **1**, **6**, **7**, **8**, **9**, and **11** with characteristic split modes for the –CH in plane bending appearing at ca. 1204 and 1214 cm^{-1} and single peak for the amide I mode at ca. 1676 cm^{-1}

modes at ca. 1204 and 1214 cm^{-1} (Table 2). This is consistent with a structural model in which $hIAPP_{22-29}$ self-assembles into a parallel β-sheet secondary structure in which π-stacking interactions occur between Phe residues on adjacent strands. The parallel arrangement of **1** and the EWG peptides observed by vibrational spectroscopy is consistent with the reported crystal structure of $hIAPP_{21-27}$ (NNFGAIL) which displays a parallel β-sheet structure [30]. An obvious narrowing of peaks was also observed with the formation of aggregates consistent with increased rigid structure formation. This establishes two particular Raman markers that interrogate the configuration of the aggregated structures, the Amide I mode at ca. 1674 cm^{-1} and some ring modes at ca. 1200–1210 cm^{-1} [18]. Aggregates exhibiting parallel β-sheet configuration display a single Amide I mode at 1674 cm^{-1} and a doublet peak in the vicinity of the 1200 cm^{-1} region. If the aggregates, on the other hand, form an antiparallel configuration, the Amide I mode at 1674 cm^{-1} plus a shoulder at around 1689 cm^{-1} is observed, while the ring mode displays a single peak at approximately 1214 cm^{-1}. Vibrational studies detected no aromatic-aromatic interactions between NYGAILS mutant and other EDG peptides.

Raman and IR spectroscopic analyses of aggregating benzene carboxylic acid conjugates indicate that these samples exhibit similar characteristics as the $hIAAP_{22-29}$ peptide mutants studied by our group and others. Regardless of the net ionic charge on the N-terminal, the aggregates yielded a similar parallel β-sheet configuration. A close inspection of Table 3 indicates **C1**, **C8**, and **C9** take on a parallel β-sheet configuration as aggregates form.

Table 3
Raman and IR peaks observed from aggregates of C1, C8, and C9 along with the apparent beta-sheet orientation

	Raman shift (cm^{-1})		IR shift (cm^{-1})	
Conjugate	Ring mode	Amide I mode	Amide I mode	Beta-sheet orientation
C1	1204 1211	1665 –	1631 –	Parallel
C8	1202 1215	1672 –	1631 –	Parallel
C9	1204 1217	1664 –	1631 –	Parallel

Conjugates **C1**, **C8**, and **C9** all present a single Amide I peak and two-peak ring modes that are ca. 10 cm^{-1} apart [19]. The net ionic charge on the N-terminal group does not influence the resulting configuration.

3.4 Effect Peptides on Amylin Self-Assembly

3.4.1 Thioflavin-T (ThT) Kinetic Aggregation Assay

To identify potential amyloid inhibitors, we screened non-aggregating EDG peptides for their ability to suppress the self-assembly of full-length $hIAPP_{1-37}$ [18]. A thioflavin-T fluorescence assay was used to monitor the self-assembly of full-length amylin in the absence and presence of non-aggregating peptides and peptide conjugates (Fig. 2). The binding of ThT to amyloid fibrils results in an increase in ThT fluorescence which is proportional to the amount of amyloid present. The final concentration of amylin, ThT, and peptide in the assay mixture is 4, 3, and 40 μM, respectively. The ThT chromophore is excited at 450 nm and the emission monitored at 482 nm as a function of time.

1. Sonicate amylin and peptide stock solutions for a minimum of 30 min (*see* **Note 5**).
2. To Tris buffer containing ThT in a quartz semi-micro cuvette, add an appropriate aliquot of peptide stock. Mix well.
3. To the resulting mixture, add an aliquot of amylin stock solution. Invert cuvette twice.
4. Prepare a control containing everything except the peptide stock solution.
5. Run the fluorescence measurement with the excitation set at 450 nm (slit 2.5 nm) and collecting emission signal at 482 nm (slit 10 nm).
6. Monitor fluorescence emission every 30 min for 24 h to generate the ThT assay curve.

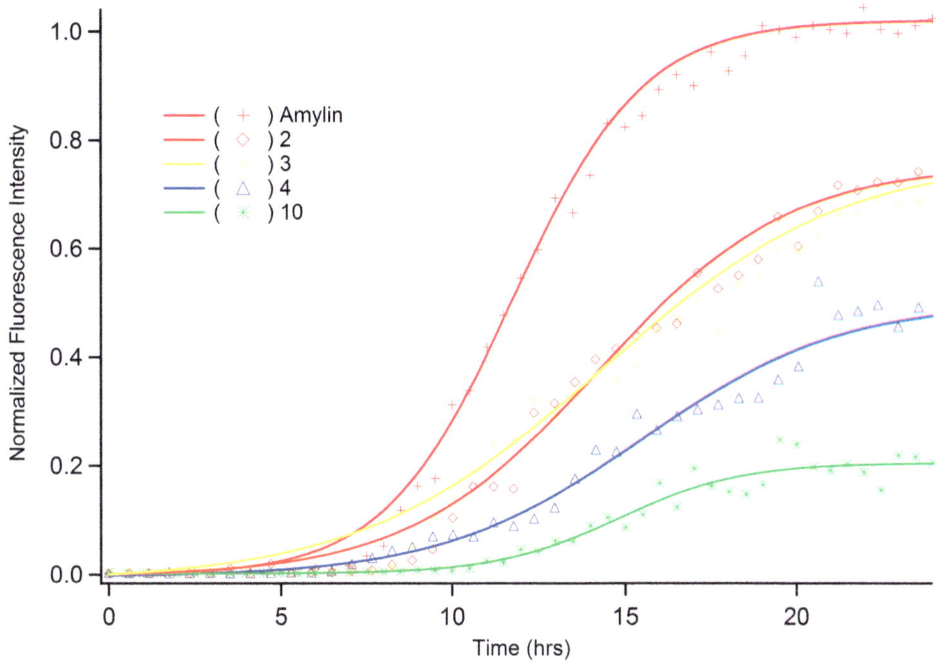

Fig. 2 ThT fluorescence assay monitoring the effects of non-aggregating electron donating group containing peptides on the amyloidogenic propensity of full-length amylin

All the EDG peptides evaluated inhibited the self-assembly of $hIAPP_{1-37}$ to varying degrees (Fig. 2). Peptides either altered lag time, the saturation phase, or the growth phase with some peptides affecting all three phases.

We also screened those non-aggregating benzoic acid peptide conjugates **C2**–**C7** for their ability to modulate the self-assembly of full-length amylin (Fig. 3). Interestingly, only a single conjugate served to completely inhibit amylin aggregation, while the others enhanced its amyloidogenic potential [19].

Conjugates **C2**, **C3**, **C4**, **C6**, and **C7** are all agonists of amylin self-assembly to varying degrees. Conjugates **C4** and **C6** virtually eliminate lag time and significantly increase the rate of fibril growth. However, these conjugates also decrease the amount of total amyloid compared to the amylin control. Conjugates **C2** and **C7** were found to slightly decrease lag time and increase the rate of fibrillization. Strikingly, these conjugates nearly doubled the total amount of amyloid produce at equilibrium compared to the amylin control. **C3** displayed only a modest increase in the rate of amylin self-assembly as well as the total amyloid produced.

The only conjugate that totally prevented amyloid formation by $hIAPP_{1-37}$ was **C5** with its 1,3,4-array of carboxylates. Also, unlike Aβ-based peptides KLVFFKKKK and KLVFFEEEE, described by Murphy et al., the EEEENFGAILSS peptide (**P8**)

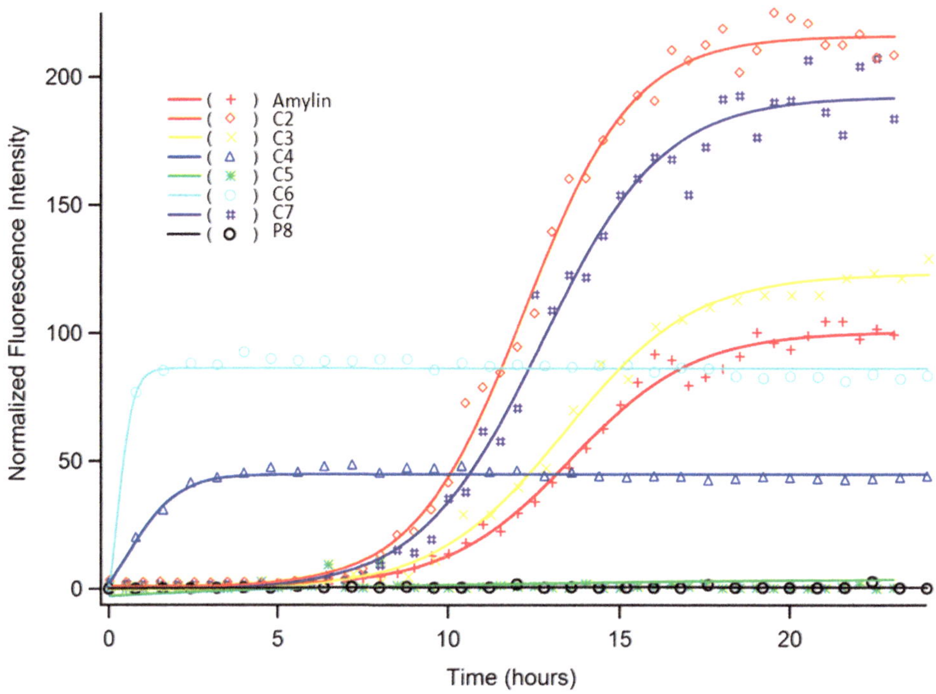

Fig. 3 Thioflavin-T fluorescence emission plot upon incubation with non-aggregating peptide conjugates

did not enhance amylin self-assembly [19, 31]. This peptide actually proved to be an effective inhibitor of amylin aggregation.

The conjugates investigated in these studies illustrate two approaches to the development of amyloid-modulating agents. **C5** and **P8** demonstrate the feasibility of employing electrostatic repulsion to prevent the self-assembly of amylin. On the other hand, charged species that are agonists of amyloid self-assembly may also be useful as they should drive amyloid formation and prevent the buildup of toxic oligomers. Importantly, compounds that significantly lengthen lag time may be the most detrimental as it is during the lag phase when soluble oligomers accumulate. Such compound could actually prolong exposure to these cytotoxic elements.

3.5 Concluding Remarks

The peptides described in this report employ π-electronic effects and electrostatic charge repulsion to modulate the aggregation propensity of human amylin. The successful application of these compounds demonstrates that both approaches are viable strategies toward the identification of peptide-based lead compounds. Through further medicinal chemistry efforts, such compounds may ultimately produce novel small molecule amyloid inhibitors.

4 Notes

1. The DMF wash may be omitted and the resin washed well with DCM.
2. Other coupling options exist, and reagents such as (benzotriazol-1-yloxy)tripyrrolidinophosphonium hexafluorophosphate (PyBOP), O-(1H-6-chlorobenzotriazole-1-yl)-1,1,3,3-tetramethyluronium hexafluorophosphate (HCTU), 1-hydroxy-7-azabenzotriazole (HOAT), and diisopropylethylamine (DIEA) may also be used.
3. Actual coupling times may vary and should be checked by Kaiser ninhydrin test. If coupling is incomplete, repeat the process with a fresh batch of activated Fmoc-amino acid. If coupling cannot be driven to completion, cap the remaining free amines by the addition of 3–5 equivalents each with acetic anhydride and pyridine (or NMM) in DMF or DCM. Confirm capping is complete by Kaiser test.
4. Crude peptides may alternatively be isolated by centrifugation.
5. Use ice to dissipate heat produced during sonication to maintain the integrity of the peptide samples.
6. For both Raman techniques, a toluene sample is used to calibrate peak positions. It is also required that spectrum of blanks be run for proper background correction.

Acknowledgments

The work presented here was supported in part by the Institute of General Medicine of the National Institutes of Health, grant # 5SC3GM89624 (to RZBD) and 1R15GM119040 (to RZBD and AAP).

References

1. Fabrizio C, Christopher MD (2006) Protein misfolding, functional amyloid, and human disease. Annu Rev Biochem 75(1):333–366. https://doi.org/10.1146/annurev.biochem.75.101304.123901
2. Buxbaum JN, Linke RPA (2012) Molecular history of the amyloidoses. J Mol Biol 421 (2):142–159. https://doi.org/10.1016/j.jmb.2012.01.024
3. Ross CA, Poirier MA (2004) Protein aggregation and neurodegenerative disease. Nat Med 10:S10–S17
4. Cao P, Marek P, Noor H et al (2013) Islet amyloid: from fundamental biophysics to mechanisms of cytotoxicity. FEBS Lett 587:1106–1118
5. Cao P, Abedini A, Raleigh DP (2013) Aggregation of islet amyloid polypeptide: from physical chemistry to cell biology. Curr Opin Struct Biol 23(1):82–89
6. Raleigh D, Zhang X, Hastoy B, Clark (2017) A the β-cell assassin: IAPP cytotoxicity. J Mol Endocrinol 59(3):R121-R140. doi:https://doi.org/10.1530/jme-17-0105
7. Jaikaran ETAS, Clark A (2001) Islet amyloid and type 2 diabetes: from molecular misfolding to islet pathophysiology. Biochim Biophys Acta 1537(3):179–203.

https://doi.org/10.1016/S0925-4439(01)00078-3
8. Westermark P, Wernstedt C, Wilander E et al (1987) Amyloid fibrils in human insulinoma and islets of Langerhans of the diabetic cat are derived from a neuropeptide-like protein also present in normal islet cells. Proc Natl Acad Sci U S A 84(11):3881–3885
9. Cooper GJS, Willis AC, Clark A et al (1987) Purification and characterization of a peptide from amyloid-rich pancreases of type 2 diabetic patients. Proc Natl Acad Sci U S A 84 (23):8628–8632
10. Clark A, Cooper GJ, Lewis CE et al (1987) Islet amyloid formed from diabetes-associated peptide may be pathogenic in type-2 diabetes. Lancet 330(8553):231–234. https://doi.org/10.1016/S0140-6736(87)90825-7
11. Westermark P, Andersson A, Westermark GT (2011) Islet amyloid polypeptide, islet amyloid, and diabetes mellitus. Physiol Rev 91 (3):795–826. https://doi.org/10.1152/physrev.00042.2009
12. Lutz TA (2012) Control of energy homeostasis by amylin. Cell Mol Life Sci 69 (12):1947–1965. https://doi.org/10.1007/s00018-011-0905-1
13. Kapurniotu A (2001) Amyloidogenicity and cytotoxicity of islet amyloid polypeptide. Pept Sci 60(6):438–459. https://doi.org/10.1002/1097-0282(2001)60:6<438::aid-bip10182>3.0.co;2-a
14. Potter KJ, Abedini A, Marek P et al (2010) Islet amyloid deposition limits the viability of human islet grafts but not porcine islet grafts. Proc Natl Acad Sci U S A 107(9):4305–4310. https://doi.org/10.1073/pnas.0909024107
15. Engel MF (2009) Membrane permeabilization by islet amyloid polypeptide. Chem Phys Lipids 160(1):1–10. https://doi.org/10.1016/j.chemphyslip.2009.03.008
16. Lin C-Y, Gurlo T, Kayed R et al (2007) Toxic human islet amyloid polypeptide (h-IAPP) oligomers are intracellular, and vaccination to induce anti-toxic oligomer antibodies does not prevent h-IAPP-induced β-cell apoptosis in h-IAPP transgenic mice. Diabetes 56 (5):1324–1332. https://doi.org/10.2337/db06-1579
17. Haataja L, Gurlo T, Huang CJ, Butler PC (2008) Islet amyloid in type 2 diabetes, and the toxic oligomer hypothesis. Endocr Rev 29 (3):303–316. https://doi.org/10.1210/er.2007-0037
18. Profit AA, Vedad J, Saleh M, Desamero RZB (2015) Aromaticity and amyloid formation: effect of π-electron distribution and aryl substituent geometry on the self-assembly of peptides derived from $hIAPP_{22-29}$. Arch Biochem Biophys 567:46–58. https://doi.org/10.1016/j.abb.2014.12.008
19. Profit AA, Vedad J, Desamero RZB (2017) Peptide conjugates of benzene carboxylic acids as agonists and antagonists of amylin aggregation. Bioconjug Chem 28 (2):666–677. https://doi.org/10.1021/acs.bioconjchem.6b00732
20. Kaiser E, Colescott RL, Bossinger CD, Cook PI (1970) Color test for detection of free terminal amino groups in the solid-phase synthesis of peptides. Anal Biochem 34(2):595–598. https://doi.org/10.1016/0003-2697(70)90146-6
21. Profit AA, Felsen V, Chinwong J et al (2013) Evidence of π-stacking interactions in the self-assembly of hIAPP22-29. Proteins 81 (4):690–703. https://doi.org/10.1002/prot.24229
22. Hunter CA, Sanders JKM (1990) The nature of .Pi.–.Pi. Interactions. J Am Chem Soc 112 (14):5525–5534. https://doi.org/10.1021/ja00170a016
23. Cockroft SL, Hunter CA, Lawson KR et al (2005) Electrostatic control of aromatic stacking interactions. J Am Chem Soc 127 (24):8594–8595. https://doi.org/10.1021/ja050880n
24. Gordy W (1946) A relation between bond force constants, bond orders, bond lengths and the electronegativities of the bonded atom. J Chem Phys 14:305–320
25. Deng H, Zheng J, Clakre A et al (1994) Source of catalysis in the lactate dehydrogenase system. Ground state interactions in the enzyme·substrate complex. Biochemistry 33 (8):2297–2305. https://doi.org/10.1021/bi00174a042
26. Getahun Z, Huang C-Y, Wang T et al (2003) Using nitrile-derivatized amino acids as infrared probes of local environment. J Am Chem Soc 125:405–411. https://doi.org/10.1021/ja0285262
27. Weeks CL, Polishchuk A, Getahun Z et al (2008) Investigation of an unnatural amino acid for use as a resonance Raman probe: detection limits and solvent and temperature dependence of the νCN band of 4-cyanophenylalanine. J Raman Spectrosc 39:1606–1613. https://doi.org/10.1002/jrs.2067
28. Schmid ED, Moschallski M, Peticolas WL (1986) Solvent effects on the absorption and raman spectra of aromatic nitro compounds. 1. Calculation of preresonance raman

intensities. J Phys Chem 90(11):2340–2346. https://doi.org/10.1021/j100402a019

29. Smith EE, Linderman BY, Luskin AC, Brewer SH (2011) Probing local environments with the infrared probe: L-4-nitrophenylalanine. J Phys Chem B 115(10):2380–2385. https://doi.org/10.1021/jp109288j

30. Wiltzius JJW, Sievers SA, Sawaya MR et al (2008) Atomic structure of the cross-beta spine of islet amyloid polypeptide (amylin). Protein Sci 17(9):1467–1474. https://doi.org/10.1110/ps.036509.108

31. Lowe TL, Strzelec A, Kiessling LL, Murphy RM (2001) Structure-function relationships for inhibitors of β-amyloid toxicity containing the recognition sequence KLVFF. Biochemistry 40(26):7882–7889. https://doi.org/10.1021/bi002734u

Chapter 3

In Silico Drug Design: Non-peptide Mimetics for the Immunotherapy of Multiple Sclerosis

Haralambos Tzoupis and Theodore Tselios

Abstract

Advances in theoretical chemistry have led to the development of various robust computational techniques employed in drug design. Pharmacophore modeling, molecular docking, and molecular dynamics (MD) simulations have been extensively applied, separately or in combination, in the design of potent molecules. The techniques involve the identification of a potential drug target (e.g., protein) and its subsequent characterization. The next step in the process comprises the development of a map describing the interaction patterns between the target molecule and its natural substrate. Once these key features are identified, it is possible to explore the map and screen large databases of molecules to identify potential drug candidates for further refinement.

Multiple sclerosis (MS) is an autoimmune disease where the immune system attacks the myelin sheath of nerve cells. The process involves the activation of encephalitogenic T cells via the formation of the trimolecular complex between the human leukocyte antigen (HLA), an immunodominant epitope of myelin proteins, and the T-cell receptor (TCR). Herein, the process for rational design and development of altered peptide ligands (APLs) and non-peptide mimetics against MS is described through the utilization of computational methods.

Key words Pharmacophore modeling, Molecular dynamics, Docking, Multiple sclerosis, Peptide mimetics

1 Introduction

Multiple sclerosis (MS) is an inflammatory disease that leads to the destruction of the myelin sheath of the central nervous system [1]. CD4$^+$ T helper (Th) cells have significant contribution during the initiation and progression of MS [2]. The triggering of the Th cells is initiated by short peptide fragments (epitopes) of more than ten amino acids, derived from the main proteins of the myelin sheath such as myelin basic protein (MBP), proteolipid protein (PLP), and myelin oligodendrocyte glycoprotein (MOG) [3–6]. The process of Th cell stimulation in MS patients is achieved via the formation of a trimolecular complex between the T-cell receptor (TCR) and the immunodominant epitope in complex

Thomas Mavromoustakos and Tahsin F. Kellici (eds.), *Rational Drug Design: Methods and Protocols*, Methods in Molecular Biology, vol. 1824, https://doi.org/10.1007/978-1-4939-8630-9_3,

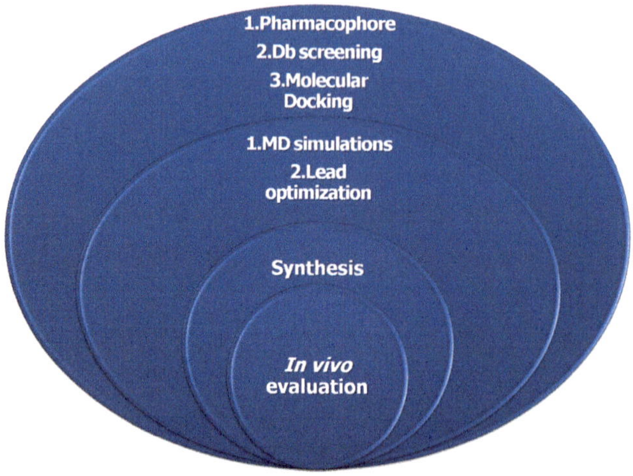

Fig. 1 Schematic representation of rational drug design process

with the major histocompatibility complex (MHC) or human lymphocyte antigen (HLA for humans) class II [4, 5]. The $MBP_{83–96}$ [7], $MOG_{1–22}$, $MOG_{35–55}$, $MOG_{61–80}$ and $MOG_{92–106}$ [8], $PLP_{40–70}$, $PLP_{100–119}$, $PLP_{139–151}$, and $PLP_{178–191}$ [9] have been identified to induce autoimmune response in MS patients. Since these epitopes elicit immune response during the progression of MS, they have been considered the main targets to develop new and potent therapeutic approaches [10–13]. The principal goal of this chapter is to highlight the steps involved in the design of potential inhibitors of the trimolecular complex formation. The process involves the breakdown of the procedure into distinct parts (Fig. 1), with the end result being the in vivo evaluation of the proposed synthesized analogues.

The application of pharmacophore modeling in the trimolecular complex (MHC/HLA–epitope–TCR) allows the researcher to differentiate between the various contributions during the epitope recognition process. Such contributions involve electrostatic, van der Waals interactions, the formation of hydrogen bonds, and hydrophobic interactions. The analysis of their variations offers the tools to screen diverse chemical databases (Db) and filter the results for identification of potential lead antagonists (Fig. 2). Following the filtering process of the databases, the potential candidate molecules are ranked as potential inhibitors by the utilization of molecular docking simulations. The best ranking hits are further submitted to molecular dynamics (MD) simulations, and the analysis of the results leads either to further optimization of the compounds or to their synthesis in the laboratory.

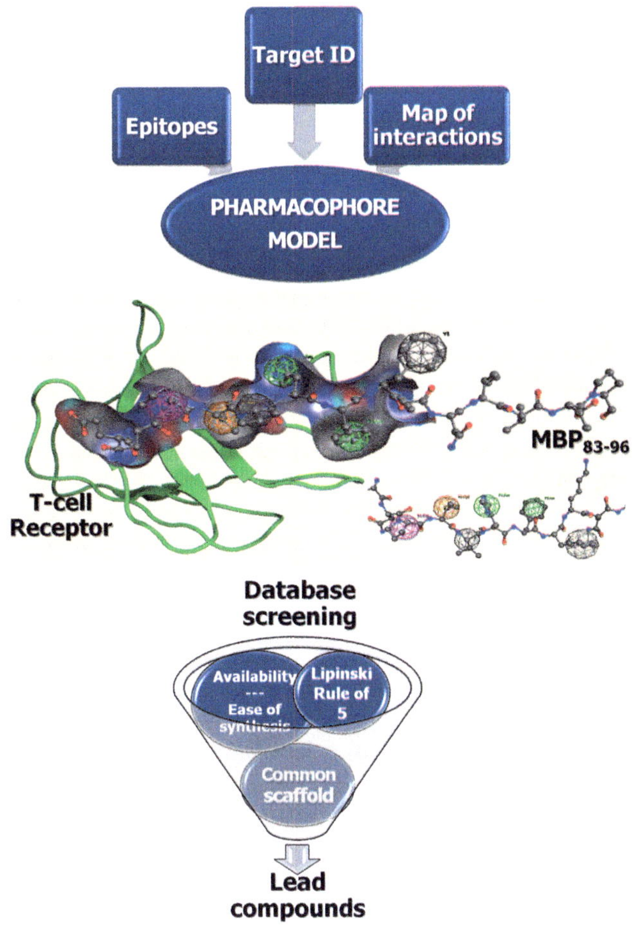

Fig. 2 Pharmacophore model (model example based on the MBP_{83-96} epitope) and its subsequent application during the screening of chemical databases [adapted by Yannakakis MP, Tselios T, et al. (2017) [22]]

2 Materials

There is an abundance of computational tools available for performing the various procedures reported in this chapter. A comprehensive list of the various databases and softwares that can be employed in drug design can be found in the following webpage (www.click2drug.org/), supported by the Swiss Institute of Bioinformatics (www.sib.swiss/, *see* **Note 1**).

The crystal structure of the trimolecular complex (HLA DR2b receptor–MBP_{83-99}–TCR) [14] was employed for all the procedures reported in this chapter. The RCSB protein databank (www.rcsb.org) [15] was the source of the initial Cartesian coordinates for the protein atoms.

2.1 Pharmacophore Modeling

The development of the pharmacophore model was performed with the use of the Molecular Operating Environment (MOE2010) software [16].

The ZINC database of small molecules (zinc15.docking.org/) [17] was employed for the screening process.

2.2 Molecular Docking

The molecular docking simulations were carried out with the respective function of the Molecular Operating Environment (MOE2010) software [16].

2.3 Molecular Dynamics Simulation

The MD simulations were carried out with the AMBER14 molecular package [18] that operates in a Linux environment.

3 Methods

The atomic information included in the crystal structures may contain missing atom information (e.g., hydrogen) or bond information. Therefore, all the issues regarding missing information should be addressed before the construction of a pharmacophore model. In our case, the MOE2010 software in combination with AMBER94 force field [16, 19] was utilized for the preparation and optimization of the protein crystal structure (*see* **Note 2**). The possible protonation states of all the His residues were evaluated with the PROpKa [20, 21] and AMBER94 tools of the MOE2010 suite [22] (*see* **Note 3**).

3.1 Pharmacophore Modeling

The development of a pharmacophore model requires the construction of a comprehensive map of interactions between the target protein and the antigen peptide (immunodominant epitope, Figs. 2 and 3). The crystal structure of the trimolecular complex (PDB entry 1YMM), along with further computational studies performed by our group [10, 12, 13, 22–24], has provided the required information. The primary contacts between the $MBP_{83–96}$ epitope (Glu^{83}-Asn-Pro-Val-Val-His-Phe-Phe-Lys-Asn-Ile-Val-Thr-Pro^{96}) and the HLA-DR2 are residues Val^{87} and Phe^{90}which anchor the peptide into pockets P1 and P4 (Fig. 3) [14]. The TCR is activated by the recognition of residues His^{88} and Phe^{89}, which are interacting with residues in pockets P2 and P3 of the TCR (Fig. 3) [14]. Finally, the secondary binding residues, Val^{86} and Lys^{91}, are oriented in pockets P-1 and P5 of the TCR [14]. The key features of the proposed pharmacophore model (Fig. 2) are based on residues His^{88} and Phe^{89} (Aro, green sphere), Val^{86} (Hyd, orange sphere), and Pro^{85} (Cat, purple sphere). The gray spheres in Fig. 2 represent residues with bulky side chains (Val^{87} and Phe^{90}) and are employed to define the volume exclusion (V) feature [22].

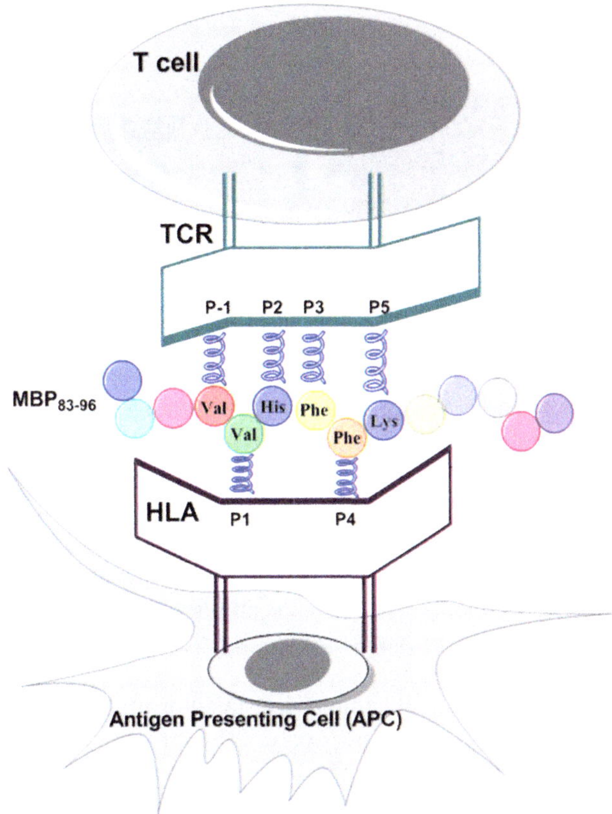

Fig. 3 Schematic depiction of the HLA/MHC–$MBP_{83–96}$–TCR trimolecular complex. The interactions between important residues of the $MBP_{83–96}$ and regions [pockets, (P)] of the two receptors are represented as coils

The next step is the application of the proposed pharmacophore model to screen databases for molecules with similar chemical features (Fig. 2). Databases, such as ZINC, contain millions of chemical compounds that would require more computational time. Hence, it is possible to impose further filters in order to minimize the required computational time. The filtering process could include criteria such as commercial availability of compounds, biologically relevant information (structural or functional similarity to known drugs), and the ease of synthesis or the presence of a common scaffold. The result of the screening process is a list of potential lead compounds (hits) that correspond to the criteria imposed by the pharmacophore model.

3.2 Molecular Docking

The molecular docking simulations are implemented to identify common substructures of the different hits (Fig. 4, left panel). Moreover, the results from the docking simulations can be implemented in order to evaluate (rank) the potential hits as antagonists (*see* **Note 4**). Subsequently, the compound with the best docking

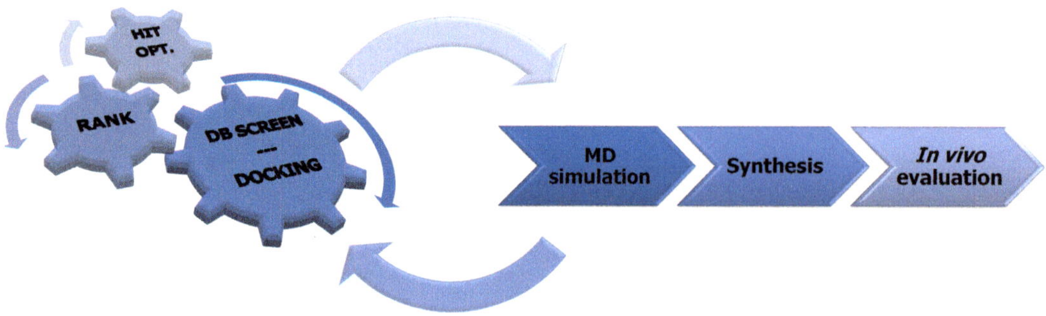

Fig. 4 Schematic representation of the pipeline employed for the rational design of non-peptide mimetics. The left panel represents the methodology of lead compound optimization (HIT OPTIMIZATION), ranking (RANK), and database screening for the discovery of potential inhibitors, while the right panel shows the process involved in the evaluation of selected inhibitors

score (lead molecule) and preferable orientation inside the protein target can be selected for optimization (Fig. 4). The optimized lead compound can either be subjected to MD simulations (Fig. 4, right panel) or be employed to screen a chemical database (Fig. 4, left panel), repeating the whole process as depicted in Fig. 4.

3.3 Molecular Dynamics Simulation

By employing an all-atom MD simulation approach, it is possible to further analyze the interactions between the epitope and the receptor [12, 23] or the potential antagonists (e.g., *antagonist14*) and the receptor [22].

The PDB file employed for the MD simulation must be thoroughly checked for any errors. This can be achieved through tools readily available by AMBER such as *pdb4amber* (*see* **Note 5**). PDB files may contain additional information that is not relevant to the MD setup process. Also, it is possible for the file to contain more than one image of our system (due to the X-ray unit cell information). In the case reported here, we have employed as a starting PDB file the best docking pose for the lead compound (*antagonist14*) labeled original.pdb. The following is the command syntax for *pdb4amber:*

pdb4amber –i original.pdb –o new.pdb –y –d

The command will remove all hydrogen atoms (*−y*) and all water molecules (*−d*), if any, from our system (original.pdb) and write a new PDB file containing only the amino acid chains (*−o new.pdb*) and the lead compound (*antagonist14*). The new PDB file will have all the residues numbered sequentially from 1 to *N* atoms. This is important because many times the files downloaded from the protein databank do not have sequential numbering. Thus, care should be taken when identifying active sites or other important residues, and the final structure (new.pdb) should be carefully examined to identify the new numbering. The program would

Table 1
Sample output for *pdb4amber*

Remarks
---------- Nonstandard residues The following nonstandard residue names in the original PDB file are not recognized by Amber and have been written to the separate file new_nonprot.pdb en2
---------- Water 0 water molecules have been removed and stored in the file new_water.pdb
---------- Histidines (renumbered residues!) The following nine histidines are found in the PDB file HIE_37 HIE_49 HIE_103 HIE_167 HIE_181 HIE_237 HIE_254 HIE_267 HIE_307 If HIS, AMBER will consider them as HIE (epsilon-HIS) by default. You might need to check their tautomerism or protonation state and change them to HID (delta-HIS) or HIP (protonated HIS)
---------- Cysteines in disulfide bonds (renumbered residues!) No disulfide bonds have been detected
---------- Gaps (renumbered residues!) Gap of 5.560313 A between TYR_90 and LYS_91 Gap of 36.469037 A between THR_96 and GLY_97 You *must* (!!!) insert a TER record between the residues listed above and consider to introduce caps (ACE and NME) at the dangling N- and C-terminals
---------- Missing heavy atoms (renumbered residues!) None

also generate a text file with the output PDB name and the label *_sslink* if *pdb4amber* has detected any disulfide bonds. The output for the complex in this case is presented in Table 1.

Based on the information from the PDB preparation output (*see* above), we can utilize a text editor (e.g., WordPad for Windows OS or vim/gedit for Linux OS) to resolve any of the issues reported in the output above and delete the connectivity records at the end of the new.pdb file (Table 2).

The resulting edited PDB file (labeled new.pdb) includes only the TCR and the lead compound (*antagonist14*). The next step in the process involves the preparation of the parameters (bond length, atomic charges) for the potential antagonist. AMBER

Table 2
Example of connectivity records at end of the PDB file

Fragment of new.pdb
CONECT 852 1318
CONECT 1614 2156
CONECT 2393 2829
CONECT 3185 3712
CONECT 3993 4561
CONECT 4980 5512

already includes the parameters for amino acids, DNA, RNA, lipids, and sugars in library files called force fields, which are periodically updated. For any other organic molecule, the user has to build the required parameters. In this case we isolate the coordinates of the lead compound from the new.pdb (produced in the previous step) using any visualization program available (*see* **Note 2**) and save it as a different PDB labeled *antagonist14.pdb*. Following this step, we can implement the *antechamber* and *parmchk2* tools from the AMBERtools package to build the parameters for the organic molecule (*see* **Note 5**).

The syntax for *antechamber* is:

antechamber –i antagonist14.pdb –fi pdb –o antagonist14.mol2 –fo mol2 –c bcc

The *antechamber* tool uses the atom information from the *antagonist14.pdb* file (*–i*) and implements the AM1BCC semi-empirical methodology (*–c bcc*) to calculate and assign the atomic charges in the output file (*–o antagonist14.mol2*). Next, with the use of the *parmchk2* tool, we further check for parameters of the *antagonist14.mol2* (*–i*) such as bond length and dihedral angles.

The syntax for *parmchk2* is:

parmchk2 –i antagonist14.mol2 –f mol2 –o antagonist14.frcmod

The output file (*–o antagonist14.frcmod*) will have information in the format presented in Table 3.

The user should check the file output (Table 3) carefully in the comment section (highlighted in Table 3) for any notes in the form of *ATTN needs revision*. If there are such comments in the particular section, the parameters should be manually inserted by the user. This process should be performed after a very extensive and careful examination of the literature regarding the values of the missing parameters.

For the final setup of the parameters for the complex (TCR–antagonist14) we will implement the *tLEAP* program of AMBER

Table 3
Output file (−*o antagonist14.frcmod*) information derived with *parmchk2*

Remarks	Comments section
MASS	
BOND	
ANGLE	
DIHE	
nh-cz-nh-c3 4 2.700 180.000 2.000	Same as X -c2-nh-X, penalty score = 462.5
nh-cz-nh-hn 4 2.700 180.000 2.000	Same as X -c2-nh-X, penalty score = 462.5
IMPROPER	
cc-cd-cc-ha 1.1 180.0 2.0	Same as X -X -ca-ha, penalty score = 38.9 (use general term))
c-cc-cc-cd 1.1 180.0 2.0	Using the default value
cc-h4-cd-na 1.1 180.0 2.0	Same as X -X -ca-ha, penalty score = 67.2 (use general term))
c3-cd-na-cd 1.1 180.0 2.0	Using the default value
ca-ca-ca-ha 1.1 180.0 2.0	Using general improper torsional angle X- X-ca-ha, penalty score = 6.0
cc-n-c-o 10.5 180.0 2.0	Using general improper torsional angle X- X- c- o, penalty score = 6.0)
cz-hn-nh-hn 1.1 180.0 2.0	Same as X -X -na-hn, penalty score = 41.2 (use general term))
nh-nh-cz-nh 1.1 180.0 2.0	Using the default value
c3-cz-nh-hn 1.1 180.0 2.0	Same as X -X -na-hn, penalty score = 41.2 (use general term))
NONBON	

(*see* **Note 5**). The functions required for the buildup of the system parameters can be inserted as a simple script (e.g., input.txt) using a text editor. In this case the script should contain the options described in Table 4.

The command to execute the above script and generate a log file (labeled leap.log) is:

tleap *-f input.txt*

By checking the log file produced by *tLEAP*, we identify any potential warnings about our system such as:

Table 4
Input file options for use in the *tLEAP* program

Options	Notes
source leaprc.ff14SB	*Upload the force field file for the amino acid parameters*
source leaprc.gaff	*Upload a generalized atom force field for all organic molecules*
loadamberparams frcmod.ionsjc_tip3p	*Upload the parameter file for the ions required for the neutralization of the system*
loadamberparams antagonist14.frcmod	*Upload the parameters for the antagonist (see parmchk2)*
en2=loadmol2 antagonist14.mol2	*Upload the charge file for the antagonist (see antecamber)*
saveoff antagonist14.lib	*Create a library file for the antagonist molecule*
complex=loadpdb new.pdb	*Upload the PDB containing the complex (see pdb4amber)*
charge complex	*Calculate the net charge of the system*
addions complex Cl– 1	*If non-zero, add the appropriate Cl^- or Na^+ to neutralize*
solvateoct complex TIP3PBOX 10.0	*Solvate the complex in water using a truncated octahedron with a cutoff of 10.0 Å*
saveamberparm complex new.top new.crd	*Save the complete parameters for the complex*
savepdb complex new_wat.pdb	*Save a new PDB file with all the changes implemented*
Quit	

Checking Unit.
Warning: There is a bond of 3.074730 angstroms between:

------- .R<TYR 90>.A<CA 3> and .R<TYR 90>.A<C 20>

These types of warnings usually reflect improper bond lengths from the X-ray crystal structure and do not pose essential problems for our calculations. The best way to resolve these issues is to impose a restraint, on the movement of atoms, during the initial steps of minimization and then gradually remove these restraints in the process. In this case the minimization was performed in two stages. In the first stage, we have placed restraints on the complex (TCR-*antagonist14*) by applying a harmonic potential constant of 500 kcal mol^{-1} $Å^{-2}$. A sample input file (created with a text editor) includes the options described in Table 5 (*see also* **Note 5**).

In the next stage of minimization, we have gradually removed the restraints in the complex and minimized the whole system for a total of 150,000 iterations. For the first 50,000 iterations, we have reduced the *restraint_wt* in the above sample input by 100.0 (for every 10,000 iterations); in the final 100,000 iterations, there were no restraints (*ntr=0*) imposed on the system.

Table 5
Input file options for minimization

Options	Notes
Minimization with solute fixed	*Remark line*
&cntrl	
imin=1,	*Perform minimization*
maxcyc=50000,	*For 50,000 iterations*
ntr=1,	*Place restraints on the system (default value ntr=0, no restraints)*
restraintmask=':1-343',	*Restraints placed on residues 1–343 (TCR–antagonist14)*
restraint_wt=500.0,	*Use a restraint constant of 500.0 kcal* mol^{-1} $Å^{-2}$
/	*End of file*

Table 6
Input file options for the heating process

Options	Notes
Heat to 300 K	*Remark line*
&cntrl	
imin=0, irest=0,	*Start a new MD simulation*
ntb=1,	*MD performed under constant volume conditions*
tempi=0.0, temp0=300.0,	*Definition of initial (0.0K) and target temperature (300.0K)*
ntt=3, gamma_ln=5.0	*Type of thermostat employed to keep temperature constant*
ntr=1,	*Place restraints on the system (default value ntr=0, no restraints)*
restraintmask=':1-343',	*Restraints placed on residues 1–343 (TCR–antagonist14)*
restraint_wt=10.0,	*Use a restraint constant of 10.0 kcal* mol^{-1} $Å^{-2}$
nstlim=50000, dt=0.002,	*No. of steps for the heating process (time duration of MD=nstlim*dt in ps)*
/	*End of file*

When the energy of the system has converged, it is safe to move to the next step of the setup process which involves the heating of the system to room temperature (where most of the in vitro experiments take place). The heating process allows the atoms to acquire momentum and start moving freely in space. As with the minimization process, it is advised to use restraints (*ntr=1*) that will be gradually abolished. A sample input file for the heating will include the options presented in Table 6 (*see* **Note 5**).

Table 7
Input file options for the pressure equilibration process

Options	Notes
Pressure equilibration at constant temp 300K	*Remark line*
&cntrl	
imin=0, irest=1, ntx=5,	*Restart (irest=1) the simulation from the last step using the velocities and coordinates from the last step (ntx=5)*
ntb=2,	*MD performed under constant pressure conditions*
ntp=1, pres0=1.0	*Keep system at constant pressure of 1.0 bar*
tempi=300.0, temp0=300.0,	*Constant temperature (300.0 K)*
ntt=3, gamma_ln=5.0	*Type of thermostat employed to keep temperature constant*
ntr=1,	*Place restraints on the system*
restraintmask=':1-343',	*Restraints placed on residues 1–343 (TCR–antagonist14)*
restraint_wt=10.0,	*Use a restraint constant of 10.0 kcal mol*$^{-1}$ *Å*$^{-2}$
nstlim=50000, dt=0.002,	*No. of steps for the process (time duration of MD=nstlim*dt in ps)*
/	*End of file*

Once the system has reached the required temperature, the following step involves the equilibration of the pressure of the system in order to create a constant pressure and temperature environment (NPT ensemble). The setup for the pressure equilibration step is similar to the heating phase above (*see* Table 7).

Finally, the production run allows the monitoring of the system under dynamic conditions and documents the changes in the conformations of both the protein and the ligand (*see* **Note 6**). The sample input for the MD production run contains the same options as above with the only difference being the *ntr* option which is now set to 0 (no restraints). The *nstlim* option for the production run defines the length of the MD simulation. An adequate simulation length for a system like the one reported here is 50 ns (*nstlim*=25,000,000). A general rule of thumb for macromolecular systems (e.g., protein–ligand complexes) is the greater the MD simulation time, the more reliable the results of the simulation will be.

As reported in the previous section (Subheading 3.2, Molecular Docking), it is advised to perform multiple runs of the same MD simulation, in order to monitor the reproducibility of the results and offer a more robust analysis regarding the potential contributions. MD simulations allow the researcher to explore the conformational space of a ligand and monitor in a dynamic environment bonding and structural characteristics such as hydrogen bond formation, electrostatic and van der Waals interactions, as well as the contributions of solvent molecules. This information can be applied to further optimize the compound and employ it for a new database screening or further move to the synthesis of the proposed compound (Fig. 4).

4 Notes

1. Before utilizing any of the tools in this diverse field, it is important to familiarize ourselves with the particulars of each software. Despite the common theoretical background, there are several small differentiations between the various tools that may affect the results of the experiment.
2. There are several softwares (free and commercial) that can be used to attend to the issues incorporated in crystal structures. A comprehensive list is reported in the webpage www.click2drug.org/.
3. The correct assignment of protonation states for residues such as His, Asp, Glu, and Lys is an integral part in the modeling process. The lack of experimental data can be approached by assigning different protonation states to the residues according to the pH environment and performing energy minimization calculations (for the whole protein) in each case. The conformation with the lowest energy may be employed in the modeling process.
4. It is ideal during molecular docking simulations to repeat the simulations in order to assess the reproducibility of the results. Depending on the software (and algorithms) employed for the docking simulations, the docking scores may vary slightly between each simulation run.
5. Refer to AMBER manual (http://ambermd.org/doc12/Amber16.pdf) for a detailed analysis of the tools employed as well as the different options for setting up input files for MD simulations.
6. Extensive tutorials for MD simulations are offered by the different softwares available. Also, depending on the desirable system to study, a careful scanning of the available literature is of paramount importance for the setup of a reliable MD simulation.

References

1. Sospedra M, Martin R (2005) Immunology of multiple sclerosis. Annu Rev Immunol 23:683–747. https://doi.org/10.1146/annurev.immunol.23.021704.115707
2. Mouzaki A, Rodi M, Dimisianos N et al (2015) Immune parameters that distinguish multiple sclerosis patients from patients with other neurological disorders at presentation. PLoS One

10(8):e0135434. https://doi.org/10.1371/journal.pone.0135434
3. Ben-Nun A, Kerlero de Rosbo N, Kaushansky N et al (2006) Anatomy of T cell autoimmunity to myelin oligodendrocyte glycoprotein (MOG): prime role of MOG44F in selection and control of MOG-reactive T cells in H-2b mice. Eur J Immunol 36(2):478–493. https://doi.org/10.1002/eji.200535363
4. Moise L, Beseme S, Tassone R et al (2016) T cell epitope redundancy: cross-conservation of the TCR face between pathogens and self and its implications for vaccines and autoimmunity. Exp Rev Vaccines 15(5):607–617. https://doi.org/10.1586/14760584.2016.1123098
5. Shahrizaila N, Yuki N (2011) Guillain-barre syndrome animal model: the first proof of molecular mimicry in human autoimmune disorder. J Biomed Biotechnol 2011:829129. https://doi.org/10.1155/2011/829129
6. Wucherpfennig KW, Catz I, Hausmann S et al (1997) Recognition of the immunodominant myelin basic protein peptide by autoantibodies and HLA-DR2-restricted T cell clones from multiple sclerosis patients—Identity of key contact residues in the B-cell and T-cell epitopes. J Clin Invest 100(5):1114–1122. https://doi.org/10.1172/Jci119622
7. Martin R, Howell MD, Jaraquemada D et al (1991) A myelin basic protein peptide is recognized by cytotoxic t cells in the context of four HLA-DR types associated with multiple sclerosis. J Exp Med 173(1):19–24
8. Pacini G, Ieronymaki M, Nuti F et al (2016) Epitope mapping of anti-myelin oligodendrocyte glycoprotein (MOG) antibodies in a mouse model of multiple sclerosis: microwave-assisted synthesis of the peptide antigens and ELISA screening. J Pept Sci 22(1):52–58. https://doi.org/10.1002/psc.2839
9. Greer JM, Sobel RA, Sette A et al (1996) Immunogenic and encephalitogenic epitope clusters of myelin proteolipid protein. J Immunol 156(1):371–379
10. Mantzourani ED, Platts JA, Brancale A et al (2007) Molecular dynamics at the receptor level of immunodominant myelin basic protein epitope 87–99 implicated in multiple sclerosis and its antagonists altered peptide ligands: triggering of immune response. J Mol Graph Model 26(2):471–481. https://doi.org/10.1016/j.jmgm.2007.02.004
11. Spyranti Z, Dalkas GA, Spyroulias GA et al (2007) Putative bioactive conformations of amide linked cyclic myelin basic protein peptide analogues associated with experimental autoimmune encephalomyelitis. J Med Chem 50(24):6039–6047. https://doi.org/10.1021/jm070770m
12. Yannakakis MP, Tzoupis H, Michailidou E et al (2016) Molecular dynamics at the receptor level of immunodominant myelin oligodendrocyte glycoprotein 35-55 epitope implicated in multiple sclerosis. J Mol Graph Model 68:78–86. https://doi.org/10.1016/j.jmgm.2016.06.005
13. Matsoukas J, Apostolopoulos V, Kalbacher H et al (2005) Design and synthesis of a novel potent myelin basic protein epitope 87-99 cyclic analogue: enhanced stability and biological properties of mimics render them a potentially new class of immunomodulators. J Med Chem 48(5):1470–1480. https://doi.org/10.1021/jm040849g
14. Hahn M, Nicholson MJ, Pyrdol J et al (2005) Unconventional topology of self peptide-major histocompatibility complex binding by a human autoimmune T cell receptor. Nat Immunol 6(5):490–496. https://doi.org/10.1038/ni1187
15. Berman HM, Westbrook J, Feng Z et al (2000) The Protein Data Bank. Nucleic Acids Res 28(1):235–242
16. Molecular Operating Environment (MOE), 2013.08 (2017). Chemical Computing Group Inc, 1010 Sherbooke St West, Suite #910, Montreal, QC, Canada, H3A 2R7
17. Sterling T, Irwin JJ (2015) ZINC 15—ligand discovery for everyone. J Chem Inf Model 55(11):2324–2337. https://doi.org/10.1021/acs.jcim.5b00559
18. Case DA, Cerutti DS, Cheatham TE et al (2017) AMBER 2017. University of California, San Francisco
19. Cornell WDCP, Bayly CI, Gould IR et al (1995) A second generation force field for the simulation of proteins, nucleic acids, and organic molecules. J Am Chem Soc 117:5179–5197
20. Jensen JH, Li H, Robertson AD et al (2005) Prediction and rationalization of protein pKa values using QM and QM/MM methods. J Phys Chem A 109(30):6634–6643. https://doi.org/10.1021/jp051922x
21. Li H, Robertson AD, Jensen JH (2005) Very fast empirical prediction and rationalization of protein pKa values. Proteins 61(4):704–721. https://doi.org/10.1002/prot.20660
22. Yannakakis MP, Simal C, Tzoupis H et al (2017) Design and synthesis of non-peptide mimetics mapping the immunodominant myelin basic protein (MBP83-96) epitope to function as T-cell receptor antagonists. Int J Mol

Sci 18(6):pii: E1215. https://doi.org/10.3390/ijms18061215

23. Laimou D, Lazoura E, Troganis AN et al (2011) Conformational studies of immunodominant myelin basic protein 1–11 analogues using NMR and molecular modeling. J Comput Aided Mol Des 25(11):1019–1032. https://doi.org/10.1007/s10822-011-9481-6

24. Ntountaniotis D, Vanioti M, Kordopati GG et al (2017) A combined NMR and molecular dynamics simulation study to determine the conformational properties of rat/mouse 35-55 myelin oligodendrocyte glycoprotein epitope implicated in the induction of experimental autoimmune encephalomyelitis. J Biomol Struct Dyn 35(7):1559–1567. https://doi.org/10.1080/07391102.2016.1188418

Chapter 4

Binding Moiety Mapping by Saturation Transfer Difference NMR

Jeffrey R. Brender, Janarthanan Krishnamoorthy, Anirban Ghosh, and Anirban Bhunia

Abstract

Saturation transfer difference (STD) NMR has emerged as one of the key technologies in lead optimization during drug design. Unlike most biophysical assays which report only on the binding affinity, STD NMR reports simultaneously on both the binding affinity and the structure of the binding ligand/protein complex. The STD experiment drives magnetization from a protein to a bound small molecule ligand which carries away the memory of the saturation signal when it dissociates. Since the transfer of saturation is distance dependent, STD NMR can be used to map the specific atoms on the ligand in contact with a protein receptor allowing the impact of any structural change in the binding site to be mapped directly on to the individual functional groups responsible when a suitable compound library is screened. Because the signal is detected from the free ligand and not the bound complex, it can be used on a much wider range of systems than protein-detected NMR and has the advantage of more directly reporting on distances than changes in chemical shifts alone. The STD experiment, while deceptively simple, is very sensitive to both sample conditions and acquisition parameters. We present a general protocol for setting up and STD NMR experiment with a particular focus on how choices in sample conditions and acquisition parameters affect the outcome of the experiment.

Key words Nuclear magnetic resonance spectroscopy, Saturation transfer difference NMR, Epitope mapping, Screening, Ligand-based NMR

1 Introduction

Small molecule binding controls many biochemical processes, either directly through the action of a protein on a small molecule substrate or indirectly through the structural changes that accompany small molecule binding. The binding of small molecules to proteins has therefore been the subject of intense focus in drug development, both as a target for intervention and due to their importance in understanding the underlying biology of the drug response [1].

Thomas Mavromoustakos and Tahsin F. Kellici (eds.), *Rational Drug Design: Methods and Protocols*, Methods in Molecular Biology, vol. 1824, https://doi.org/10.1007/978-1-4939-8630-9_4, © Springer Science+Business Media, LLC, part of Springer Nature 2018

Characterization of receptor/ligand interactions often focuses on two questions: how tightly the ligand binds and what chemical features control its specificity and affinity. While there are many analytical techniques to characterize the binding affinity [2–5], there are far fewer tools to identify the contribution of specific chemical features to binding for structure activity relationships. NMR is the most prominent among these [6, 7]. Every proton on a ligand can give rise to a distinct peak in an NMR spectrum. The effect of binding can therefore be probed for every atom individually. How this influence is manifested is dependent on the exact NMR sequence. The simplest experiment is to observe the changes in the chemical shift of the ligand upon titration with the protein [8]. Although these experiments are easy to set up, they are relatively insensitive and may be difficult to interpret due to the complexity of underlying chemical shift changes. The chemical shift is fundamentally a quantum mechanical property [9] that responds nonlinearly and anisotropically to environmental changes [10]. The nonlinear dependence means a large change in chemical shift for a particular ligand atom does not guarantee that the atom is in close proximity to the receptor.

In theory, the same principle used to derive protein structures in NMR can be applied to determine the structure of the receptor-ligand complex. The nuclear Overhauser effect (NOE) between two nuclei is, to a reasonable approximation, inversely dependent on the sixth power of the distance between them when short mixing times are used. Since the NOESY effect is a through-space interaction, in theory, the formation of a receptor-ligand complex will give rise to intermolecular cross-peaks in a 2D NOESY spectrum. In practice, a number of obstacles prevent the routine use of intermolecular NOE cross-peaks for epitope mapping. The NOESY effect is only quantitatively distance dependent for short mixing times, which limits the sensitivity of the method as the spin populations do not reach equilibrium. A high concentration of protein is needed to reach detectable levels in this experiment, which can be problematic when the protein is difficult to express or purify. More seriously, the targets of drug discovery are often large or membrane-bound proteins that have wide, poorly resolved spectra in which the weak intermolecular NOEs are obscured by the much larger intramolecular NOE peaks from the ligand [11]. As a result receptor-ligand intermolecular NOESY cross-peaks are only observed under very favorable conditions [12].

However, NOESY cross-peaks are not needed to derive intermolecular distance constraints from the NOE effect. Magnetization decays slowly in small molecules due to their small T_1 relaxation times. For K_D values in the micromolar to millimolar range, the k_{off} value is usually fast enough that the ligand will dissociate before the magnetization is lost. By rapidly repeating the saturation pulse, new ligands are also saturated with every binding event. The result is that magnetization spreads throughout the entire ligand pool, both bound and free. Rather than trying to observe the difficulty to detect bound complex, the memory of the bound state in the ligand can be detected free in solution where it is much easier to observe. The transfer of magnetization to the entire ligand pool also gives a significant amplification of the signal when compared to techniques that directly detect only the bound complex. One practical consequence is that only a small concentration of protein needs to be used, which is often a significant advantage when the protein is difficult to express or purify.

The saturation transfer difference (STD) NMR experiment is based on this principle [13, 14]. The receptor is saturated at a frequency where there is a broad underlying protein peak but no ligand resonances. The spin polarization induced by the saturation pulse spreads in all directions, including to any attached ligands (within 5 Å distance), such that when the ligand detaches its binding site, it carries bulk-induced spin polarization from the receptor (Fig. 1). The saturation pulse equalizes spin populations. Since the intensity of a peak is proportional to the difference in spin populations, the groups/atoms closest to the receptor will be less intense due to more efficient saturation transfer. This is easiest to see when plotted as a difference spectrum by subtracting out a spectrum taken with the saturation pulse off-resonance in a completely empty region of the spectrum (Fig. 2).

The ability to map binding epitopes and its relatively high sensitivity has made STD NMR a popular tool for studying receptor binding [15]. STD NMR first found widespread application in studies of protein carbohydrate interactions, where its ability to overcome problems of poor spectral dispersion and weak binding proved essential [16]. Starting from interactions of carbohydrates with soluble proteins [13], it has found widespread application for other protein-small molecule interactions. Variants of the STD NMR technique [15, 17] have been developed to study the interaction of small molecules with membrane proteins [18], viruses [19, 20], DNA [21], RNA [20], and nanoparticles [22]. The STD NMR method has even been extended to work as an in vivo technique for cells in suspension [21, 23].

Within the pharmaceutical industry, the ability of STD NMR to pick up essential information from a very low concentration of unlabeled macromolecule ($\leq$1 nmol) without upper limits on size and its sensitivity to a broad range of binding affinity (K_D = mM to nM) has found a particular niche within the lead optimization process [24], particularly with fragment-based approaches [25–27]. Although the technique is slow in comparison to non-NMR techniques, it can be used simultaneously with multicomponent mixtures or used in a flow through mode with the protein immobilized on a substrate [28]. The distance constraints from STD can be used as restraints for docking [29–31], by quantitative analysis of the relaxation matrix through the CORCEMA-STD procedure [32].

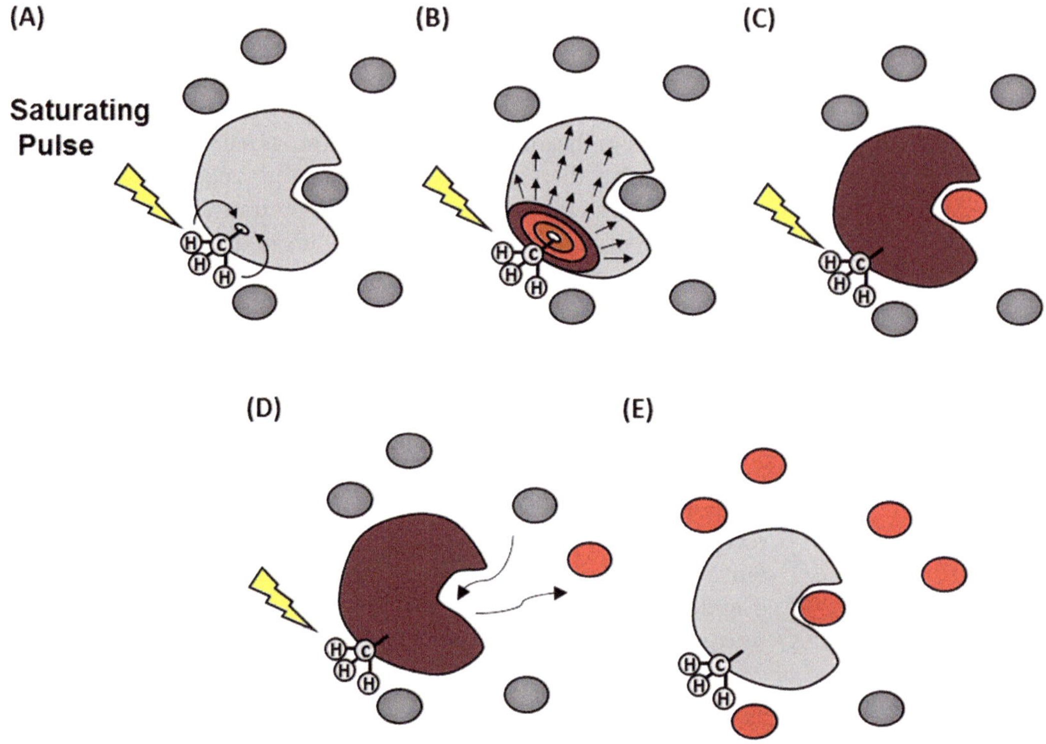

Fig. 1 Cartoon of the STD NMR experiment. (**a**) A long RF pulse (here centered on the methyl groups) selectively saturates the protein, equalizing the spin populations and driving the signal to zero. (**b**) The saturation spreads through the protein by spin diffusion. (**c**) Bound ligand becomes saturated by virtue of being in close proximity to the protein. (**d**) The ligand dissociates from the protein and a new one takes its place. Once bound, the new ligand is also saturated by the magnetization propagating through the protein. (**e**) The saturation spreads in this manner throughout the ligand pool, both bound and free. An equilibrium is established as ligand saturation is lost through T_1 relaxation and gained by fresh binding to the protein

2 Materials

1. **NMR Tube**: A standard 5 mm NMR tube can be used if necessary. To reduce sample volume, enhance sensitivity, and increase resolution, a susceptibility-matched NMR tube with a plunger can also be used such as those sold by Shigemi. These NMR tubes come in two parts: a thin-walled glass tube and a glass plunger. To take advantage of the improved shimming possible on a Shigemi tube, the glass plunger must be in contact with the solution, and any air interfaces must be eliminated. Any air bubbles will decrease the field homogeneity, increase linewidth, and lead to poor resolution. Total volume should be 600 μL for an ordinary NMR tube or 300 μL for a Shigemi tube.
2. **Phosphate Buffer or Fully Deuterated Tris or Hepes Buffer**: As with all NMR experiments, buffers with high ionic

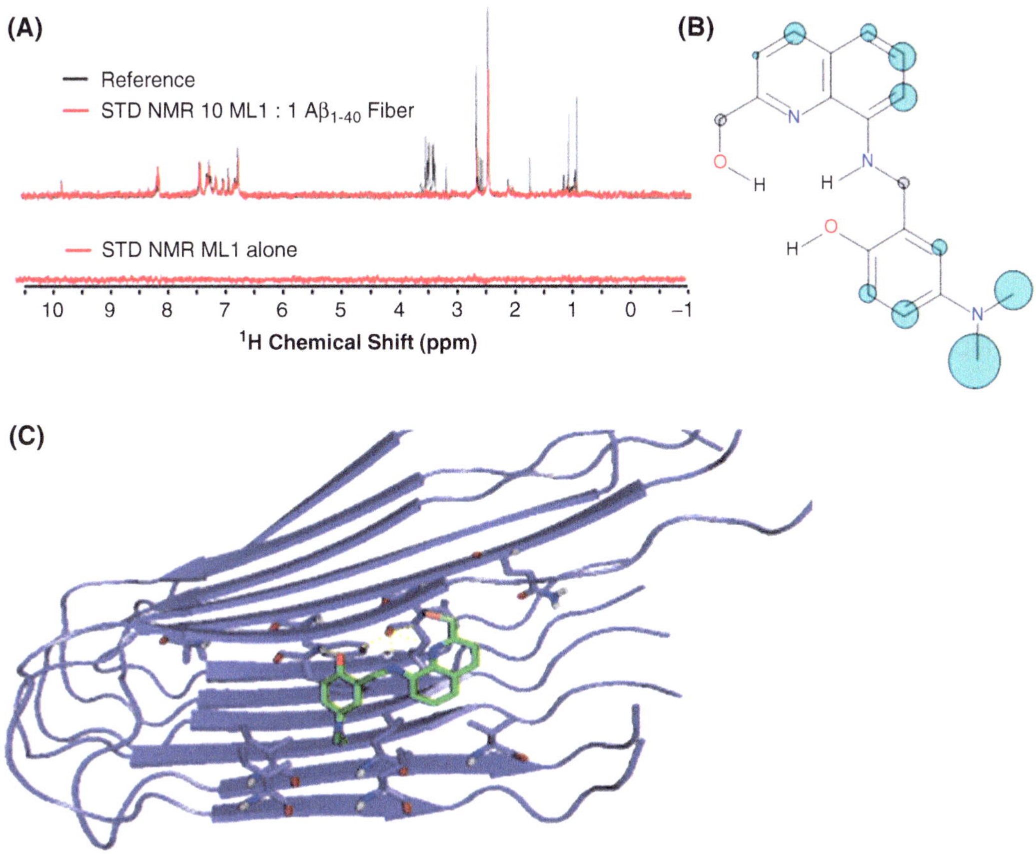

Fig. 2 (**a**) Example STD spectrum from a potential small molecule binder ("ML") to $A\beta_{1-40}$ amyloid fibers. The ordinary 1D reference spectrum is shown in black on top with the STD spectrum in red. The peaks in the STD spectrum correspond to the protons in close proximity to the fiber. (**b**) Fractional STD effect mapped onto the structure. (**c**) Docking of the ML ligand to the amyloid fiber in the absence of restraints. Note that the protons showing the largest STD effect are in closest proximity to the fiber. The dimethylamino group, which shows the largest effect, is packed tightly between the sidechains within the fiber, while the edge of the heteroaromatic quinoline pointed away from the fiber shows relatively little STD signal

strength are to be avoided if possible to limit resistive losses from conductivity in the sample (*see* **Note 1**). Typical salt concentrations are usually around 50 mM, which represents a compromise between probe performance and physiological relevance. If phosphate buffer is incompatible with the protein, Tris or Hepes can be used but should be deuterated to prevent buffer resonances from obscuring ligand peaks (Hepes has peaks at 3.85, 3.15, 3.06, 2.85, and 2.94 ppm and Tris at 3.92 and 3.40 ppm).

3. **Deuterium Oxide**: The STD experiment is run in 100% D_2O. The STD signal is usually very weak, which requires an accurate baseline to quantify correctly. The residual water signal is usually the largest obstacle to obtaining a flat baseline. For

this reason, STD experiments on ligands without exchangeable protons (or where the exchangeable protons are not of interest) are usually performed in 100% D_2O. Use of D_2O also has the advantage of preventing loss of the saturated signal by transfer to water.

4. **Deuterated DMSO**: Most ligands are more soluble in DMSO than water. DMSO is therefore useful in preparing a stock solution.

3 Methods

A number of protocols have been published for running STD experiments on specific systems [16, 18], including step-by-step instructions for setting up the STD experiment [33, 34]. Rather than duplicating these efforts, we will take a more general approach and outline the critical sample conditions and acquisition parameters that influence STD experiments.

3.1 Preparing the NMR Sample

Create the sample by dissolving at ligand to 1 mM concentration and the protein to 10 μM concentration in 50 mM phosphate buffer prepared in 100% D_2O. Exchanging the protein buffer to D_2O is usually not practical as it is an expensive procedure. Assuming a buffer exchange cannot be performed by gel filtration, the easiest way to prepare this sample is to make a 100 μM stock solution of the protein in the expression buffer and dissolve the protein directly in the 50 mM buffer/D_2O solution.

The concentrations above are meant as a guide and may need to be adjusted depending on the strength of the STD signal and ligand aggregation. Sample concentration is one of the most critical parameters in a saturation transfer experiment. The STD response is proportional to the fraction of ligand bound to the receptor. Under high ligand excess and fast exchange $k_{\mathrm{off}} \gg T_1$, a relationship similar to a binding isotherm can be derived linking the proportional STD response $\frac{I_0 - I_{\mathrm{SAT}}}{I_0}$ to the total ligand and protein concentrations L_{T} and P_{T} as $\frac{I_0 - I_{\mathrm{SAT}}}{I_0} \approx \frac{T_1 R_{\mathrm{SAT}} P_{\mathrm{T}}}{(L_{\mathrm{T}} + K_{\mathrm{D}})}$, where R_{SAT} is the magnetization transfer rate from the protein to the ligand and T_1 is the longitudinal relaxation time of the free ligand [35]. From this equation, it can be seen that:

1. The STD response in absolute terms increases with increasing ligand concentration.
2. The marginal effect of adding more ligand decreases as the ligand concentration increases.

This suggests that, other things being equal, the ligand concentration should be as high as possible to maximize the STD signal. However, many ligands have limited solubility, which can introduce numerous complications in analysis. First, the formation of aggregates reduces the effective ligand concentration, which can reduce the accuracy of determining binding constants. Colloidal aggregates also decrease the field homogeneity broadening lines and negating the sensitivity increase from increasing ligand concentration. The decrease in resolution may also potentially obscure peaks for group epitope mapping. More seriously, the formation of aggregates can create a binding surface that can bind proteins non-specifically, resulting in false-positive results [36, 37]. This is a well-known problem in drug screening [38, 39]. In many screening libraries, between 1% and 3% of molecules aggregate at low micromolar concentrations [40]. At NMR concentrations, the number will be higher. Ligand aggregation is probably the most common if often unrecognized artifact in STD NMR-based experiments.

3.2 Loading the Sample

An ordinary NMR tube can be loaded with no special precautions except tapping the tube to dislodge any air bubbles adhering to the walls of the NMR tube. A special loading procedure must be applied with Shigemi tubes to remove air bubbles before the sample can be used:

1. Degas the sample beforehand if possible by leaving it in open Eppendorf tube in an empty desiccator under slight vacuum for 5 min.
2. Pipette the degassed sample as close to the bottom of the tube as possible. Avoid making a tight seal with mouth of the tube with the pipette to prevent the introduction of additional bubbles from trapped air at the interface.
3. Wait until all the liquid has settled to the bottom of the tube and any foam generated during the pipetting process has disappeared.
4. Once the liquid has settled, slowly push the plunger down rotating it in order to eliminate trapped air pockets. Stop once the plunger has fully passed the meniscus of the sample.
5. Bubbles will likely have formed between the sample and the bottom of the plunger. To remove the bubbles, push the plunger down roughly 1 cm with a quick jerking motion, taking care not to extend the plunger so far that sample escapes out the top of the NMR tube.
6. Slowly push the plunger up to the original position, rotating it on the way up. Do not extend past the meniscus as more air will be introduced into the sample.
7. Repeat **steps 4** and **5** until the bubbles disappear. It may help to tap the tube a few times after each cycle to dislodge bubbles from the sides of the tube and prevent them from adhering strongly to the bottom of the plunger.
8. Wrap parafilm along the top of the tube to hold the plunger in place and prevent it from sliding in under the force of gravity.

3.3 NMR Acquisition

Because the exact procedures will vary with the particular manufacturer, this protocol assumes you are familiar with the basic operation of the instrument at least to the level of being able to take a 1D NMR spectrum [41, 42]. Specifically, you will need to be able to tune the probe, shim the magnet, adjust the frequency length, and calibrate power of 90° pulse for each ligand (*see* **Note 1**) [33]. The exact procedure for doing this will depend on the spectrometer manufacturer.

The simplest STD pulse sequence consists of only a frequency selective 90° pulse to saturate the protein signal for a specific saturation time before acquisition of the signal and a normal 90° pulse to record the signal. Because even the weak residual water signal from 99% D_2O can affect the baseline complicating the analysis of weak peaks, a water suppression sequence is usually included to suppress the solvent signal. Finally, a T_1 filter is usually added to suppress any signal from direct excitation of the protein. A standard 1D STD pulse sequence incorporating these elements is *stddiffesgp.3* on Bruker spectrometers and *1D-3 STD* for Varian spectrometers, found under the **DPFGSE 1D menu in water suppression experiments in VnmrJ BioPack.**

3.3.1 Determining the Parameters for the Solvent Suppression Block

Solvent suppression can be achieved by either excitation sculpting [43] or the 3–9–19 WATERGATE [44] sequence block (*stddiffesgp.3* on Bruker spectrometers). Excitation sculpting is generally preferred as it gives excellent water suppression if calibrated correctly and usually results in clean baselines, which are essential for the detection of weak peaks [43]. The excitation sculpting technique is largely dependent on two parameters, the frequency offset **o1** and the power level for the shaped pulse **sp1**.

1. Record a 1D NMR spectrum without water suppression (*zg30* on Bruker spectrometers) to find the frequency of the water peak. The frequency offset **o1** should be close to this value.
2. Set the power of the shaped selective excitation pulse. Select the selective 1H pulse calibration sequence (*selzg* on Bruker spectrometers). Set the pulse length **p11** to 2 ms and the relaxation delay to 1 s. Leave the other parameters as is. Click on the filename box with the right mouse button to call up the menu of possible shape files. From this list, select **Sincl.1000**. After setting the receiver gain with the "rga" command, start data acquisition in "zg" mode. Execute the "paraopt" macro to scan the pulse power variable **sp1** from 60 to 80 dB in 21 steps.

Enter parameter to modify: sp1

Enter initial parameter value: 60

Enter parameter increment: 1

Enter # of experiments: 21

The value of sp1 with the maximum signal is the power for a 90° pulse. This value may be easier to determine by finding the power for the minimum signal and dividing by two. The value for the shaped pulse power level will also be used for the saturation pulse.

3.3.2 Finding the Optimal Saturation Frequency

The saturation frequency should be placed in the vicinity of the protein peaks but far enough from a ligand peak to avoid direct saturation of the ligand peak (at least 1.8 ppm away from the nearest ligand peak) [45]. For this reason, it is helpful to have a 1D NMR of both the ligand and protein separately to place the saturation pulse before starting the STD experiment.

1. Record a 1D spectrum of the ligand with water suppression at the same concentration that will be used in the STD experiment. The peaks should be intense, sharp, and ideally well-resolved. If the intensity or resolution of the peaks is less than expected, the ligand may be aggregating at this concentration. If available, dynamic light scattering can be useful to detect the formation of colloidal aggregates. If dynamic light scattering is not available, reduce the concentration tenfold, and repeat the experiment after spinning down the sample. A concentration-dependent change in chemical shifts or the presence of additional or broader peaks at higher concentration indicates the presence of aggregates and an unsuitably high ligand concentration.
2. If enough protein is available, record a 1D spectrum of the protein alone with water suppression to assist in placement of the saturation frequency (*see* Subheading 3.1). If not enough protein is available to get a quality NMR, the region around 6–8 ppm corresponding to the aromatic side chains is usually a good choice for the on-resonance saturation frequency provided the ligand lacks aromatic groups. If ligand peaks are present in this region, folded proteins often possess a peak near 0.5–0 ppm corresponding to strongly shielded aliphatic groups buried in the interior of the protein [46]. This peak is usually distinct from those arising from aliphatic groups on the ligand, as aliphatic groups in small molecules are not shielded from solvent and usually resonate further downfield closer to 1–1.5 ppm. The off-resonance saturation frequency must be far from both the ligand and protein peak. Usually −50 ppm is sufficient for all except the very largest of proteins such as amyloid fibers.

3.3.3 Setting Up the Saturation Transfer Experiment

1. Set the relaxation delay **d1** to 5.5 s. **d1** should be 1–5 times the T_1 value of the ligand. Shorter times decrease acquisition time but can skew intensities toward protons with shorter relaxation

times. The relaxation delay must be long enough to allow the entire pulse sequence to complete. A relaxation time of 5.5 s allows the same relaxation time to be used for every experiment.

2. Set the spinlock time **d29** to 10 ms. The spinlock is a sequence of closely spaced 180° pulses that continually refocus the magnetization, locking the magnetization along one axis of the rotating frame for the duration of the spinlock. The 180° pulse suppresses T_2 relaxation while allowing $T_{1\rho}$ relaxation to take place. The spinlock sequence therefore serves as $T_{1\rho}$ filter to suppress unwanted protein signals from direct excitation of the protein from the saturation pulse. Longer spinlock times may be needed for smaller proteins (*see* **Note 2**). The spinlock time **d29** can be set to zero for maximum sensitivity if there is no background signal from the protein evident in the STD spectrum.
3. Set the length of the pulse for solvent suppression **p11** to 2 ms. Shorter pulses have wider excitation profiles and are more efficient at solvent suppression, while a longer pulse can be used to avoid suppressing ligand resonances near the water peak. The power level **sp1** and frequency offset **o1** for solvent suppression was determined in Subheading 3.3.1. Copy the parameters from the solvent suppression experiment.
4. Set the total number of scans to 256. The number of scans is determined by two parameters: the number of blocks **l4** and the number of scans per block **ns**. The total number of scans is equal to 2 × **l4** × **ns**. The spectrometer will run **ns** scans on-resonance followed by ns scans off-resonance, repeating the cycle **l4** times. Dividing the experiment into blocks has the advantage of mitigating any instability of the magnet. Set the number of scans per block **ns** to 32 and the number of blocks **l4**. If 256 scans are insufficient, increase the number of blocks **l4,** or consider decreasing the length of the saturation pulse as described below.
5. Set the saturation pulse shape to Gaussian1.1000. Gaussian pulses have smaller sidelobes outside the main pulse, which leads to narrower excitation profiles [47]. Alternatively, the saturation pulse shape can be set to Eburp2.1000 for a wider excitation profile.
6. Set the saturation power **sp13** to 50 db. The saturation power, along with the saturation time, controls the degree of saturation. A higher saturation power generally results in higher saturation efficiency (the power is on an attenuation scale and smaller values of **sp13** correspond to higher power levels) [48]. However, the reflected power from an excessively high power pulse can damage the receiver, particularly if the probe is

not tuned exactly. 50 db is usually a good compromise between saturation efficiency and reflected power [33].

7. Set the length of the saturation pulse **p13** to 50 ms. The saturation block is made of a train of saturation pulses. The length of each saturation pulse within the block, along with the pulse shape, determines the excitation profile of excitation. For the same saturation power **sp13**, a shorter saturation pulse will yield a narrower excitation profile, while a longer pulse will excite resonances over a greater ppm range. The excitation profile of a shaped pulse corresponding to 70% excitation efficiency is equal to a constant, the bandwidth factor, divided by the pulse length. The bandwidth factor for a Gaussian pulse is 2.122 (EBURP pulses have longer tails and a higher bandwidth factor of 4.952) [49]. A 50 ms Gaussian pulse therefore excites an approximately 42 Hz range, or 0.1 ppm on a 400 MHz spectrometer. Shorter pulses, down to 2.5 ms, can be used to increase saturation efficiency, provided no ligand signals are within this range [45].
8. Define the frequency list. Type ".freqlist" on the command line to define the frequencies for the on- and off-resonance saturation pulses. Choose FQ1LIST and give the list a name. Make sure the "Don't sort frequencies" button is on. A window will open with the last spectrum acquired (ideally the protein 1H spectrum). Place the cursor on the protein peak you want to saturate and right click. Move the cursor to the off-resonance frequency and left click. Save. Type "ased" on the command line to bring up the parameter editor. Go to "lists." Under FQLIST set the newly created list as FQ2LIST, and then click "edit." Remove the first line, which defines the central ^{1}H resonance. The on-resonance frequency in Hz should be on the first line and the off-resonance frequency on the second line.
9. Type *rga* to automatically adjust the receiver gain.
10. The remainder of the parameters can be left to the default values.
11. Define the first saturation time **D$_2$O** as 0.5 s. Longer saturation times generally result in a stronger STD signal but may give rise to artifacts in group epitope mapping [50]. Protons with significantly longer T_1 times like aromatic groups will accumulate saturation more efficiently than those with shorter T_1 times. The result is that the relative STD signals at long saturation times will be skewed toward the protons with strongest longitudinal relaxation, which will disproportionately weight the epitope map toward those groups.
12. Create the next experiment by typing *iexpno*. Set **D$_2$O** to 0.75 s for this experiment. Type *rga* to automatically adjust the receiver gain.

13. Repeat **step 11** setting **D_2O** to 1.00, 1.25, 1.50, 2.00, 2.50, 3.00, 4.00, and 5.00 s.
14. Once all the experiments are created, open the first one, and in the command line, type *multizg 10* to specify the number of experiments as 10. This will start serial acquisition for each experiment.
15. Type *efp* in the command line to Fourier transform the on-resonance spectrum for the first saturation time.
16. Repeat for the corresponding off-resonance spectra. Phase and integrate each peak to obtain I_0.
17. Type *.md* and the command line to bring up the multispectrum display window. Drag the on- and off-resonance spectra files onto the spectrum window.
18. Click the button with the delta sign to calculate the difference spectrum. *See* **Note 3** if the difference spectrum is much weaker than anticipated.
19. Phase and integrate each peak in the difference spectrum to obtain I_{SAT}.
20. Repeat **steps 14–18** for the remainder of the saturation times.
21. Plot the fractional STD effect $\frac{I_0 - I_{SAT}}{I_0}$ for each saturation time. The saturation time with the largest dispersion in fractional STD effect gives the most informative binding epitope map as the magnetization has reached the protons on the ligand closest to the protein but has not spread to the ones more distant from the binding site. A more accurate answer can be obtained by dividing by the T_1 value for each ligand proton, if known [50].

4 Notes

1. **Pulse Length Exceeds Recommended Values**: High salt concentrations can affect probe performance by introducing resistance into the coil. Increasing resistance has two effects, both originating from the increased conductivity of the sample [51]. On the receive side, the electrical losses from increased resistance decrease sensitivity by reducing the detection efficiency of the induced current. On the transmission side, solutions with higher salt concentrations interfere with power transmission, meaning that higher power levels are needed to generate equivalent 90° excitation and saturation pulses [52]. The increase in pulse length is particularly problematic [52] for STD experiments which use spinlocks as a T_1 filter to suppress the residual signal from direct excitation of the receptor [15]. The effect is particularly prominent with cryoprobes,

whose signal enhancement originates from cooling the sample down to liquid nitrogen or liquid helium temperatures. The heating associated with resistive power losses eliminates this advantage.

If the protein is stable at lower salt concentrations, a simple solution is to simply use a lower ionic strength solution. However, while this solves the problem from the technical side, a nonphysiological ionic strength can alter the K_D by increasing the strength of ionic interactions and altering the hydrophobic ones. In some situations, it can even change the binding mode. One solution is to use a buffer with a lower conductivity than phosphate, which limits the induced resistance [51]. This method has the disadvantage of receiving a strong signal from the buffer unless fully deuterated buffers are used. Since the induced resistance is dependent on the total amount of the salt within the active volume, not just the concentration, reducing the sample volume by using a 3 mm NMR tube instead of the standard 5 mm size and increasing the concentration can also be used for samples that require high amount of salt [52]. Detuning the coil slightly to lower the Q-factor can also reduce pulse length.

2. **The Off-Resonance Signal Shows Detectable Saturation**: No protein peaks should be resonating 30 ppm. A loss of signal when a saturation pulse is applied at this frequency indicates a severely broadened peak, which implies the existence of either protein or ligand aggregates. Beyond the difficulty of interpreting STD spectra when off-resonance saturation effects are present, aggregates reduce the effective population of interacting molecules and reduce the accuracy of quantitative analysis. More seriously, protein aggregates are likely in a different conformation than the native protein and may inappropriately expose hydrophobic surfaces that act as alternative sites for ligand binding.

   Three alternatives exist for reducing protein aggregation. First, try reducing the protein concentration. If the off-resonance still shows detectable saturation, try increasing the salt concentration, keeping in mind that higher salt concentrations affect probe performance (*see* **Note 1**). As a last resort, protein aggregation can be reduced in some cases with nonionic detergents. The detergent must be deuterated to eliminate interfering signals. This is referred to as a last resort because detergents will also mask ligand aggregation giving rise to the possibility of false positives.

3. **STD Signal Is Small with a Ligand Known to Have High-Affinity Receptor**: The STD experiment relies on the slow relaxation of the saturation signal relative to a rebinding event. When relaxation is slow and exchange is rapid, every

ligand molecule makes several trips back and forth to the receptor before the saturation signal decays due to T_1 relaxation. Small ligand molecules have long T_1 times in their free states due to their fast rotational correlation times. When bound to a large receptor, however, the rotational correlation time of the ligand is much slower than in the free state, and relaxation is consequently much faster. As a consequence if k_{off} is small (tight binding, usually less than low micromolar or less [53]), the magnetization from the saturation pulse may be lost due to relaxation before the ligand leaves the receptor. Although it is sometimes possible in specific instances to increase k_{off} by manipulating the salt concentration, in general ligands with nanomolar or less affinity require indirect techniques to study by STD NMR. A reporter molecule with moderate affinity can be used in a competition assay to determine the apparent K_D by techniques similar to those used for high-affinity compounds in isothermal calorimetry. The tight-binding ligand displaces the reporter molecule from the receptor, allowing K_D to be estimated by the decrease in the STD signal of the reporter molecule with increasing ligand concentrations even if the STD signal of the ligand molecule cannot be observed directly [54–56]

References

1. Meyer B, Peters T (2003) NMR spectroscopy techniques for screening and identifying ligand binding to protein receptors. Angew Chem Int Ed Eng 42(8):864–890. https://doi.org/10.1002/anie.200390233
2. Groftehauge MK, Hajizadeh NR, Swann MJ, Pohl E (2015) Protein-ligand interactions investigated by thermal shift assays (TSA) and dual polarization interferometry (DPI). Acta Crystallogr D Biol Crystallogr 71 (Pt 1):36–44. https://doi.org/10.1107/S1399004714016617
3. Jerabek-Willemsen M, André T et al (2014) MicroScale Thermophoresis: interaction analysis and beyond. J Mol Struct 1077(Supplement C):101–113. https://doi.org/10.1016/j.molstruc.2014.03.009
4. Carpenter JW, Laethem C, Hubbard FR et al (2002) Configuring radioligand receptor binding assays for HTS using scintillation proximity assay technology. Methods Mol Biol 190:31–49. https://doi.org/10.1385/1-59259-180-9:031
5. Patching SG (2014) Surface plasmon resonance spectroscopy for characterisation of membrane protein-ligand interactions and its potential for drug discovery. Biochim Biophys Acta 1838(1 Pt A):43–55. https://doi.org/10.1016/j.bbamem.2013.04.028
6. Shuker SB, Hajduk PJ, Meadows RP, Fesik SW (1996) Discovering high-affinity ligands for proteins: SAR by NMR. Science 274 (5292):1531–1534
7. Stockman BJ, Dalvit C (2002) NMR screening techniques in drug discovery and drug design. Prog Nucl Magn Reson Spectrosc 41 (3–4):187–231. https://doi.org/10.1016/S0079-6565(02)00049-3
8. Pellecchia M, Bertini I, Cowburn D et al (2008) Perspectives on NMR in drug discovery: a technique comes of age. Nat Rev Drug Discov 7(9):738–745. https://doi.org/10.1038/nrd2606
9. Jameson CJ (1996) Understanding NMR chemical shifts. Annu Rev Phys Chem 47:135–169. https://doi.org/10.1146/annurev.physchem.47.1.135
10. de Dios AC, Jameson CJ (2012) Recent advances in nuclear shielding calculations. Annu Rep Nmr Spectro 77:1–80. https://doi.org/10.1016/B978-0-12-397020-6.00001-5
11. Anglister J, Srivastava G, Naider F (2016) Detection of intermolecular NOE interactions in large protein complexes. Prog Nucl Magn

Reson Spectrosc 97:40–56. https://doi.org/10.1016/j.pnmrs.2016.08.002

12. Post CB (2003) Exchange-transferred NOE spectroscopy and bound ligand structure determination. Curr Opin Struct Biol 13 (5):581–588. https://doi.org/10.1016/j.sbi.2003.09.012
13. Mayer M, Meyer B (1999) Characterization of ligand binding by saturation transfer difference NMR spectroscopy. Angew Chem Int Ed 38 (12):1784–1788. https://doi.org/10.1002/(Sici)1521-3773(19990614)38:12<1784::Aid-Anie1784>3.0.Co;2-Q
14. Mayer M, Meyer B (2001) Group epitope mapping by saturation transfer difference NMR to identify segments of a ligand in direct contact with a protein receptor. J Am Chem Soc 123(25):6108–6117. https://doi.org/10.1021/ja0100120
15. Bhunia A, Bhattacharjya S, Chatterjee S (2012) Applications of saturation transfer difference NMR in biological systems. Drug Discov Today 17(9–10):505–513. https://doi.org/10.1016/j.drudis.2011.12.016
16. Haselhorst T, Lamerz AC, Itzstein M (2009) Saturation transfer difference NMR spectroscopy as a technique to investigate protein-carbohydrate interactions in solution. Methods Mol Biol 534:375–386. https://doi.org/10.1007/978-1-59745-022-5_26
17. Wagstaff JL, Taylor SL, Howard MJ (2013) Recent developments and applications of saturation transfer difference nuclear magnetic resonance (STD NMR) spectroscopy. Mol BioSyst 9(4):571–577. https://doi.org/10.1039/c2mb25395j
18. Venkitakrishnan RP, Benard O, Max M et al (2012) Use of NMR saturation transfer difference spectroscopy to study ligand binding to membrane proteins. Methods Mol Biol 914:47–63. https://doi.org/10.1007/978-1-62703-023-6_4
19. Benie AJ, Moser R, Bauml E et al (2003) Virus-ligand interactions: identification and characterization of ligand binding by NMR spectroscopy. J Am Chem Soc 125(1):14–15. https://doi.org/10.1021/ja027691e
20. Harris KA, Shekhtman A, Agris PF (2013) Specific RNA-protein interactions detected with saturation transfer difference NMR. RNA Biol 10(8):1307–1311. https://doi.org/10.4161/rna.25948
21. Di Micco S, Bassarello C, Bifulco G et al (2006) Differential-frequency saturation transfer difference NMR spectroscopy allows the detection of different ligand-DNA binding modes. Angew Chem Int Ed 45(2):224–228. https://doi.org/10.1002/anie.200501344
22. Hens Z, Martins JC (2013) A solution NMR toolbox for characterizing the surface chemistry of colloidal nanocrystals. Chem Mater 25 (8):1211–1221. https://doi.org/10.1021/cm303361s
23. Claasen B, Axmann M, Meinecke R, Meyer B (2005) Direct observation of ligand binding to membrane proteins in living cells by a saturation transfer double difference (STDD) NMR spectroscopy method shows a significantly higher affinity of integrin alpha(IIb)beta3 in native platelets than in liposomes. J Am Chem Soc 127(3):916–919. https://doi.org/10.1021/ja044434w
24. Dias DM, Ciulli A (2014) NMR approaches in structure-based lead discovery: recent developments and new frontiers for targeting multi-protein complexes. Prog Biophys Mol Biol 116(2–3):101–112. https://doi.org/10.1016/j.pbiomolbio.2014.08.012
25. Ma R, Wang P, Wu J, Ruan K (2016) Process of fragment-based lead discovery-a perspective from NMR. Molecules 21(7). https://doi.org/10.3390/molecules21070854
26. Cala O, Krimm I (2015) Ligand-orientation based fragment selection in STD NMR screening. J Med Chem 58(21):8739–8742. https://doi.org/10.1021/acs.jmedchem.5b01114
27. Kim HY, Wyss DF (2015) NMR screening in fragment-based drug design: a practical guide. Methods Mol Biol 1263:197–208. https://doi.org/10.1007/978-1-4939-2269-7_16
28. Vanwetswinkel S, Heetebrij RJ, van Duynhoven J et al (2005) TINS, target immobilized NMR screening: an efficient and sensitive method for ligand discovery. Chem Biol 12 (2):207–216. https://doi.org/10.1016/j.chembiol.2004.12.004
29. Jayalakshmi V, Krishna NR (2005) Determination of the conformation of trimethoprim in the binding pocket of bovine dihydrofolate reductase from a STD-NMR intensity-restrained CORCEMA-ST optimization. J Am Chem Soc 127(40):14080–14084. https://doi.org/10.1021/ja054192f
30. Jayalakshmi V, Biet T, Peters T, Krishna NR (2004) Refinement of the conformation of UDP-galactose bound to galactosyltransferase using the STD NMR intensity-restrained CORCEMA optimization. J Am Chem Soc 126(28):8610–8611. https://doi.org/10.1021/ja048703u
31. Zhang W, Li R, Shin R, Wang Y et al (2013) Identification of the binding site of an allosteric ligand using STD-NMR, docking, and CORCEMA-ST calculations. ChemMedChem 8(10):1629–1633. https://doi.org/10.1002/cmdc.201300267

32. Jayalakshmi V, Krishna NR (2002) Complete relaxation and conformational exchange matrix (CORCEMA) analysis of intermolecular saturation transfer effects in reversibly forming ligand-receptor complexes. J Magn Reson 155(1):106–118. https://doi.org/10.1006/jmre.2001.2499
33. Quiros MT, Macdonald C, Angulo J, Munoz MP (2016) Spin saturation transfer difference NMR (SSTD NMR): a new tool to obtain kinetic parameters of chemical exchange processes. J Vis Exp 117. https://doi.org/10.3791/54499
34. Viegas A, Manso J, Nobrega FL, Cabrita EJ (2011) Saturation-transfer difference (STD) NMR: a simple and fast method for ligand screening and characterization of protein binding. J Chem Educ 88(7):990–994. https://doi.org/10.1021/ed101169t
35. Kemper S, Patel MK, Errey JC et al (2010) Group epitope mapping considering relaxation of the ligand (GEM-CRL): including longitudinal relaxation rates in the analysis of saturation transfer difference (STD) experiments. J Magn Reson 203(1):1–10. https://doi.org/10.1016/j.jmr.2009.11.015
36. McGovern SL, Caselli E, Grigorieff N, Shoichet BK (2002) A common mechanism underlying promiscuous inhibitors from virtual and high-throughput screening. J Med Chem 45(8):1712–1722
37. Coan KE, Shoichet BK (2008) Stoichiometry and physical chemistry of promiscuous aggregate-based inhibitors. J Am Chem Soc 130(29):9606–9612. https://doi.org/10.1021/ja802977h
38. Aldrich C, Bertozzi C, Georg G et al (2017) The ecstasy and agony of assay interference compounds. J Med Chem 60(6):2165–2168. https://doi.org/10.1021/acs.jmedchem.7b00229
39. Feng BY, Shelat A, Doman TN et al (2005) High-throughput assays for promiscuous inhibitors. Nat Chem Biol 1(3):146–148. https://doi.org/10.1038/nchembio718
40. Feng BY, Simeonov A, Jadhav A et al (2007) A high-throughput screen for aggregation-based inhibition in a large compound library. J Med Chem 50(10):2385–2390. https://doi.org/10.1021/jm061317y
41. Harwood JS, Mo H (2016) Practical NMR spectroscopy laboratory guide using Bruker spectrometers. Academic Press, London
42. Berger S, Braun S (2004) 200 and more NMR experiments: a practical course. 3rd rev. and expanded edn. Wiley, Leipzig
43. Hwang TL, Shaka AJ (1995) Water suppression that works. Excitation sculpting using arbitrary wave-forms and pulsed-field gradients. J Magn Reson Ser A 112(2):275–279. https://doi.org/10.1006/jmra.1995.1047
44. Piotto M, Saudek V, Sklenar V (1992) Gradient-tailored excitation for single-quantum NMR spectroscopy of aqueous solutions. J Biomol NMR 2(6):661–665
45. Ley NB, Rowe ML, Williamson RA, Howard MJ (2014) Optimising selective excitation pulses to maximise saturation transfer difference NMR spectroscopy. RSC Adv 4(14):7347–7351. https://doi.org/10.1039/C3RA46246C
46. Mitra P, Shultis D, Brender JR et al (2013) An evolution-based approach to De novo protein design and case study on mycobacterium tuberculosis. PLoS Comput Biol 9(10):e1003298. https://doi.org/10.1371/journal.pcbi.1003298
47. Bauer C, Freeman R, Frenkiel T et al (1984) Gaussian pulses. J Magn Reson 58(3):442–457. https://doi.org/10.1016/0022-2364(84)90148-3
48. Cutting B, Shelke SV, Dragic Z et al (2007) Sensitivity enhancement in saturation transfer difference (STD) experiments through optimized excitation schemes. Magn Reson Chem 45(9):720–724. https://doi.org/10.1002/mrc.2033
49. Claridge TDW, ScienceDirect (Online service) (2009) High-resolution NMR techniques in organic chemistry. Elsevier, Amsterdam
50. Yan J, Kline AD, Mo H et al (2003) The effect of relaxation on the epitope mapping by saturation transfer difference NMR. J Magn Reson 163(2):270–276
51. Kelly AE, Ou HD, Withers R, Dotsch V (2002) Low-conductivity buffers for high-sensitivity NMR measurements. J Am Chem Soc 124(40):12013–12019
52. Voehler MW, Collier G, Young JK et al (2006) Performance of cryogenic probes as a function of ionic strength and sample tube geometry. J Magn Reson 183(1):102–109. https://doi.org/10.1016/j.jmr.2006.08.002
53. Lepre CA, Moore JM, Peng JW (2004) Theory and applications of NMR-based screening in pharmaceutical research. Chem Rev 104(8):3641–3676. https://doi.org/10.1021/cr030409h
54. Dalvit C, Flocco M, Knapp S et al (2002) High-throughput NMR-based screening with competition binding experiments. J Am Chem Soc 124(26):7702–7709
55. Jahnke W, Floersheim P, Ostermeier C et al (2002) NMR reporter screening for the detection of high-affinity ligands. Angew Chem Int Ed Eng 41(18):3420–3423. https://doi.org/

10.1002/1521-3773(20020916)41:18<3420::AID-ANIE3420>3.0.CO;2-E

56. Siriwardena AH, Tian F, Noble S, Prestegard JH (2002) A straightforward NMR-spectroscopy-based method for rapid library screening. Angew Chem Int Ed Eng 41(18):3454–3457. https://doi.org/10.1002/1521-3773(20020916)41:18<3454::AID-ANIE3454>3.0.CO;2-L

Chapter 5

Protein-Ligand Docking in Drug Design: Performance Assessment and Binding-Pose Selection

Flavio Ballante

Abstract

Main goal in drug discovery is the identification of drug-like compounds capable to modulate specific biological targets. Thus, the prediction of reliable binding poses of candidate ligands, through molecular docking simulations, represents a key step to be pursued in structure-based drug design (SBDD). Since the increasing number of resolved three-dimensional ligand-protein structures, together with the expansion of computational power and software development, the comprehensive and systematic use of experimental data can be proficiently employed to validate the docking performance. This allows to select and refine the protocol to adopt when predicting the binding pose of trial compounds in a target. Given the availability of multiple docking software, a comparative docking assessment in an early research stage represents a must-use step to minimize fails in molecular modeling. This chapter describes how to perform a docking assessment, using freely available tools, in a semiautomated fashion.

Key words Drug design, Drug discovery, Molecular docking, Molecular modeling, Docking assessment, Structure-based drug design (SBDD)

1 Introduction

Molecular recognition (generally referred as the non-covalent interactions between two or more molecules) is a key event in many biological systems, and its optimization represents one of the most challenging problems in drug discovery when targeting a certain protein by using small molecules [1]. Prediction or analysis of ligand-protein interactions can be performed with different computer-aided drug design (CADD) tools, generally classified as ligand-based (LB, which depend on the information of diverse molecules that bind to the biological target) and structure-based (SB, which rely on knowledge of three-dimensional structural information from biological targets) methods [2]. Among others, molecular docking is one of the most used structure-based drug design (SBDD) tools in medicinal chemistry to predict ligands' binding pose in a protein, allowing to evaluate molecular

Thomas Mavromoustakos and Tahsin F. Kellici (eds.), *Rational Drug Design: Methods and Protocols*, Methods in Molecular Biology, vol. 1824, https://doi.org/10.1007/978-1-4939-8630-9_5,

interactions, induced conformational changes, and binding energetics, as well as to perform virtual screening applications [3]. In addition, docked poses can be proficiently used in classic (ligand-based) [4] or per-residue (structure-based) [5] three-dimensional quantitative structure-activity relationship (3D QSAR) studies [6, 7]. When ligand-protein structural data from experimental methods (such as X-ray crystallography or NMR spectroscopy) are available, assessment of the docking protocol is required to estimate the reliability of the designed procedure in predicting compounds' binding pose without experimental information, for a selected target. Different strategies can be adopted to evaluate a docking procedure: docking accuracy (DA) calculation [8], enrichment factor (EF) analysis [9], correlation between experimental and predicted binding affinities [10], and distance between a metal ion in the active site (if present) and the ligands' metal-binding moieties [11], among others.

This chapter describes how to benchmark and evaluate a docking method by:

1. Performing re-docking (or self-docking) and cross-docking (or ensemble docking) simulations
2. Computing the relative docking accuracies based on root-mean square deviation (RMSD) values between the predicted (docked) and the experimental binding poses

The protocol is characterized by four steps:

1. Setup of working directories
2. Preparation of the structures and input files
3. Docking simulation, cluster analysis, and DA calculation
4. Analysis of the results

UCSF Chimera [12], LigandBox, and MGLTools [13] are used to perform **step 2**, AutoDock Vina [14] to perform molecular docking on a small set of human coagulation factor Xa (FXa) inhibitor complexes [15–19], and Clusterizer-DockAccessor [20] to perform cluster analysis and DA calculation (**step 3**). The whole protocol is intended to run on a Linux environment: a series of basic shell commands to be written in the Linux terminal are provided, step-by-step, to semiautomate the process (*see* **Note 1**).

2 Materials

1. **AutoDock Vina (Version 1.1.2)**. Download AutoDock Vina [14] (for Linux, version 1.1.2) from http://vina.scripps.edu/download.html. For installation instructions, *see* http://vina.scripps.edu/manual.html#linux (*see* **Note 2**).

2. **AutoDockTools (version 1.5.6)**. Go to the "MGLTools Web Portal" website (http://mgltools.scripps.edu/downloads), and download MGLTools [13] (MGLTools version 1.5.6; 32 or 64 bit, according to the Linux system in use). Install following the instructions available from http://mgltools.scripps.edu/downloads/instructions/linux (*see* **Note 3**).
3. **Clusterizer-DockAccessor (Version 1.1)**. Download Clusterizer-DockAccessor [20] from http://cheminf.com/software/clusterizer_dockaccessor/. Select "Clusterizer-DockAccessor 1.1 Software," fill the registration form, and click "Send." An e-mail will be sent reporting a link for downloading the software. To install the software, follow the instructions reported in the user manual available from http://cheminf.com/software/clusterizer_dockaccessor/ (*see* **Note 4**).
4. **DOCK 6 (version 6.8)**. Request DOCK 6 [21] license from the UCSF DOCK website (http://dock.compbio.ucsf.edu/Online_Licensing/index.htm). An e-mail will be sent when the DOCK 6 license is accepted. Follow the instructions provided in the received e-mail to download the last release of DOCK 6. Follow the installation instructions available from the DOCK 6 manual (http://dock.compbio.ucsf.edu/DOCK_6/dock6_manual.htm, *see* **Note 5**).
5. **LigandBox**. Download LigandBox from http://cheminf.com/software/ligandbox; fill the registration form and click "Send." An e-mail will be sent reporting a link for downloading the software. Follow the installation instructions available from http://cheminf.com/software/ligandbox (*see* **Note 6**).
6. **Open Babel (Version 2.4.1)**. Download Open Babel [22, 23] (stable release for Linux), and follow the installation instructions (http://openbabel.org/wiki/Get_Open_Babel, *see* **Note** 7).
7. **UCSF Chimera**. Download the latest Linux release of UCSF Chimera [12] (32 or 64 bit, according to the Linux system in use) from https://www.cgl.ucsf.edu/chimera/download.html. Click the relative "Instructions" link from the same web page for installation instructions (*see* **Note 8**).
8. **Human Coagulation Factor Xa (FXa) PDB Files**. 6 FXa co-crystal structures (PDB codes: 1EZQ, 1F0S, 1XKA, 2BOK, 2CJI, and 2FZZ) have been selected for this exercise (*see* **Note 9**). The complexes can be downloaded from the Protein Data Bank (PDB) (https://www.rcsb.org/) [24]. A convenient way to retrieve the structures is through the Linux command line interface (terminal). Open the Linux terminal. Type into the terminal the code shown in Table 1 to create a parent directory ("FXA") containing a child folder ("00_PDB"), and download the PDB files in there.

Table 1
Command line sequence 1: retrieve structures from PDB

```
mkdir  -p FXA/00_PDB
cd FXA/00_PDB
wget http://www.rcsb.org/pdb/files/1EZQ.pdb
wget http://www.rcsb.org/pdb/files/1F0S.pdb
wget http://www.rcsb.org/pdb/files/1XKA.pdb
wget http://www.rcsb.org/pdb/files/2BOK.pdb
wget http://www.rcsb.org/pdb/files/2CJI.pdb
wget http://www.rcsb.org/pdb/files/2FZZ.pdb
cd ..
```

3 Methods

The protocol is characterized by four steps (Fig. 1):

1. Set the working directories to store the input/output files.
2. Prepare the PDB structures and input files for molecular docking: PDB structures are "cleaned" from solvent molecules and non-interacting ions and then superimposed and protonated at physiological pH (using UCSF Chimera); unwanted lines from the PDB files are also removed (using Linux shell command lines). From each cleaned PDB complex, the relative protein ("lock") and ligand ("key") structures are extracted; then randomized keys' conformations are derived (through Open Babel) to perform the subsequent "random conformation docking simulations" (*see* **Note 10**). The obtained PDBs are then converted into PDBQT format (as input files for AutoDock Vina) using Python scripts available from MGLTools. Afterward, the grid box center coordinates and dimensions are computed using LigandBox and placed into the AutoDock Vina configuration file (*see* **Note 9**).
3. Experimental/random conformation re-docking and cross-docking simulations (ECRD, RCRD, ECCD, and RCCD, respectively) through AutoDock Vina, followed by cluster analysis and DA calculation using Clusterizer-DockAccessor.
4. Analysis of the results.

   Before starting the protocol, it is advisable to test the system (*see* **Notes 2–8**).

3.1 Setting the Working Directories

A series of directories will now be set to store input/output files during the protocol (run the code shown in Table 2).

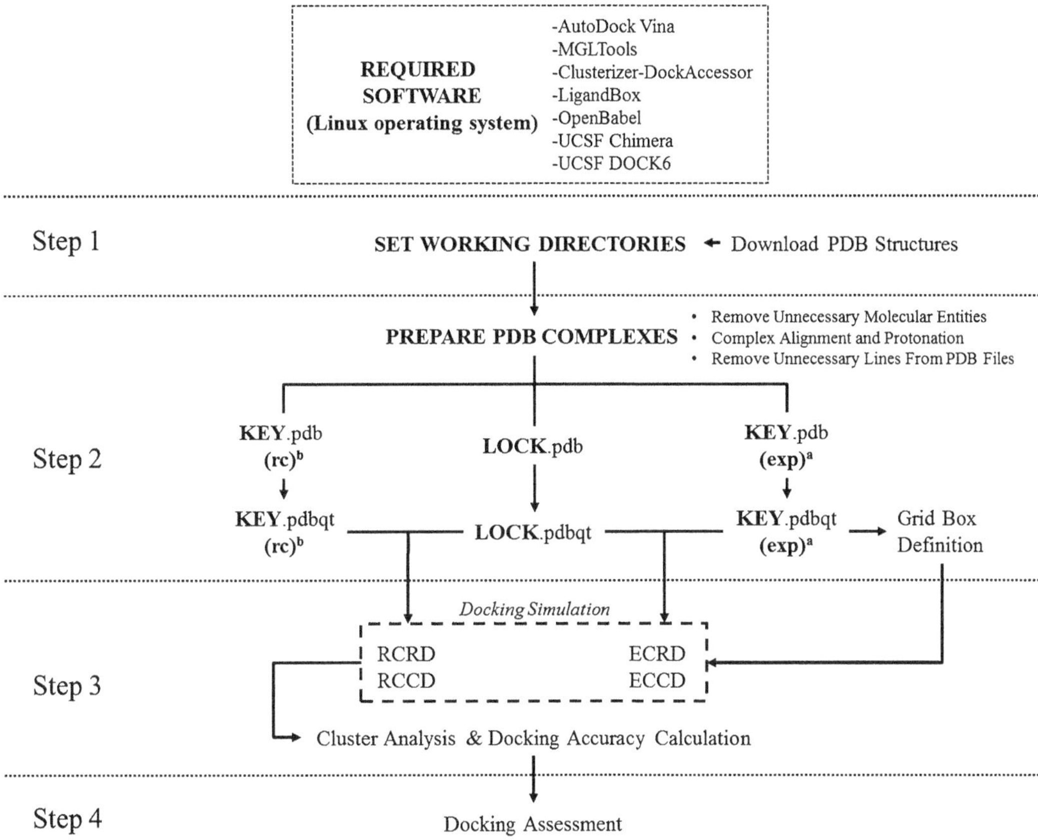

Fig. 1 Top, required software; bottom, schematized procedure. The protocol is characterized by four main steps for setting the working directories (step 1); preparing the docking input files (step 2); running the experimental conformation re-docking (ECRD), random conformation re-docking (RCRD), experimental conformation cross-docking (ECCD), and random conformation cross-docking (RCCD) simulations (step 3); and assessing the docking performance (step 4). [a]*Exp* Experimental, [b]*RC* randomized starting conformer

Table 2
Command line sequence 2: set working directories

```
1. mkdir 01_PDB_ALIGNED
2. mkdir 02_PDB_CLEANED_ALIGNED
3. mkdir 03_LOCK_KEY
4. mkdir 04_PDBQTs
5. mkdir -p 05_DOCKING/VINA/ECRD
6. mkdir 05_DOCKING/VINA/RCRD
7. mkdir 05_DOCKING/VINA/ECCD
8. mkdir 05_DOCKING/VINA/RCCD
```

3.2 Preparing PDB Structures and Input Files

3.2.1 Preparing the PDB Complexes

To prepare the PDB complexes (*see* **Note 11**), launch UCSF Chimera from the "00_PDB" folder (Table 3).

All the downloaded complexes are now opened in UCSF Chimera and shown in the main graphic window (*see* Fig. 2, left). Click *Favorites* → *Command Line* to start the command line tool; then click *Favorites* → *Model Panel* to list all the models loaded in the Chimera session (*see* Fig. 2, right).

(a) **Removing Unnecessary Chains**

Unnecessary chains in the PDBs can be removed from the native structure (*see* **Note 11**). Write "split" into the Chimera command line to partition each model into separate sub-models; the Model Panel will show all the different models according to the chain (*see* Fig. 3, left). In this exercise, six models (*see* below) can be removed from the Chimera session since secondary chains are

Table 3
Command line sequence 3: launch UCSF Chimera from "00_PDB"

```
1. cd 00_PDB
2. chimera *.pdb
```

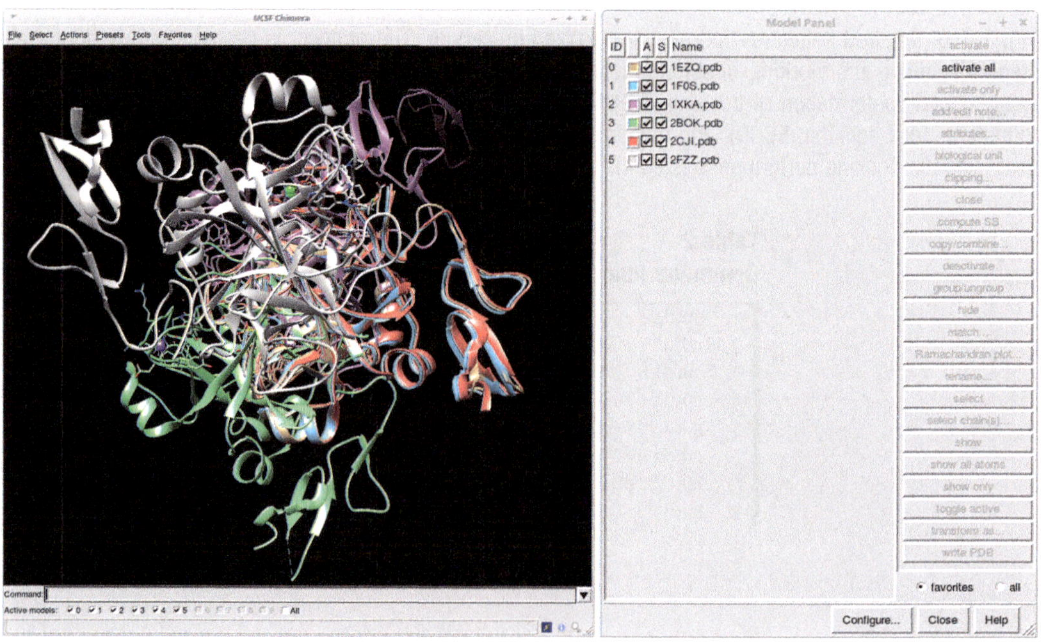

Fig. 2 UCSF Chimera. Left, graphic window (molecular structures are shown and the command line is turned on); right, "Model Panel"

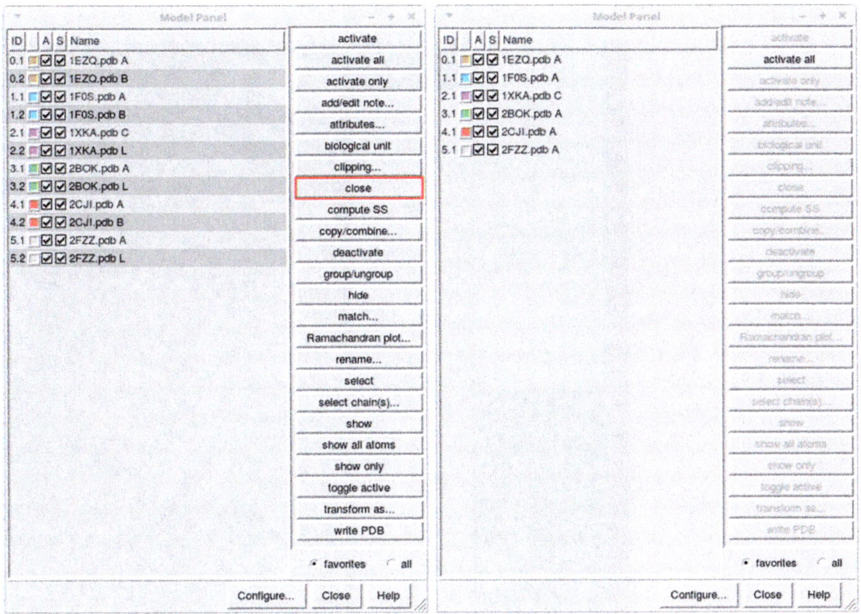

Fig. 3 UCSF Chimera: "Model Panel." Left, selected models to be removed; right, models to maintain in the session

unnecessary for the docking simulation. Go to the Model Panel, hold Ctrl key and click "1EZQ.pdb B," "1F0S.pdb B," "1XKA. pdb L," "2BOK.pdb L," "2CJI.pdb B," and "2FZZ.pdb L" to select the models to be removed, then release the Ctrl key (selected models are highlighted as shown in Fig. 3, left), and click the "close" button placed on the right side panel (the one enclosed in the red box in Fig. 3, left) to remove the selected models from the Chimera session. Now, only proteins' chains comprising the active site are listed (*see* Fig. 3, right).

(b) **Removing Solvent and Non-interacting Ions**

Solvent molecules and non-interacting ions will be now removed (*see* **Note 11**).

Click *Select* → *Residue* to show standard amino acids, ligands ("4PP," "5QC," "784," "GSK," "PR2," "RPR"), solvent molecules ("HOH"), and ions ("CA" and "NA") codes characterizing the models (*see* Fig. 4, *see* **Note 11**).

In the empty Chimera command line write "select #:HOH,CA, NA" and then press enter (or return); H_2O molecules, Ca^{2+}, and Na^{+} ions from all the loaded models are now selected (green highlighted from the graphic window). While the selection is active, write in the empty command line "delete selection," and then press enter (or return). Water molecules, Ca^{2+}, and Na^{+} ions are now removed from the session.

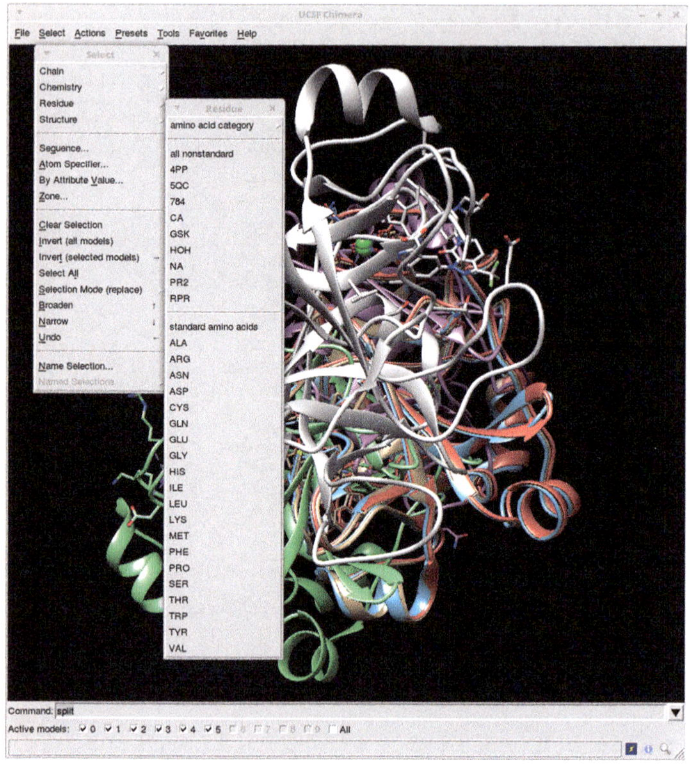

Fig. 4 UCSF Chimera: "Residue" window

(c) **Complex Alignment**

Complex structures can be superimposed upon each other using the structure with the highest resolution and no gaps as reference.

In Chimera, click *Tools* → *Structure Comparison* → *MatchMaker* to open the MatchMaker tool. As "Reference structure" (left panel of the dialog window), select "2CJI.pdb A" (characterized by the highest resolution, 2.1 Å, and without missing non-terminal residues), and as "Structure(s) to match" (right panel of the dialog window), select all the structures except "2CJI.pdb A" (as depicted in Fig. 5). Click *OK* to start MatchMaker.

Complexes are now superimposed (Fig. 6).

(d) **Structure Protonation**

Complexes can now be protonated, through Chimera, considering the physiological pH (pH 7.4, *see* **Note 12**). Click *Tools* → *Structure Editing* → *AddH* (check that "Consider each model in isolation from all others," "also consider H-bonds," and "Residue-name-based" options are selected) → *Click OK*. Structures are now protonated (*see* **Note 13**).

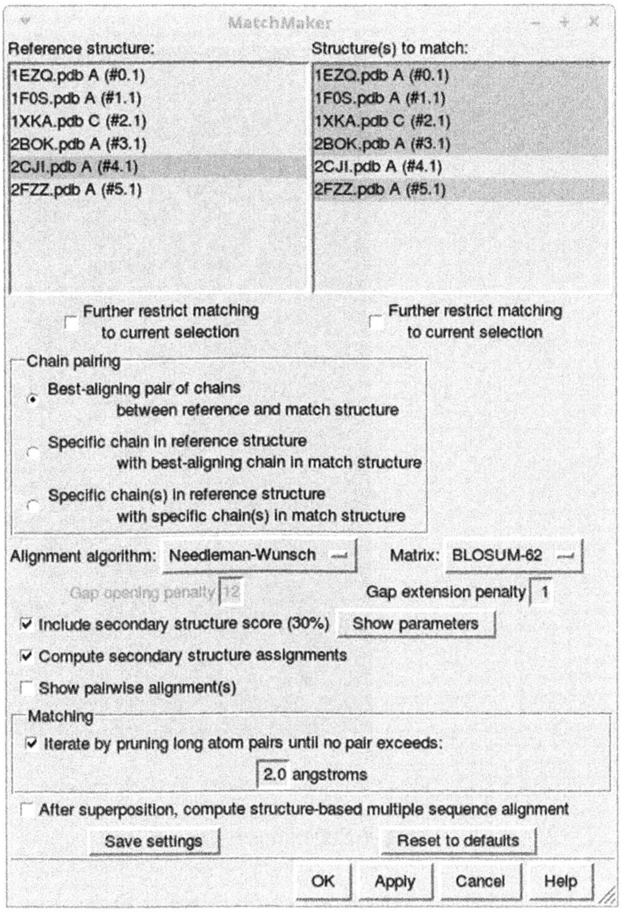

Fig. 5 UCSF Chimera: "MatchMaker" dialog box

(e) **Renaming and Saving the PDB Structures**

Models need to be renamed: click *Favorites* → *Model Panel* → *1EZQ.pdb A*, and then click *rename* ...; a dialog window will open showing the actual model's name ("1EZQ.pdb A") which should be modified to "1EZQ.A.pdb"; then click *OK*. In a similar way, rename all the other complexes (*see* **Note 11**). A list of renamed models as shown in Fig. 7 (left) should be obtained and ready to be saved: click *File* → *Save PDB* ...; a new window will open; click "01_PDB_ALIGNED" folder, check that "Save relative to model" is set to "2CJI.A.pdb" and "Save multiple models in" is set to "multiple files [file name must contain $name or $number]"; then write "$name" in the "File name" field, and deselect "Add . pdb suffix if non given" (*see* Fig. 7, right).

Click *Save*. The new PDB files are now saved in the "01_PDB_ALIGNED" folder. Exit from Chimera by clicking *File* → *Quit*.

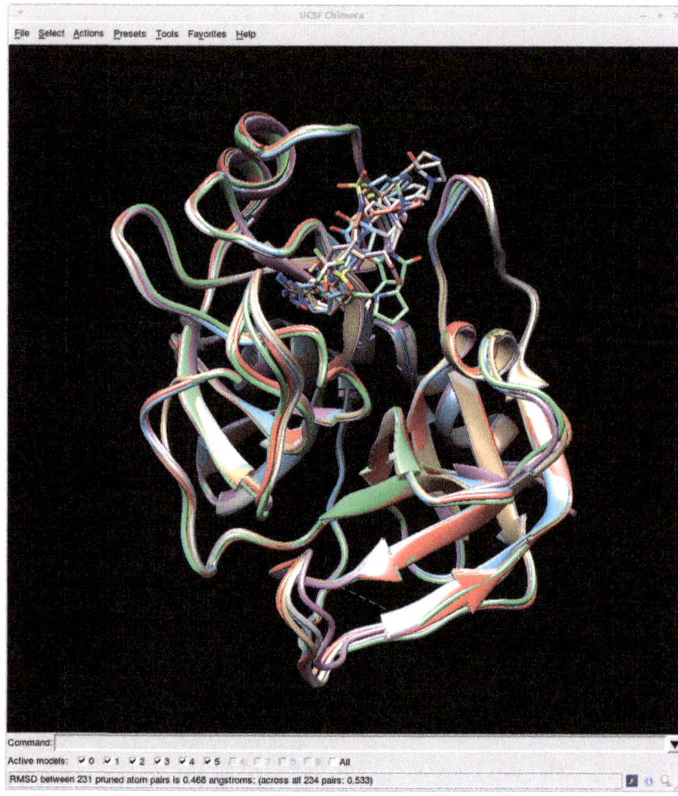

Fig. 6 Superimposed complexes

(f) **Extracting Useful Data from PDB Files**

Since unnecessary information is still present in the PDB files, additional cleaning is required (run the code shown in Table 4).

3.2.2 Extrapolating Locks and Keys

Now, proteins ("locks") and ligands ("keys") can be extracted from the cleaned complexes (run the code shown in Table 5).

In "03_LOCK_KEY" folder, a total of six lock and six key PDB files are now available.

3.2.3 Preparing Ligand Random Conformation

Open Babel will be employed to center the ligands (XYZ = 0,0,0) and perform conformational analysis to generate conformers to be used as input structures for the random conformation docking simulations (run the code shown in Table 6).

Six new PDB files are now saved in "03_LOCK_KEY" folder.

3.2.4 Preparing PDBQT Input Files for AutoDock Vina

Next, two Python scripts ("prepare_ligand4.py" and "prepare_receptor4.py") available from MGLTools will be used to format (PDBQT format) the ligand and receptor files for AutoDock Vina (run the code shown in Table 7, *see* **Note 3**).

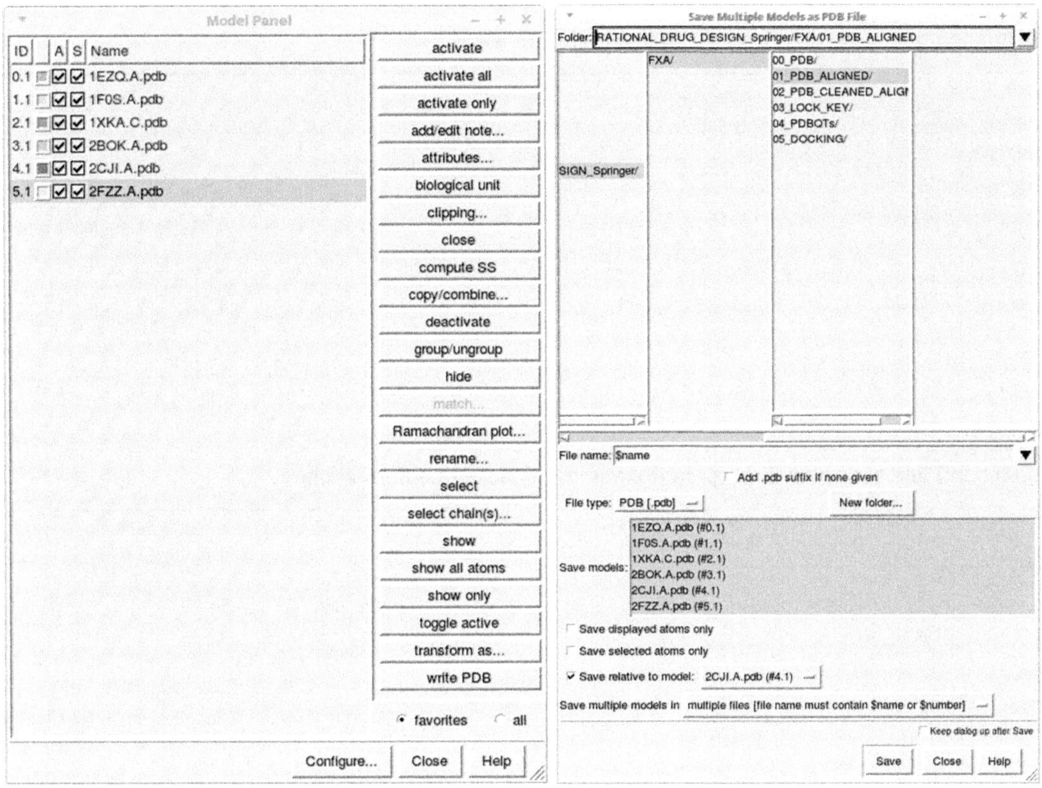

Fig. 7 Left, renamed models in "Model Panel"; right, "Save PDB. . ." dialog box

Table 4
Command line sequence 4: enter the "01_PDB_ALIGNED" folder and clean the PDB files

```
cd ../01_PDB_ALIGNED
ls -1 *.pdb > PDB.list
for PDBcode in `cat PDB.list`
do
   egrep -w 'ATOM|TER|HETATM|END' ${PDBcode}|grep -v REMARK>../02_PDB_CLEANED_ALIGNED/${PDBcode}
done
cd ..
```

3.2.5 Setting the Grid Box

LigandBox can be used to calculate the box center and size (run the code shown in Table 8). Since a unique grid box is required, a multi-PDBQT file needs to be created. The box center is computed by considering the center of mass of the ensemble of co-crystallized ligands, while each edge length is derived in order to enclose all the ligands with additional 10 Å from each XYZ dimension (*see* **Notes 6** and **9**).

A message with the grid box center XYZ coordinates, dimensions, and number of points (with a default grid points spacing of 0.375 Å) will be displayed (Fig. 8, *see* **Note 9**).

Table 5
Command line sequence 5: save LOCK and KEY PDBs

```
cd 02_PDB_CLEANED_ALIGNED
ls -1 *.pdb|sed 's/.pdb//'>PDB.list
for PDBcode in `cat PDB.list`
do
  grep  HETATM ${PDBcode}.pdb>../03_LOCK_KEY/${PDBcode}.key.pdb
done
for PDBcode in `cat PDB.list`
do
  grep -v HETATM ${PDBcode}.pdb>../03_LOCK_KEY/${PDBcode}.lock.pdb
done
cd ..
```

Table 6
Command line sequence 6: prepare ligands' randomized conformations

```
cd 03_LOCK_KEY
cp ../02_PDB_CLEANED_ALIGNED/PDB.list .
for PDBcode in `cat PDB.list`
do
  obabel -c -ipdb ${PDBcode}.key.pdb -opdb -O ${PDBcode}.key.c.pdb
  obconformer 250 250 ${PDBcode}.key.c.pdb > ${PDBcode}.key.cc.pdb
  egrep 'HETATM|END' ${PDBcode}.key.cc.pdb > ${PDBcode}.key.rc.pdb
  rm ${PDBcode}.key.c.pdb ${PDBcode}.key.cc.pdb
done
```

Table 7
Command line sequence 7: prepare PDBQT files

```
for PDBcode in `cat PDB.list`
do
  prepare_ligand4.py -l ${PDBcode}.key.pdb -o ../04_PDBQTs/${PDBcode}.key.pdbqt
done
for PDBcode in `cat PDB.list`
do
  prepare_ligand4.py -l ${PDBcode}.key.rc.pdb -o ../04_PDBQTs/${PDBcode}.key.rc.pdbqt
done
for PDBcode in `cat PDB.list`
do
  prepare_receptor4.py -r ${PDBcode}.lock.pdb -o ../04_PDBQTs/${PDBcode}.lock.pdbqt
done
cd ..
```

The resulting grid box can be explored through AutoDock-Tools (ADT).

Launch ADT, and then open all the experimental PDBQT files (keys + locks): click *File* → *Read Molecule*. A new window will open, double click the "04_PDBQTs" folder, select only the experimental PDBQT files (as shown in Fig. 9, top left), and then click *Open*. Now ligands and proteins are loaded into ADT (Fig. 9, top right).

Table 8
Command line sequence 8: enter the "04_PDBQTs" folder and launch LigandBox

```
cd 04_PDBQTs
cat *.key.pdbqt > all.keys.pdbqt
LigandBox.sh all.keys.pdbqt
cd ..
```

```
BOX center    (XYZ coords): 7.987 5.753 21.795
BOX dimension (XYZ Å):      21.099 23.517 25.471
BOX dimension (XYZ npts):   56 63 68
```

Fig. 8 Grid box parameters

To facilitate the visualization, display the proteins as ribbon and the ligands as ball-and-stick using the dashboard widget panel on the left (Fig. 9, top right). Click *Grid* → *Grid Box* → *Set Dimensions*, and then insert the previously obtained box parameters (from LigandBox, *see* **Note 9**) in the "Grid Options" panel to show the resulting grid box (Fig. 9, bottom).

Click *File* → *Exit* to close ADT.

3.2.6 Setting the AutoDock Vina Configuration File

The grid box parameters can now be included in the AutoDock Vina configuration file:

By using a text editor, create a configuration file as depicted in Fig. 10 (*see* **Note 9**), and save as "conf" in the "05_DOCKING" directory.

3.3 Docking Simulations and Assessment

Go to the parent directory "FXA" (*see* Subheading 2, **item 8**) to start the docking simulations and assessment (using AutoDock Vina and Clusterizer-DockAccessor, respectively).

To automatize the simulations, a series of list files must be created by typing the code shown in Table 9.

3.3.1 Re-docking Simulations and Assessment

Experimental conformation re-docking (ECRD) and cluster analysis can be launched by typing the code shown in Table 10.

Once calculations are finished, random conformation re-docking (RCRD) and relative cluster analysis can be started by typing the code shown in Table 11.

After completion of the calculations, it's possible to compute the ECRD and RCRD docking accuracies (using DockAccessor) by typing in the terminal the code shown in Table 12.

3.3.2 Cross-docking Simulations and Assessment

Experimental and random conformation cross-docking (ECCD and RCCD, respectively) can be performed by typing sequentially the codes from Tables 13, 14, and 15. Cross-docking demands higher computational time.

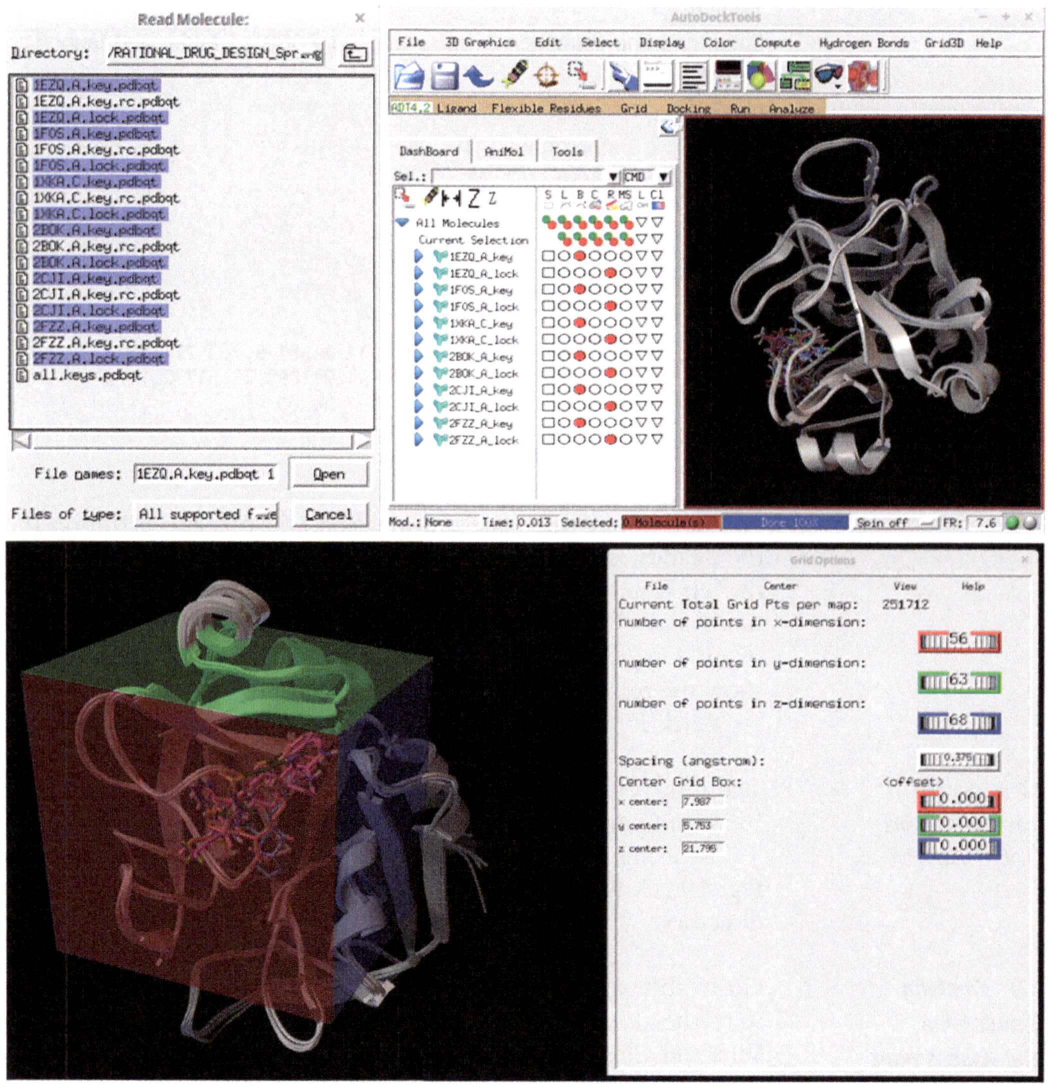

Fig. 9 AutoDockTools (ADT). Top left, Read Molecule dialog window; top right, ADT GUI; bottom, ADT 3D-viewer and Grid Options panel

3.4 Analysis of the Results

In the "VINA" folder, four log files can be found, reporting the docking accuracy values as well as the relevant RMSDs (*see* **Notes 14** and **15**). Let's start considering the results from re-docking simulations:

Open with a text editor "ECRD.DOCKING.ACCURACY.HA.RMSDh.log" and "RCRD.DOCKING.ACCURACY.HA.RMSDh.log" files (Fig. 11), which report the docking accuracies from best docked (BD), best cluster (BC), and best fit (BF) poses (previously extrapolated through Clusterizer).

```
receptor
ligand

center_x = 7.987
center_y = 5.753
center_z = 21.795

size_x = 21.099
size_y = 23.517
size_z = 25.471

energy_range = 10
exhaustiveness = 8
num_modes = 20

log
out
```

Fig. 10 AutoDock Vina configuration file

Table 9
Command line sequence 9: set list files for iterative ECRD and RCRD docking simulations

```
cp 03_LOCK_KEY/PDB.list 05_DOCKING/key.list
cp 03_LOCK_KEY/PDB.list 05_DOCKING/lock.list
cp 03_LOCK_KEY/PDB.list 05_DOCKING/VINA/PDB.list
```

Table 10
Command line sequence 10: ECRD (AutoDock Vina) and cluster analysis (Clusterizer)

```
WD=$PWD
cd 05_DOCKING
for PDBcode in `cat key.list`
do
  mkdir ${WD}/05_DOCKING/VINA/ECRD/${PDBcode}
  ln -sf ${WD}/04_PDBQTs/${PDBcode}.lock.pdbqt ${WD}/05_DOCKING/VINA/ECRD/${PDBcode}
  ln -sf ${WD}/04_PDBQTs/${PDBcode}.key.pdbqt ${WD}/05_DOCKING/VINA/ECRD/${PDBcode}
  cp ${WD}/05_DOCKING/conf ${WD}/05_DOCKING/VINA/ECRD/${PDBcode}
  cd ${WD}/05_DOCKING/VINA/ECRD/${PDBcode}
  sed -i "s/receptor/receptor = ${PDBcode}.lock.pdbqt/" conf
  sed -i "s/ligand/ligand = ${PDBcode}.key.pdbqt/" conf
  sed -i "s/out/out = ${PDBcode}.key_${PDBcode}.lock.pdbqt/" conf
  sed -i "s/log/log = ${PDBcode}.key_${PDBcode}.lock.log/" conf
  vina --config conf
  cd ..
  Clusterizer.1.1.VINA.sh ${PDBcode}.key ${PDBcode}.lock ${PDBcode}.key ${PDBcode} h
  cd $WD
done
```

Table 11
Command line sequence 11: RCRD (AutoDock Vina) and cluster analysis (Clusterizer)

```
cd 05_DOCKING
for PDBcode in `cat key.list`
do
  mkdir ${WD}/05_DOCKING/VINA/RCRD/${PDBcode}
  ln -sf ${WD}/04_PDBQTs/${PDBcode}.lock.pdbqt ${WD}/05_DOCKING/VINA/RCRD/${PDBcode}
  ln -sf ${WD}/04_PDBQTs/${PDBcode}.key*.pdbqt ${WD}/05_DOCKING/VINA/RCRD/${PDBcode}
  cp ${WD}/05_DOCKING/conf ${WD}/05_DOCKING/VINA/RCRD/${PDBcode}
  cd ${WD}/05_DOCKING/VINA/RCRD/${PDBcode}
  sed -i "s/receptor/receptor = ${PDBcode}.lock.pdbqt/" conf
  sed -i "s/ligand/ligand = ${PDBcode}.key.pdbqt/" conf
  sed -i "s/out/out = ${PDBcode}.key.rc_${PDBcode}.lock.pdbqt/" conf
  sed -i "s/log/log = ${PDBcode}.key.rc_${PDBcode}.lock.log/" conf
  vina --config conf
  cd ..
  Clusterizer.1.1.VINA.sh ${PDBcode}.key.rc ${PDBcode}.lock ${PDBcode}.key ${PDBcode} h
  cd $WD
done
```

Table 12
Command line sequence 12: ECRD/RCRD docking assessment (Dock-Accessor)

```
cd 05_DOCKING/VINA
DockAccessor.1.1.sh ECRD PDB.list h
DockAccessor.1.1.sh RCRD PDB.list h
cd $WD
```

The analysis of the results (Fig. 11) shows that:

- BF DA value is 100% from ECRD and RCRD. This indicates that even starting from a randomized ligand conformer (RCRD simulation), the docking sampling algorithm is capable to explore efficiently the search space.
- BD poses give the highest DA value (83.33%) compared to BC (66.67% and 50% from ECRD and RCRD, respectively).
- Discrepancy between the BD (or BC) and the BF docking accuracy values reflects the limitation of the scoring function.

To analyze results from cross-docking simulations:

Open with a text editor "ECCD.DOCKING.ACCURACY.HA.RMSDh.log" and "RCCD.DOCKING.ACCURACY.HA.RMSDh.log" files (Fig. 12).

As expected, when performing cross-docking, the docking performance results get worse as the structures of the receptor with diverse ligands can be rather different. Indeed, this is demonstrated by the lower docking accuracy values from BF poses (since the increased difficulty to sample the experimental conformer of a ligand when considering non-cognate protein structures).

Table 13
Command line sequence 13: ECCD (AutoDock Vina) and cluster analysis (Clusterizer)

```
cd 05_DOCKING
for KEY in `cat key.list`
do
  for LOCK in `cat lock.list`
  do
    if [ $KEY == $LOCK ]; then continue; else
    mkdir ${WD}/05_DOCKING/VINA/ECCD/${KEY}_${LOCK}
    ln -sf ${WD}/04_PDBQTs/${LOCK}.lock.pdbqt ${WD}/05_DOCKING/VINA/ECCD/${KEY}_${LOCK}
    ln -sf ${WD}/04_PDBQTs/${KEY}.key.pdbqt ${WD}/05_DOCKING/VINA/ECCD/${KEY}_${LOCK}
    cp ${WD}/05_DOCKING/conf ${WD}/05_DOCKING/VINA/ECCD/${KEY}_${LOCK}
    cd ${WD}/05_DOCKING/VINA/ECCD/${KEY}_${LOCK}
    sed -i "s/receptor/receptor = ${LOCK}.lock.pdbqt/" conf
    sed -i "s/ligand/ligand = ${KEY}.key.pdbqt/" conf
    sed -i "s/out/out = ${KEY}.key_${LOCK}.lock.pdbqt/" conf
    sed -i "s/log/log = ${KEY}.key_${LOCK}.lock.log/" conf
    vina --config conf
    cd ..
    Clusterizer.1.1.VINA.sh ${KEY}.key ${LOCK}.lock ${KEY}.key ${KEY}_${LOCK} h
    cd $WD/05_DOCKING
    fi
  done
done
cd $WD
```

Table 14
Command line sequence 14: RCCD (AutoDock Vina) and cluster analysis (Clusterizer)

```
cd 05_DOCKING
for KEY  in `cat key.list`
do
  for LOCK in `cat lock.list`
  do
    if [ $KEY == $LOCK ]; then continue; else
    mkdir ${WD}/05_DOCKING/VINA/RCCD/${KEY}_${LOCK}
    ln -sf ${WD}/04_PDBQTs/${LOCK}.lock.pdbqt ${WD}/05_DOCKING/VINA/RCCD/${KEY}_${LOCK}
    ln -sf ${WD}/04_PDBQTs/${KEY}.key*.pdbqt ${WD}/05_DOCKING/VINA/RCCD/${KEY}_${LOCK}
    cp ${WD}/05_DOCKING/conf ${WD}/05_DOCKING/VINA/RCCD/${KEY}_${LOCK}
    cd ${WD}/05_DOCKING/VINA/RCCD/${KEY}_${LOCK}
    sed -i "s/receptor/receptor = ${LOCK}.lock.pdbqt/" conf
    sed -i "s/ligand/ligand = ${KEY}.key.rc.pdbqt/" conf
    sed -i "s/out/out = ${KEY}.key.rc_${LOCK}.lock.pdbqt/" conf
    sed -i "s/log/log = ${KEY}.key.rc_${LOCK}.lock.log/" conf
    vina --config conf
    cd ..
    Clusterizer.1.1.VINA.sh ${KEY}.key.rc ${LOCK}.lock ${KEY}.key ${KEY}_${LOCK} h
    cd $WD/05_DOCKING
    fi
  done
done
cd $WD
```

Moreover, BD poses still outperform the BC ones in terms of docking accuracy values (Fig. 12), suggesting to consider (in this instance) the BD poses when docking ligands with no experimental pose information.

Table 15
Command line sequence 15: ECCD/RCCD docking assessment (DockAccessor)

```
cd 05_DOCKING/VINA
ls -1 ECCD/ |grep -v CD.list >CD.list
DockAccessor.1.1.sh ECCD CD.list h
DockAccessor.1.1.sh RCCD CD.list h
```

```
Selected RMSD: Hungarian (symmetry-corrected) heavy-atom RMSD (HA_RMSDh)
*
*
BEST.BINDING.POSES  *   DOCKING  ACCURACY  DOCKING  ACCURACY.(extended)
*
*
BEST.DOCKED         =>  83.33    %         83.33    %
BEST.CLUSTER        =>  66.67    %         66.67    %        ECRD
BEST.FIT            =>  100.00   %         100.00   %
*
*
```

```
Selected RMSD: Hungarian (symmetry-corrected) heavy-atom RMSD (HA_RMSDh)
*
*
BEST.BINDING.POSES  *   DOCKING  ACCURACY  DOCKING  ACCURACY.(extended)
*
*
BEST.DOCKED         =>  83.33    %         83.33    %
BEST.CLUSTER        =>  50.00    %         50.00    %        RCRD
BEST.FIT            =>  100.00   %         100.00   %
*
*
```

Fig. 11 Re-docking: docking accuracy values. ECRD results (top) and RCRD results (bottom)

4 Notes

1. Command lines may be written line by line (press enter or return at the end of each line) as reported in the tables (without the line number). Since temporary environment variables are set during the computation, the same Linux terminal window must be used.
2. AutoDock Vina program files ("vina" and "vina_split") must be executable throughout the whole system (e.g., copied or linked to /usr/local/bin). Test: open a terminal, write "vina"

```
Selected RMSD: Hungarian (symmetry-corrected) heavy-atom RMSD (HA_RMSDh)
*
*
BEST.BINDING.POSES  *   DOCKING  ACCURACY  DOCKING  ACCURACY.(extended)
*
*
BEST.DOCKED         =>  43.33    %         45.83    %
BEST.CLUSTER        =>  21.67    %         25.00    %          ECCD
BEST.FIT            =>  60.00    %         66.67    %
*
*
```

```
Selected RMSD: Hungarian (symmetry-corrected) heavy-atom RMSD (HA_RMSDh)
*
*
BEST.BINDING.POSES  *   DOCKING  ACCURACY  DOCKING  ACCURACY.(extended)
*
*
BEST.DOCKED         =>  31.67    %         37.50    %
BEST.CLUSTER        =>  24.14    %         29.31    %          RCCD
BEST.FIT            =>  65.00    %         67.50    %
*
*
```

Fig. 12 Cross-docking: docking accuracy values. ECCD results (top) and RCCD results (bottom)

or "vina_split," and then press enter (or return). Both programs should run.

3. Some Python scripts from the MGLTools "Utilities24" folder (http://autodock.scripps.edu/faqs-help/faq/where-can-i-find-the-python-scripts-for-preparing-and-analysing-autodock-dockings) must be executable throughout the whole system (e.g., copied or linked to /usr/local/bin), in particular "write_conformation_from_dlg.py," "prepare_ligand4.py," and "prepare_receptor4.py". Test: open a terminal, write "write_conformation_from_dlg.py" or "prepare_ligand4.py" or "prepare_receptor4.py," and then press enter (or return). All the programs should run.
4. Clusterizer-DockAccessor programs must be executable throughout the whole system (e.g., copied or linked to /usr/local/bin). Test: open a terminal, write "Clusterizer.1.1.VINA.sh" or "DockAccessor.1.1.sh," and then press enter (or return). All the programs should run.
5. After installing DOCK6.8, an environment variable called "DOCKPATH" (specifying the absolute path in which DOCK6 is installed) must be set: i.e., write "export DOCKPATH=/SOFTWARE/dock6" if DOCK6 is installed in /SOFTWARE/dock6. The DOCKPATH variable must be set before starting the protocol.

6. LigandBox program must be executable throughout the whole system (e.g., copied or linked to /usr/local/bin). Test: open a terminal, write "LigandBox.sh," and then press enter (or return). The program should run.
7. Open Babel program must be executable throughout the whole system. Test: open a terminal and write "obabel", and then press enter (or return). The program should run.
8. UCSF Chimera program may be executable throughout the whole system. Test: open a terminal and write "chimera", and then press enter (or return). The program should run.
9. A reduced set of FXa co-crystal structures was selected for the purpose of this exercise. Since the crystal structures of PDB entries can be revised during the time, current atomic coordinates can differ from those actually used when preparing this chapter; as a consequence, the grid box center XYZ coordinates and size can differ from those herein reported.
10. The use of input ligand structures with randomized conformation is preferred, since it prevents biases toward the starting conformation in the sampling algorithm.
11. Because of the variability of the PDB files, preparation of other PDBs may differ from the one herein described. Thus, a preventive inspection of the considered PDB files is generally necessary.
12. UCSF Chimera assigns protonation states at physiological pH. However, a visual inspection of the protonated ligands and proteins is always recommended. If protonation at different pH is required, Open Babel is a valid alternative to be considered.
13. Energy minimization of 3D structures solved by X-ray crystallography is generally carried out (before docking simulation) to reduce nonphysical contacts or interactions and optimize molecular geometry. In the present exercise, energy minimization is not addressed since it is beyond the scope of this work.
14. Since AutoDock Vina uses a random seed for the search algorithm, a certain variability of the docking results is expected.
15. Extensive analyses (not discussed in this exercise) can be performed by considering the RMSD values from each docked ligand, from re-docking and cross-docking results. For example, it is possible to detect if: 1) the simulation fails when docking a certain ligand scaffold (i.e., when higher RMSD values are obtained by docking a congeneric series of compounds); 2) a representative structure from the protein ensemble can be used proficiently to dock new ligands (i.e., when from cross-docking simulations lower RMSDs are obtained by docking different ligands in a same protein conformer from the

ensemble). Also, quantification of the DA results can help the user in tuning the docking parameters (e.g. AutoDock Vina's exhaustiveness) to achieve optimal performance.

Acknowledgments

F.B. thanks Prof. Garland R. Marshall (Washington University School of Medicine in St. Louis, MO) for supporting and funding the design and development of the Clusterizer-DockAccessor protocol; Dr. Chris M. W. Ho (Drug Design Methodologies, LLC, St. Louis, MO) and Ms. Mariama Jaiteh (Uppsala University, Uppsala, Sweden) for providing insightful comments.

References

1. Persch E, Dumele O, Diederich F (2015) Molecular recognition in chemical and biological systems. Angew Chem Int Ed Eng 54(11):3290–3327. https://doi.org/10.1002/anie.201408487
2. Yu W, MacKerell AD Jr (2017) Computer-aided drug design methods. Methods Mol Biol 1520:85–106. https://doi.org/10.1007/978-1-4939-6634-9_5
3. Tang YT, Marshall GR (2011) Virtual screening for lead discovery. Methods Mol Biol 716:1–22. https://doi.org/10.1007/978-1-61779-012-6_1
4. Ballante F, Ragno R (2012) 3-D QSAutogrid/R: an alternative procedure to build 3-D QSAR models. Methodologies and applications. J Chem Inf Model 52(6):1674–1685. https://doi.org/10.1021/ci300123x
5. Ballante F, Reddy DR, Zhou NJ et al (2017) Structural insights of SmKDAC8 inhibitors: targeting schistosoma epigenetics through a combined structure-based 3D QSAR, in vitro and synthesis strategy. Bioorg Med Chem 25 (7):2105–2132. https://doi.org/10.1016/j.bmc.2017.02.020
6. Kubinyi H (1993) 3D QSAR in drug design. Volume 1: theory methods and applications. Three-dimensional quantitative structure activity relationships, Vol. 1. Springer, Berlin
7. Oprea TI, Waller CL (1997) Theoretical and practical aspects of three-dimensional quantitative structure-activity relationships. In: Reviews in computational chemistry. Wiley, Hoboken, NJ, pp 127–182. https://doi.org/10.1002/9780470125885.ch3
8. Bursulaya BD, Totrov M, Abagyan R et al (2003) Comparative study of several algorithms for flexible ligand docking. J Comp Aided Molec Design 17(11):755–763. https://doi.org/10.1023/B:Jcam.0000017496.76572.6f
9. Stahl M (2000) Modifications of the scoring function in FlexX for virtual screening applications. Perspect Drug Discov Design 20 (1):83–98. https://doi.org/10.1023/A:1008724921888
10. Wang R, Lu Y, Fang X et al (2004) An extensive test of 14 scoring functions using the PDBbind refined set of 800 protein-ligand complexes. J Chem Inf Comput Sci 44 (6):2114–2125. https://doi.org/10.1021/ci049733j
11. Reddy DR, Ballante F, Zhou NJ et al (2017) Design and synthesis of benzodiazepine analogs as isoform-selective human lysine deacetylase inhibitors. Eur J Med Chem 127:531–553. https://doi.org/10.1016/j.ejmech.2016.12.032
12. Pettersen EF, Goddard TD, Huang CC et al (2004) UCSF Chimera—a visualization system for exploratory research and analysis. J Comput Chem 25(13):1605–1612. https://doi.org/10.1002/jcc.20084
13. Morris GM, Huey R, Lindstrom W et al (2009) AutoDock4 and AutoDockTools4: automated docking with selective receptor flexibility. J Comput Chem 30(16):2785–2791. https://doi.org/10.1002/jcc.21256
14. Trott O, Olson AJ (2010) AutoDock Vina: improving the speed and accuracy of docking with a new scoring function, efficient optimization, and multithreading. J Comput Chem 31 (2):455–461. https://doi.org/10.1002/jcc.21334
15. Maignan S, Guilloteau JP, Pouzieux S et al (2000) Crystal structures of human factor Xa complexed with potent inhibitors. J Med Chem 43(17):3226–3232

16. Kamata K, Kawamoto H, Honma T et al (1998) Structural basis for chemical inhibition of human blood coagulation factor Xa. Proc Natl Acad Sci U S A 95(12):6630–6635
17. Scharer K, Morgenthaler M, Paulini R et al (2005) Quantification of cation-pi interactions in protein-ligand complexes: crystal-structure analysis of Factor Xa bound to a quaternary ammonium ion ligand. Angew Chem Int Ed Eng 44(28):4400–4404. https://doi.org/10.1002/anie.200500883
18. Watson NS, Brown D, Campbell M et al (2006) Design and synthesis of orally active pyrrolidin-2-one-based factor Xa inhibitors. Bioorg Med Chem Lett 16(14):3784–3788. https://doi.org/10.1016/j.bmcl.2006.04.053
19. Pinto DJ, Orwat MJ, Quan ML et al (2006) 1-[3-Aminobenzisoxazol-5'-yl]-3-trifluoromethyl-6-[2'-(3-(R)-hydroxy-N-pyrrolidin yl) methyl-[1,1']-biphen-4-yl]-1,4,5,6-tetrahydropyrazolo-[3,4-c]-pyridin-7-one (BMS-740808) a highly potent, selective, efficacious, and orally bioavailable inhibitor of blood coagulation factor Xa. Bioorg Med Chem Lett 16(15):4141–4147. https://doi.org/10.1016/j.bmcl.2006.02.069
20. Ballante F, Marshall GR (2016) An automated strategy for binding-pose selection and docking assessment in structure-based drug design. J Chem Inf Model 56(1):54–72. https://doi.org/10.1021/acs.jcim.5b00603
21. Allen WJ, Balius TE, Mukherjee S et al (2015) DOCK 6: Impact of new features and current docking performance. J Comput Chem 36 (15):1132–1156. https://doi.org/10.1002/jcc.23905
22. O'Boyle NM, Banck M, James CA et al (2011) Open Babel: an open chemical toolbox. Aust J Chem 3:33. https://doi.org/10.1186/1758-2946-3-33
23. The Open Babel Package. 2.4.1 http://openbabel.org. Accessed June 2017. edn.
24. Berman HM, Westbrook J, Feng Z et al (2000) The protein data bank. Nucleic Acids Res 28 (1):235–242

Chapter 6

Rational Drug Design Using Integrative Structural Biology

Magda S. Chegkazi, Michael Mamais, Anastasia I. Sotiropoulou, and Evangelia D. Chrysina

Abstract

Modern drug discovery and design approaches rely heavily on high-throughput methods and state-of-the-art infrastructures with robotic facilities and sophisticated platforms. However, the anticipated research output that would eventually lead to new drugs with minimal or no side effects to the market has not been achieved. Despite the vast amount of information generated, very little is converted to knowledge and even less is capitalized for cross-discipline research actions. Therefore, the need for re-launching rational approaches has become apparent. Here we present an overview of the new trends in rational drug design using integrative structural biology with emphasis on X-ray protein crystallography and small molecules as ligands. With the aim to increase researchers' awareness on the available possibilities to perform front line research, we also underline the benefits and enhanced prospects offered to the scientific community, through access to research infrastructures.

Key words Structure-based drug design, Structural biology, Bioinformatics, X-ray protein crystallography

Abbreviations

3D	Three dimensional
DLS	Dynamic light scattering
DMSO	Dimethyl sulfoxide
EM	Electron microscopy
HPLC	High-performance liquid chromatography
HR-MS	High-resolution mass spectrometry
MALLS	Multi-angle laser light scattering
NMR	Nuclear magnetic resonance
RI	Research infrastructure
SAXS	Small-angle X-ray scattering
SEC	Size exclusion chromatography
SRS	Synchrotron radiation source

Thomas Mavromoustakos and Tahsin F. Kellici (eds.), *Rational Drug Design: Methods and Protocols*, Methods in Molecular Biology, vol. 1824, https://doi.org/10.1007/978-1-4939-8630-9_6,

1 Introduction

The origins of structural biology stretch back to the beginning of the twentieth century, when the first structures were determined by X-ray crystallography. The growing collection of protein crystal structures, coupled with the advances in computer graphics at the time, was the driving force for providing an open-access central repository for structural data sharing [1]. One hundred years later, the data entries at the protein data bank are still on the rise following a logarithmic scale. The number of structural biologists has also grown considerably and now includes experts in X-ray crystallography, nuclear magnetic resonance (NMR) spectroscopy, and during the last 20 years small-angle X-ray scattering (SAXS) and electron microscopy (EM). The structural biology community is expanding fast; similar to neural networks, today, it is organized into interconnected layers, involving scientists with complementary expertise in biology, chemistry, physics, informatics, and engineering. The challenge that this new generation of structural biologists faces is to traverse the frontiers of their discipline in order to both contribute and make use of the deposited protein structures for the benefit of other researchers and the society. The information derived from the three-dimensional (3D) structure of protein molecules has enabled researchers to convert it to knowledge by elucidating the underlying mechanisms of protein function and understanding structure-function relationships. Out of this process, the medicinal chemists were the first to gain maximum benefit, investing on drug design and discovery following rational approaches. The latest technological advances, comprising high-performance equipment, robotic devices, and sophisticated software and hardware, have contributed significantly to this direction, and this is reflected on the rapidly increasing number of protein structures deposited with the protein data bank; however, the number of the new drugs that have been developed by the structure-based drug design approach and are launched to the market, is significantly low. Considering the competitive advantage that structural biology can offer for the development of new drugs with high specificity for the target, minimizing if not eliminating side effects, it has become apparent that concentrated efforts are required towards increasing the synapses between the expanding community of structural biologists and other scientists working in biomedical sciences. Nonetheless, a review, presented by Scannel and coworkers in 2012, discussed the decline in pharmaceutical R&D efficiency [2]. Their work was followed by a recent interesting analysis on the predictive validity of the different models employed that influence the decisions made in R&D departments based on disease models and drugs available for each disease. The paper also summarizes nicely the imbalance between the investment that has been made on drug discovery and the output of this effort, despite the improvements, introduced by the high-throughput screening approaches [3]. Some of the questions that researchers working in the field of drug discovery and design have to answer, include whether they have produced enough data to make a decision and, if not, there are open-access data that can be used for validation purposes and how long should one work on a drug target before it gets abandoned for a new one. One of the questions that are also yet to be answered is what would one need so as to be able to provide some kind of "guarantee" that the research conducted has increased chances to lead to a "good" or at least improved potential drug. Is it innovative research that is missing or tools and new targets, or is it a matter of maturity of the projects and osmosis between the information and knowledge space? These are questions that one cannot provide a unique answer, but every scientist is trying to mimic a "tunable monochromator" filtering the available information so as to transform it to knowledge, unwinding Ariadne's thread of druggable targets and ligands. To this end, structural biology has made an outstanding contribution in enhancing the knowledge derived by the ligand binding to protein structures, fostering rational drug design. A recent work on opioid analgesics [4] reveals the power of the knowledge derived from the 3D protein structure, when applying a structure-based ligand discovery on GPCR. This finding is complemented by the structural insights that LSD, a well-known hallucinogen, provides upon binding to human serotonin receptor, explaining its action based on the crystal structure of the complex [5]. Structural vaccinology is also one of the emerging fields that gives emphasis on the structural design of immunoreagents and vaccines with tailor-made antigens/epitopes that would allow explaining how the 3D structure affects immunogenicity and immunodominance of epitopes [6, 7].

Here we shall focus on presenting the workflow from sample preparation to complex formation and structure determination of a known protein target when the ligand is a small molecule giving emphasis on X-ray protein crystallography.

2 Methods

2.1 Molecular Biology

2.1.1 Molecular Cloning

Assuming that the target selection of the protein of interest has been made, the design of the relevant construct follows in order to proceed with further studies. Construct design is considered a crucial step, since it plays a key role in determining the stability of the macromolecular target, its proper folding, and possibly its ability to crystallize. If the protein structure is known, then the sequence design focuses on particular regions of the protein that are important for ligand binding, i.e., residues at the catalytic or the allosteric site of an enzyme or loop regions or domains that might be implicated in ligand binding. For example, lid domains in lipases or esterases are significant for the activity of the enzymes (e.g., *Thermomyces lanuginosus* lipase or *Rhodothermus marinus* esterase) [8, 9]. Otherwise, sequence design is based on existing targets using tools that predict secondary structure elements by submitting the sequence of the target of interest to servers such as PSIPRED (Protein Sequence Analysis Workbench); correct protein folding is then verified by biophysical and biochemical experiments (*see* **Note 1**).

Preparation of the target is performed by isolating it from the organism of interest, directly with biochemical methods or through cDNA and genomic libraries or *via* recombinant DNA. Molecular cloning is the most widely used method for producing recombinant proteins because it allows the preparation of the desired protein and is modular. Based on the properties of the protein target, a variety of model expression systems can be used. The advantage of heterologous expression is that a plethora of human protein targets can be studied avoiding sacrificing animals, and at the same time, working in compliance with the rule of three Rs (*see* **Note 2**) for this step, since there is a palette of cell lines available in the market. The cloning steps involve:

1. Design of protein construct
2. Selection of a suitable expression system according to known properties of the protein, based on the literature, handling limitations, post-translational modifications, and location in the cell and function (e.g. bacteria, yeast, mammalian hosts, insect-based cells, or cell-free systems)
3. Selection of a suitable cloning vector for the expression host system
4. Ligation of the gene in the cloning vector, using restriction enzymes
5. Transformation of the recombinant vector that contains the gene, into the cells (host), in the presence of a suitable antibiotic
6. Sequencing of selected colonies to validate the correct gene insertion
7. Protein expression using the previously selected colonies having the gene of interest

2.1.2 Protein Expression

The expression system is selected by taking into consideration several variables such as the physiological environment of the native protein, its function, its location in the cell, and the interactions that it performs with neighboring molecules (e.g. proteins, nucleic molecules, enzymes, or ligands). The recombinant protein is then expressed using certain strains that have been carefully modified for increasing protein expression levels [10, 11]. Common challenges that one usually faces in *E. coli* host cells concern the formation of inclusion bodies during expression; these need to be disrupted under rather harsh conditions (e.g. chaotropic agents like urea and guanidine hydrochloride) that result in protein unfolding, followed by refolding of the denaturing protein and purification using chromatographic techniques. A major drawback, in this procedure, is that the protein might aggregate during refolding; therefore, new methods have been developed that include mild solubilization processes [12] and increase the protein yields.

Even a single mutation in the protein might affect its solubility, an important factor especially if the protein will be used for structural studies (*see* **Note 3**). Proteins are charged molecules consisting of a combination of aliphatic, aromatic, polar, and nonpolar amino acids. Their solubility in aqueous solutions is directly correlated with the proportion of the area comprising charged residues [13]. In cases where the target protein precipitates or is insoluble in water-based media, protein engineering might be considered to overcome this issue, by modifying certain hydrophobic or aliphatic amino acids. The protein expression stage involves the following steps:

1. Literature research on the molecular target properties, its taxonomy, family, function, whether it is involved in particular metabolic pathways or associated with other proteins in the cell, etc. (*see* **Note 4**)
2. Examination of the stability of the protein to decide whether the presence of cofactors (in the case of enzymes), metal ions, ligands, or other proteins are required for correct folding and function
3. Investigation of different expression systems and different cell lines to ensure that the optimum expression profile is achieved

2.1.3 Protein Purification

Protein purification is a method of isolating the protein of interest from a pool of other proteins that are present during expression, by employing liquid chromatography techniques. The biophysical properties of the protein (e.g. protein size, physicochemical properties, binding affinity, total charge, etc.) will navigate the researcher across different approaches. These involve immobilized metal affinity chromatography, size exclusion and ion exchange chromatography or pH gradient techniques, reverse-phase and hydrophobic interaction chromatography [14].

The protein purification stage involves the following steps:

1. Calculation of the theoretical isoelectric point of the protein using in silico tools such as *ExPASy* (http://web.expasy.org/compute_pi/) [15].

2. Identification of possible glycosylation sites (if applicable) using servers like *NetNGlyc* (http://www.cbs.dtu.dk/services/NetNGlyc/) [16] or *NetOGlyc* (http://www.cbs.dtu.dk/services/NetOGlyc/) [17] depending on the type of glycosylations (e.g. C-linked, N-linked, O-linked, or S-linked).
3. Evaluation of the protein solubility at different ionic strengths, buffer composition, etc.
4. Introduction of tags that will facilitate purification in positions that will not interfere with the binding site of interest (e.g. His-tag, glutathione S-transferase tag, streptavidin / biotin-based tags either at the N- or C-terminus of the protein, etc.) [18].
5. Use of light scattering methods and, more specifically, multi-angle laser light scattering (MALLS) or dynamic light scattering (DLS) detectors in line of SEC-UV or refractive index to assess polydispersity and to provide molecular weight and size determination [19].
6. It is likely that complex formation might not be possible if preformed crystals are used due to crystal packing interactions that do not allow the ligand to access the binding site (e.g. ligand soaking technique).
7. The purity of the protein has to be >98% (assessed by SDS-PAGE) and of low polydispersity (validated by light scattering methods), so as to proceed to crystallization (*see* **Note 5**).

2.2 Working at the Interface of Chemistry and Biology in 3D

2.2.1 From Proteins to Crystals

Protein samples of high purity (>98%) are subjected to crystallization trials using either conditions previously established by in-house or commercial screens. The primary aim is to obtain crystals of the native protein and then proceed to complex formation using either preformed crystals, employing the soaking method prior to X-ray data collection, or co-crystallization (Fig. 1).

More specifically, the steps for setting up a crystallization plate include:

- Preparation of a registry with all the details for the protein. This comprises the following:
  1. Details on how the protein was cloned, expressed, and purified with emphasis on the environment of the eluted samples after purification, along with an SDS-PAGE that will assess the purity of the protein and the presence of potential protein degradation.
  2. The results from biophysical characterization of the sample, i.e. light-scattering methods and circular dichroism spectroscopy (to determine the secondary structure of the protein and its folding properties [20]).

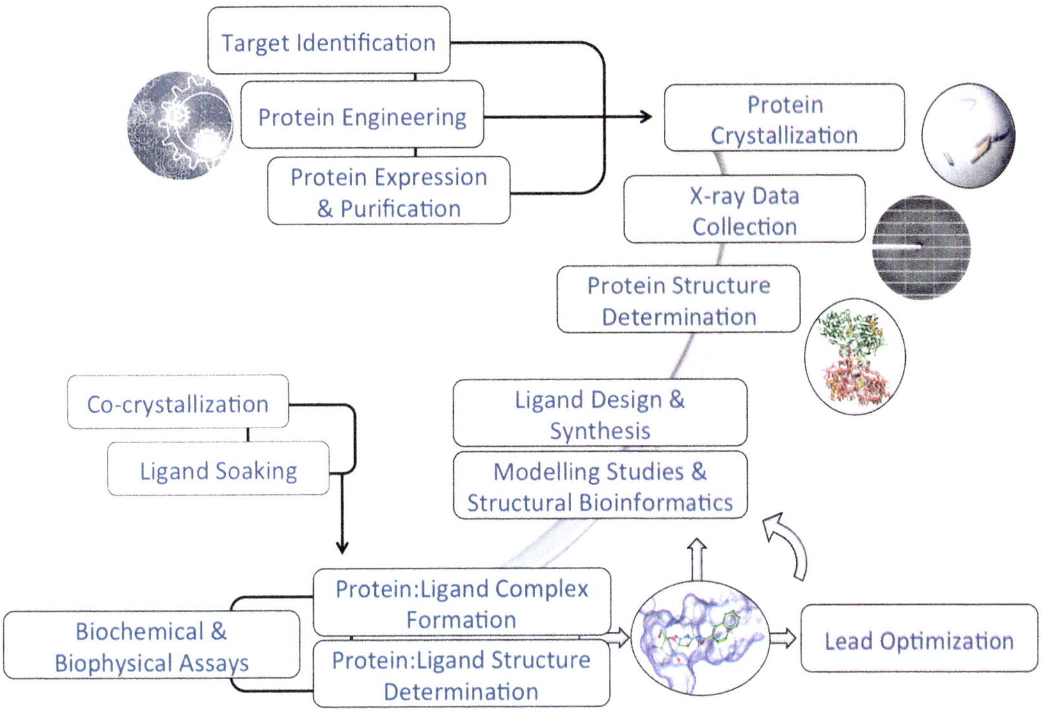

Fig. 1 Workflow of the rational drug design approach from sample preparation to complex formation and protein structure determination by X-ray protein crystallography

3. Determination of protein absorbance is performed with microvolume spectrophotometers, using just 1 μL of protein or with the use of other methods like Bradford or BSA assay. For assessment of the protein concentration, the theoretical extinction coefficient can be calculated from *ExPASy* server (http://web.expasy.org/protparam/).
4. Protein concentration used for crystallization trials ranges from 5 to 20 mg/mL. Usually pre-crystallization tests are performed to estimate the starting protein concentration.
5. Excessive increase of protein concentration might lead to precipitation and should be avoided.
6. The sample should be ideally used immediately after its preparation; however if storage is required for longer periods, the protein should be kept at 4, −20, or −80 °C in the presence of common cryoprotectants such as glycerol, unless flash-freezing is performed (*see* **Note 6**).

2.2.2 Protein-Ligand Complex Preparation

Protein-ligand complex formation is a rather challenging process especially when there is limited information about the ligand properties or its affinity for the target. A registry of the ligand is prepared providing details and spectra about the chemical composition and its purity such as HPLC, HR-MS, or NMR, from the synthetic chemist. If the ligand is commercially available, then this information is provided directly from the company purchased. The ligand solution preparation involves the following steps:

1. Preparation of a ligand-stock solution taking into account the hydrophobicity or hydrophilicity of the compound according to its chemical structure.
   (a) If the compound is hydrophilic, an aquatic solution of the ligand is prepared as a stock solution at high concentration. Instead of water, the buffer that the crystals were grown could be used (*see* **Note 7**).
   (b) If the compound is partially soluble in water, a mixture of dimethyl sulfoxide (DMSO) in water or crystallization buffer can be used as solvent (*see* **Note 8**).
   (c) Initially, the pH of the ligand solution is adjusted to a value similar to the pH of the crystal mother liquor so as not to damage the crystal. This step is not essential if the ligand is successfully dissolved in the crystallization buffer (*see* **Note 9**).
   (d) If the compound exhibits decreased solubility forming a suspension in water, then heat is applied until it becomes completely dissolved (*see* **Note 10**).
   (e) Fresh ligand solutions are used immediately, or they are stored in sealed vessels at low temperature (around 4 °C). If the compounds are easily oxidized or hydroscopic, the vessel can be flushed with argon before closing and sealing the lid (*see* **Note 11**).
2. For complex formation using preformed crystals of the protein soaked in the ligand solution (*see* **Note 12**):
   (a) If the crystals were grown using the vapor diffusion technique, the ligand solution is preferably added to an empty well of the same plate, and one or more crystals are soaked into it.
   (b) The well is sealed, and the ligand is allowed to diffuse in the crystal and reach the binding site. Monitoring of the crystals every 5–10 min is essential to observe whether any cracks appear. If this is the case, then the crystal is frozen immediately. Depending on the ligand and crystal availability, the ligand concentration and soaking time are optimized accordingly.
3. For co-crystallization experiments:
   (a) The ligand solution is prepared following the approach described in Subheading 2.2.2. Co-crystallization is affected by temperature, protein concentration, ligand concentration, use of specific additives to promote ligand binding, etc.

(b) The protein solution is mixed with the ligand solution preferably above 1:2 in molar ratio so as to ensure that the ligand is in excess and binding will occur. The solution is left to equilibrate prior to crystallization (*see* **Note 13**).

2.2.3 From Crystal to Structure

(*a*) *Data collection and 3D structure determination of the protein-ligand complex*: Data collection can be performed either in-house or at synchrotron radiation sources (SRS). Today, there is a significant number of such large-scale facilities worldwide (http://www.lightsources.org/regions) that one could collect data at high resolution if quality crystals have been produced. For this purpose, protein crystals of the complex are cryoprotected prior to data collection, to avoid ice formation on the crystal during data collection at 100 °K. The advantage of data collection at cryo-conditions instead of room temperature is that it reduces the effect of radiation damage on the crystal and it also decreases the effects of thermal motion of the molecules in the crystal lattice [21]. However, the cryoprotectant sometimes interacts with the protein molecules in the crystal, by forming non-specific interactions, disrupting eventually the crystal lattice. Therefore, it is advisable the cryoprotectant is included in the crystallization medium, as soon as the conditions are optimized. Otherwise, the ligand is added in the cryoprotectant solution to ensure that it will remain bound, when the crystal is transferred to it. There are crystals, though, that "prefer" to be exposed at room temperature, and the significant reduction of the detectors' readout time along with automated tools that move the crystal, while getting exposed (helical data collection) has made it possible to collect a full data set from just one crystal [22]. To overcome cryoprotection or the stage of crystal mounting, during the last years, in situ data collection has been possible at large-scale facilities such as Diamond Light Source (http://www.diamond.ac.uk/Beamlines/Mx/Equipment-on-Demand/In-situ-Data-Collection.html), EMBL Hamburg Petra III (https://www.embl-hamburg.de/services/mx/P14/), etc.

A number of fully automated pipelines that produce straightway the electron density maps are nowadays available on site. Details on the available or recommended software are provided at the facility. The user, however, should know the basic principles behind the processing of data collection, so as to evaluate the quality of the diffraction data and most importantly to interpret correctly additional portions of density that might be observed and will be allocated to the ligand under study. Selected software for both SRS and in-house users includes:

1. *XDS* [23], *MOSFLM* [24] and DIALS (https://dials.github.io) convert the intensity of the diffracted beam to structure factors taking into account the geometry of the experimental setup for data collection, the wavelength of the beam, and the sample to detector distance.

2. *CCP4* suite [25] is then used for merging and scaling of the collected data.
3. 3D structure determination follows by molecular replacement if there is a previously determined structure with high sequence or structural homology. For this purpose, modules in *CCP4* suite [25] are available such as *AMoRe* [26], *PHASER* [27], and *MOLREP* [28], while other software like *PHENIX* [29] or online severs like *BALBES* can also be used. Usually, for protein-ligand complexes, the structure of the protein is already known.
4. Calculation of the difference electron density maps $2F_o$-F_c and F_o-F_c.
5. Visual inspection of the difference maps with the molecular graphics program *Coot* [30] will verify the presence of an additional portion of density that could be assigned to the ligand.
6. Alternate cycles of manual building and refinement with *Coot* and programs like *REFMAC* [31, 32] or *PHENIX* [29] are used to prepare the final model of the structure taking care of possible changes in the side chains of the residues lining the ligand binding. Solvent molecules that form direct or water-mediated hydrogen bond interactions with the protein are added with *Coot* avoiding though to incorporate any of them at the site of interest.
7. The final geometry of the model including the geometry of the peptide bonds is validated with *MolProbity* [33].

(*b*) *Building the ligand*: The geometry of the protein structure can be easily validated because the amino acids are already known. The geometry of the peptide bond is also well studied and depicted in various dictionaries and libraries. In addition, the conformers that amino acids adopt are also described in detail through the rotamers emerging from the number of rotatable bonds of the side chain. There are other, computational mainly, challenges that one has to face in this case, if it is to perform, for example, molecular dynamic simulations. What is difficult to know in advance, though, is the chemical structure of the compound that the medicinal chemists will synthesize. The most common approach to assess the stereochemistry of a small molecule is *via* X-ray diffraction studies. This information is incorporated in the protein-ligand complex structure as well. Otherwise, only some of the compound features could be determined from previously described small molecules, whose structure has been determined, and their ideal stereochemistry is described in different dictionaries for commonly used moieties. Selected information that is available in these dictionaries includes ideal bond lengths, stereochemistry of sugar moieties (glucose, lactose, etc.), geometry of aromatic rings, and atom types when atoms are part of a 6-member ring or a 5-member ring or when it is bonded to a nitrogen, a carbon, an oxygen atom, etc. Today there are databases that one can find the ideal values of commonly used compounds/ligands along with repositories like Ligand Expo (http://ligand-expo.rcsb.org) that is available through the Protein Data Bank (PDB, http://www.rcsb.org) and comprises ligands that have been deposited with the PDB.

The steps that one follows so as to prepare a model of a new ligand and a topology file that will describe its geometry and will be used by software that performs the protein-ligand complex refinement, are summarized below:

1. Drawing of the ligand using *ChemDraw* (http://www.cambridgesoft.com/software/overview.aspx), *Avogadro* (http://avogadro.cc/) [34], or similar chemical drawing software, e.g. in *CCP4* suite (http://www.ccp4.ac.uk) [25] or *Schrödinger's* suite (https://www.schrodinger.com/).
2. Energy minimization is performed to find the most stable ligand conformation in the free state.
3. The Dundee server is used (http://davapc1.bioch.dundee.ac.uk/cgi-bin/prodrg) [35] to prepare the topology of the ligand that also includes all the stereochemistry parameters (.cif file). This then has to be given as input along the default library files used by the refinement software.

   For example, in the case of *REFMAC* as implemented in the *CCP4* suite, a module that merges the existing .cif files for the amino acids with the new one of the ligand has to run first and then the merged .cif file to be given as input to *REFMAC* to run the refinement taking into account the ligand coordinates (*see* **Note 14**).
4. Once the ligand coordinates and .cif file are available, then the ligand is manually built in the difference electron density map by adjustment of its rotatable bonds and dihedral angles if required. For example, in *Coot*, the options for *tor_residue* or *tor_general* are used to define those four atoms that determine the torsion angle, which can be modified. Unless a torsion angle is changed to variable in the .cif file, no modification is allowed. Also the *reverse* option defines the part of molecule around the rotatable bond, which the torsion angle will change. The ligand is fitted to continuous portions of density where there is clear indication that it has been bound.
5. Examination of the overall structure of the protein and identification of all the possible binding sites follows. It is rather common compounds to bind to more than one sites of the protein (*see* **Note 15**).

(*c*) *Crystal structure interpretation: insights on the complex formation*: Once the protein-ligand structure is determined, analysis follows so as to proceed with the structure interpretation. This involves the following steps:

1. Record the hydrogen bond and *van der Waals* interactions upon binding of the ligand at the protein site. Almost all molecular graphics programs perform this task automatically and show the bonds as well for visual inspection; however, since only some but not all of them take into account the geometry of the hydrogen bond, it is better to carefully examine how the software calculates these bonds (for hydrogen bonds both the distance and the angle of the relevant atoms should be considered). Selected applications for this purpose are: *Contact* as implemented in *CCP4* suite [25]; *LigPlot* [36] and *Chimera* [37], *Coot* [30], *Schrödinger* (https://www.schrodinger.com/), etc. that take into account both the distance and the angle of the interacting molecules.
2. Superposition of the native protein structure onto the protein structure when in complex with the ligand follows, in order to monitor:
   (a) The number of the water molecules that have been replaced by the ligand atoms, or have been displaced upon ligand binding, or those that have appeared to interact with the ligand and enhance binding through either a direct solvent network or through water-mediated protein-ligand interactions.
   (b) Changes in the conformation or shifts observed in the backbone atoms of residues at the site of interest or in the vicinity upon ligand binding.
   (c) The orientation of the functional groups of the ligand, i.e., aromatic rings tend to intercalate with residues like phenylalanine, tyrosine, or tryptophan forming π-π stacking interactions. Aryl-containing amino acids (Trp, Phe, Tyr, and His) commonly expose their aromatic side chain to the protein binding site. Two aromatic π systems may undergo hydrophobic interaction in two ways: the T-shaped edge-to-face and the parallel stacking interaction. Although the latter appears to be more frequent in proteins, according to theoretical calculations, the two interaction modes are almost isoenergetic [38].
   (d) The affinity of ligands for such stacking interactions with aromatic amino acids depends on the comparative electron availability of the two aromatic systems. Generally, interaction is stronger between an electron-rich and an electron-poor aromatic system and between electron-poor systems. Trp and Tyr have electron-rich aromatic systems,

compared to Phe. In this context, rendering the aromatic ring of the ligand electron poor by inserting electron withdrawing groups such as carbonyl or nitro groups may increase the alkyl stacking strength of interaction [39].

(e) On the other hand, T-shaped edge-to-face interactions are favored when the interacting hydrogen is rendered more acidic, by insertion of electron withdrawing groups in *ortho-* and *para*-position relative to the aforementioned hydrogen atom [38].

(f) The ligand interactions with residues from protein molecule or secondary interactions with symmetry-related molecules that might either mimic the physiological dimer or be induced only due to crystal contacts.

2.2.4 Structure-Based/Ligand-Based Drug Design

The structural determinants for ligand binding have to be identified. To this end, a selected list of the actions followed is presented:

1. Evaluation of the solvent content in cooperation with medicinal chemists, and assessment of whether the remaining solvent molecules are ordered waters and their structure give insights on new compounds that could be prepared, using this one as a lead molecule.
2. Use of advanced mathematical tools, some of which are already implemented in software like *Chimera* [37] or servers like the one of European Bioinformatics Institute (EBI) to calculate the protein accessibility as compared to the physiological assembly, analyzing the protein interfaces and determining the accessible areas (*PISA* server). The topology diagram of the protein structure is also useful.
3. Mapping of the binding site of a protein molecule can be performed with rather sophisticated geometry algorithms using α-shapes and different geometrical schemes (some of these with curvatures) to allow detailed mapping of the protein interactions (*see* **Note 16**).

   (a) A broad range of computational approaches has been generated utilizing geometrical algorithms and mathematics with the aim to either detect new or delineate known binding sites of a protein target. Structural bioinformatics provide tools for this purpose, enhancing the potential to produce valuable results from such analysis. The number of these new tools is growing fast, underlying clearly the scope and importance of synergistic actions that are absolutely essential to be developed at the interface of disciplines in the fields of mathematics, informatics, and engineering with biology, chemistry, and biomedicine. The use of geometrical aspects of a binding site, statistical analysis of the trajectories of the amino acid rotamers that build this site, along with clustering algorithms and scoring functions utilizing data from in silico and in vitro results can give new insights in the structure-function relationships that underlie the protein mechanisms of action, as well as the structural evolution of proteins. Selected software that has been developed to this end includes *Fpocket* (http://fpocket.sourceforge.net) [40], *CASTp* (http://sts.bioe.uic.edu/castp/) [41], and *TRAPP* (http://trapp.h-its.org) [42]. Similarly, data management and data analytics have promoted the construction of databases and repositories that facilitate focused studies, e.g., the *Catalytic Site Atlas* (*CSA*) (http://www.ebi.ac.uk/thornton-srv/databases/CSA/index.html) [43] including a library of structural templates to recognize catalytic sites [44], the kinase database (http://kinbase.com) along with the kinase-ligand interaction space (http://klifs.vu-compmedchem.nl) [45, 46], etc. Analysis of protein-ligand interactions by *Relibase+* (https://www.ccdc.cam.ac.uk/solutions/csd-discovery/Components/Relibase/) [47] is one of the typical examples of such software. In the case of enzymes, particular emphasis is given on ligand-substrate analogues; however, cofactors and additional ligands such as metal ions are also vital for correct protein function, and their role in the structure-function integrity should be taken into consideration [48]. The role of the solvent structure also requires to be taken into account [49–51].

(b) Once one or more lead molecules are identified, pharmacophore modelling then enables the optimization of the ligand proposing a number of derivatives to be prepared employing different functional groups the properties of which will promote binding.

(c) The more data is provided, the better the rational design process that will be performed. Additional analyses of the microenvironment of the binding site of interest using tools such as *DEPTH* (http://cospi.iiserpune.ac.in/depth/htdocs/index.html) [52] are also beneficial since beyond size, shape complementary, and stereochemical restraints, the charge of the residues in the vicinity, as compared to the charge or tautomeric/protonation state of the ligand in the free state, provides a wealth of information that could be further exploited for the rational design of the ligand derivatives or analogues.

Other approaches give emphasis on the ligand, the scaffold of which is treated as a template that will be matched by screening libraries of compounds and the hits will be exploited as lead molecules. Both the ligand-based and the structure-based approaches improve daily and are unique tools both for experimental and computational scientists working at the interface of biology, chemistry, and informatics.

3 Notes

1. For the design of a protein sequence that folds to a target structure, a sequence prediction tool is employed that uses an algorithm based on the target fold and takes into consideration all the possible conformations of the amino acids. Finally the sequences are ranked according to the lowest energy conformation. A number of tools are also available regarding tertiary and quaternary protein structure and function prediction, e.g., *PHYRE2* [53], *i-TASSER* [54], *Swiss-Model* [55], *Robetta* [56] etc., which generate 3D protein models and most of which also predict protein ligand binding sites, based on homology modelling formulas. These tools provide an automated user-friendly interface by employing advanced algorithms for computational biology.
2. The principles of three *R*s have been incorporated in the legislation of international research organizations and set the framework for more humane experimental techniques. These include the following: *Replace* or *Reduce* the use of animals where possible but still obtain valid experimental results (e.g., statistical significance), and *Refine* the way that the experiments are carried out to ensure minimal animal suffering.
3. Introduction of the right mutations, toward increasing solubility, is a rather demanding process; residues such as alanine or glycine are usually selected for this purpose to replace the amino acids of interest. Protein engineering might lead to the desired result, i.e. soluble protein in aqueous solutions; however it might affect its folding and as a consequence its function. In addition, the amino acids that will be mutated should be carefully selected, since this might affect the structure of the area of interest or it might produce correctly folded but inactive proteins (e.g. in the case of enzymes). Overall, the major pitfall of this approach is that it is a time-consuming trial and error method, which should be carefully considered at the stage of construct design.
4. An important factor that one should take into consideration when choosing the expression host is the folding properties of the protein of interest. Some proteins might require assistance from other molecules to perform their proper folding and function or might require post-translational modifications

that not all the hosts are able to provide. Therefore, in order to increase the rate of success, one should explore different approaches and possibly a range of expression systems and different cell lines.

5. After protein purification, if the eluted protein contains increased salt concentration or agents such as imidazole, or phosphate, a dialysis step is usually required to remove these components that might either interfere with crystallization or affect the protein stability. For detailed protocols on protein expression and purification, *see* [57].
6. The amount of protein available is decisive for the variety of conditions that will be explored. The classical method of vapor diffusion using sitting/hanging drops is commonly used with either 24- or 96-well crystallization plates if there is an in-house robotic crystallization facility. For reviews on this, *see* [58]. If the protein has already been crystallized, then repeating the published conditions might require some variations in the pH or the concentration of the precipitant agents or use of additives. In the case of a mutant, the conditions established for the wild type could be initially explored; however, new screening might be also required. Ideally, crystallization trials are set from the same protein batch.
7. Dissolving the ligand in the crystallization buffer is usually advantageous compared to water. This surpasses the need of pH adjustments, which might be required for crystal soaking. In addition, it is preferable to offer the crystal a more "familiar" environment that would maintain its integrity during longer periods of soaking.
8. Although polar compounds can be easily dissolved in water, most drug-like compounds exhibit limited water solubility, when they contain aliphatic or hydrophobic groups. To counter that, a water miscible organic solvent, such as dimethyl sulfoxide (DMSO), can be used. The aforementioned solvent can dissolve most compounds regardless of polarity and is nontoxic, and, most importantly, macromolecules can tolerate it up to a certain concentration. The compound is usually mixed with 100% DMSO and is stirred until it is completely dissolved (stock solution). Then water or buffer is added with the aim to prepare dilutions of the stock solution, at the desired volume.
9. It should be noted that the order that the solvents are added is crucial, i.e. addition of DMSO, followed by water, might not lead to the same result as the one that would be obtained if the same steps in the reverse order are performed. This is due to the hydration sphere of the protein molecule and the number of water or other polar molecules of the solvent that will interact

with the residues lining the protein surface. If light precipitation or suspension of the ligand is observed in solution, rigorous stirring (for a long time) might lead to complete dilution. This could also be facilitated by using ultrasound baths. When the ligand is used for co-crystallization studies, common practice has also shown that ideally the ligand solution should be used immediately after dissolving it, since the heat released upon dilution could facilitate complex formation.

10. The suspension is heated initially approximately 10 °C above room temperature for 10 min, followed by stirring using a vortex. If required, this process is repeated in alternate steps of 10 °C and stirring in between until complete dissolution is achieved. Although drug-like organic compounds generally tolerate temperatures as high as 100 °C, it is advisable to consult the synthetic chemist about possible instability of the compound due to heating.
11. pH adjustment is a crucial step when the ligand has strong acidic or basic groups, since when it is dissolved in an aquatic solution, the compound might be ionized. This should be kept in mind during analysis of the ligand binding mode. Furthermore, there are many cases where the microenvironment inside the active site of the macromolecule has a pH much different than in the bulk solution, and it is actually this pH that will dictate the protonation state of the ligand [59]. If no solubility issues are encountered, compound solutions can be stored for longer periods at 4 or −20 °C, to ensure optimal stability in aquatic solutions. This is especially the case for compounds containing sensitive to oxidation groups such as hydroxyls or aldehydes. However, in cases of poor solubility, storage at low temperature is not recommended, since irreversible precipitation might occur.
12. It has also been shown that using preformed crystals might not be desirable, since the energy cost required for the ligand to leave the bulk solvent and access the binding site might induce significant conformational changes, which might outweigh its affinity for the target. In addition, the binding site might be buried with limited accessible surface area, due to the packing of the molecules in the crystal. In cases where the solubility of the ligand is extremely low, a droplet of the ligand solution, after intensive stirring, is used for crystal soaking. It might not be possible to calculate accurately the ligand concentration; however what is known is that the soaking takes place using a saturated solution and if binding is observed, then the required concentration is much less than the one in the saturated solution. Additional data available from assays will allow the calculation of the protein-ligand binding affinity in solution. Depending on their affinity, binding might occur from minutes

to several hours or even days, until the ligand is settled in the binding site.

13. In case the ligand has poor solubility and it is in powder form, the protein solution might be used as a solvent of the ligand. It is not very common to use this as an option, though.
14. Extra attention should be taken at the minimization step because different software "destroy" the geometry of the ligand in an effort to achieve the minimum energy. This might be correct numerically, but it is not possible to ignore the stereochemical restraints imposed, e.g. in sugar rings like glucopyranose. In case that the geometry of the ligand changes upon minimization or refinement, then the ideal values are manually introduced in the .cif file, and if required constraints are also applied.
15. The solvent molecules of the protein structure need to be excluded from the model to make sure that the additional density that will appear at the site of interest could be attributed to the ligand. The geometry of a small molecule might be slightly different when bound compared to the free state. Although no huge differences are expected to be encountered, it is normal to observe deviations of certain bond angles of the ligand, from the ideal values. These deviations appear after performing energy minimization of the ligand inside the binding pocket. In this case, the actual bond angles result from the electron density (experimental data), while the ideal values are theoretical.
16. Commercial, virtual, and natural substances and combinatorial chemistry libraries can be used to probe the huge chemical space available (estimated up to 10^{100} possibilities) for compound-potential binders to the protein (high-throughput screening, HTS). Although such a screen may reveal hundreds of thousands of hits of modest binding affinity, the ligand efficiency is usually low, since the ligand may grossly fit in the protein cavity, forming a number of non-optimized interactions. A rather well-known free database for commercially available ligand screening is *ZINC* database (http://zinc.docking.org) [60]. During the last two decades, there is an increasing interest on fragment-based discovery (FBD) as an alternative approach for initial hits. The basic principle is to identify fragments that bind to sub-pockets of a cavity that will elaborate to larger-molecule lead compounds introducing suitable linkers [61]. Fragments are also organized in libraries that will be exploited for screening purposes. Although it is not expected to exhibit high affinity for the target (i.e., low mM range), they probe binding sites and might provide significant information on shape complementarity and affinity. After

generating the virtual library, several filters can be applied to decrease the number of compounds to a manageable number of hits. Initially it is explored whether a compound meets drug-likeness criteria, a number of rules that it has been observed to apply in most drugs. One example of such a restraint is the Lipinski's "rule of 5," according to which a potential drug should have molecular weight less than 500 Da, an octanol water partition coefficient calculated using the Hansch and Leo approach should be in a range of −5 to 5, the number of hydrogen bond donors calculated simply as the sum of the number of oxygens and nitrogens with a hydrogen attached should be <5, and the sum of oxygens and nitrogens without hydrogen attached should be <1. Other rules that have been used include the existence of less than 10 rotatable bonds and the total polar surface area not to exceed 140 A^2 [62]. After applying these initial filters, the remaining compounds undergo molecular docking, which is a computational technique that predicts the binding mode and affinity of a small molecule on a particular binding site of the protein. The process can be computationally demanding, especially if blind docking is carried out, that is, using the entire protein structure. There are several factors to be taken into consideration, with regard both to the target and the ligand. Concerning the target, the input is usually a file with coordinates for every atom of the protein but lacks information about its flexibility. Since a protein is not frozen, various techniques can be utilized, at the expense of computational power, to take into consideration flexible regions of the protein. Concerning the ligand, an ensemble of conformers rather than a single structure should be used as input for docking. Furthermore, issues such as different stereoisomers, protonation, and tautomeric states should be addressed, and corresponding ensembles of structures for such ligands should be taken into account during docking.

4 Conclusions

The future in rational drug design using integrative structural biology, but also other approaches, is very well-described in a recent review by de Vrueh and Crommelin [63], who discuss pharmaceutical public-private partnerships while commenting on all the key players in the field, including health foundations, research and academic organizations, patient organizations, and individual scientists. Further discussion on this is beyond the scope of this chapter. However, attention should be drawn to the development of synergies and the boost that innovative integrative structural biology approaches have provided to drug discovery. During the last decade, international initiatives such as the Structural Genomics Consortium Initiative and the European Strategic Forum for Research Infrastructures (ESFRI) in the field of biomedical sciences have promoted the establishment of dedicated, yet complementary RIs, enabling the smooth transfer from molecules to medicines by applying high-throughput approaches. For example, target and drug discovery can be accelerated by the access to RIs focusing on genome analysis, proteomics, and systems biology (like ELIXIR, EATRIS-ERIC, ISBE, etc.), followed by those that give emphasis on structural biology and chemical screening (like INSTRUCT-ERIC, EU-OPENSCREEN, etc.). Similarly, the drug development process, including drug validation, has been facilitated through RIs dedicated on animal models and imaging technologies to visualize potential drug action (e.g., INFRAFRONTIER, Euro-BIOIMAGING, etc.) and clinical testing using samples from biobanks, through the corresponding RIs (e.g., ECRIN-ERIC, BBMRI-ERIC). A complete roadmap on the landscape of the RIs in Europe can be found at the following links http://www.esfri.eu/roadmap-2016 and https://ec.europa.eu/research/infrastructures. A common aim of all these RIs is to adopt international standards; hence they give particular emphasis on international outreach by expanding and making international agreements with non-EU countries and industry users to endorse innovative approaches and tools in the drug discovery and development process. These infrastructures provide unique services to the scientific community, including access to cutting-edge technologies, large-scale facilities, and high-quality expertise that would not be possible to be offered by individual laboratories. The diversity of the RIs is not limited in the same thematic area but concerns cross-discipline RIs that have initially developed for material sciences but have significant applications in biomolecules and maximum benefit for the drug design and discovery process. These include X-FEL (https://www.xfel.eu), in Hamburg, Germany, that generates intense X-ray flashes and the European Spallation Source (ESS) in Lund, Sweden (https://europeanspallationsource.se), both with a broad range of applications. Through these powerful energy sources, the 3D protein structure determination is possible at high resolution; especially in the case of neutrons, mapping of detailed hydrogen bond interactions is enabled giving unique insights on the structural determinates that dictate protein-ligand complex formation. These findings can be associated to targeted communities beyond structural biologists, like medical doctors or funders through Open Science Services, already developed and available like OpenAIRE (https://www.openaire.eu). Therefore, integrative structural biology can play a leading role in rational drug design enhancing the researchers' potential to increase their competitiveness at international level, with a clear socioeconomic impact.

References

1. Berman HM (2008) The protein data bank: a historical perspective. Acta Crystallogr A 64 (Pt 1):88–95. https://doi.org/10.1107/S0108767307035623
2. Scannell JW, Blanckley A, Boldon H et al (2012) Diagnosing the decline in pharmaceutical R&D efficiency. Nat Rev Drug Discov 11 (3):191–200. https://doi.org/10.1038/nrd3681
3. Scannell JW, Bosley J (2016) When quality beats quantity: decision theory, drug discovery, and the reproducibility crisis. PLoS One 11(2): e0147215. https://doi.org/10.1371/journal.pone.0147215
4. Manglik A, Lin H, Aryal DK et al (2016) Structure-based discovery of opioid analgesics with reduced side effects. Nature 537 (7619):185–190. https://doi.org/10.1038/nature19112
5. Wacker D, Wang S, McCorvy JD et al (2017) Crystal structure of an LSD-bound human serotonin receptor. Cell 168(3):377–389.e12. https://doi.org/10.1016/j.cell.2016.12.033
6. Dormitzer PR, Grandi G, Rappuoli R (2012) Structural vaccinology starts to deliver. Nat Rev Microbiol 10(12):807–813. https://doi.org/10.1038/nrmicro2893
7. Gourlay L, Peri C, Bolognesi M et al (2017) Structure and computation in immunoreagent design: from diagnostics to vaccines. Trends Biotechnol 35(12):1208–1220. https://doi.org/10.1016/j.tibtech.2017.06.018
8. Khan FI, Lan D, Durrani R et al (2017) The lid domain in lipases: structural and functional determinant of enzymatic properties. Front Bioeng Biotechnol 5:1–13. https://doi.org/10.3389/fbioe.2017.00016
9. Jensen MBV, Horsfall LE, Wardrope C et al (2016) Characterisation of a new family of carboxyl esterases with an OsmC domain. PLoS One 11(11):e0166128. https://doi.org/10.1371/journal.pone.0166128
10. Scholz J, Besir H, Strasser C et al (2013) A new method to customize protein expression vectors for fast, efficient and background free parallel cloning. BMC Biotechnol 13(1):12. https://doi.org/10.1186/1472-6750-13-12
11. Owens RJ (ed) (2015) Structural proteomics: high-throughput methods. Humana Press, Totowa, NJ. https://doi.org/10.1007/978-1-4939-2230-7
12. Singh A, Upadhyay V, Upadhyay AK et al (2015) Protein recovery from inclusion bodies of Escherichia coli using mild solubilization process. Microb Cell Factories 14:2–10. https://doi.org/10.1186/s12934-015-0222-8
13. Malissard M, Berger EG (2001) Improving solubility of catalytic domain of human beta-1,4-galactosyltransferase 1 through rationally designed amino acid replacements. Eur J Biochem 268(15):4352–4358. https://doi.org/10.1046/j.1432-1327.2001.02357.x
14. Janson J-C (ed) (2011) Protein purification: principles, high resolution methods and applications. Wiley, Hoboken. https://doi.org/10.1002/9780470939932
15. Gasteiger E, Hoogland C, Gattiker A et al (2005) Protein identification and analysis tools on the ExPASy server. In: Walker J (ed) The proteomics protocols handbook. Humana Press, Totowa, NJ
16. Gupta R, Brunak S (2002) Prediction of glycosylation across the human proteome and the correlation to protein function. Pac Symp Biocomput 7:310–322
17. Steentoft C, Vakhrushev SY, Joshi HJ et al (2013) Precision mapping of the human O-GalNAc glycoproteome through SimpleCell technology. EMBO J 32(10):1478–1488. https://doi.org/10.1038/emboj.2013.79
18. Kimple ME, Brill AL, Pasker RL (2015) Overview of affinity tags for protein purification. Curr Protoc Protein Sci Unit-9.9:1–26. https://doi.org/10.1002/0471140864.ps0909s73
19. Sahin E, Roberts CJ (2012) Size-exclusion chromatography with multi-angle light scattering for elucidating protein aggregation mechanisms. In: Voynov V, Caravella J (eds) Therapeutic proteins. Methods in molecular biology (methods and protocols), vol 899. Humana Press, Totowa, NJ
20. Greenfield NJ (2006) Using circular dichroism spectra to estimate protein secondary structure. Nat Protoc 1(6):2876–2890. https://doi.org/10.1038/nprot.2006.202
21. Macchi P (2011) Cryo-crystallography: diffraction at low temperature and more. In: Rissanen K (ed) Advanced X-ray crystallography. Topics in current chemistry, vol 315. Springer, Berlin, Heidelberg
22. Krojer T, Pike ACW, Von Delft F (2013) Squeezing the most from every crystal: the fine details of data collection. Acta Crystallogr Sect D Biol Crystallogr 69:1303–1313. https://doi.org/10.1107/S0907444913013280
23. Kabsch W (2010) XDS. Acta Crystallogr D Biol Crystallogr 66(Pt2):125–132. https://doi.org/10.1107/S0907444909047337
24. Leslie AGW, Powell HR (2007) Processing diffraction data with mosflm. In: Read RJ, Sussman JL (eds) Evolving methods for

macromolecular crystallography. NATO Science Series, vol 245. Springer, Dordrecht

25. Winn MD, Ballard CC, Cowtan KD et al (2011) Overview of the CCP4 suite and current developments. Acta Crystallogr Sect D Biol Crystallogr 67(Pt.4):235–242. https://doi.org/10.1107/S0907444910045749
26. Navaza J, Saludjian P (1997) *AMoRe*: an automated molecular replacement program package. Methods Enzymol 276:581–594. https://doi.org/10.1016/S0076-6879(97)76079-8
27. McCoy AJ, Grosse-Kunstleve RW, Adams PD et al (2007) Phaser crystallographic software. J Appl Crystallogr 40(Pt.4):658–674. https://doi.org/10.1107/S0021889807021206
28. Vagin A, Teplyakov A (1997) MOLREP: an automated program for molecular replacement. J Appl Crystallogr 30:1022–1025. https://doi.org/10.1107/S0021889897006766
29. Adams PD, Afonine PV, Bunkóczi G et al (2010) PHENIX: a comprehensive python-based system for macromolecular structure solution. Acta Crystallogr Sect D Biol Crystallogr 66(Pt.2):213–221. https://doi.org/10.1107/S0907444909052925
30. Emsley P, Lohkamp B, Scott WG et al (2010) Features and development of coot. Acta Crystallogr Sect D Biol Crystallogr 66 (Pt.4):486–501. https://doi.org/10.1107/S0907444910007493
31. Murshudov GN, Vagin AA, Dodson EJ (1997) Refinement of macromolecular structures by the maximum-likelihood method. Acta Crystallogr D Biol Crystallogr 53(Pt.3):240–255. https://doi.org/10.1107/S0907444996012255
32. Murshudov GN, Skubák P, Lebedev AA et al (2011) *REFMAC* 5 for the refinement of macromolecular crystal structures. Acta Crystallogr Sect D Biol Crystallogr 67:355–367. https://doi.org/10.1107/S0907444911001314
33. Chen VB, Arendall WB, Headd JJ et al (2010) MolProbity: all-atom structure validation for macromolecular crystallography. Acta Crystallogr Sect D Biol Crystallogr 66(Pt.1):12–21. https://doi.org/10.1107/S0907444909042073
34. Hanwell MD, Curtis DE, Lonie DC et al (2012) Avogadro: an advanced semantic chemical editor, visualization, and analysis platform. Aust J Chem 4(1):17. https://doi.org/10.1186/1758-2946-4-17
35. Schüttelkopf AW, Van Aalten DMF (2004) PRODRG: a tool for high-throughput crystallography of protein-ligand complexes. Acta Crystallogr Sect D Biol Crystallogr 60 (Pt.8):1355–1363. https://doi.org/10.1107/S0907444904011679
36. Laskowski RA, Swindells MB (2011) LigPlot+: multiple ligand-protein interaction diagrams for drug discovery. J Chem Inf Model 51(10):2778–2786. https://doi.org/10.1021/ci200227u
37. Pettersen EF, Goddard TD, Huang CC et al (2004) UCSF chimera—a visualization system for exploratory research and analysis. J Comput Chem 25(13):1605–1612. https://doi.org/10.1002/jcc.20084
38. Bissantz C, Kuhn B, Stahl M (2010) A medicinal chemist's guide to molecular interactions. J Med Chem 53(14):5061–5084. https://doi.org/10.1021/jm100112j
39. Meyer EA, Castellano RK, Diederich F (2003) Interactions with aromatic rings in chemical and biological recognition. Angew Chem Int Ed 42(11):1210–1250. https://doi.org/10.1002/anie.200390319
40. Le Guilloux V, Schmidtke P, Tuffery P (2009) Fpocket: an open source platform for ligand pocket detection. BMC Bioinformatics 10:168. https://doi.org/10.1186/1471-2105-10-168
41. Dundas J, Ouyang Z, Tseng J et al (2006) CASTp: computed atlas of surface topography of proteins with structural and topographical mapping of functionally annotated residues. Nucleic Acids Res 34:W116–W118. https://doi.org/10.1093/nar/gkl282
42. Stank A, Kokh DB, Horn M et al (2017) TRAPP webserver: predicting protein binding site flexibility and detecting transient binding pockets. Nucleic Acids Res 45(W1):W325–W330. https://doi.org/10.1093/nar/gkx277
43. Porter CT (2004) The catalytic site atlas: a resource of catalytic sites and residues identified in enzymes using structural data. Nucleic Acids Res 32:129D–133D. https://doi.org/10.1093/nar/gkh028
44. Torrance JW, Bartlett GJ, Porter CT et al (2005) Using a library of structural templates to recognise catalytic sites and explore their evolution in homologous families. J Mol Biol 347(3):565–581. https://doi.org/10.1016/j.jmb.2005.01.044
45. Van Linden OPJ, Kooistra AJ, Leurs R et al (2014) KLIFS: a knowledge-based structural database to navigate kinase-ligand interaction space. J Med Chem 57(2):249–277. https://doi.org/10.1021/jm400378w
46. Kooistra AJ, Kanev GK, Van Linden OPJ et al (2016) KLIFS: a structural kinase-ligand interaction database. Nucleic Acids Res 44:D365–D371. https://doi.org/10.1093/nar/gkv1082

47. Hendlich M, Bergner A, Günther J et al (2003) Relibase: design and development of a database for comprehensive analysis of protein-ligand interactions. J Mol Biol 326(2):607–620. https://doi.org/10.1016/S0022-2836(02)01408-0
48. Verma R, Mitchell-Koch K (2017) In silico studies of small molecule interactions with enzymes reveal aspects of catalytic function. Catalysts 7(7):212. https://doi.org/10.3390/catal7070212
49. Lu Y, Wang R, Yang CY et al (2007) Analysis of ligand-bound water molecules in high-resolution crystal structures of protein-ligand complexes. J Chem Inf Model 47(2):668–675. https://doi.org/10.1021/ci6003527
50. Spyrakis F, Ahmed MH, Bayden AS et al (2017) The roles of water in the protein matrix: a largely untapped resource for drug discovery. J Med Chem 60(16):6781–6828. https://doi.org/10.1021/acs.jmedchem.7b00057
51. Mavrokefalos N, Myrianthopoulos V, Chajistamatiou AS et al (2015) Discovery of the glycogen phosphorylase-modulating activity of a resveratrol glucoside by using a virtual screening protocol optimized for solvation effects. Planta Med 81(6):507–516. https://doi.org/10.1055/s-0035-1545910
52. Tan KP, Nguyen TB, Patel S et al (2013) Depth: a web server to compute depth, cavity sizes, detect potential small-molecule ligand-binding cavities and predict the pKa of ionizable residues in proteins. Nucleic Acids Res 41: W314–W321. https://doi.org/10.1093/nar/gkt503
53. Kelly LA, Mezulis S, Yates C et al (2015) The Phyre2 web portal for protein modelling, prediction, and analysis. Nat Protoc 10(6):845–858. https://doi.org/10.1038/nprot.2015.053
54. Zhang Y (2008) I-TASSER server for protein 3D structure prediction. BMC Bioinformatics 9:40. https://doi.org/10.1186/1471-2105-9-40
55. Biasini M, Bienert S, Waterhouse A et al (2014) SWISS-MODEL: modelling protein tertiary and quaternary structure using evolutionary information. Nucleic Acids Res 42: W252–W258. https://doi.org/10.1093/nar/gku340
56. Kim DE, Chivian D, Baker D (2004) Protein structure prediction and analysis using the Robetta server. Nucleic Acids Res 32:526–531. https://doi.org/10.1093/nar/gkh468
57. Koehn J, Hunt I (2009) High-throughput protein production (HTPP): a review of enabling technologies to expedite protein production. In: Doyle SA (ed) High throughput protein expression and purification. Methods in molecular biology, vol 498. Humana Press, Totowa, NJ
58. McPherson A, Gavira JA (2014) Introduction to protein crystallization. Acta Crystallogr Sect F Structural Biol Commun 70(Pt.1):2–20. https://doi.org/10.1107/S2053230X13033141
59. Mamais M, Degli Esposti A, Kouloumoundra V et al (2017) A new potent inhibitor of glycogen phosphorylase reveals the basicity of the catalytic site. Chem—A Eur J 23(37):8800–8805. https://doi.org/10.1002/chem.201701591
60. Irwin JJ, Shoichet BK (2005) ZINC—a free database of commercially available compounds for virtual screening. J Chem Inf Model 45(1):177–182. https://doi.org/10.1021/ci049714+
61. Blundell TL, Jhoti H, Abell C (2002) High-throughput crystallography for lead discovery in drug design. Nat Rev Drug Discov 1(1):45–54. https://doi.org/10.1038/nrd706
62. Cavasotto CN (ed) (2017) In silico drug discovery and design theory, methods, challenges, and applications. CRC Press, Boca Raton
63. de Vrueh RLA, Crommelin DJA (2017) Reflections on the future of pharmaceutical public-private partnerships: from input to impact. Pharm Res 34(10):1985–1999. https://doi.org/10.1007/s11095-017-2192-5

Chapter 7

Enalos+ KNIME Nodes: New Cheminformatics Tools for Drug Discovery

Dimitra-Danai Varsou, Spyridon Nikolakopoulos, Andreas Tsoumanis, Georgia Melagraki, and Antreas Afantitis

Abstract

In this chapter we present and discuss Enalos+ nodes designed and developed by NovaMechanics Ltd. for the open-source KNIME platform, as a useful aid when dealing with cheminformatics and nanoinformatics problems or medicinal applications. Enalos+ nodes facilitate tasks performed in molecular modeling and allow access, data mining, and manipulation for multiple chemical databases through the KNIME interface. Enalos+ nodes automate common procedures that greatly facilitate the rapid workflow prototyping within KNIME. Methods and techniques that are included in Enalos+ nodes are presented in order to offer a deeper understanding of the theoretical background of the incorporated functionalities. An emphasis is given to demonstrate the usefulness of Enalos+ nodes in different cheminformatics applications by presenting four indicative case studies. Specifically, we present case studies that underline the value and the effectiveness of the nodes for molecular descriptors calculation and QSAR predictive model development. In addition, case studies are also presented demonstrating the benefits of the use of Enalos+ nodes for database exploitation within a drug discovery project.

Key words Nanoinformatics, Computational nanotoxicology, QSAR, Cheminformatics, Virtual screening

1 Introduction

Within a drug discovery, toxicity assessment, or environmental chemistry study, scientists need to get a detailed insight in the structural characteristics of the molecules in order to understand their activity mechanisms and to point out those properties that render some molecules as the ideal candidates for pharmaceutical or other applications [1]. Current efforts in the field of drug design include high-throughput screening (HTS) and combinatorial chemistry methodologies that produce a significant number of data. The abundance of experimental data and the need for a sustainable exploitation led to the development of well-structured online databases like PubChem or ChEMBL that contain chemical

Thomas Mavromoustakos and Tahsin F. Kellici (eds.), *Rational Drug Design: Methods and Protocols*, Methods in Molecular Biology, vol. 1824, https://doi.org/10.1007/978-1-4939-8630-9_7,

substances and their (bio)activity information [2]. New tools to handle experimental big data are highly desired, and this considerably boosted in silico methods within cheminformatics [3].

Cheminformatics involves several computational methods and strategies, including data mining and modeling approaches, to deal with a wide range of problems arising within a drug discovery or material design framework [4]. In a cheminformatics context, the structural information of the molecules needs to be transformed into mathematical representations that can be used as inputs to the cheminformatics tools. These representations—referred as molecular descriptors—are useful in data mining, diversity analysis, virtual screening, modeling, etc. [5]. In a next step, ligand based on in silico methods such as quantitative structure-activity relationship (QSAR) modeling can be used to correlate the structural properties of the molecules with their properties or biological activities [5, 6]. These models can be a very useful aid in highlighting the critical parameters that explain the behavior of the molecules and on top of that can be used to obtain reliable predictions of molecular properties or activities of uncharacterized molecules [1, 5]. QSAR model development includes several crucial steps to afford robust models with high predictive power. The QSAR workflow mainly includes data curation, modeling, internal and external validation, and definition of the domain of their applicability [6].

The above steps for model development can be performed employing a multitude of tools and software. While researchers can create custom scripts to automate common procedures, this solution is less than ideal when projects demand rapid workflow prototyping, interactive data analysis, and robust, appropriately validated models. KNIME open-source [7] software is considered ideal when dealing with cheminformatics problems, given that it provides access to several analysis tools such as Enalos, *CDK*, *RDKit*, *EMBL-EBI* nodes, Chemical Identifier Resolver, etc. [2]. In addition, KNIME provides many modeling options offering a wide variety of machine learning algorithms including Weka tools. However, there are still some functionality gaps to be filled in KNIME, mainly concerning the calculation of molecular descriptors, data handling, model validation, domain of applicability definition, data mining, and extraction from popular databases. Enalos + nodes were developed to fill these gaps within the open-source KNIME interface [8]. Enalos+ nodes, described in this chapter, are designed to help the user with data preprocessing, descriptors' calculation, and model validation and allow easy access to multiple chemical databases for data mining and manipulation through KNIME interface.

1.1 KNIME as a Tool for Data Analysis

Analysis of large experimental data usually requires a series of complex processing steps (statistical analysis, descriptors calculation, modeling, image analysis, exploitation of large databases, etc.) that can be performed using a wide variety of computational tools and programming scripts. However, the need for a systematic, automated approach of each analysis and the need of exporting reproducible results demand the unification of the above processing steps under a common platform, where different data manipulation tools can be used [9].

KNIME (Konstanz Information Miner) is a user-friendly and open-source platform that combines various software tools for data integration, processing, analysis, and exploitation. The user can create interactive workflows composed of processing nodes that analyze the data and share the results through a system of "pipelines" (connections) [10]. Data, models, and produced results can be presented via interactive tables and plots, and reports can be extracted. The user can create a network of nodes that gives the flexibility to interact easily with the workflow, experiment with different methodologies in short time, compare the results, and—most importantly—have the complete supervision of the analysis process, using only one file [11].

One of the major advantages of KNIME is that it can bridge, under the same interface, different software tools that can be compatible with each other. Especially in the field of life sciences (cheminformatics, nanoinformatics, etc.), there is a wide variety of nodes that can be used for molecules' handling such as the *Chemistry Development Kit* (*CDK*), the *Indigo* software for organic chemistry, *RDKit*, *ChEMBL*, etc. [2, 9]. It is also possible to extend the capabilities of KNIME by creating custom-made nodes or by integrating scripts implemented in different programming languages and take advantage of their capabilities. It is possible to integrate R scripts and use R packages for statistical computing, visualization, and analysis of biological data. It is also possible to integrate scripts from MATLAB or Python programming languages for data processing and modeling [9]. The modeling capabilities of KNIME can be also highly extended using the Weka nodes that give access to the various machine learning algorithms for data mining (regression and classification) [9–11].

The present chapter is devoted in the presentation of Enalos+ KNIME nodes developed by NovaMechanics Ltd. [8]. Enalos+ nodes are associated with data preprocessing and analysis, modeling, data mining of chemical databases (PubChem, UniChem, NCI, etc.), and molecular descriptors' calculation. Especially for PubChem, Enalos+ includes a full and complete range of nodes: search for similar compounds, search for patents, extract compounds from patents, search for vendors, extract compounds from assays, etc. All these nodes are under the same interface with the option to apply in real time a predictive model or other analysis tools.

2 Enalos+ Nodes

Enalos and Enalos+ KNIME nodes are designed and developed by NovaMechanics Ltd. [8] with the aim to facilitate the robust and accurate model development, as well as to perform data analysis and curation for cheminformatics and nanoinformatics. The Enalos+ family nodes contain *Modeling*, *Molecular Descriptors*, *NCI*, *PubChem*, and *UniChem* nodes and significantly increase the number of the available KNIME nodes and extend the capabilities of the users [2, 10].

We have selected and highlighted below several Enalos+ nodes together with case studies explaining key inputs and steps required to execute the corresponding cheminformatics tasks.

2.1 Create New Molecules

Create New Molecules Enalos+ node enables the user to create a list of molecules by combining a series of substituents with a main scaffold. All the possible combinations of molecules can be then used as inputs to other KNIME nodes, such as Valence Checker (to check the feasibility of molecules), Molecule to CDK (to visualize the structures), etc.

2.1.1 Case Study 1: Using Create New Molecules Enalos+ Node

This case study describes the generation of molecules with different substituents through *Create New Molecules* Enalos+ node combined with *Molecule to CDK* node in KNIME interface (Figs. 1 and 2). The SMILES notation of a main scaffold with two positions for substitution, namely, R_1 and R_2, is presented below:

$$[R_1]C1 = C([R_2])C = CC = C1$$

Create New Molecules node requires as input a table containing different substituents at the indicated positions of the basic scaffold. Each column represents the position for the substituents, and each row must contain only one substituent. In example, random substituents are presented in Table 1.

Using Table 1 as input, the *Create New Molecules* node will produce a table with all possible nine combinations of substitution:

In order to visualize all the created new molecules, the user can utilize the existing *Molecule to CDK* KNIME node. This node takes

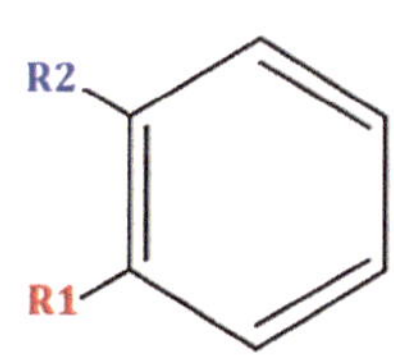

Fig. 1 Core molecule

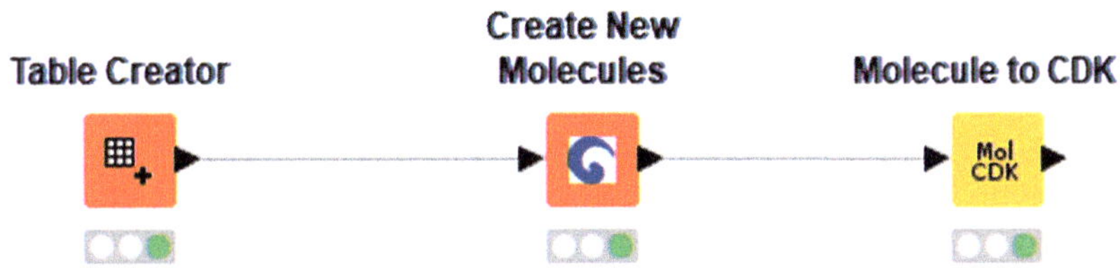

Fig. 2 KNIME workflow using create new molecules

Table 1
Input table substituents for the core molecule

R_1	R_2
O	C
CO	O
C	CO

Table 2
Output table new molecules

R_1	R_2	New molecule
O	C	OC1 = C(C)C = CC = C1
O	O	OC1 = C(O)C = CC = C1
O	CO	OC1 = C(CO)C = CC = C1
CO	C	COC1 = C(C)C = CC = C1
CO	O	COC1 = C(O)C = CC = C1
CO	CO	COC1 = C(CO)C = CC = C1
C	C	CC1 = C(C)C = CC = C1
C	O	CC1 = C(O)C = CC = C1
C	CO	CC1 = C(CO)C = CC = C1

as input the table containing the molecules to be parsed (the output of the *Create New Molecules* nodes Table 2) and outputs a table with the parsed molecules (Table 3).

2.2 Molecular Descriptors

Molecular descriptors are essential in various fields of scientific research such as health and pharmaceutical sciences, toxicology, and environmental Chemistry, since they convey molecular structure key data [1]. Molecular descriptors attempt to describe with

Table 3
Parsed new molecules

R_2 R_1	C	O	CO
O	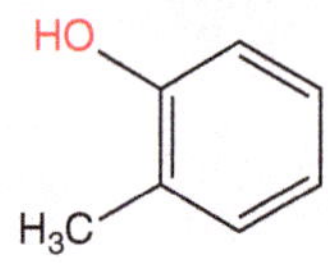	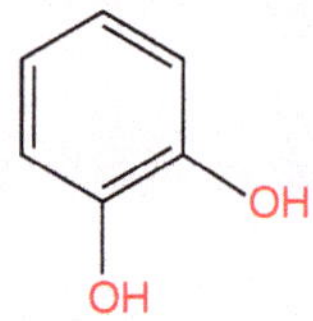	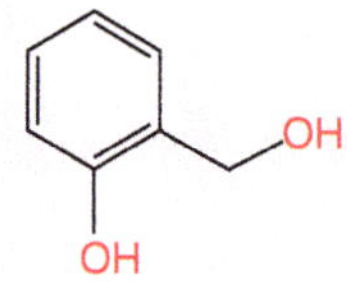
CO	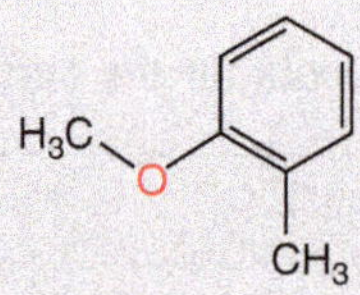	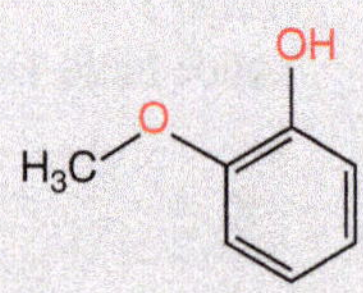	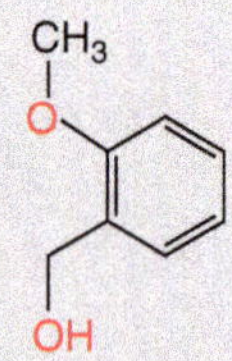
C	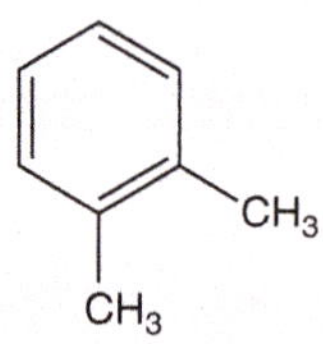	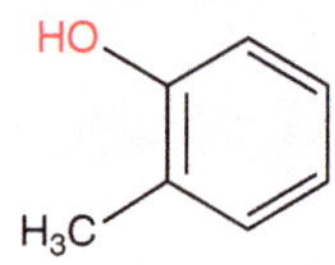	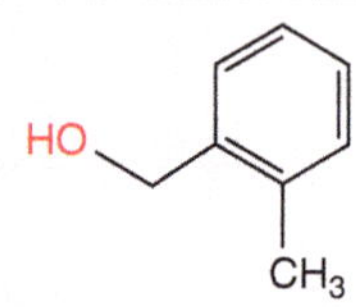

numerical values the structural features and properties of the molecules; thus the chemical information contained in the molecule can be treated mathematically and can be used for QSAR model development [5, 11, 12]. In that way the structural characteristics can be directly linked with the biological or physicochemical properties of chemical compounds [5].

Molecular descriptors can be calculated or derived based on different theories including organic and quantum chemistry, graph theory, etc. [1]. Mold2 freely available software, designed and produced by the National Center for Toxicological Research of FDA, can be used for the calculation of a large and diverse set of molecular descriptors, encoding two-dimensional chemical structure information, including topological, geometric, and structural characteristics of compounds [5]. It is demonstrated, using several published datasets, that this software produces sufficient structural information and that the developed models using Mold2 descriptors are of high quality [2, 5].

The calculation of molecular descriptors using the Mold2 software through KNIME was made available via the *EnalosMold2* node [13]. An example of its use is demonstrated below.

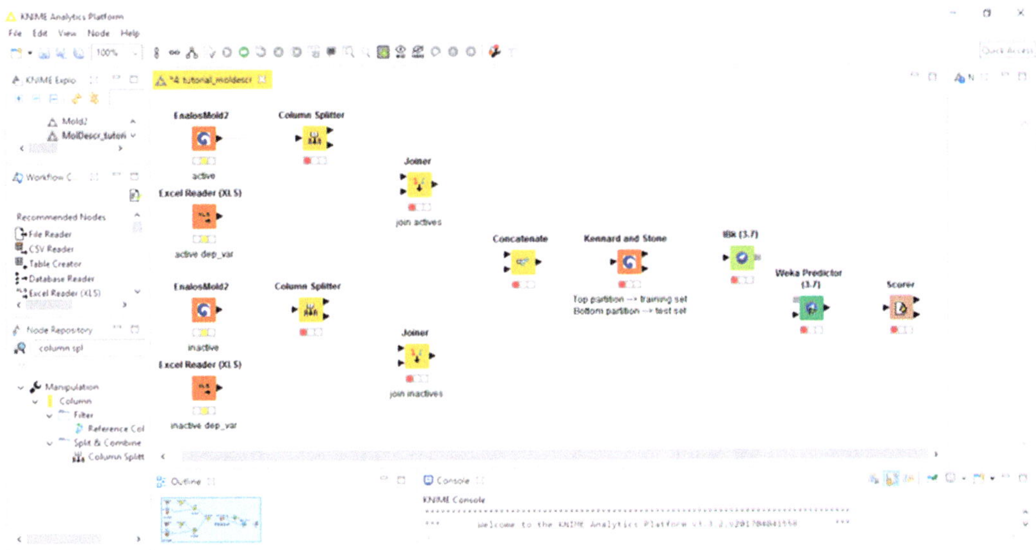

Fig. 3 Basic workflow using molecular descriptors

2.2.1 Case Study 2: Using Enalos+ Molecular Descriptors

The current case study is designed to help the interested reader in going step-by-step through the process of building a KNIME workflow, using the Molecular Descriptor Enalos+ nodes of Nova-Mechanics Ltd. This case study deals with a Luminescence Cell-Based Counter screen to Identify Inhibitors of A1 Apoptosis (AID 449761 in PubChem). Figure 3 illustrates the KNIME workflow that allows the descriptors calculation for this case study.

With the aid of Enalos+ KNIME nodes, the user can download from PubChem small molecules screened for a specific assay (in our case study assay AID 449761—Inhibitors of A1 Apoptosis).

The Kennard and Stone method used in this case study allows the selection of two representative subsets (as training and test sets) with a uniform distribution over an initial dataset. *Kennard and Stone* node takes as input the table that is going to be partitioned and outputs the two partitions (training and test set). *Kennard and Stone* node is configured by defining the "Target column" which refers to the depended variable and the "Model percentage." In general, the test set should be about 15–20% of the entire dataset. For this case study, a value of 80% was selected as a "Model percentage."

IBk node includes the *k*-nearest neighbor (*k*NN) classifier. In the configuring menu, the user can select an appropriate value of *k* based on cross-validation and do distance weighting. The *Weka Predictor* node takes a model generated in a Weka node and classifies the test data. The output is given in Fig. 4 together with the confusion matrix, and accuracy statistics are shown in Figs. 5 and 6.

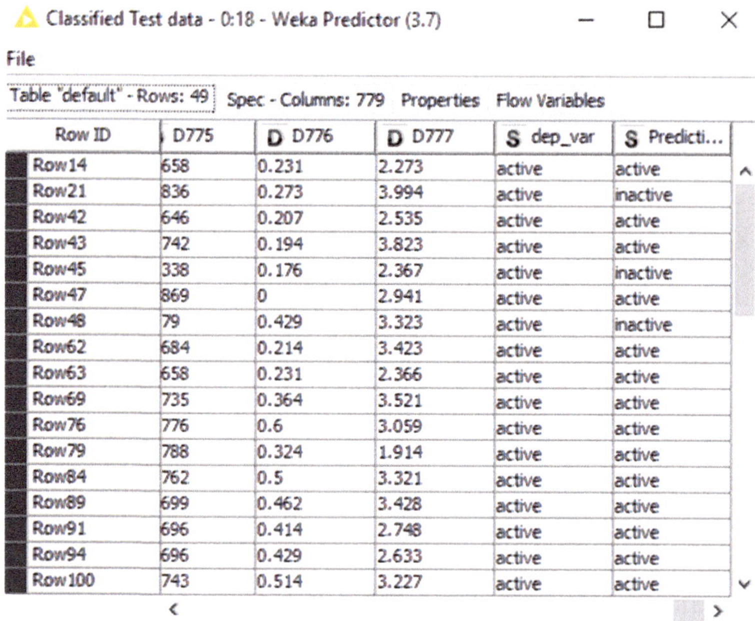

Row ID	D775	D776	D777	dep_var	Predicti...
Row14	658	0.231	2.273	active	active
Row21	836	0.273	3.994	active	inactive
Row42	646	0.207	2.535	active	active
Row43	742	0.194	3.823	active	active
Row45	338	0.176	2.367	active	inactive
Row47	869	0	2.941	active	active
Row48	79	0.429	3.323	active	inactive
Row62	684	0.214	3.423	active	active
Row63	658	0.231	2.366	active	active
Row69	735	0.364	3.521	active	active
Row76	776	0.6	3.059	active	active
Row79	788	0.324	1.914	active	active
Row84	762	0.5	3.321	active	active
Row89	699	0.462	3.428	active	active
Row91	696	0.414	2.748	active	active
Row94	696	0.429	2.633	active	active
Row100	743	0.514	3.227	active	active

Fig. 4 Weka prediction node outputs the classified test data

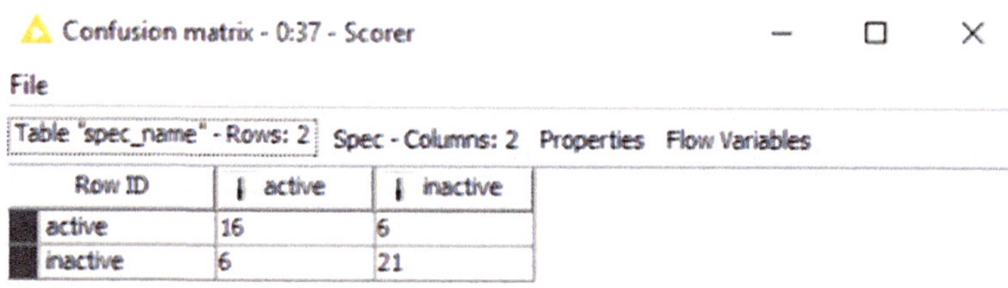

Row ID	active	inactive
active	16	6
inactive	6	21

Fig. 5 Scorer node exports the confusion matrix (1)

In order to increase the accuracy of the model, the main workflow can be extended in the following ways:

- Adding the Enalos+ *Remove Column* node. This node removes the selected input columns of the table that contain the same

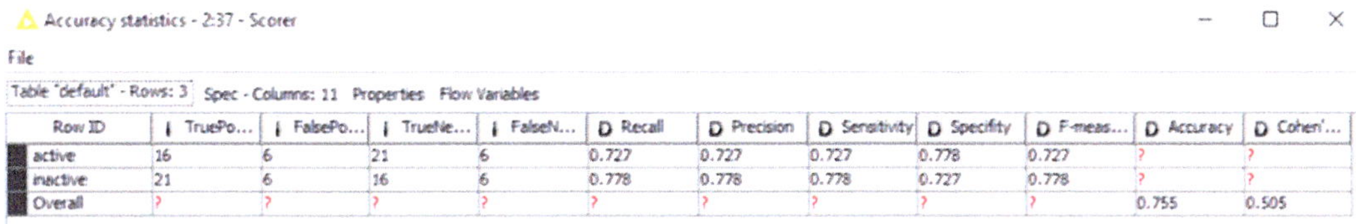

Accuracy statistics - 2:37 - Scorer

File

Table "default" - Rows: 3 Spec - Columns: 11 Properties Flow Variables

Row ID	TruePo...	FalsePo...	TrueNe...	FalseN...	Recall	Precision	Sensitivity	Specifity	F-meas...	Accuracy	Cohen'...
active	16	6	21	6	0.727	0.727	0.727	0.778	0.727	?	?
inactive	21	6	16	6	0.778	0.778	0.778	0.727	0.778	?	?
Overall	?	?	?	?	?	?	?	?	?	0.755	0.505

Fig. 6 Scorer node exports the accuracy statistics table (2)

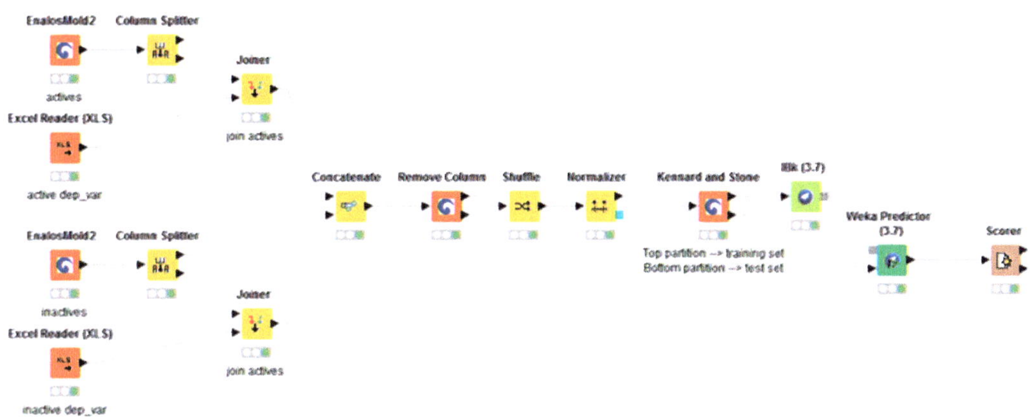

Fig. 7 Updated workflow (1)

values at a percentage equal or higher than a specific cutoff limit. In the configuring menu, remove the column containing the depended variable and set 10% as threshold.

- Data normalization. The user can also add *Normalizer* node, which normalizes the values of all (numeric) columns. In the dialog, the user can choose the desired columns to work on and set a method of normalization, for example, *Z*-score normalization.

The updated workflow is depicted in Fig. 7.

The new classified test data from the *Weka Predictor* node are displayed in Fig. 8. Concerning the *Scorer* node's output ports, the 1st one exports the confusion matrix (Fig. 9) and the second the accuracy statistics (Fig. 10).

2.3 Modeling Nodes

Within Life Sciences and especially in drug discovery processes, emphasis is given to substitute the expensive and the labor-intensive procedures of in vivo and in vitro experiments with the in silico testing. In silico testing includes computational approaches, such as quantitative structure-activity/toxicity relationships (QSAR/QSTR), and is used as an alternative to the experimental methods. Modeling techniques address the needs of exploring the

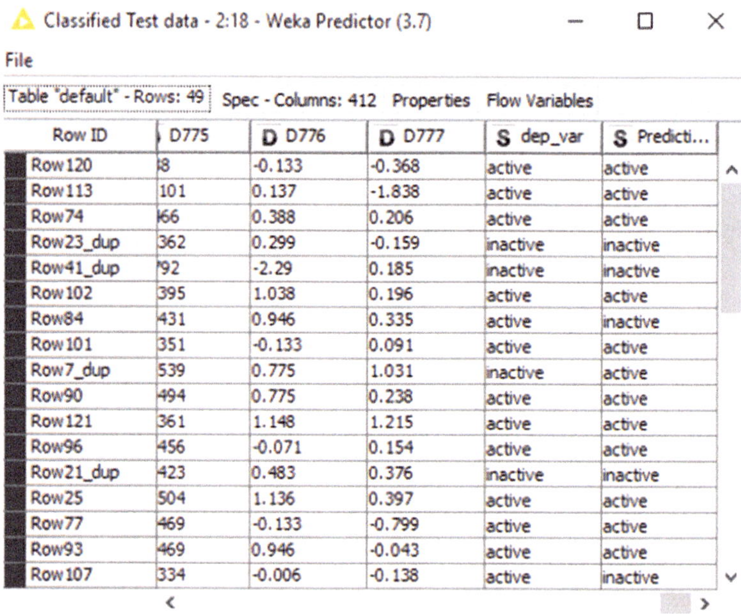

Classified Test data - 2:18 - Weka Predictor (3.7)

File

Table "default" - Rows: 49 Spec - Columns: 412 Properties Flow Variables

Row ID	D775	D D776	D D777	S dep_var	S Predicti...
Row120	8	-0.133	-0.368	active	active
Row113	101	0.137	-1.838	active	active
Row74	66	0.388	0.206	active	active
Row23_dup	362	0.299	-0.159	inactive	inactive
Row41_dup	92	-2.29	0.185	inactive	inactive
Row102	395	1.038	0.196	active	active
Row84	431	0.946	0.335	active	inactive
Row101	351	-0.133	0.091	active	active
Row7_dup	539	0.775	1.031	inactive	active
Row90	494	0.775	0.238	active	active
Row121	361	1.148	1.215	active	active
Row96	456	-0.071	0.154	active	active
Row21_dup	423	0.483	0.376	inactive	inactive
Row25	504	1.136	0.397	active	active
Row77	469	-0.133	-0.799	active	active
Row93	469	0.946	-0.043	active	active
Row107	334	-0.006	-0.138	active	inactive

Fig. 8 Weka predictor results

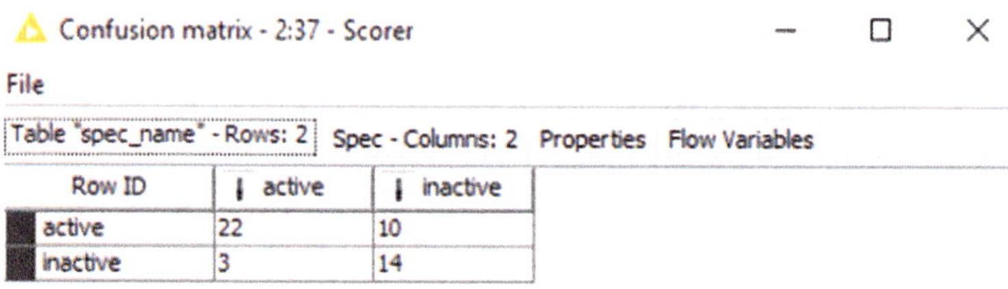

Confusion matrix - 2:37 - Scorer

File

Table "spec_name" - Rows: 2 Spec - Columns: 2 Properties Flow Variables

Row ID	I active	I inactive
active	22	10
inactive	3	14

Fig. 9 Scorer results (1)

relationships between experimental data and an activity profile, seeking strong patterns among them and using these relationships for making accurate predictions in future data. As part of building a robust model, the input is filtered following a variable selection

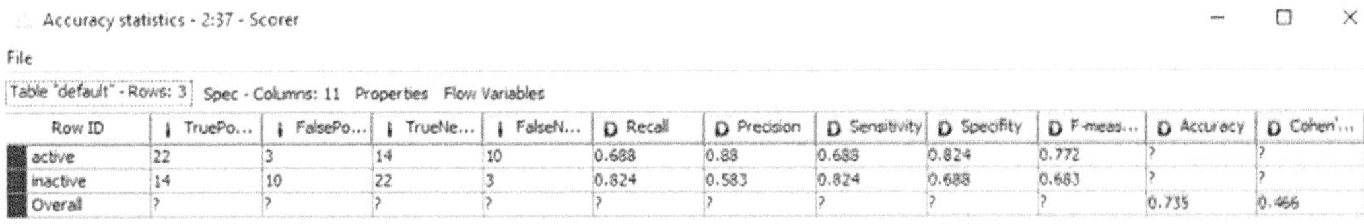
Accuracy statistics - 2:37 - Scorer

File

Table "default" - Rows: 3 Spec - Columns: 11 Properties Flow Variables

Row ID	TruePo...	FalsePo...	TrueNe...	FalseN...	Recall	Precision	Sensitivity	Specifity	F-meas...	Accuracy	Cohen'...
active	22	3	14	10	0.688	0.88	0.688	0.824	0.772	?	?
inactive	14	10	22	3	0.824	0.583	0.824	0.688	0.683	?	?
Overall	?	?	?	?	?	?	?	?	?	0.735	0.466

Fig. 10 Scorer results (2)

procedure to exclude the ones that do not significantly contribute to the data analysis. It is also of outmost importance to evaluate the model's performance and accuracy to ensure that trustworthy predictions are delivered.

The Enalos+ *Modeling* group contains eleven nodes specified for data handling and preprocessing as well as model validation.

2.3.1 Preprocessing Nodes

The preprocessing nodes perform some simple but crucial procedures for data handling and preprocessing. Especially when large datasets are analyzed, time-consuming procedures can be automated, eliminating significantly the effort and time required. The preprocessing nodes include *Create New Molecules*, *Int 2 Double*, *Remove Column*, and *Remove Duplicates.*

Create New Molecules node, as explicitly presented above, enables the user to create a list of molecules by combining a series of substituents with a main scaffold, reducing therefore the time spent to produce molecules with every combination of given substituents.

Int 2 Double converts the selected integer values of an input table to double values. In that way, many problems that may occur due to the format of the values can be avoided.

Remove Column node removes the selected input columns of the table that contain the same values at a percentage equal or higher than a specified cutoff limit. As the repetition of data can be a source of error in modeling and biases the results, this node can be used as a cleaning step in model building.

Remove Duplicates is also a filtering node that enables the user to remove the rows of the input table that contains the same values in selected columns. The filtered table contains all rows that are unique and the first one of each repeated row.

2.3.2 Partitioning Nodes

Data mining performed on large datasets often requires a reduction of data by dividing the initial dataset in smaller but representative subsets [14, 15]. Moreover, within the model validation process, two representative subsets are often required, and for that the initial dataset is divided into training and test sets. Objects within the test set are not used during model development but are left out for validation purposes [16]. Within Enalos+ nodes two algorithms for selecting representative objects from an initial dataset are included, namely, Kennard and Stone and sphere exclusion. These methods are briefly described below.

Kennard and Stone Method

The Kennard and Stone method allows the selection of a representative subset with a uniform distribution over an initial dataset. At first a central object is selected from the initial dataset, and then extreme objects from the data space border are introduced to the training set [17]. This method starts by calculating the mean of the dataset (Eq. 1). The closest object to it, which is the most representative object, is assigned as the first object to the subset, and it is removed from the initial dataset. The second object included in the subset is the most distant from the first one, and it is removed from the initial dataset as well. Then, according to the algorithm, the remaining objects are introduced to the subset by computing the Euclidean distance between each unassigned object and selected objects and finding the object which is the farthest from its closest neighbors in the subset, until the desired number of objects has been reached in the subset [13].

$$d_{ij}^2 = ||x_i, -, x_j|| = \sum_k (x_{ik} - x_{jk})^2 \tag{1}$$

Sphere Exclusion Method

The sphere exclusion method attempts to specify compounds which most effectively cover the available data space. The algorithm starts by scaling the values of each of the available variables between -1 and 1. Then, the starting compound for the analysis, which can be the most representative compound of the initial dataset, is assigned as the first object to the subset, and it is removed from the initial dataset. The minimum exclusion radius is selected as the desired percentage of the maximum Euclidean distance from the starting compound (center). All compounds closer to the starting compound than the exclusion radius are excluded from the subset. The remaining compound which is closest to the starting compound is assigned to the subset and is removed from the initial dataset. The latter compound is now the center of the new sphere, and all the remaining compounds closer to the new center than the exclusion radius are excluded from the subset. Then, the centroid of the selected compounds of the subset is calculated, and the remaining compound which is closest to this centroid is selected and assigned to the subset. This compound is also the new center. This process is repeated until no compounds remain to the initial dataset [15].

As already mentioned, the partitioning Enalos+ nodes are *Kennard and Stone* and *sphere exclusion* and are suitable for the selection of two representative subsets with a uniform distribution over an initial dataset using the methods described above.

2.3.3 Modeling Nodes

Multiple linear regression (MLR) is a method used to model the linear relationship between a dependent variable (target) and one or more independent variables (predictors). Multiple linear regression modeling is made available in KNIME through the Enalos+ MLR node, in order to model the relationships between a scalar dependent variable y and two or more independent variables denoted as *X*. The node produces, apart from the predicted values, the model coefficients and the coefficient of determination (R^2) in order to evaluate the modeling.

2.3.4 Testing Modeling Nodes

Model validation is a critical step during model development in order to evaluate whether the generated predictions are reliable or not. The quality of fit and the predictive power of a continuous QSAR model, as proposed by Tropsha et al. [12, 18–20], can be examined by testing the following criteria:

1. $q^2 > 0.5$
2. $R^2 > 0.6$
3. $(R^2 - R_0^2)/R^2 < 0.1 \ \vee \ \left(R^2 - R'^2_0\right)/R^2 < 0.1$
4. $0.85 \leq k \leq 1.15 \ \vee \ 0.85 \leq k' \leq 1.15$

Where:

q^2 is the external cross-validation coefficient.

R^2 is the correlation coefficient between the predicted and observed values.

R_0^2 is the coefficient of determination (predicted vs. observed activities).

R'^2_0 is the coefficient of determination (observed vs. predicted activities).

k is the slope of the regression lines through the origin (predicted vs. observed values).

k' is the slope of the regression lines through the origin (observed vs. predicted values).

The *Y*-randomization or *Y*-scrambling method ensures the robustness and the statistical significance of a QSAR model and is usually performed to eliminate the possibility of chance correlation. In this method, the dependent variable vector is randomly shuffled, and all modeling calculations are repeated using the original independent variable matrix. After several repetitions the derived models are expected to have less significant correlation coefficient values than the ones of the original model, and, if this is the case, the original model is considered reliable. Otherwise, an acceptable predictive model cannot be produced for both modeling methodologies and original data set [10, 18, 21, 22].

The above validation tests are available through KNIME via Enalos+ *Model Acceptability Criteria* and *Y-Randomization* nodes.

2.3.5 Domain Nodes

Even if a model is fully validated and proven robust, it cannot produce reliable predictions for all input data that may be provided [23]. For example, in a toxicology assessment in silico model, the predictions of the model cannot be reliable for all the compounds of the chemical space. Especially within a virtual screening framework, it is very important to indicate whether a prediction can be considered reliable or not. For this purpose, it is necessary that the limits of the domain of applicability of the model are determined. Predictions for only those compounds that fall into this domain may be considered reliable [6].

Two approaches for defining the domain of applicability are included in Enalos+ nodes. First, the domain of applicability can be calculated using similarity measurements based on the Euclidean distance among all training and test compounds. The distance of each test compound to its nearest neighbor in the training set is compared to the predefined applicability domain (APD) threshold (Eq. 2). The prediction is considered unreliable when the distance is higher than the APD [10, 22].

$$\mathrm{APD} = \langle d \rangle + Z\sigma \tag{2}$$

Where:

$<d>$ is the average of all distances included in the subset of distances that are lower than the mean value of all distances.

σ is the standard deviation of all distances included in the subset of distances that are lower than the mean value of all distances.

Z is an empirical cutoff value (usually is chosen equal to 0.5).

Extent of extrapolation is another simple approach to define the applicability of the domain. It is based on the calculation of the leverage h_i for each chemical, where the QSAR model is used to predict its activity:

$$h_i = x_i^T \left(X^T X\right) x_i \tag{3}$$

Where:

x_i is the descriptor-row vector of the query compound.

X is the $k \times n$ matrix containing the k descriptor values for each one of the n training compounds.

A leverage value greater than $3k/n$ is considered large, and it means that the predicted response is the result of a substantial extrapolation of the model and may not be reliable [10, 21].

The KNIME user has the possibility to employ both the above methodologies through two Enalos+ nodes: *Domain APD* enables the user to define the domain of applicability of the model using the method based on the Euclidean distances, and *Domain Leverage* enables the user to define the domain of applicability of the model using the method based on the extent of extrapolation.

2.4 Case Study 3: Using Modeling Enalos + Nodes

This case study deals with the development of a linear quantitative structure-activity relationship (QSAR) model for modeling and predicting the inhibition of CXCR3 receptor.

To achieve this goal, KNIME workflow was built including the necessary Enalos+ nodes in interaction with other existing KNIME nodes.

With the aid of *Excel Reader* (*XLS*) nodes and Enalos+ Modeling nodes, the following workflow was constructed (Fig. 11).

In order to inspect the data and the results, two output ports exist in *MLR* node. The first one extracts a table containing the coefficient of determination (R squared), the constant y-intercept, and the regression coefficients for each independent variable of the multiple linear model. The second exports the experimental and the predicted values of the dependent variable y (Table 4).

Model Acceptability Criteria node exports the quality of fit and predictive ability statistics of a continuous QSAR model (Table 5).

The previous workflow can be extended by adding other Enalos + Modeling nodes:

In order to define the model applicability domains, the user can add *Domain-APD* and *Domain-Leverage* nodes. These two nodes take as input the training test and the test set not including the depended variable.

Υ-Randomization node could also be included. *Υ*-randomization (or *Υ*-scrambling) is a technique, applied to ensure a QSAR model's robustness. This test consists of repeating all the calculations with scrambled values of the response variable of the training set. In this case a *Column Splitter* needs to be connected to the

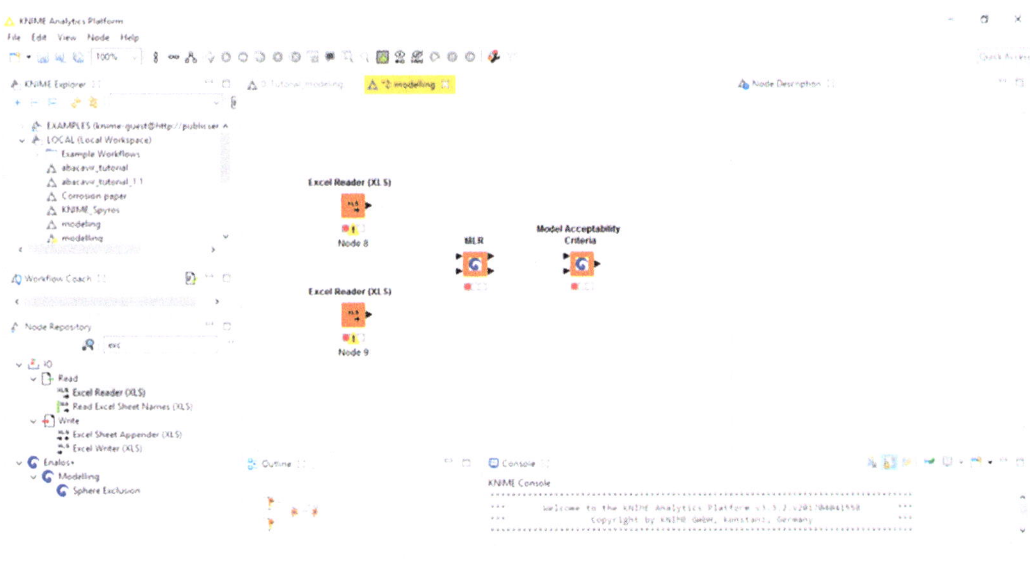

Fig. 11 Basic workflow using modeling Enalos+ nodes

Table 4
MLR results—experimental vs. predictive values

Row ID	Value	Experimental values	Predictive values
R^2	0.748	0.155	0.175
Epsilon	3.991	1.222	0.797
Mdescr1	−2.584	0.194	0.474
Mdescr2	−2.354	0.921	0.729
Mdescr3	−0.009	0.602	0.525
Mdescr4	0.787	1.222	1.259
Mdescr5	0.194	0.051	0.416

Table 5
Model acceptability criteria results

Row ID	Results
R^2	0.748
$R_{cvext}{}^2$	0.721
$R_0{}^2$	0.519
$R'_0{}^2$	0.722
$(R^2 - R_0{}^2)/R^2$	0.306
$(R^2 - R'_0{}^2)/R^2$	0.035
$\|R_0{}^2 - R'_0{}^2\|$	0.203
k	1.053
k'	0.854

output of *Y-Randomization* node in order to include only one randomization per time.

The updated workflow is depicted in Fig. 12.

As already described above, for validation purposes, the experimental data are split in training and test sets using the appropriate algorithms such as Kennard and Stone and sphere exclusion. These algorithms can also be included given that the workflow is modified accordingly.

For example, the *Kennard and Stone* node can be included where the depended variable and the "Model percentage" must be specified. In general, the test set should be about 15–20% of the entire dataset and, i.e., 80% can be selected as a "Model percentage."

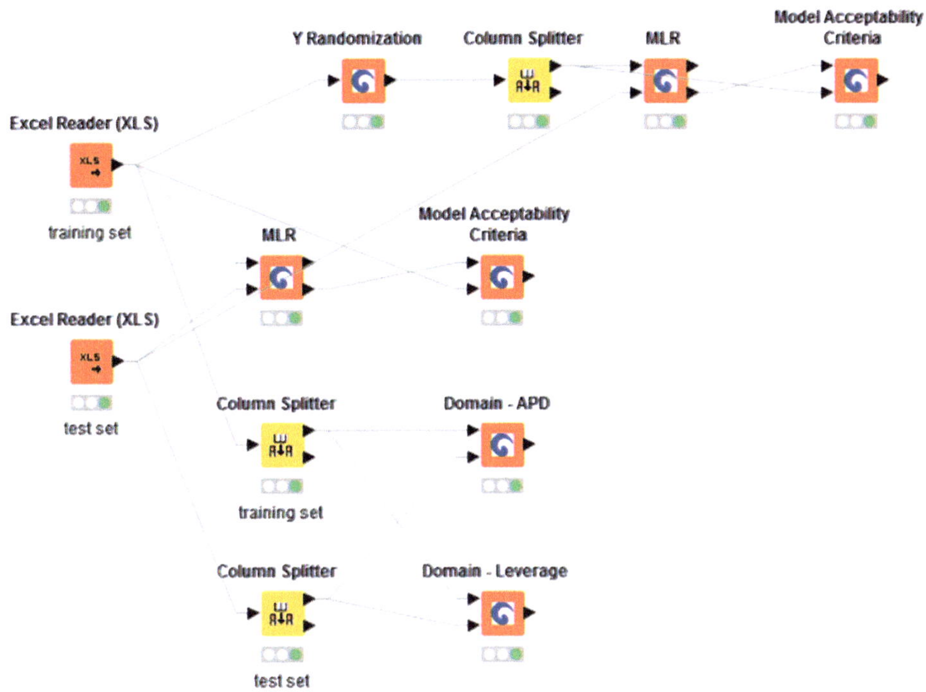

Fig. 12 Updated workflow (2)

Then, *MLR* and *Model Acceptability Criteria* nodes can be added, connected, configured, and executed. Given the aforementioned modifications of the workflow, results of the *MLR* and *Model Acceptability Criteria* nodes are depicted in Table 6 and Fig. 13.

If a different algorithm is selected for data separation, another branch can be constructed, by connecting the *Excel Reader* (*XLS*) output with *sphere exclusion* node instead of *Kennard and Stone* node. This will change the results of the new pipeline as shown below (Table 7 and Fig. 14). The new, converted workflow is depicted in Fig. 15.

2.5 Databases Nodes

Research in cheminformatics is mainly based in the availability of large collections of data that permit the extraction of useful conclusions from their statistical analysis. Data are necessary for the development of predictive models that eliminate the time and resources spent on experiments. To exploit data available for modeling purposes, direct access and a subsequent refinement and analysis are required. This process may be rather complicated—especially when different analytic and modeling tools and platforms are involved—and data and time may be lost while dealing with compatibility problems.

Database Enalos+ nodes contain *NCI*, *PubChem*, and *UniChem* related nodes that give access to NCI, PubChem, and

Table 6
MLR results—experimental vs. predictive values (Kennard and Stone)

Row ID	Value	Experimental values	Predictive values
R^2	0.797	0.31	0.541
Epsilon	5.24	0.469	0.470
Mdescr1	−3.49	0.292	0.386
Mdescr2	−2.358	1.222	1.081
Mdescr3	−0.01	1.222	0.765
Mdescr4	0.838	0.921	0.745
Mdescr5	0.173		

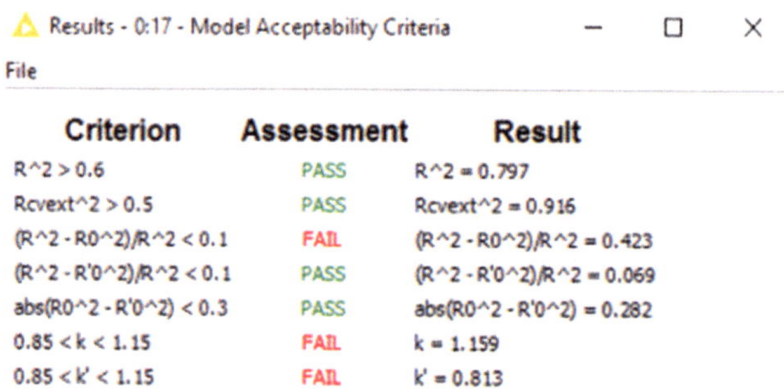

Fig. 13 Model acceptability criteria results (Kennard and Stone)

Table 7
MLR results—experimental vs. predictive values (sphere exclusion)

Row ID	Value	Experimental values	Predictive values
R^2	0.948	0.538	0.312
Epsilon	5.366	0.469	0.271
Mdescr1	−3.44	0.469	0.452
Mdescr2	−2.661	0.155	0.096
Mdescr3	−0.011	1.222	1.278
Mdescr4	0.926		
Mdescr5	0.174		

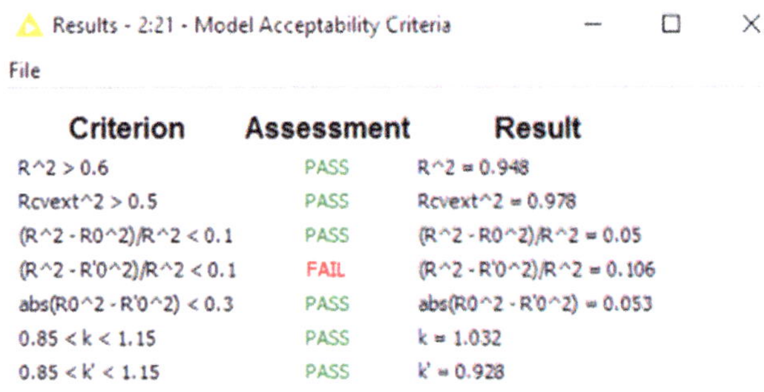
Results - 2:21 - Model Acceptability Criteria

File

Criterion	Assessment	Result
R^2 > 0.6	PASS	R^2 = 0.948
Rcvext^2 > 0.5	PASS	Rcvext^2 = 0.978
(R^2 - R0^2)/R^2 < 0.1	PASS	(R^2 - R0^2)/R^2 = 0.05
(R^2 - R'0^2)/R^2 < 0.1	FAIL	(R^2 - R'0^2)/R^2 = 0.106
abs(R0^2 - R'0^2) < 0.3	PASS	abs(R0^2 - R'0^2) = 0.053
0.85 < k < 1.15	PASS	k = 1.032
0.85 < k' < 1.15	PASS	k' = 0.928

Fig. 14 Model acceptability criteria results (sphere exclusion)

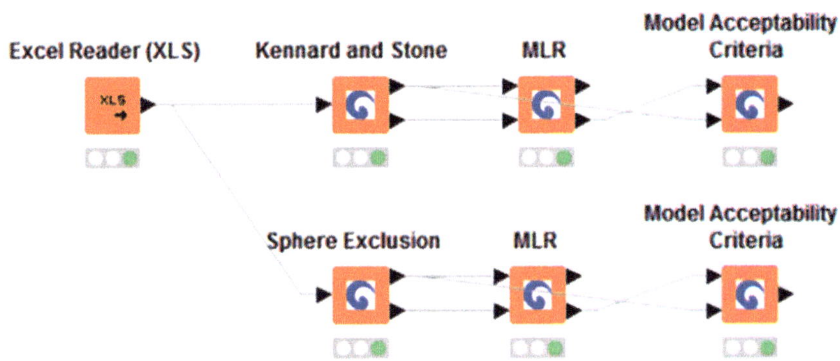

Fig. 15 Converted workflow

UniChem chemical databases. Importing data from databases via KNIME offers a great flexibility as permits their direct analysis and handling and offers fast and automated modeling.

2.5.1 NCI Nodes

The *NCI* group of nodes contains *CIR* node which enables the user to get direct access to CIR (Chemical Identifier Resolver) through KNIME. CIR works as a resolver for different chemical structure identifiers and allows one to convert a given structure identifier into another representation or structure identifier. The user has the option to select several output formats through a GUI menu.

2.5.2 PubChem Nodes

PubChem (https://pubchem.ncbi.nlm.nih.gov) is an open repository for chemical structures and their biological activities, hosted by the US National Institutes of Health (NIH), and it is administered as part of the Molecular Libraries Roadmap Initiative (MLI) [20]. PubChem is currently one of the largest publicly available molecular databases which is still expanding, offering to the researchers' community, at the time of writing, information for more than 93 million compounds. The repository includes data, which are not limited to small molecules, but also includes information for iRNAs, lipids, peptides, carbohydrates, and so on, from different sources including university laboratories, chemical vendors, assay providers, pharmaceutical companies, publishers, etc. [11, 24].

It consists of three main "parts": Bio-Assays, where bioactivity data of compounds or RNAi are stored, and Substances and Compounds that form the chemical-oriented part [25]. Apart from being a well-organized database, PubChem offers the user a series of web tools in order to refine and analyze the stored substances and assays, provides links to patents, and is a resource of secondary databases and web services, contributing in this way to drug discovery process [26].

The *PubChem* Enalos+ nodes contain eight nodes that give direct access to PubChem database through KNIME in order to extract useful information:

- The *Assay* node gives the user access to PubChem database via substance or compound IDs (SID and CID, respectively), to retrieve the Assays where a particular compound is tested. Using this node, the user can download within a KNIME workflow, information about the Assay and the Assay outcome.
- The *Assay Class* node allows PubChem database search according to one or more given AIDs (Bio-Assay identification numbers) and displays only the active or inactive compounds.
- The *Main PubChem* node enables the user to search the PubChem database and obtain information for thousands of compounds with one request. The node exports for each query compound the PubChem CID, the IUPAC name, the InChI, the InChIKey, its molecular formula and molecular weight, the canonical SMILES, and the direct PubChem URL.
- The *Patent* node gives the user straight access to the PubChem database to obtain information about the patent coverage for thousands of compounds with one request.
- The *Patent to Sid* node helps the user to search the PubChem database and obtain the SIDs of the compounds covered by the patents in request.
- The *Sid* node exports the CIDs of a given list of SIDs, searching the PubChem database.

- Via *Similarity* node, the user can search the whole PubChem database for similar compounds (Tanimoto similarity) and obtain the PubChem CID, the molecular formula and weight, and the number of rotatable bonds of the similar compounds to the query compound.
- The *Vendor* node enables the user to search the PubChem database and obtain information about the commercial availability for thousands of compounds.

2.5.3 UniChem Nodes

UniChem is a very simple, large-scale nonredundant database of pointers between chemical structures and EMBL (European Molecular Biology Laboratory)-EBI (European Bioinformatics Institute) chemistry resources. The advantage of UniChem is that it implements an easily scalable and maintainable system of chemical structure integration within the EBI-Search infrastructure, allowing future new chemistry resources within the EBI to be included with minimal effort. Interestingly, centralized mapping for external resources such as PubChem, ZINC, etc. is also straightforward and economical and provides a wider cross-referencing service. The recent exposure of UniChem externally to EMBL-EBI provides these same mapping benefits to resources outside of EMBL.

The *UniChem* group of Enalos+ nodes contains two nodes for accessing UniChem databases:

- The *UniChem* node gives the user direct access to UniChem databases through KNIME. UniChem is a "superset" of all 27 available databases, separated in five friendly and easily recognizable categories.
- The *UniChem Connectivity* is an expanded version of the standard UniChem tool that allows the user to find related molecules. Connectivity Search allows molecules to be first matched on the basis of complete identity between the connectivity layer of their corresponding Standard InChIs and the remaining layers and then compared to highlight stereochemical and isotopic differences.

2.6 Case Study 4: Using Databases Enalos+ Nodes

This case study demonstrates the process of building a KNIME workflow, using the Databases Enalos+ nodes. This case study deals with the chemical compound abacavir, which is a medication used to prevent and treat HIV/AIDS.

At first a *Table Creator* node is required in order to enter the name of the chemical compound in interest (abacavir). Then *Main PubChem*, *Similarity*, *Assay*, *Patent*, and *Vendor* nodes are connected (Fig. 16) to complete a basic simple workflow.

Main PubChem helps the user to search the PubChem database and obtain useful information for thousands of compounds such as

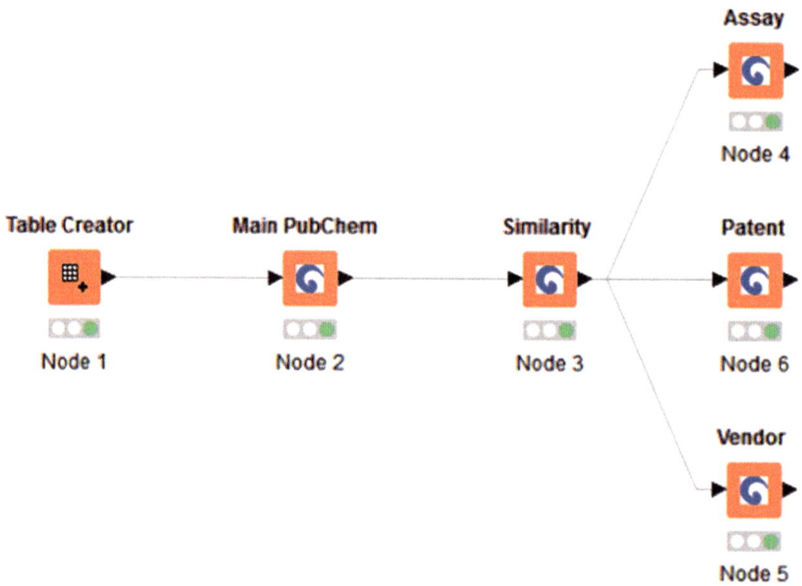

Fig. 16 Basic workflow using databases Enalos+ nodes

PubChem CID (Compound ID), IUPAC name, InChI, InChIKey, molecular formula, molecular weight, canonical SMILES, and the direct PubChem URL. Via *Similarity* node, the user can search the whole PubChem database for similar compounds. Consequently, *Assay* node gives the user the chance to find the Assays where a particular compound (abacavir) is tested. *Patent* node gives the user straight access to the PubChem database in order to obtain information about the patent coverage for a compound of interest. *Vendor* node enables the user to obtain information about the commercial availability of the compound.

The previous workflow can be extended by adding other NCI, PubChem, and UniChem nodes. The user can connect the *Main PubChem*'s output with *CIR*, *UniChem*, and *UniChem Connectivity* nodes. *CIR* node enables the user to get direct access to CIR (Chemical Identifier Resolver) and select several output formats through a GUI menu. *UniChem* and *UniChem Connectivity* nodes give the user access to UniChem databases through KNIME. UniChem is a superset of all 27 available databases, separated in five friendly and easily recognizable categories.

Other Enalos+ nodes can also be included:

Remove Duplicates node removes the rows of the input table that contain the same values in selected columns. In this case the CID column can be selected in the configuring menu. *Assay Class* nodes (active and inactive) display both active and inactive compounds. In *Patent to Sid* node, the user gives the Patent's ID as input, in order to obtain compounds' SIDs that are covered by the

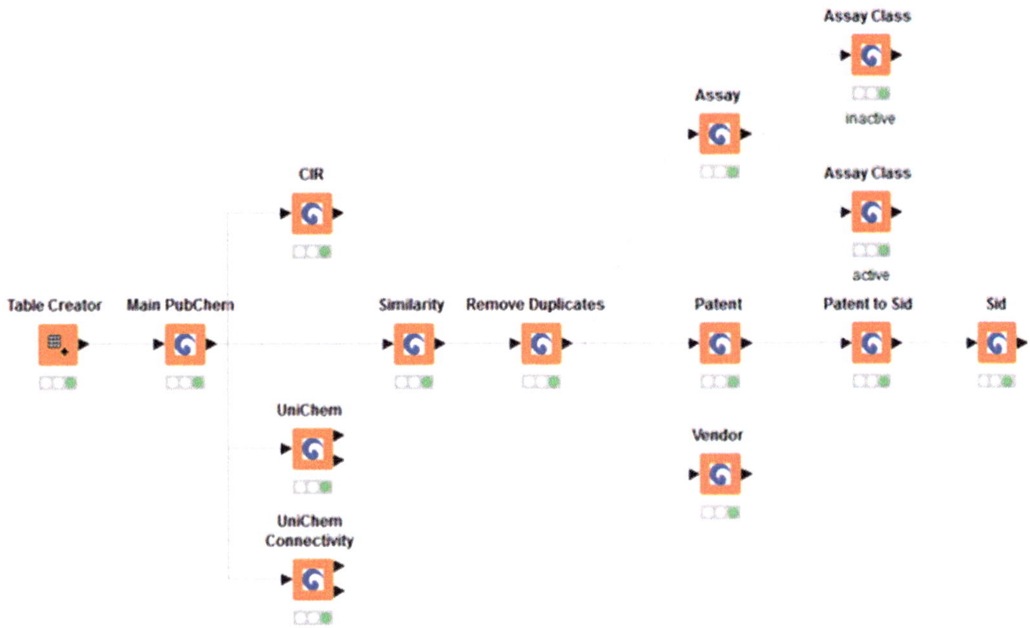

Fig. 17 Extended version of the main workflow

patents in request. The *Sid* node exports the CIDs and synonyms of a given list of SIDs, searching the PubChem database (Fig. 17).

In order to control easily the data flow, the user can add *Column Splitter* and *Row Splitter* nodes. The *Column Splitter* has to be connected to the output of *Remove Duplicates*, *Assay*, *Patent*, and *Patent to Sid* nodes. For the top partition, only one column can be selected and all the other columns for the bottom partition. The top partition column will be used as input to the following nodes. For example, CS4 top partition ("SID") is used as *SID* node input. The user can also connect *Row Splitter* to the output of *Assay* and *Patent* nodes, in order to export a data table with less rows meeting the specified criteria. The converted workflow, using the *Column Splitter* and *Row Splitter* nodes, is depicted in Fig. 18.

Concerning the results of the new added Enalos+ nodes, *CIR* node exports a table with all pre-requested representations. *UniChem* and *UniChem Connectivity* nodes output the InChiKeys that were found in the preselected UniChem databases and the InChiKeys that were not found in these databases. *Assay Class* nodes export a table with information from PubChem about PubChem SIDs (Substance IDs) of compounds that are active or inactive. *Patent to Sid* extracts a table with information from PubChem about PubChem SIDs of compounds that are covered by the patents in request. In case that no compounds are found under a patent, the number −1 is assigned as SID of this patent. Finally, *Sid* outputs information from PubChem about CIDs and synonyms.

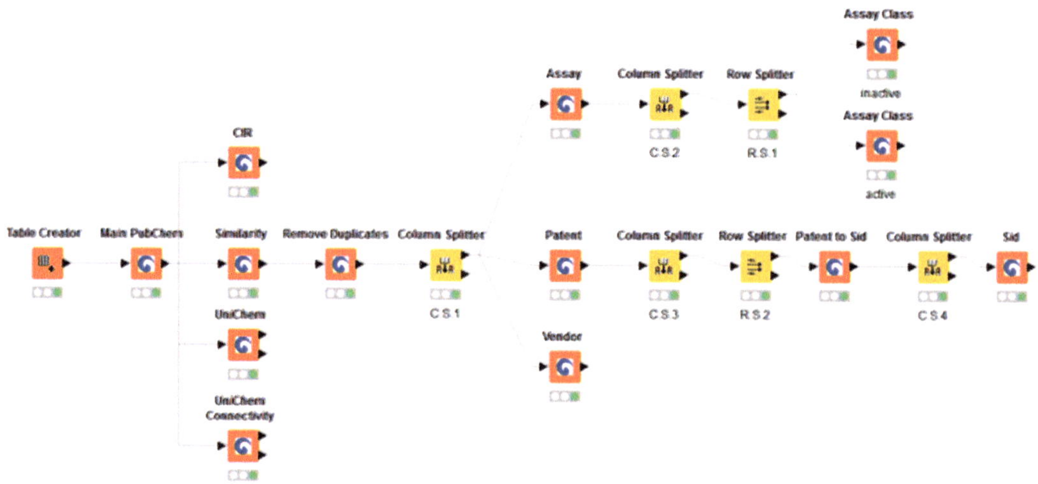

Fig. 18 Final version of the workflow

3 Conclusions

Real-world research seldom involves a single question being answered by means of a single operation, and the fields of molecular modeling, cheminformatics, and nanoinformatics are no exception. While researchers can create custom scripts to automate common procedures, this solution is less than ideal when projects demand rapid workflow prototyping, interactive data analysis, and robust, appropriately validated models.

Enalos+ nodes within the open-source KNIME interface are specifically useful in the field of molecular modeling and data mining and manipulation and offer several unique advantages. The Molecular Descriptors Enalos+ node offers new features in transforming the structural information of the molecules into mathematical representations that can be used as inputs to the cheminformatics tools. These representations are useful in data mining, diversity analysis, virtual screening, modeling, etc. Enalos + nodes also offer new innovative tools that give straight access to multiple chemical databases for data mining and manipulation. Database Enalos+ nodes contain NCI, PubChem, and UniChem groups of nodes that give access to NCI, PubChem, and UniChem chemical databases. Importing data from databases via KNIME permits their direct analysis and handling within KNIME interface and offers a great support to the fast and automated modeling. The Enalos+ Modeling group contains nodes specified for data handling and preprocessing, testing the robustness of modeling and the accuracy of predictions.

In conclusion, the new Enalos+ nodes, developed by Nova-Mechanics Ltd. [8], are a very useful aid in the field of cheminformatics, bioinformatics, and nanoinformatics as they significantly increase the number of the available KNIME nodes that allow data handling and analysis, fill the gaps, and bridge different and innovative cheminformatics and modeling tools upon the KNIME interface.

References

1. Todeschini R, Consonni V (eds) (2010) Molecular descriptors for chemoinformatics, vol 2. Wiley, Weinheim, pp 1–252
2. Leonis G et al (2016) Open source chemoinformatics software including KNIME analytics. In: Leszczynski J (ed) Handbook of computational chemistry. Springer, New York, pp 1–48
3. Willett P (2002) Chemistry plans a structural overhaul the rising tide of data being generated by high-throughput. Nature 419:4–7. https://doi.org/10.1038/nj6903-04a
4. Leach AR, Gillet VJ (2007) An introduction to chemoinformatics. Revised Ed. Springer, New York; 260 p
5. Hong H, Xie Q, Ge W et al (2008) Mold2, molecular descriptors from 2D structures for chemoinformatics and toxicoinformatics. J Chem Inf Model 48(7):1337–1344. https://doi.org/10.1021/ci800038f
6. Tropsha A (2010) Best practices for QSAR model development, validation, and exploitation. Mol Inform 29(6–7):476–488. https://doi.org/10.1002/minf.201000061
7. Melagraki G, Afantitis A (2016) Editorial: towards open access for cheminformatics. Comb Chem High Throughput Screen 19 (4):260–261. https://doi.org/10.2174/138620731904160413183904
8. http://enalosplus.novamechanics.com/
9. Fillbrunn A, Dietz C, Pfeuffer J et al (2017) KNIME for reproducible cross-domain analysis of life science data. J Biotechnol 261:149–156. https://doi.org/10.1016/j.jbiotec.2017.07.028
10. Melagraki G, Afantitis A (2013) Enalos KNIME nodes: exploring corrosion inhibition of steel in acidic medium. Chemom Intell Lab Syst 123:9–14. https://doi.org/10.1016/j.chemolab.2013.02.003
11. Melagraki G, Afantitis A (2015) A risk assessment tool for the virtual screening of metal oxide nanoparticles through enalos insiliconano platform. Curr Top Med Chem 15 (18):1827–1836. https://doi.org/10.2174/1568026615666150506144536
12. Ojha PK, Roy K (2016) Development of a robust and validated 2D-QSPR model for sweetness potency of diverse functional organic molecules. Food Chem Toxicol. https://doi.org/10.1016/j.fct.2017.03.043
13. Melagraki G, Ntougkos E, Rinotas V et al (2017) Cheminformatics-aided discovery of small-molecule protein-protein interaction (PPI) dual inhibitors of tumor necrosis factor (TNF) and receptor activator of NF-κB ligand (RANKL). PLoS Comput Biol 13(4): e1005372. https://doi.org/10.1371/journal.pcbi.1005372
14. Daszykowski M, Walczak B, Massart DL (2002) Representative subset selection. Anal Chim Acta 468(1):91–103. https://doi.org/10.1016/S0003-2670(02)00651-7
15. Hudson BD, Hyde RM, Rahr E et al (1996) Parameter based methods for compound selection from chemical databases. Quant Struct Relationships 15(4):285–289. https://doi.org/10.1002/qsar.19960150402
16. Melagraki G, Afantitis A, Makridima K et al (2006) Prediction of toxicity using a novel RBF neural network training methodology. J Mol Model 12(3):297–305. https://doi.org/10.1007/s00894-005-0032-8
17. Kennard RW, Stone LA (1969) Computer aided design of experiments. Am Soc Qual 3 (2):167–190. https://doi.org/10.2307/1266770
18. Tropsha A, Gramatica P, Gombar V (2003) The importance of being earnest: validation is the absolute essential for successful application and interpretation of QSPR models. QSAR Comb Sci 22(1):69–77. https://doi.org/10.1002/qsar.200390007
19. Golbraikh A, Tropsha A (2002) Beware of q^2! J Mol Graph Model 20(4):269–276. https://doi.org/10.1016/S1093-3263(01)00123-1
20. Golbraikh A, Tropsha A (2000) Predictive QSAR modeling based on diversity sampling of experimental datasets for the training and test set selection. Mol Divers 5(4):231–243. https://doi.org/10.1023/A:1021372108686
21. Afantitis A, Melagraki G, Sarimveis H et al (2009) A novel QSAR model for predicting the inhibition of CXCR3 receptor by 4-N-aryl-[1,4] diazepane ureas. Eur J Med Chem

44(2):877–884. https://doi.org/10.1016/j.ejmech.2008.05.028

22. Melagraki G, Afantitis A (2014) Enalos InSilicoNano platform: an online decision support tool for the design and virtual screening of nanoparticles. RSC Adv 4(92):50713–50725. https://doi.org/10.1039/C4RA07756C
23. Schrey AK, Nickel-Seeber J, Drwal MN et al (2017) Computational prediction of immune cell cytotoxicity. Food Chem Toxicol 107:150–166. https://doi.org/10.1016/j.fct.2017.05.041
24. Chen B, Wild DJ (2010) PubChem BioAssays as a data source for predictive models. J Mol Graph Model 28(5):420–426. https://doi.org/10.1016/j.jmgm.2009.10.001
25. Kim S, Thiessen PA, Bolton EE et al (2016) PubChem substance and compound databases. Nucleic Acids Res 44(D1):D1202–D1213. https://doi.org/10.1093/nar/gkv951
26. Cheng T, Pan Y, Hao M et al (2014) PubChem applications in drug discovery: a bibliometric analysis. Drug Discov Today 19(11):1751–1756. https://doi.org/10.1016/j.drudis.2014.08.008

Chapter 8

Bioguided Design of Trypanosomicidal Compounds: A Successful Strategy in Drug Discovery

Guzmán Ignacio Álvarez Touron

Abstract

Drug development is a long and expensive process that takes about 15 years and is mostly carried out by the pharmaceutical industry. In the case of the diseases produced by trypanosomatids, this development is poorly performed by the pharmaceutical industry. As a result the academia is the one that take a leading role with the drug development process. More effective and economic methodologies to obtain safe compounds and with strong trypanosomicidal activity are urgently needed. In this work, a series of methods are described to obtain bioactive molecules with antiparasitic activity and good pharmacological profiles.

Key words Targeted and phenotypic screening, Toxicology, Oral formulations, Preclinical studies, Trypanosomiasis, Bioguided design

1 Introduction

Trypanosomatidae parasites, transmitted by blood-feeding insects, cause three major groups of human diseases around the world: sleeping sickness caused by *Trypanosoma brucei*, Chagas disease caused by *Trypanosoma cruzi*, and Leishmaniasis a group of different diseases caused by *Leishmania spp.* [1]. Chemotherapy remains the only way for the control of all of these diseases, as effective vaccines have yet to be developed [2]. The currently used drugs were all derived empirically, mainly decades ago, and, for the majority, little is known about their modes of action. The search for new drugs continues, albeit at a low level; although the diseases are major, they affect mainly the poor of the world and so are not afforded high priority by pharmaceutical companies [3]. Phylogenetic information suggests that trypanosomatids are relatively early-branching eukaryotic cells. Biochemical pathways present in trypanosomatids but absent from their hosts should, in theory, provide excellent targets for rational drug design. Several of these pathways are common to all of the pathogenic trypanosomatids, so a

Thomas Mavromoustakos and Tahsin F. Kellici (eds.), *Rational Drug Design: Methods and Protocols*, Methods in Molecular Biology, vol. 1824, https://doi.org/10.1007/978-1-4939-8630-9_8,

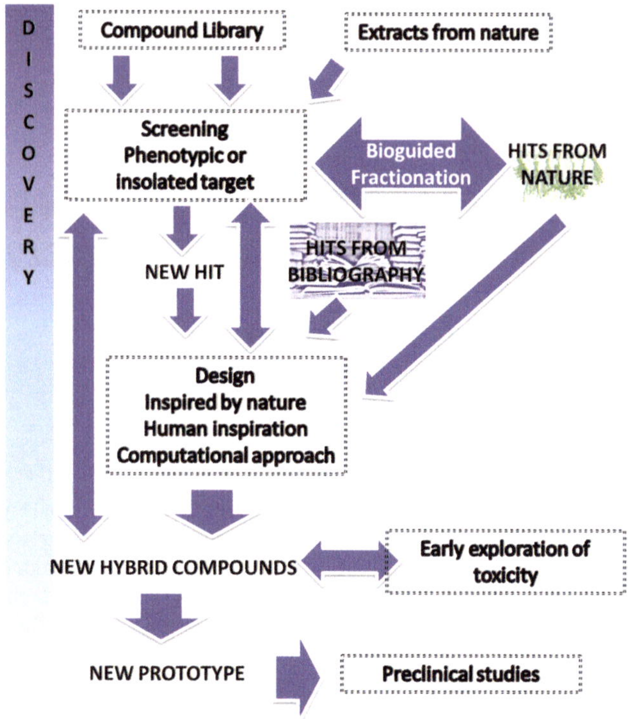

Fig. 1 Workflow to a successfully obtain a novel drug prototype. The discovery process starts with a screening using the parasites in culture or an isolated essential protein. The identified Hits could be used to redesign new molecules combining another pharmacophore previously reported in bibliography. Three approaches could be used to redesign new molecules: inspired by nature, when the pharmacophore is from a natural resource; human inspiration, when the organic chemist uses his imagination to design the new molecules; and computational approach, when the computational model guides the structural modification to obtain theoretically better activities with the studied target. The new compounds obtained are assayed again with the parasites or the target to find the new Hit. In a bioguided design process, you can repeat this process several times to obtain better molecules. With the active molecules, explore in one in vitro model the toxicity and choose the drug prototype [5]

broad-spectrum of clinically useful drugs against all three diseases is theoretically possible [4].

In this section we describe easy workflow to successfully obtain bioactive molecules with trypanosomicidal activity. We divide the process in two steps, the discovery of the bioactive molecule (*see* Fig. 1) and the preclinical studies (*see* Fig. 2). The most important consideration in this process is the bioguided design and the early exploration of the toxicity. In the bioguided design process, a reevaluation of a reduced group of new molecules from the first design is crucial. With the structural activity relationship information of the first group of molecules, a new round of synthesis is

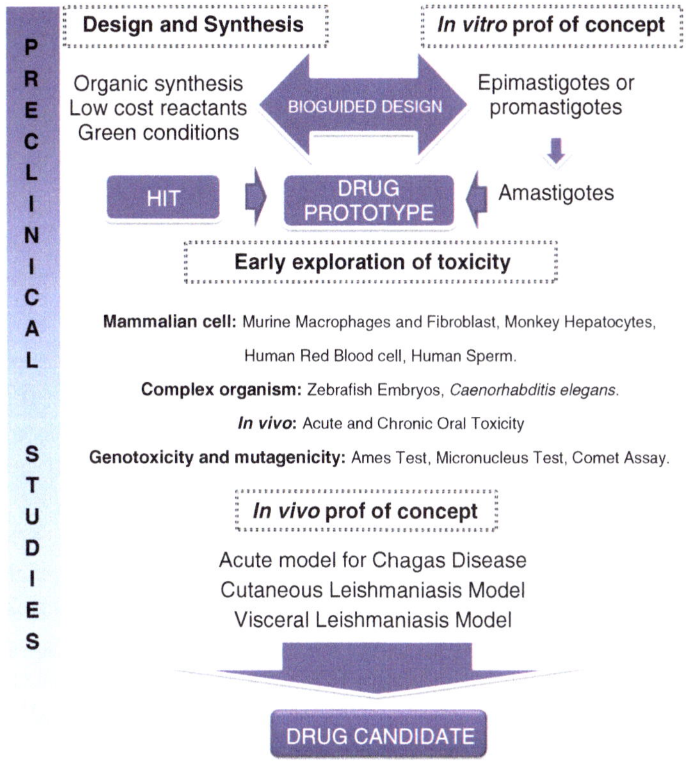

Fig. 2 Workflow to successfully obtain a novel drug candidate. When a series of Hits are identified, it is time to start the preclinical studies. In the case of the neglected diseases is good to tend to use of low cost reactions and green chemistry beginnings. A high-cost drug will be not useful for the affected people. In the in vitro toxicology, we expect more than 10 times activity compared with the parasites. In complex models, it is good to see another type of toxicity like cardiotoxicity. In the in vivo toxicology, we define the therapeutic window for the in vivo proof of concept. Also at this time of development, it is recommended to explore pharmacokinetic and pharmacodynamics aspects

performed and again the in vitro evaluation on the parasites. This iterative process yields better molecules with robust biological activities and good pharmacological profiles.

An early look at the toxicology aspect of the new molecules could be useful to decide better structural modifications. It is generally recognized that early evaluation of new drug candidates is necessary to improve the process. Building in vitro datasets that can accurately predict adverse effects in vivo would allow compounds with high-risk profiles to be deprioritized, while those that possess the requisite drug attributes and a lower-risk profile are brought forward. In vitro cytotoxicity assays have been used for decades as a tool to understand hypotheses-driven questions regarding mechanisms of toxicity [6].

2 Materials

2.1 Isolated Target Screening in Triosephosphate Isomerase

1. Lysis-equilibration-wash buffer (LEW buffer, 1 L): Mix this entire component in 800 mL of pure water: 50 mM NaH_2PO_4 weigh 7.8 g $NaH_2PO_4 \times 2H_2O$ (MW = 156.01 g/mol) and 300 mM NaCl weigh 17.5 g NaCl (MW = 58.44 g/mol). Adjust pH to 8.0 using NaOH. Add enough water to get a final volume of 1 L of solution.
2. Elution buffer (1 L): Mix this entire component in 800 mL of pure water: 50 mM NaH_2PO_4 weigh 7.8 g $NaH_2PO_4 \times 2H_2O$ (MW = 156.01 g/mol), 300 mM NaCl weigh 17.5 g NaCl (MW = 58.44 g/mol), and 250 mM imidazole weigh 17.0 g imidazole (MW = 68.08 g/mol). Adjust pH to 8.0 using NaOH. Add enough water to get a final volume of 1 L of solution.
3. Preparation of a solution of DL-glyceraldehyde-3-phosphate (*see* **Note 1**). A package of specially washed DowexÒ 50 × 4-200R resin is included with this product for preparing the solution.
   - (a) Suspend 1.5 g (wet weight) of Dowex-50 hydrogen form (product code 50 × 4200R) in 6.0 mL of water in a PyrexÒ test tube.
   - (b) Add 100 mg of *DL*-glyceraldehyde-3-phosphate, diethyl acetal, and monobarium salt to the test tube.
   - (c) Place the test tube into a boiling water bath for 3 min and shake intermittently.
   - (d) Quickly chill the solution by transferring the test tube to an ice bath.
   - (e) Centrifuge, decant the solution, and save the supernatant.
   - (f) Resuspend the resin in approximately 2 mL of water, centrifuge again, and decant. Resuspend the resin in approximately 2 mL of water, centrifuge again, and decant. Combine the supernatants from **steps e** and **f**.
   - (g) Repeat the resin washing (in **step f**) several times with water for complete extraction of the free DL-glyceraldehyde-3-phosphate into the supernatant fluid. If hydrolysis and washing are substantially complete, the combined supernatants will contain ~200 mmoles of *DL*-glyceraldehyde-3-phosphate (100 mmoles of the enzymatically active *D*-isomer). The pH of the solution will be approximately 2.4. Based upon enzymatic assay, this solution appears to be stable at 25 °C for at least 4 days. Freezing is recommended for prolonged storage.

2.2 Antiparasitic Test In Vitro

2.2.1 In Promastigotes of Leishmania spp.

1. A culture of promastigotes of *L. braziliensis* (MHOM/BR/75/M2904) and *L. infantum* (MHOM/FR/91/LEM2259V).
2. Schneider's Drosophila medium: (a) Suspend 26.2 mg in 900 mL tissue culture grade water with constant, gentle stirring. Material will not go completely in the solution. Do not heat the water. (b) Add 0.4 g of $NaHCO_3$ powder or 5.3 mL of 7.5% $NaHCO_3$ solution for each liter of the final volume of the medium being prepared. Stir until dissolved. (c) Adjust the pH to 9.2 ± 0.2 with 1 N NaOH with constant stirring. Solution may become turbid. (d) Adjust the pH to 6.7 ± 0.2 with 1 NaCl, with constant stirring. Solution will become clear. (e) Add 0.6 g of anhydrous CaCl per liter of the medium. Prepare a solution by dissolving 0.6 g of anhydrous CaCl in 50 mL of tissue culture grade water. Add the solution slowly with constant stirring to avoid precipitate formation.
3. Solution of resazurin: Resazurin sodium salt was obtained from Sigma-Aldrich (St. Louis, MO, USA) and stored at 4 °C protected from light. Resazurin sodium salt 1.25 mg/mL in sterile phosphate buffer saline (137 mM NaCl, 2.7 mM KCl, 10 mM Na_2HPO_4, 1.76 mM KH_2PO_4, pH 7.6).
4. Preparation of phosphate buffer saline: Dissolve 1.44 g of Na_2HPO_4 anhydrous, 0.24 g of KH_2PO_4 anhydrous, 8 g of NaCl, and 0.2 g of KCl in 800 mL of pure water. Adjust the pH to 7.6 ± 0.2 with 1 N NaOH, with constant stirring and go to 1 L of final volume.

2.2.2 In Epimastigotes of Trypanosoma cruzi

1. *Trypanosoma cruzi* strains, epimastigotes Tulahuen 2 and Y.
2. BHI-tryptose: For 1 L of culture medium, dissolve 33 g of brain-heart infusion, 3 g of tryptose, 6.2 g of NaCl (106 mM), 5 g of $H_2K_2PO_4$ (29 mM), and 4 g of HK_2PO_4 (23 mM), and sterilize for 20 min in autoclave.
3. Dissolve 0.02 g/L hemin, 0.3 g/L D-(+)-glucose, 200,000 units/L penicillin, and 0.2 g/L streptomycin, and sterilize by 22 μ filter.
4. Add the solution in 3 to the solution in 2, adjust the pH to 7·2 ± 0.2 with constant stirring, and go to 1 L of final volume.

2.2.3 In Amastigotes of Trypanosoma cruzi

1. A culture in monolayer of Vero cell (3×10^5 cells/mL in RPMI 1640 milieu +10% FCS) on 8-well cell culture slides.
2. Giemsa-stained slides: (a) Fix slides in methanol 5–7 min. (b) Leave to dry on air. (c) Dilute Giemsa stain 1:20 with deionized water. Color can be varied by diluting in buffer. (d) Stain film for 15–60 min. Rinse in deionized water. (e) Air-dry and evaluate.

2.3 Cytotoxicity Test In Vitro

2.3.1 In Monkey Hepatic Cell

1. Ninety-six-well plates with a monolayer culture of 5×10^5 of Vero cell per well in DMEM.
2. MTT (3-(4,5-dimethylthiazol-2-yl)-2,5-diphenyltetrazolium bromide): Prepare a 12 mM MTT stock solution by adding (a) 1 mL of sterile PBS to 5 mg of MTT (Component A). (b) Mix by vortexing or sonication until dissolved. Occasionally there may be some particulate material that will not dissolve; this can be removed by filtration or centrifugation.
3. Using 10 μL of the stock solution per well. Once prepared, the MTT solution can be stored for 4 weeks at 4 °C protected from light.
4. Add 10 mL of 0.01 M HCl to one tube containing 1 mg of SDS (Component B). Mix the solution gently by inversion or sonication until the SDS dissolves. Once prepared, the solution should be used promptly.
5. Each tube makes sufficient solution for 100 tests, using 100 μL per well.

2.3.2 Cytotoxicity Tests In Vitro In Murine Macrophages

1. A culture of J774.1 murine macrophage cells (ATCC, USA) in a 96-well plate (5.00×10^4 cells in 200 μL culture medium)
2. Use the same solution than in Subheading 2.4.2. to 2.4.5.

2.3.3 In Murine Fibroblast

1. Use the same solution than in solution of resazurin: Subheading 2.4.2 to 2.4.5.

2.3.4 In Human Red Blood Cell

1. Human blood from National Blood Bank. Usually is descanted blood, not useful for transfusion.
2. Carefully made PBS for 1 L of 1× PBS is prepared as follows: Start with 800 mL of distilled water. Dissolve 8 g of NaCl, 0.2 g of KCl, 1.44 g of Na_2HPO_4, and 0.24 g of KH_2PO_4. Adjust the pH to 7.4 with HCl.
3. Add distilled water to a total volume of 1 L. Dispense the solution into aliquots and sterilize by autoclaving (20 min, 121 °C, liquid cycle). Store at room temperature.

2.3.5 In Human Sperm

1. Semen samples were obtained from a healthy fertile volunteer man and kept frozen in 0.5 mL straws (extended in Andromed, Minitube, Germany) under liquid nitrogen until use.
2. Use the same solution of PBS than in Subheading 2.5.2, **item 2**.

2.4 Zebrafish Embryo Toxicity Test to Lipophilic Drugs

1. Fish maintenance and embryo production: Zebrafish lines were kept under controlled conditions, in an automated ZebTec (Tecniplast, Milan, Italy) stand-alone system at 28 °C, 500 μS/cm² conductivity, pH 7.5, and fed with dry and live food (*Artemia salina*) three times a day, following accepted

protocols and under the approval of the local and national ethical committees.

2. The SAT (Sanger AB Tübingen) wild-type line used for most experiments was obtained from Zebrafish International Resource Center (http://zebrafish.org) (Eugene, OR, USA).
3. Embryos obtained from natural crossings were cultured at 28.5 °C in system water and methylene blue (1 ppm) as a fungistatic. 1-Phenyl-2-thiourea (PTU, 0.003%) was added to system water to inhibit melanogenesis in embryos destined for microscopic imaging.

2.5 In Vivo Formulation for Lipophilic Compound

1. The lipophilic compound (Log$P > 3$) was disposed in lipidic suspension, composed of a surfactant (10%), containing Eumulgin HRE 40 (polyoxyl-40 hydrogenated castor oil), sodium oleate, and soya phosphatidylcholine (8:6:3), and an oil phase (10%) containing cholesterol and PBS (pH 7.4) (80%).
2. PBS idem Subheading 2.5.2, **item 2**.

2.6 Acute Oral Toxicity in Mouse

1. Healthy adult male B6D2F1 mice (30 days old, 25–30 g) were used in this study. The initial number of mice is eight (for one compound, could be more if the compound is toxic at the initial test dose).
2. Keep the animals in chambers on a controlled condition, with food and water at free demand. The animal was fasted, maintained, and observed for 14 days according to the OECD guidelines.
3. Initial dose of the compound in the lipophilic formulation is at 2000 mg/kg.

2.7 Genotoxicity in Mouse

1. For the in vivo micronucleus test, approximately 3-month-old CD-1 male mice were housed in polycarbonate cages at an ambient temperature of 25 °C and a photoperiod of 12 h throughout the study. Total numbers of animals for assay eight including controls.
2. The study compound at dose of 200 mg/kg of body weight.
3. For the positive control, a solution of cyclophosphamide dissolved in sterile PBS to get 50 mg/kg of body weight per dose.

2.8 Mutagenicity Prediction (AMES Test)

1. Culture of *Salmonella enterica serovar Typhimurium* TA98, TA100, TA102, TA1535, and TA1537 strains in the agar minimum glucose medium-agar solution, 50_Vogel-Bonner E, and 40% glucose solution.
2. Minimum of 50 petri plates for compound tested.
3. The S9 fraction of mouse liver treated with Aroclor, obtained from Moltox, Inc. (Annapolis, MD, USA). Positive controls of

4-nitro-*o*-phenylenediamine (20 μg/plate, in the run without S9 activation) and 2-aminofluorene (10 μg/plate, in the case with S9 activation) for TA98, 4-nitro-o-phenylenediamine (20 μg/plate, in the run without S9 activation) and 2-aminofluorene (10 μg/plate, in the run with S9 activation) for TA100, or sodium azide (2 μg/plate, in the run without S9 activation) and 2-aminoanthracene (2 μg/plate, in the run with S9 activation) for TA102, TA1535, and TA1537.

3 Methods

3.1 Isolated Target Screening in Triosephosphate Isomerase [7, 8]

1. Expression and purification of proteins: *Tc*TIM, *Lm*TIM, and *Hs*TIM were expressed in *Escherichia coli* and purified as described. The pCR I1 vector containing the gene was treated with Ndel and BamHI, and the released gene was ligated to the PET vector (Novagen). Expression of the triosephosphate isomerase was accomplished in *E. coli* cells strain BL23 (DE3) pLysS following the PET system manual instructions (Novagen). Expression was induced in bacterial cultures at A_{600} 0.6 arbitrary units of absorption at 600 nm by adding 0.4 mM isopropyl thio-β-D-galactoside and culturing the cells for an additional 3 h. After this incubation, cells were harvested by centrifugation at 5000 × *g* for 10 min and processed immediately or frozen at -70 °C until used.
2. Protein was purified by nickel affinity chromatography. Briefly, 10 g of frozen cell pellet was resuspended in 10 mL of LEW buffer (50 mM NaH_2PO_4, 300 mM NaCl), pH 8, with lysozyme (Sigma) at a final concentration of 1 mg/mL and anti-protease cocktail 16 (Halt™ Protease Inhibitor Cocktail, Thermo Scientific) and DNase I (Sigma) at a final concentration of 2 U/mL, followed by 1 h on ice. The resuspended pellet was lysed by sonication during 3 × 3 min, using a SONIFIER 250 (Branson). The bacterial lysate was clarified by centrifugation at 10,000 × *g* for 20 min, before the supernatant was filtered through a 0.45 μm membrane. The supernatant was loaded onto a gravity column packed with 2 g of Ni^{2+-} TED resin (Macherey-Nagel) and eluted with LEW buffer containing 50 mM of imidazole after three washes with LEW buffer.
3. After purification, the enzyme was dissolved in 100 mM triethanolamine, 10 mM EDTA, and 1 mM dithiothreitol (pH 8) and precipitated with ammonium sulfate (75% saturation) and stored at 4 °C.
4. Before use, extensive dialysis against 100 mM triethanolamine/10 mM EDTA (pH 7.4) was performed. Protein concentration was determined by absorbance at 280 nm

($\varepsilon = 36{,}440\ M^{-1}\ cm^{-1}$) TcTIM and LmTIM ($\varepsilon = 33{,}460\ M^{-1}\ cm^{-1}$) for HsTIM.

5. Enzymatic activity was determined following the conversion of glyceraldehyde 3-phosphate into dihydroxyacetone phosphate. The decrease in absorbance at 340 nm was followed in a multicell Cary spectrophotometer at 25 °C. The reaction mixture (1 mL, pH 7.4) contained 100 mM triethanolamine, 10 mM EDTA, 0.2 mM NADH, 1 mM glyceraldehyde 3-phosphate, and 0.9 units of α-glycerol phosphate dehydrogenase. The reaction was initiated by the addition of 5 ng/mL of the TcTIM.
6. For the inhibition studies, TcTIM, LmTIM, and HsTIM were incubated at a concentration of 5 mg/mL in a buffer containing 100 mM triethanolamine, 10 mM EDTA, pH 7.4, and 10% of DMSO at 37 °C for 1 h. The mixture also contained the compounds at the indicated concentrations. Compounds were dissolved in DMSO. After 1 h, 10 μL was withdrawn and added to a final volume of 100 μL of the reaction mixture for the activity assay. The inhibition assay was performed in a 96-well microplate in a Varioskan spectrophotometer. None of the molecules tested here affected the activity of α-glycerol phosphate dehydrogenase, the enzyme used for trapping the product. The IC_{50} value was taken as the concentration of drug needed to reduce the enzymatic activity to 50%. The experiments were performed in triplicate.

3.2 Antiparasitic Test In Vitro in Promastigotes of Leishmania spp. [9]

1. The promastigotes were grown at 26 °C in Schneider's Drosophila medium supplemented with 20% FBS in a 25 mL sterile bottles (*see* **Note 2**). Count the number of parasites in a Neubauer chamber. Dispense 2×10^6 parasites/well in 96-well plastic plates in a final volume of 200 μL. Dissolve the compounds in a 100% of dimethyl sulfoxide (DMSO). Dispense different dilutions of the compounds for triplicate (*see* **Note 3**) but leaving the first column of the plate with only parasite with 0.5% DMSO and the last column only with culture media without parasites.
2. After 72 h at 26 °C, 20 μL of a 2 mM resazurin solution is added. Then after 6 h, the oxidation-reduction is quantified at 570 and 600 nm (Varioskan spectrophotometer).
3. The solution of resazurin was prepared at 2.5 mM in a phosphate-buffered solution (PBS), pH 7.4, and filtered through 0.22 μm membranes prior to use. All tests were carried out in triplicate. The efficacy of each compound was estimated by calculating the IC_{50} values. Each antiproliferative experiment was done in duplicate, and each concentration was tested in triplicate.

3.3 Antiparasitic Test In Vitro in Epimastigotes of Trypanosoma cruzi *[10]*

1. For the in vitro anti-*T. cruzi* activity (*see* **Note 2**), we used epimastigotes of the Tulahuen 2 strain (genotype TcVI) grown in an axenic milieu (BHI-tryptose) at 28 °C. Cells from a 5–7-day-old culture were inoculated in fresh culture milieu to give an initial concentration of 1×10^6 cells/mL.
2. Count the number of parasites in a Neubauer chamber and adjust the concentration to dispense 1×10^6 parasites/well in 96-well plastic plates in a final volume of 200 μL. Dissolve the compounds in a 100% of dimethyl sulfoxide (DMSO).
3. Dispense different dilutions of the compounds for triplicate (*see* **Note 3**) but leaving the first column of the plate with only parasite with 0.5% DMSO and the last column only with culture media without parasites.
4. After 72 h at 28 °C, 20 μL of a 2 mM resazurin solution is added. Then after 6 h, the oxidation-reduction is quantified at 570 and 600 nm (Varioskan spectrophotometer).
5. The solution of resazurin was prepared at 2.5 mM in a phosphate-buffered solution (PBS), pH 7.4, and filtered through 0.22-μm membranes prior to use. All tests were carried out in triplicate. The efficacy of each compound was estimated by calculating the IC50 values. Each antiproliferative experiment was done in duplicate, and each concentration was tested in triplicate.

3.4 Antiparasitic Test In Vitro in Amastigotes of Trypanosoma cruzi *[11]*

1. Amastigotes of Sylvio X-10 strain, DTU TcI, was used. Briefly, Vero cells, 3×10^5 cells/mL in RPMI 1640 milieu +10% FCS, were infected with tissue derived trypomastigotes at a ratio of parasites to cells of 10:1 for 24 h (*see* **Note 2**).
2. After 24 h the infected cells were treated twice with serial dilutions of each evaluated compound (*see* **Note 3**) and reference drugs (Nfx and Bnz). The second dose of compound or reference drugs was added 48 h after the first addition. Control cells were maintained without compound, only with 0.5% of DMSO. The incubation times of the drug with the parasites were 72 h.
3. After incubation remove the well to get the slice free, put a drop of menthol onto the cells and leave dry and then a drop of stain solution with Giemsa 1 min, and wash with water.
4. The percentage of infected cells was determined by counting infected and non-infected cells on methanol-fixed and Giemsa-stained slides on 300 cells in a 40× optical microscopy with focus randomly. Each parasite experiment was tested in duplicate and each concentration for triplicate.
5. An image of the resulting material in a 100× optical microscopy is shown in Fig. 3 (showing infected and non-infected cell (black star)). This is the resultant preparation to count the 300 cell.

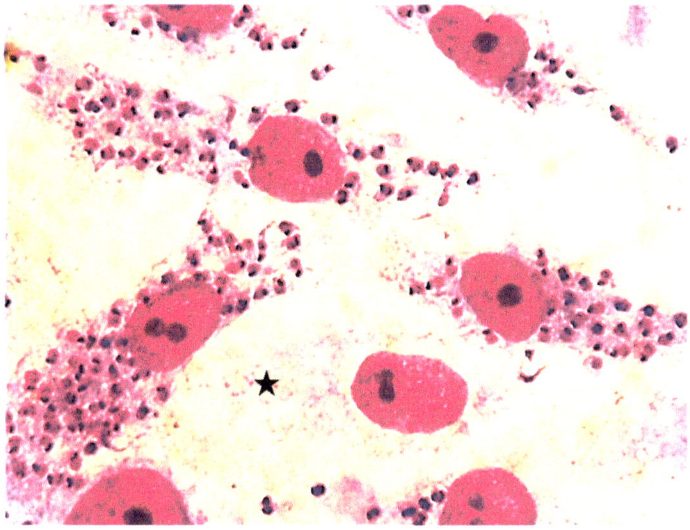

Fig. 3 Figure of the resulting material in a 100× optical microscopy (showing infected and not infected cell (black star). This preparation is used to count the number of cells infected at 40× magnification, but also you can analyze the number of amastigotes in the cell

3.5 Cytotoxicity Test In Vitro in Monkey Hepatic Cell [12]

1. Vero cell lines were cultivated in Dulbecco's modified Eagles medium (DMEM) with 10% FCS in a humid atmosphere of 5% CO_2 at 37 °C (*see* **Note 2**).
2. The cytotoxicity of the compounds was evaluated by MTT reduction assays. Vero cells were seeded in 96-well plates at an initial density of 5×10^3 cells per well. The cells were incubated with increasing concentrations of the compounds (*see* **Note 3**) for 48 h at 37 °C and 5% CO_2.
3. MTT solution (5 mg/mL) was added to the cells, which were further incubated for 4 h. MTT was removed, and 100 μL of DMSO were added for 5 min. The optical density was measured at 570 nm (Microplate Autoreader Varioskan spectrophotometer).
4. Each experiment was performed in triplicate, and experiments were repeated at least two times. The cytotoxicity was expressed as the IC50, which was the concentration of the test substances that inhibited the growth of Vero cells by 50% compared with the growth of the untreated cells.

3.6 Cytotoxicity Test In Vitro in Murine Macrophages [10]

1. J774.1 murine macrophage cells (ATCC, USA) were grown in DMEM culture milieu containing 4 mM L-glutamine and supplemented with 10% FCS (*see* **Note 2**). The cells were seeded in a 96-well plate (5.00×10^4 cells in 200 μL culture medium) and incubated at 37 °C in a 5% CO_2 atmosphere for 48 h, to allow cell adhesion prior to drug testing.

2. Afterwards, cells were exposed for 48 h to the compounds (25–400 μM, *see* **Note 3**) or the vehicle for control (0.4% DMSO), and additional controls (cells in medium) were used in each test. Cell viability was then assessed by measuring the mitochondria-dependent reduction of MTT to formazan.
3. For this purpose, MTT in sterile PBS (0.2% glucose), pH 7.4, was added to the macrophages to achieve a final concentration of 0.1 mg/mL, and the cells were incubated at 37 °C for 3 h. After removing the medium, formazan crystals were dissolved in 180 μL of DMSO and 20 μL of MTT buffer (0.1 M glycine, 0.1 M NaCl, 0.5 mM EDTA, pH 10.5), and the absorbance at 560 nm was measured.
4. The IC_{50} was defined as the drug concentration at which 50% of the cells were viable, relative to the control (no drug added), and was determined by analysis using OriginLab8.5® sigmoidal regression (% of viable cells vs. the logarithm of the compound concentration). Tests were performed in triplicate.

3.7 Cytotoxicity Test In Vitro in Murine Fibroblast [13]

1. NCTC-Clone 929 were grown in minimal essential medium (Sigma) supplemented with 10% heat-inactivated FBS, penicillin G (100 U/mL), and streptomycin (100 μg/mL). Cell cultures were maintained at 37 °C in a humidified 5% CO_2 atmosphere (*see* **Note 2**).
2. The procedure for cell viability measurement was evaluated with resazurin by a colorimetric method.
3. The cells were plated in 96-microtiter plates at 3×10^4 cells/well in 100 μL growth medium. The cells were grown overnight at 37 °C, 5% CO_2.
4. Thereafter, the medium was removed, and the compounds were added to 200 μL of medium for 48 h (*see* **Note 3**), leaving the first column of the plate with only cells with 0.5% DMSO and the last column only with culture media without cells.
5. After incubation, 20 μL of a 2 mM resazurin solution were added to each well. The plates were incubated for 3 h to allow optimal oxidation-reduction. The reduction of resazurin was determined by dual wavelength absorbance measurement at 490 and 595 nm (*see* Fig. 4).
6. The background was subtracted. Each concentration was assayed three times. Medium and drug controls were used in each test as blanks.
7. The IC_{50} was defined as the drug concentration at which 50% of the cells were viable, relative to the control (no drug added), and was determined by analysis using OriginLab8.5® sigmoidal regression (% of viable cells vs. the logarithm of the compound concentration).

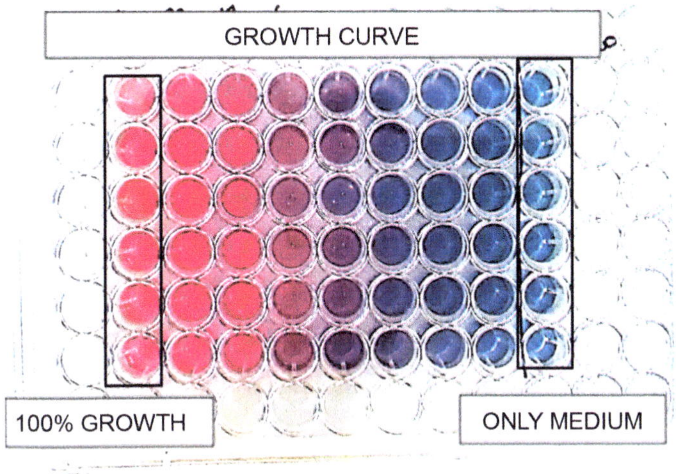

Fig. 4 Cell culture plate. Resazurin assay with different concentration of parasites, you can see the color solution pink (maximum grown) and blue (no grown)

3.8 Cytotoxicity Test In Vitro in Human Red Blood Cell [14]

1. Human blood collected in sodium citrate solution (3.8%) was centrifuged at 200 × *g* for 10 min at 4 °C (*see* **Note 4**). The plasma supernatant was removed, and the erythrocytes were suspended under ice with cold PBS.
2. The cells were again centrifuged at 200 × *g* for 10 min at 4 °C. This procedure was repeated two more times to ensure the removal of any released hemoglobin.
3. Once the supernatant was removed after the last wash, the cells were suspended in PBS to 2% w/v red blood cell solution. A volume of 400 μL of compound to be analyzed (*see* **Note 3**), in PBS (final doses 50, 100, and 200 μM), negative control (solution of PBS), or AmpB (final dose 1.5 μM), was added to the 2% w/v red blood cell solution.
4. Ten replicates for each concentration were done and incubated for 24 h at 37 °C prior to analysis. Complete hemolysis was attained using neat water yielding the 100% control value (positive control).
5. After incubation, the tubes were centrifuged, and the supernatants were transferred to new tubes.
6. The release of hemoglobin into the supernatant was determined spectrophotometrically at 405 nm (Microplate Autoreader Varioskan spectrophotometer), or an ELISA standard rider could be useful (*see* Fig. 5).
7. Results are expressed as percentage of total hemoglobin released in the presence of the compounds. This percentage was calculated using the equation percentage hemolysis (%) = [(A1 − A0)/(A1water)] × 100, where A1 is the

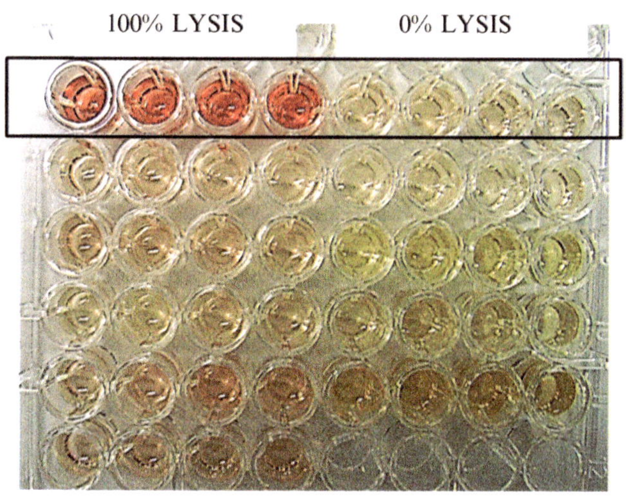

Fig. 5 Red blood cell incubation in 96-well plates. You can see the positive control (toxic effect or lysis) in the red solution, when the hemoglobin is free

absorbance at 405 nm of the test sample at $t = 24$ h, A0 is the absorbance at 405 nm of the test sample at $t = 0$ h, and A1water is the absorbance at 405 nm of the positive control (water) at $t = 24$ h.

8. The experiments were done by quintuplicate. AmpB was used as positive control. The IC50 was defined as the drug concentration at which 50% of the cells were viable, relative to the control (no drug added), and was determined by analysis using OriginLab8.5 sigmoidal regression (% of viable cells vs. the logarithm of the compound concentration).

3.9 Cytotoxicity Test In Vitro in Human Sperm [15]

1. Samples from three different men were thawed, a sperm pool was prepared in PBS at a concentration of 40 million spermatozoa per mL (*see* **Note 4**), and then 50 μL of this sperm suspension was carefully mixed with 50 μL of the studied compound diluted (*see* **Note 3**) to 100, 50, 25, 12.5, and 6.25 μM or with 1% DMSO in control experiments.
2. Each condition was assayed by duplicate in 96-well plates, and controls were assayed by triplicate. Plates were incubated at 37 °C for 1 h with moderate shaking.
3. The motility analysis was carried out using a CASA (Computer Assisted Semen Analyzer) system Androvision (Minitube, Tiefenbach, Germany) with an Olympus BX 41 microscope (Olympus, Japan) equipped with a warm stage at 37 °C.
4. Each sample (10 μL) was placed onto a Makler counting chamber (depth 10 μm, Sefi-Medical Instruments, Israel), and the following parameters were evaluated: percentage of total motile spermatozoa (motility >5 μm/s) and velocity curved line (VCL, >24 μm/s).

5. At least 400 spermatozoa were analyzed from each sample from at least four microscope fields. The IC50 was defined as the drug concentration at which 50% of the cells were viable, relative to the control (no drug added), and was determined by analysis using OriginLab8.5® sigmoidal regression (% of viable cells vs. the logarithm of the compound concentration).

3.10 Zebrafish Embryo Toxicity Test to Lipophilic Drugs [13]

1. For the assay, six hpf embryos were dechorionated in agarose-bottom dishes. Only embryos that were clearly undamaged after 60 min of observation were kept and subsequently used (*see* **Note 5**).
2. Dechorionated embryos were further manipulated using flame-rounded tip glass Pasteur pipettes. Dechorionated embryos (20 per condition) were then transferred to round-bottom 96-well plates (1 embryo/well) for incubation with drugs.
3. In all cases, the embryos were incubated in system water with 1% DMSO (negative control) and the compound at different doses (*see* **Note 3**) between 8 and 72 hpf. The treatment solution was changed daily.
4. As a positive control, we used 2.4 mM caffeine (*see* Fig. 6 shows the characteristic morphology for this treatment), and the negative control was 1% DMSO in system water.
5. The embryos were placed at 28.5 ± 0.5 °C in a 96-well round bottom plate. At selected time points, namely, 24, 48, and 72 hpf, embryotoxicity (mortality) and morphological characteristics of the embryos were evaluated using a Nikon SMZ800 stereomicroscope. The embryos were evaluated for the presence and morphological development (as appropriate) of somites, tail detachment, eyes, heartbeat, and blood circulation. All individuals were evaluated at all-time points.
6. For each group of treatment, we register the mortality to construct the dose response curves. The LD50 was defined as the drug dose at which 50% of the embryos were viable, relative to the control (no drug added), and was determined by analysis using OriginLab8.5® sigmoidal regression (% of viable embryo vs. the logarithm of the compound doses).

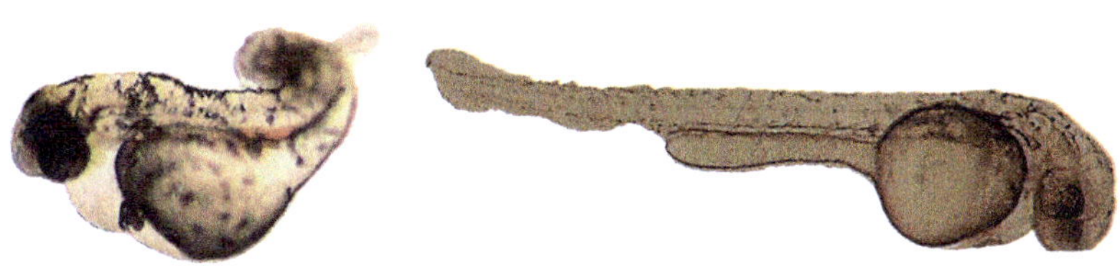

Fig. 6 Figure showing the effect of 2.4 mM of caffeine as a control to validate the assay; the normal stage is shown at the right for 48 hpf

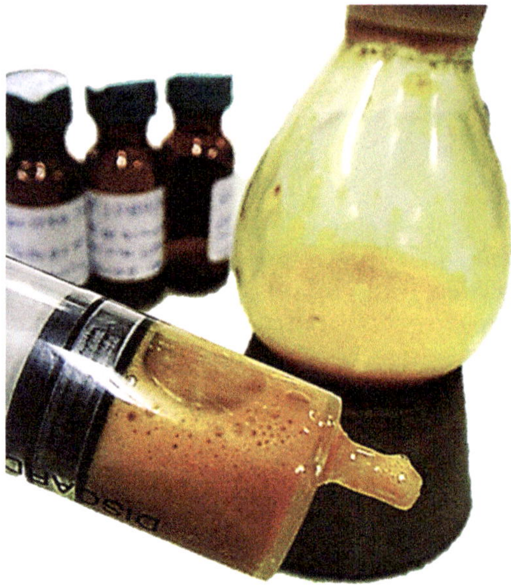

Fig. 7 Appearance of the vehicles for lipophilic or not water-soluble compounds. The solution in the picture is a lipids emulsion (liposomal like solution), when the compound is in the lipid face, the body absorption is enhanced compared with a saline solution vehicle

3.11 In Vivo Formulation for Lipophilic Compound [16]

1. The lipophilic compound (Log$P > 3$) was disposed in lipidic suspension, composed of a surfactant (10%), containing Eumulgin HRE 40 (polyoxyl-40 hydrogenated castor oil), sodium oleate, and soya phosphatidylcholine (8:6:3), and an oil phase (10%) containing cholesterol and phosphate buffer (pH 7.4) (80%).
2. For the preparation of the formulation, the compound, previously pulverized in a mortar, cholesterol, Eumulgin HRE 40, and phosphatidylcholine were dissolved in chloroform, and the solvent was evaporated under vacuum to dryness (executive elimination).
3. In parallel, sodium oleate was dissolved in phosphate buffer and left in an orbital shaker for 12 h at room temperature.
4. The oleate buffer solution was then added to the evaporated residue, and the mixture was homogenized and placed in an ultrasonic bath at full power for 30 min, four times (*see* Fig. 7).

3.12 Acute Oral Toxicity in Mouse [17]

1. Healthy adult male B6D2F1 mice (30 days old, 25–30 g) were used in this study. Initially, the compound in the lipophilic formulation at 2000 mg/kg was administrated by orogastric cannula, to one animal. The animal was fasted, maintained, and observed for 14 days according to the OECD guidelines (TG425 guideline for the up-and-down procedure).

2. If the mice survived for the first 48 h, another animal received the same dose. If this repeated, a third animal was dosed with 2000 mg/kg. When the three animals survive for 14 days the experiment is finish and the animals were euthanized.
3. If some animals die, follow the instruction on the software recommended by OECD. The AOT425 Statistical Program gives the different dosage to the next animal to completed six animals and then get the LD_{50} value.
4. Dosing continues depending on the fixed-time interval (e.g., 48 h) outcomes of all the animals up to that time. The testing stops when one of the following stopping criteria first is met: (a) three consecutive animals survive at the upper bound; (b) five reversals occur in any six consecutive animals tested; and (c) at least four animals have followed the first reversal, and the specified likelihood ratios exceed the critical value.
5. For a wide variety of combinations of LD_{50} and slopes, stopping rule (c) will be satisfied with four to six animals after the test reversal. In some cases for chemicals with shallow-slope dose response curves, additional animals (up to a total of 15 tested) may be needed.
6. The following statistical details may be helpful in implementing the maximum likelihood calculations suggested (with an assumed sigma). All deaths, whether immediate or delayed or humane kills, are incorporated for the purpose of the maximum likelihood analysis. The likelihood function is written as follows: $L = L_1, L_2, \ldots, L_n$,

where L is the likelihood of the experimental outcome, given *mu* and *sigma*, and n is the total number of animals tested.

$L_{i=1}$ - $F(Zi)$ if the ith animal survived, or $L = F(Zi)$ if the ith animal died.

$F =$ cumulative standard normal distribution.

$Z_i = [\log(d_i) - mu]/sigma$.

$d_i =$ dose given to the ith animal, and sigma = standard deviation in log units of dose (which is not the log standard deviation).

7. An estimate of the true LD_{50} is given by the value of mu that maximizes the likelihood L.
8. An estimate of sigma of 0.5 is used unless a better generic or case-specific value is available.
9. In any case when the initial dose of 2000 mg/kg is toxic, follow the instruction given in the software AOT425 Statistical Program.

3.13 Genotoxicity in Mouse [18]

1. For the in vivo micronucleus test, approximately 3-month-old CD-1 male mice were housed in polycarbonate cages at an ambient temperature of 25 °C and a photoperiod of 12 h throughout the study.
2. The compound at doses of 200 mg/kg of body weight and the vehicle were orally administered two times, days 1 and 2, two groups of five mice.
3. Mice were sacrificed 24 h after the last administration, and the bone marrow was prepared for evaluation: before the animals are killed, a 5 mL centrifuge tube is filled with fetal calf serum for each individual.
4. From the freshly killed animal, both femora are removed in toto, which means that one is cutting through pelvis and tibia. The muscle is separated from the bone using tweezers and scalpel. By gentle traction the distal epiphyseal portion is torn off together with the rest of the tibia and the surrounding muscle. The proximal end of the femur is carefully shortened with scissors until a small opening to the marrow canal becomes visible.
5. With the needle of appropriate size mounted, about 0.2 mL serum is pulled from the tube into a disposable plastic syringe. Then the needle is inserted a few mm into the proximal part of the marrow canal which is still closed at the distal end.
6. Next, the femur is submerged completely in the serum and squeezed against the tube to prevent the bone from slipping off the needle. Subsequently, the marrow is aspirated; should the needle have become obstructed, the serum in the syringe is first pressed out. After several gentle aspirations and flushings, the process is repeated from the distal end of the femur. The bone marrow cells should get into the serum as a fine suspension and not in the form of gross particles.
7. The tube is centrifuged at 1000 × *g* for 5 min. The supernatant is removed with a Pasteur pipette. If the sediment is large, half a drop of serum is left; if it is minute, all the supernatant is drawn off.
8. The cells in the sediment are carefully mixed by aspiration into the capillary part of a fresh siliconized Pasteur pipette. A small drop of the viscous suspension is put on the end of a slide and spread by pulling the material behind a polished cover glass held at an angle of 45°. The size of the droplet is chosen so that all material is used up at a distance of 2–3 cm. The preparations are then air-dried.
9. At least two slides of the cell suspension per animal were made. The air-dried slides were stained with Giemsa stain (5% in phosphate buffer, pH 7.4). Slides were then examined at 1000 magnification. Small round or oval bodies, the size of

which ranged from about 1/5 to 1/20 of the diameter of a polychromatic erythrocyte (PCE), were counted as micronuclei. A total of 1000 PCEs were scored per animal by the same observer for determining the frequencies of micronucleated polychromatic erythrocytes (MNPCEs).

10. Cyclophosphamide, 50 mg/kg, administered intraperitoneally (i.p.) 24 h before mouse sacrifice, was used as a positive control. For statistical analysis, the homogeneity of variances of data was tested by the analysis of variance (ANOVA) test (*P* _ 0.05) using Epi Info (3.5.1) software.

3.14 Mutagenicity Prediction (AMES Test) [19, 20]

1. For the mutagenicity assay, the method of direct incubation in the plate was performed. Culture of *Salmonella enterica* serovar Typhimurium TA98, TA100, TA102, TA1535, and TA1537 strains in the agar minimum glucose medium-agar solution, 50_Vogel-Bonner E, and 40% glucose solution were used.
2. First, the direct toxicity of the compounds against the bacteria was assayed. DMSO solutions of the studied compounds at five consecutive dilutions (1/3) were assayed in triplicate. The highest dose without toxic effects was used as the starting one for the Ames test.
3. Prepare melt top agar supplemented with 0.05 mM histidine and biotin, and maintain at 43–48°C.
4. Use 10 × 75 mm sterile glass tubes maintained at 43 °C, add in the following order with mixing, (e.g., vortexing) after each addition: (a) 2 mL of molten top agar, (b) 0.50 mL of metabolic activation (S-9) mix or buffer, (c) 0.05 mL of the test chemical dilution, and (d) 0.05–0.10 mL overnight culture of the *Salmonella* strain (about 1–2 × 10^8 bacteria per tube).
5. The contents of the test tubes are then mixed and poured onto the surface of glucose minimal agar medium-agar plates.
6. When the top agar has hardened (2–3 min), the plates are inverted and placed in a 37 °C incubator for 48 h.
7. The colonies are then counted, and the results are expressed as the number of revertant colonies per plate.
8. The influence of the metabolic activation was tested by adding 500 μL of the S9 fraction of mouse liver treated with Aroclor, obtained from Moltox, Inc. (Annapolis, MD, USA). Positive controls of 4-nitro-*o*-phenylenediamine (20 μg/plate, in the run without S9 activation) and 2-aminofluorene (10 μg/plate, in the case with S9 activation) for TA98, 4-nitro-*o*-phenylenediamine (20 μg/plate, in the run without S9 activation) and 2-aminofluorene (10 μg/plate, in the run with S9 activation) for TA100, or sodium azide (2 μg/plate, in the run without S9 activation) and 2-aminoanthracene (2 μg/plate, in the run with

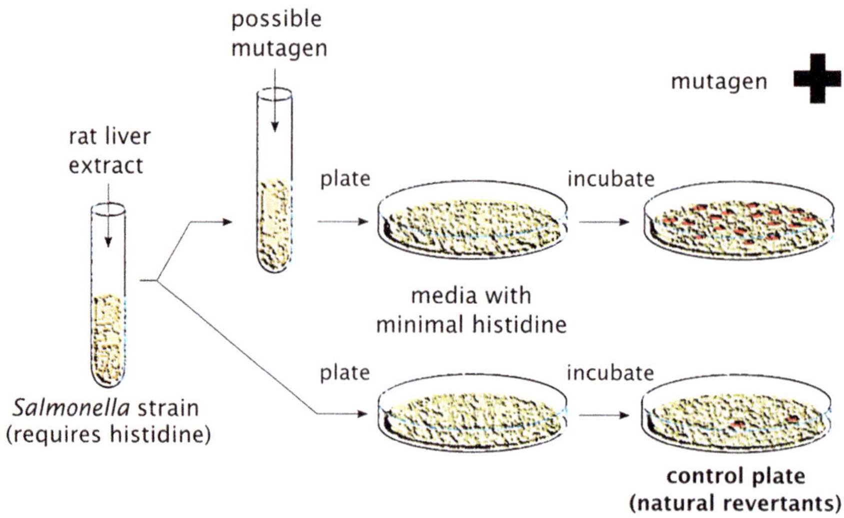

Fig. 8 Ames test schematization: In this case is the S9 proof (hepatic metabolization), there are the tubes with the salmonella culture in agar incubated with the compound and S9. The next step is plateing the culture solution and incubates again for bacteria grown. Finally if the bacteria grown, the result is mutagenic, the compounds or their metabolites are mutagens. The bacteria colonies are in red

S9 activation) for TA102, TA1535, and TA1537 and a negative control of DMSO were run in parallel. The revertant number was counted manually.

9. The sample was considered mutagenic when the number of revertant colonies was at least twice the negative control for at least two consecutive dose levels (*see* Fig. 8).

3.15 In Vivo Anti-T. cruzi Studies (Acute Model) [11, 16]

1. For the acute model of Chagas disease, A statistical numero (usualy 6 to 8 per sample) of BALB/c male mice (30 days old, 25–30 g) bred under specific pathogen-free conditions were infected by intraperitoneal injection with 1×10^3 blood trypomastigotes of the Y strain.
2. The mice were divided into three groups. One group of eight animals was used as a control (treated orally with the vehicle), and two groups of eight animals were treated with compound and Bnz, respectively.
3. Initial parasitemias were counted 5 days post-infection (week 1), and the treatment was begun the following day (sixth day; *see* **Note 6**). Bnz (at 50 mg/kg body weight [BW]/day, for 14 days) or compound (at 50, 100, or 200 mg/kg BW/day, for 14 days) was administered orally.
4. Parasitemias in the control and treated mice were determined once a week after the first administration, for 60 days after beginning of treatment, in tail vein blood.

5. Additionally, the mortality rate was recorded. For IgG antibody detection, all the sera obtained after centrifugation of the blood that were extracted from infected mice were tested twice by enzyme-linked immunosorbent assay (ELISA) at 30 and 60 days after the start of treatment. An in-house ELISA kit (Chagas' disease test; Instituto de Investigaciones en Ciencias de la Salud [IICS], Asunción, Paraguay) was used according to the procedure recommended by the manufacturer (IICS Production Department, Asunción, Paraguay). The optical density values were obtained in an ELISA plate reader (Titerek Unistan I). The Wilcoxon test was used in order to compare the levels of anti-T. cruzi antibodies between experimental groups.
6. Histopathology. At the end of the experiments, samples of the tissues of the heart, skeletal muscle, intestine, and urinary bladder were taken and stored in 10% formaldehyde.
7. Followed by dehydration in alcohol solutions and xylol and embedment in paraffin. Each organ was embedded separately in paraffin and cut in a microtome set at 6 μm.
8. Slides were stained with hematoxylin-eosin and observed under a Zeiss microscope at ×10, ×40, and ×100 magnifications. Photographs were taken at all of these magnifications with an Olympus X-785 digital camera coupled to the microscope (*see* Fig. 9).
9. The experimental protocols with animals were evaluated and supervised by the local ethics committee and the research adhered to the Principles of Laboratory Animal Care.

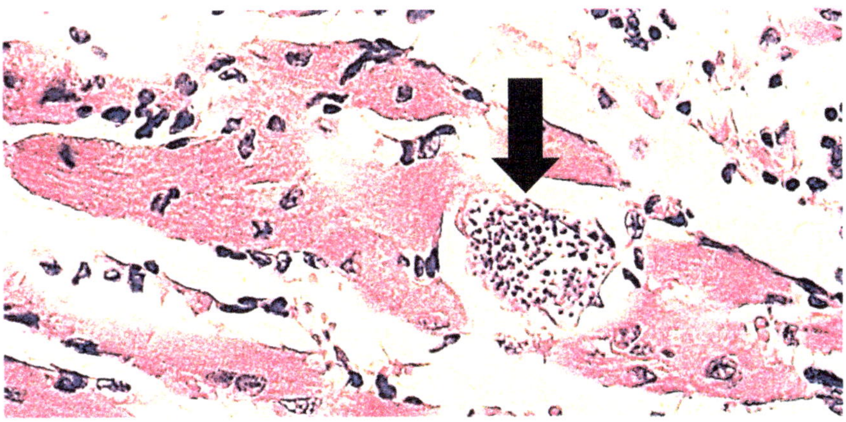

Fig. 9 Figure of amastigote nest in the mouse heart tissue. Histopathology analysis and histology preparation. This analysis is used to compare the organ damage between treated and non-treated animals

3.16 In Vivo Anti-Leishmania Studies (Cutaneous Model) [9]

1. Female and male BALB/c 6–8 weeks of age were used. Golden hamsters (Mesocritus auratus) were used to maintain the parasites. The animals were sacrificed by cervical dislocation following international recommendations at the end of the study.
2. Infection: *L. amazonensis* MHOM/IFLA/BR/67/PH8 is used and identified by isoenzyme analysis. The strain was maintained by passage every 6–8 weeks in hamsters.
3. BALB/c ($n = 8$) were inoculated in the right hind footpad with 2×10^6 amastigotes obtained from donor hamsters. The parasites were delivered in 100 mL of phosphate buffered saline (PBS).
4. Disease progression was monitored by the measurement of lesion diameters weekly for 10 weeks.
5. Drug treatment: The treatment was initiated 6 weeks after inoculation when the infection was well established, and lesions were obvious. Two days before administration of drug, the mice were randomly divided into groups of eight. N-methylglucamine antimonate was dissolved in 50 mL of PBS and administered to BALB/c mice in regimens of 100 mg per kg of body weight daily for 15 days by subcutaneous route. Compound (at 50, 100, or 200 mg/kg BW/day, for 14 days) was administered orally in the selected vehicle.
6. Effect of treatment: The animals were sacrificed 1 week after cessation of treatments to assess parasitological loads in the infected footpad.
7. Briefly, the mice were killed, and the lesions of the infected footpad were excised, weighed, and homogenized in a glass Teflon (Potter, OSI) homogenized in 5 mL of RPMI 1640 (Gibco, France) tissue culture medium supplemented with 10% fetal calf serum, 1 mL of glutamine (GIBCO, France) (29.4 mg/L), penicillin (100 U/mL), and streptomycin (100 mg/mL).
8. Plates were examined, and the number of amastigotes per host lesion cell nucleus was counted. The number of amastigotes per lesion per nucleus × lesion weight or spleen weight in gram is approximately equal to the total number of amastigotes per organ.
9. Parasite suppression was calculated from the ratio of the mean lesion amastigote counts of drug-treated mice and the mean lesion amastigote counts of untreated mice multiplied by 100 to obtain the percentage of parasite suppression.
10. Statistical analysis using the program JMP 3.2.2 (version 3.2.2, ASA Institute Inc., Cary, NC) was used to calculate the means standard deviations (Sds). The differences between groups were determined by using Student's t-test or the Kruskal–Wallis nonparametric analysis of variance test. Significance was established for a *P* value of <0.05.

4 Notes

1. In the triosa fosfato enzymatic activity, the limitation is the glyceraldehyde 3 phosphate preparation. This compound is not easy to find, and the commercial presentation is in a DL-Glyceraldehyde 3-phosphate diethyl acetal barium salt. It is an expensive reagent, then the best to handle it is preparing small amount of stocks solution before use. In the preparation procedure when the acetal salt is in the heating water, be exhaustive in the agitation. Because the salt is not soluble, but when the total white powder disappears in the solution, the hydrolysis is total. This is the perfect time to finalize the procedure, to get the highest yields. In this time is when the Glyceraldehyde 3-phosphate is free.
2. In all of the assays with living cells, work all the time in a type 2 laminar flow chamber in aseptic conditions. Remember to use a small amount of media culture and the solutions to minimize the contamination problems.
3. When using an organic compound in the in vitro test, generally the dissolution is a problem. The organic compound has poor solubility in aqueous solutions as all of the solutions utilized in biological assays. Usually in a large screening of compound, the concentrations used are high, 100 μM for example. This concentration would be suitable to see a biological activity, but sometime the compound precipitates in the assay conditions. If you have a precipitation in the assay, the result is not useful. To manage this matter, you can use small concentration of the compound, or to get the needed concentration, dilute the compound in a DMSO gradient. You can decrease sequentially, taking the DMSO concentration off to get a gradient of DMSO concentration, at the final useful concentration in a biological condition. First dilute the highest stock solution of the compound two times in a 50% final concentration of DMSO, then do the same to get a 25% final concentration of DMSO, and repeat that to get the final useful concentration in a biological condition. Try to resolve the precipitation problem, but do not discard the compound, could be a leader.
4. Red blood cells and sperm are very sensible to the manipulation; be careful and avoid sudden movements. Also if the buffer is not perfectly isotonic, the cell damage is high.
5. Minimal stress to embryos was achieved by slightly pinching the chorion at two points, followed by slowly tearing the chorion by two points and pressing it down, until the embryo slowly gently slides off the chorion (like when the grape skin is removed to get the pulp but without smashing the pulp). Only embryos that were clearly undamaged after 60 min of

observation were kept and subsequently used. Dechorionated embryos were further manipulated using only flame-rounded tip glass Pasteur pipettes.

6. In the acute model of Chagas disease in mice, generally you choose one fixed dose, and the treatment is once a day. But you can change this thinking, because there are no compound usually biodistributed 24 h, for example. Also the parasitemia peak is at 30 days around, but if the treatment finalizes before, and the next parasitemia is positive, of course the parasite will be there longer. Then you can change the duration of the treatment or change the beginning of the administration. Another issue is the effect of the immune system around 30 days, when the parasitemia decreases to zero; but this is not a cure. The parasite is there in somewhere, also in this type of assay you can not said the animal is cured. Only if an immunosuppressed animal survives one week after treatment and the parasite do not emerge in blood at this time, then it is ok say the animal is cured.

Acknowledgments

This work was supported by CSIC I+D 2016 grant #435.

References

1. Cavalli A, Bolognesi ML (2009) Neglected tropical diseases: multi-target-directed ligands in the search for novel lead candidates against Trypanosoma and Leishmania. J Med Chem 52:7339–7359. https://doi.org/10.1021/jm9004835
2. Renslo AR, McKerrow JH (2006) Drug discovery and development for neglected parasitic diseases. Nat Chem Biol 2:701–710. https://doi.org/10.1038/nchembio837
3. Papadopoulou MV, Bloomer WD, Rosenzweig HS et al (2016) Nitrotriazole-based acetamides and propanamides with broad spectrum antitrypanosomal activity. Eur J Med Chem 123:895–904. https://doi.org/10.1016/j.ejmech.2016.08.002
4. Barrett MP, Mottram JC, Coombs GH (1999) Recent advances in identifying and validating drug targets in trypanosomes and leishmanias. Trends Microbiol 7:82–88
5. Bettiol E, Samanovic M, Murkin AS et al (2009) Identification of three classes of heteroaromatic compounds with activity against intracellular Trypanosoma cruzi by chemical library screening. PLoS Negl Trop Dis 3:e384. https://doi.org/10.1371/journal.pntd.0000384
6. McKim JM (2010) Building a tiered approach to in vitro predictive toxicity screening: a focus on assays with in vivo relevance. Comb Chem High Throughput Screen 13:188–206. https://doi.org/10.2174/138620710790596736
7. Alvarez G, Aguirre-López B, Varela J et al (2010) Massive screening yields novel and selective Trypanosoma cruzi triosephosphate isomerase dimer-interface-irreversible inhibitors with anti-trypanosomal activity. Eur J Med Chem 45:5767–5772. https://doi.org/10.1016/j.ejmech.2010.09.034
8. Olivares-Illana V, Pérez-Montfort R, López-Calahorra F et al (2006) Structural differences in triosephosphate isomerase from different species and discovery of a multitrypanosomatid inhibitor. Biochemistry 45:2556–2560. https://doi.org/10.1021/bi0522293
9. Ferreira ME, Rojas de Arias A, Yaluff G et al (2010) Antileishmanial activity of furoquinolines and coumarins from Helietta apiculata. Phytomedicine 17:375–378. https://doi.org/10.1016/j.phymed.2009.09.009
10. Aguilera E, Varela J, Birriel E et al (2016) Potent and selective inhibitors of trypanosoma cruzi triosephosphate isomerase with

concomitant inhibition of cruzipain: inhibition of parasite growth through multitarget activity. ChemMedChem 11:1328–1338. https://doi.org/10.1002/cmdc.201500385

11. Álvarez G, Varela J, Márquez P et al (2014) Optimization of antitrypanosomatid agents: identification of nonmutagenic drug candidates with in vivo activity. J Med Chem 57:3984–3999. https://doi.org/10.1021/jm500018m
12. Liao TT, Jia RW, Shi YL et al (2011) Propidium iodide staining method for testing the cytotoxicity of 2,4,6-trichlorophenol and perfluorooctane sulfonate at low concentrations with Vero cells. J Environ Sci Health A Tox Hazard Subst Environ Eng 46:1769–1775. https://doi.org/10.1080/10934529.2011.624016
13. Álvarez G, Perdomo C, Coronel C et al (2017) Multi-anti-parasitic activity of arylidene ketones and thiazolidene hydrazines against Trypanosoma cruzi and Leishmania spp. Molecules 22(5):pii: E709. https://doi.org/10.3390/molecules22050709
14. Gerpe A, Alvarez G, Benítez D et al (2009) 5-Nitrofuranes and 5-nitrothiophenes with anti-Trypanosoma cruzi activity and ability to accumulate squalene. Bioorg Med Chem 17:7500–7509. https://doi.org/10.1016/j.bmc.2009.09.013
15. Ferraro F, Merlino A, dell'Oca N et al (2016) Identification of chalcones as fasciola hepatica cathepsin L inhibitors using a comprehensive experimental and computational approach. PLoS Negl Trop Dis 10:e0004834. https://doi.org/10.1371/journal.pntd.0004834
16. Álvarez G, Varela J, Cruces E et al (2015) Identification of a new amide-containing thiazole as a drug candidate for treatment of chagas' disease. Antimicrob Agents Chemother 59(3):1398–1404. https://doi.org/10.1128/AAC.03814-14
17. OECD (2001) OECD Guidelines for the Testing of Chemicals, Section 4, Test No. 425: Acute Oral Toxicity—Up-and-Down Procedure. Guidel Test Chem 26. https://doi.org/10.1787/9789264071049-en
18. Schmid W (1975) The micronucleus test. Mutat Res Mutagen Relat Subj 31:9–15. https://doi.org/10.1016/0165-1161(75)90058-8
19. Mortelmans K, Zeiger E (2000) The Ames Salmonella/microsome mutagenicity assay. Mutat Res 455:29–60
20. Cabrera M, Lavaggi ML, Hernández P et al (2009) Cytotoxic, mutagenic and genotoxic effects of new anti-T. cruzi 5-phenylethenylbenzofuroxans. Contribution of phase I metabolites on the mutagenicity induction. Toxicol Lett 190:140–149. https://doi.org/10.1016/j.toxlet.2009.07.006

Chapter 9

A Hybrid Virtual Screening Protocol Based on Binding Mode Similarity

Andrew Anighoro and Jürgen Bajorath

Abstract

In structure-based virtual screening (SBVS), a scoring function is usually applied to rank a database of docked compounds. Docking programs are often successful in reproducing experimental binding modes; however, the estimation of binding affinity still is the Achilles' heel of docking. The integration of SB and ligand-based (LB) methods is considered a promising strategy to increase hit rates in VS. Herein, we describe a hybrid protocol that is based on the assessment of binding mode similarity between docked compounds and a bound reference ligand. In this context, both experimental and computationally modeled poses have been successfully used as references for three-dimensional (3D) similarity calculations. In this chapter, the methods applied in recent validation studies are described.

Key words Virtual screening, Compound ranking, Molecular docking, Binding mode, 3D similarity, Protein–ligand interaction fingerprints, Homology modeling

1 Introduction

Virtual screening (VS) is widely applied in pharmaceutical research as a tool to identify new hit compounds [1, 2]. In a typical VS campaign, a large database of compounds is ranked according to an estimated probability to display a given biological activity. In a prospective application, the most promising candidates are selected among the top-ranking compounds and experimentally tested for activity. By limiting the number of experiments, VS has the potential to save considerable time and resources. The methods typically applied to VS can roughly be divided into structure (SB)- and ligand-based (LB) approaches. SBVS make use of the structure of the biological target to predict compounds that are likely to form favorable interactions in the binding site. Computational docking is the premier approach applied to SBVS [3, 4]. When a suitable conformation of the target is available, binding mode prediction (posing) performed by docking is often successful; however, an accurate estimation of the binding affinity (scoring) by force

Thomas Mavromoustakos and Tahsin F. Kellici (eds.), *Rational Drug Design: Methods and Protocols*, Methods in Molecular Biology, vol. 1824, https://doi.org/10.1007/978-1-4939-8630-9_9, © Springer Science+Business Media, LLC, part of Springer Nature 2018

field-based functions remains elusive [5]. Ligand-based (LB) methods, on the other hand, aim at identifying compounds having structural features and properties related to known actives [6]. The integration of LBVS and SBVS methods is regarded as a viable strategy to further improve hit rates [7]. A number of such hybrid approaches have been reported in literature [7].

Herein, we describe a hybrid VS protocol aiming to improve the recall of actives by molecular docking [8–10]. Following this protocol, a binding mode similarity measure is used to rank the database by comparing docked compounds to a bound reference ligand. A schematic representation of the protocol is provided in Fig. 1. The reference binding mode is typically provided by a cocrystallized ligand [8, 9]. However, we have shown that computationally modeled complexes (i.e., known active compounds docked into a homology model) can also be successfully used [10]. In this contribution, we will describe the application of two binding mode similarity measures, i.e., whole-ligand three-dimensional (3D) similarity [11] and protein–ligand interaction fingerprint (PLIF)-based similarity [12]. The protocol described herein was assessed and validated by performing VS benchmark calculations on a variety of target proteins belonging to different families (Table 1). Investigated targets included dihydrofolate reductase (DHFR), glucocorticoid receptor (GR), HIV-1 protease (HIV1PR), vascular endothelial growth factor receptor-2 (VEGFR2), adenosine A_{2A} (A_{2A}) receptor, and β_2 adrenergic (β_2) receptor [8–10]. As target structures, both X-ray complexes and homology models of GPCRs [10] were used, which are premier drug targets with still limited structural information, despite substantial progress made in GPCR structural biology over the past decade.

This approach discussed herein represents a potential alternative to conventional scoring schemes. In principle, 3D similarity calculations may be applied to reevaluate existing rankings because they are independent of the method used to generate the docking poses. Going forward, the anticipated increase in available crystallographic complexes will boost the applicability of knowledge-based approaches such as the one described herein. New complexes will provide more reference structures for 3D similarity calculations as well as templates for comparative modeling.

We found that recall rates of known active compounds obtained on the basis of binding mode similarity calculations were often superior to those of traditional force field-based scoring methods. Therefore, this protocol is thought to be a viable alternative to traditional SBVS. For a detailed report and extended discussion of the results obtained in each study case (Table 1), we refer to previous publications reports [8–10], while here we focus on describing the applied computational methods.

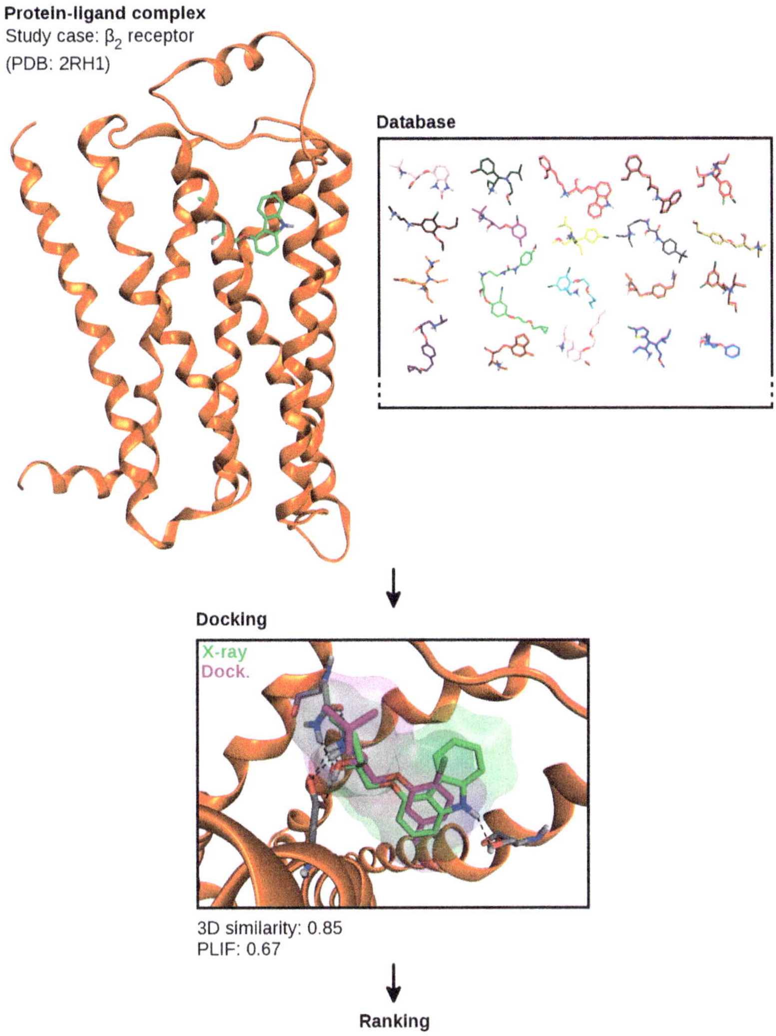

Fig. 1 The scheme summarizes the VS protocol including the selection of a target complex and compound database. Each compound is docked into the chosen binding site, and the predicted pose (magenta) is compared to a reference binding mode (green) on the basis of 3D similarity or a protein–ligand interaction fingerprint (PLIF). Finally, docked compounds are ranked using a selected similarity metric

2 Materials

2.1 Protein Structures

The initial step is downloading a structure of the target protein from the Protein Data Bank (PDB) (*see* **Notes 1** and **2**) [19]. When an experimental structure of the target is not available, one may try extracting a homology model from publicly available databases [20, 21]. For G-protein-coupled receptors (GPCRs), we typically rely on the GPCRdb [21]. Alternatively, one may build homology model in-house, which often provides higher confidence (*see* Subheading 3).

Table 1
Target proteins from previous validation studies and reference ligands are listed

Protein	Method	Source	Reference ligand	Method	Reference
DHFR	X-ray	PDB: 1KMV [13]	SRI-9662	3D similarity	[8]
GR	X-ray	PDB: 1NHZ [14]	Mifepristone	3D similarity	[8]
HIV1PR	X-ray	PDB: 3NU3 [15]	Amprenavir	3D similarity	[8]
VEGFR2	X-ray	PDB: 3VO3 [16]	Imidazo[1,2-*b*]pyridazine derivative	3D similarity	[8]
A_{2A}	X-ray	PDB: 4EIY [17]	ZM241385	3D similarity and PLIF	[9]
β_2	X-ray	PDB: 2RH1 [18]	Carazolol	3D similarity and PLIF	[10]
A_{2A}	Model	Built with MODELLER	ZM241385	3D similarity and PLIF	[10]
β_2	Model	Built with MODELLER	Carazolol	3D similarity and PLIF	[10]
5-HT_6	Model	GPCRdb	Ro 04-6790	3D similarity	[10]

For each target, structural information is provided and preferred similarity measures for compound ranking are given

2.2 Compound Set

Virtual screening benchmark sets for selected targets may be obtained from databases such as DEKOIS 2.0 (*see* **Note 3**) [22]. Other popular alternatives are DUD [23] and its successor DUD-E [24] or use a set of active compounds selected from ChEMBL [25] or BindingDB [26]. We have also used the IUPHAR/BPS Guide to Pharmacology database (GtoPdb) [27] to extract GPCR agonists or antagonists. Then, molecular decoys can be automatically generated with the DUD-E webserver (http://dude.docking.org/generate) [24].

3 Methods

3.1 Homology Modeling

If an experimental or modeled structure is not available from public repositories, an in-house homology model must be built (*see* **Note 4**) [10]. We have used MODELLER version 9.17 to model the structure of two GPCRs (Table 1) [28]. An initial sequence alignment with the template can be generated, for example, using Clustal Omega [29]. It is strongly advised to examine the computed alignment for local errors (misalignments) (*see* **Note 5**). MODELLER can generate an ensemble of plausible models (e.g., 500). The model with the most favorable DOPE score is usually selected. To adjust side chain positions of residues in the modeled binding site in a ligand-assisted manner, one selects a known active compound and applies an induced fit docking protocol. For this purpose, we have used the Dock module of MOE [12], permitting flexibility of side chains within a 6 Å distance of the ligand atoms. Typically, on the order of 100,000 poses are initially generated to finally retain 100 for scoring with the GBVI/WSA dG function implemented in MOE (using default parameter settings). The best-scoring pose is ultimately selected.

3.2 Protein Structure Preparation

The protein structure is prepared for docking by adding hydrogen atoms, computing protonation states and tautomers, assigning partial charges, and carrying out limited energy minimization of the binding site residues and the ligand (e.g., until a root mean square (RMS) gradient of 0.1kcal/mol/Å^2 is obtained). These steps are performed with the LigX tool of MOE [12]. We typically use the MMFF94* force field. Only for GPCRs, Amber10 with AM1-BCC partial charges for the ligand is used. The same protocol is applied to both X-ray and modeled structures.

3.3 Ligand Preparation

Ligands are prepared by calculating protonation states, assigning partial charges, and generating initial 3D conformations (*see* **Note 6**). These steps are also conveniently carried out with MOE. In addition, MMFF94* charges are used for all compound sets except GPCR ligands, for which AM1-BCC charges are calculated (for consistency with target charge settings).

3.4 Docking

We first generate a preferred docking pose for each database compound using the "rigid receptor" protocol implemented in the Dock module of MOE [12]. The coordinates of the cocrystallized or docked (in the case of homology models) ligand are used to center the calculations on the binding site. The triangle matcher algorithm is applied to generate 1000 docking poses. Then the 30 best-scoring solutions, according to the London dG function, are selected and further refined using force field calculations and subjected to rescoring using the GBVI/WSA dG scoring function. Then, the best-scoring pose is selected for each compound.

3.5 Binding Mode Similarity Assessment

The binding mode similarity of each docked compound to a reference ligand (cocrystallized or docked) is quantified using alternative measures including whole-molecule 3D similarity [11] or PLIF calculations [12] (*see* **Note 7**).

3.5.1 3D Ligand Similarity

3D similarity is assessed by means of a previously developed 3D similarity function that compares compound binding modes using property density functions taking conformational, positional, and atomic property differences into account [11]. Pair-wise ligand binding mode similarity is assessed by comparing the generated docking pose for each compound to reference ligand binding modes. Relative ligand positions for 3D similarity calculation are provided by computed docking poses. The normalized overlap of property density functions is calculated and used as a measure of 3D similarity. Therefore, each ligand atom is represented as a spherically symmetric Gaussian density function centered on the position of the nucleus with a width determined by the van der Waals radius of the atom. A global density function is defined for different atomic properties by calculating the sum of the density functions of all atoms of a ligand. For a detailed description of the formalism, we refer to a previous report [11]. This 3D similarity approach has previously been shown to be a sensitive measure of positional, conformational, and chemical property differences between compound binding modes [11, 30]. For X-ray complexes, the reference binding mode is provided by the coordinates of the cocrystallized ligand. For homology models, the three poses with largest RMSD values among 30 pre-computed binding modes are selected for 1-NN 3D similarity calculations by applying the diverse subset tool of MOE [12] (*see* **Note 8**). The similarity values (percentages) are used for compound ranking instead of docking scores.

3.5.2 Protein–Ligand Interaction Fingerprints

Based on the PLIF implementation of MOE [12], protein–ligand interactions are classified into different categories including side chain-mediated hydrogen bonds (donor and acceptor), backbone-mediated hydrogen bonds (donor and acceptor), ionic interactions, and surface interactions. PLIFs are calculated with default settings and compared using the conventional Tanimoto coefficient.

3.6 Performance Evaluation

We evaluate the overall performance of VS benchmark calculations by generating receiver operator characteristic (ROC) plots and calculating the area under the ROC curve (AUC). We note that AUC values of 0.5 correspond to random distribution of active compounds and decoys in rankings, whereas increasing AUC values greater than 0.5 indicate increasing enrichment of active compounds at high rank positions. Accordingly, an AUC value of 1 would be produced by a ranking in which all active compounds would be ranked higher than the best-scoring decoys. We determine AUC values by applying the composite trapezoidal rule. Furthermore, the factor for enrichment factor (E_f) in rankings (e.g., 1%, 2%, and 10%) is calculated [31]. The Rocker webserver (http://users.jyu.fi/~pentikai/rocker/) can be used to automatically generate ROC plots and calculate AUC and E_f values [32].

3.7 Results Summary

Ranking by whole-ligand 3D similarity calculations was found to outperform force field-based ranking in essentially all case studies both on the basis of AUC and early enrichment factor values [8–10]. Perhaps surprisingly, the resolution of the structure providing the reference binding mode was not found to represent a bottleneck for this approach. Furthermore, even “artificial” references such as GPCR agonists transferred by structural superposition from an active into an inactive conformation of the receptor (*see* **Note 2**) [9] and fuzzy docking poses of known ligands in a homology model [10] were found to be effective starting points for 3D similarity-based ranking, perhaps unexpectedly. On the other hand, in the case of A_{2A} receptor, it was observed that a ligand was less suitable as a reference for 3D similarity calculations if it contained large exposed groups not directly interacting with the target. This specific problem was overcome by applying PLIF-based similarity ranking (*see* **Note 1**). It was also shown that in 2D fingerprint-based and 3D similarity values in general correlated only poorly [8, 10], in accord with other studies. PLIF-based similarity ranking was meaningful as long as accurate binding modes were predicted for docked compounds, for example, in the case of the A_{2A} receptor [9]. By contrast, in the case of the β_2 receptor, including its X-ray structure and several differently constructed homology models, missing key interactions in docked complexes impaired the detection of PLIF-based similarity of binding modes. In most cases, this resulted in AUC values comparable to or lowers than obtained on the basis of force field docking scores [10]. In these cases, 3D similarity-based scoring was superior (*see* **Note 7**).

4 Notes

1. If multiple X-ray complexes are available as potential docking templates and reference binding modes for 3D similarity calculations, ligands with large groups that are solvent-exposed and not directly interacting with the target are deprioritized. We have shown that modeled core fragments involved in putative key interactions within the binding site may even be more effective references for 3D similarity assessment than native ligands [9]. For 3D similarity-based ranking, an important aspect is that reference ligands should as much as possible engage in interactions within the binding site. On the other hand, PLIF scoring may overcome difficulties associated with exposed ligand fragments because they do not contribute to calculated interactions (Fig. 2) [9].
2. In our experience, the crystallographic resolution of reference ligands and binding modes is not a limiting factor as long as the pose is overall correct. Even the assessment of fuzzy 3D similarity on the basis of modeled binding modes yields promising results in compound ranking [10].
3. This protocol has not yet been evaluated in prospective applications. Reference ligands for such applications may be obtained from vendor catalogs or in-house libraries.
4. In our experience, sequence identity as low as 30% is sufficient for homology modeling of GPCRs.

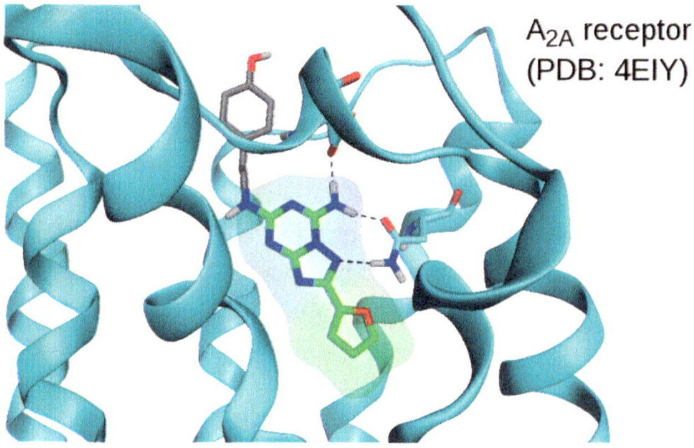

Fig. 2 A core fragment of the crystallographic A_{2A} receptor ligand ZM241385 (highlighted in green), which was most intimately involved in the interaction with A_{2A}, was a more effective reference for 3D similarity calculations than complete ZM241385. By contrast, PLIF calculations based upon the fragment or ZM241385 gave similar results [9]

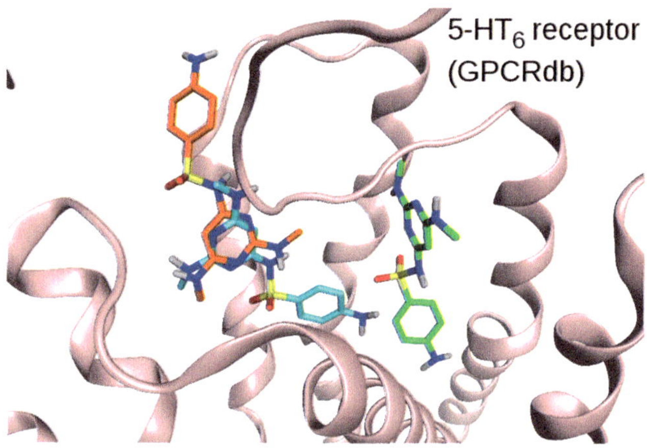

Fig. 3 Shown are three docking poses of the 5-HT_6 receptor antagonist Ro 04-6790 (orange, cyan, and green) in a homology model of 5-HT_6. When using homology models, a "fuzzy" subset of three different reference binding modes used for 3D similarity assessment improved compound recall compared to an individual prioritized ligand pose

5. Sequence alignments should best be manually adjusted for homology modeling in order to match known conserved structural motifs and appropriately place insertions and deletions in variable regions.

6. For ligands for which an initial 3D conformation is provided (e.g., DEKOIS 2.0), energy minimization to an RMS gradient of 0.1 kcal/mol/Å^2 is usually sufficient. Otherwise, a conformational search protocol should be applied to generate

preferred low energy conformers. For example, the MOE Dock module includes a conformational search option prior to placement of ligands into binding sites; however, an initial reasonable 3D conformation is required [12].

7. PLIF-based ranking proved to be very sensitive to correct posing of database compounds. On the other hand, 3D similarity calculations were much more robust and yielded high ranks for actives as long as docking poses were at least approximately correct. Importantly, 3D similarity calculations following our approach quantify whole-molecule resemblance by comparing atomic property density functions but are insensitive to interaction differences. For example, if ligand-receptor interactions are mainly formed by a large rigid (aromatic) ring system, posing tends to be reliable and stable. Consequently, in such cases, PLIF-based compound ranking is often successful. However, in the presence of approximate poses, 3D similarity assessment is more effective [10].
8. For homology models, we have compared the use of both single and multiple reference binding modes. Providing larger coverage of a binding site by using multiple-related putative binding modes often compensates for their approximate nature. This strategy often outperforms similarity calculations using single reference binding modes (Fig. 3) [10].

Acknowledgment

We thank OpenEye Scientific Software, Inc., for a free academic license of the OpenEye Toolkit and Chemical Computing Group, Inc., for academic teaching licenses of the Molecular Operating Environment.

References

1. Heikamp K, Bajorath J (2013) The future of virtual compound screening. Chem Biol Drug Des 81:33–40. https://doi.org/10.1111/cbdd.12054
2. Lavecchia A, Di Giovanni C (2013) Virtual screening strategies in drug discovery: a critical review. Curr Med Chem 20:2839–2860. https://doi.org/10.2174/09298673113209990001
3. Kitchen DB, Decornez H, Furr JR, Bajorath J (2004) Docking and scoring in virtual screening for drug discovery: methods and applications. Nat Rev Drug Discov 3:935–949. https://doi.org/10.1038/nrd1549
4. Irwin JJ, Shoichet BK (2016) Docking screens for novel ligands conferring new biology. J Med Chem 59:4103–4120. https://doi.org/10.1021/acs.jmedchem.5b02008
5. Gathiaka S, Liu S, Chiu M et al (2016) D3R grand challenge 2015: evaluation of protein--ligand pose and affinity predictions. J Comput Aided Mol Des 30:651–668. https://doi.org/10.1007/s10822-016-9946-8
6. Ripphausen P, Nisius B, Bajorath J (2011) State-of-the-art in ligand-based virtual screening. Drug Discov Today 16:372–376. https://doi.org/10.1016/j.drudis.2011.02.011
7. Drwal MN, Griffith R (2013) Combination of ligand- and structure-based methods in virtual

screening. Drug Discov Today Technol 10: e395–e401. https://doi.org/10.1016/j.ddtec.2013.02.002
8. Anighoro A, Bajorath J (2016) Three-dimensional similarity in molecular docking: prioritizing ligand poses on the basis of experimental binding modes. J Chem Inf Model 56:580–587. https://doi.org/10.1021/acs.jcim.5b00745
9. Anighoro A, Bajorath J (2016) Binding mode similarity measures for ranking of docking poses: a case study on the adenosine A2A receptor. J Comput Aided Mol Des 30:447–456. https://doi.org/10.1007/s10822-016-9918-z
10. Anighoro A, Bajorath J (2017) Compound ranking on the basis of fuzzy 3D similarity improves the performance of docking into homology models of G-protein coupled receptors. ACS Omega 2:2583–2592. https://doi.org/10.1021/acsomega.7b00330
11. Peltason L, Bajorath J (2007) Molecular similarity analysis uncovers heterogeneous structure-activity relationships and variable activity landscapes. Chem Biol 14:489–497. https://doi.org/10.1016/j.chembiol.2007.03.011
12. Molecular Operating Environment (MOE), 2014.09; Chemical Computing Group Inc., 1010 Sherbooke St. West, Suite #910, Montreal, QC, Canada, 2014.
13. Klon AE, Héroux A, Ross LJ et al (2002) Atomic structures of human dihydrofolate reductase complexed with NADPH and two lipophilic antifolates at 1.09 a and 1.05 a resolution. J Mol Biol 320:677–693. https://doi.org/10.1016/S0022-2836(02)00469-2
14. Kauppi B, Jakob C, Färnegårdh M et al (2003) The three-dimensional structures of antagonistic and agonistic forms of the glucocorticoid receptor ligand-binding domain: RU-486 induces a transconformation that leads to active antagonism. J Biol Chem 278:22748–22754. https://doi.org/10.1074/jbc.M212711200
15. Shen C-H, Wang Y-F, Kovalevsky AY et al (2010) Amprenavir complexes with HIV-1 protease and its drug-resistant mutants altering hydrophobic clusters. FEBS J 277:3699–3714. https://doi.org/10.1111/j.1742-4658.2010.07771.x
16. Miyamoto N, Sakai N, Hirayama T et al (2013) Discovery of N-[5-({2-[(cyclopropylcarbonyl)amino]imidazo[1,2-b]pyridazin-6-yl}oxy)-2-methylphenyl]-1,3-dimethyl-1H-pyrazole-5-carboxamide (TAK-593), a highly potent VEGFR2 kinase inhibitor. Bioorg Med Chem 21:2333–2345. https://doi.org/10.1016/j.bmc.2013.01.074
17. Liu W, Chun E, Thompson AA et al (2012) Structural basis for allosteric regulation of GPCRs by sodium ions. Science 337:232–236. https://doi.org/10.1126/science.1219218
18. Cherezov V, Rosenbaum DM, Hanson MA et al (2007) High-resolution crystal structure of an engineered human β2-adrenergic G protein-coupled receptor. Science 318:1258–1265. https://doi.org/10.1126/science.1150577
19. Berman HM, Westbrook J, Feng Z et al (2000) The protein data bank. Nucleic Acids Res 28:235–242. https://doi.org/10.1093/nar/28.1.235
20. Bienert S, Waterhouse A, de Beer TAP et al (2017) The SWISS-MODEL repository-new features and functionality. Nucleic Acids Res 45:D313–D319. https://doi.org/10.1093/nar/gkw1132
21. Isberg V, Mordalski S, Munk C et al (2016) GPCRdb: an information system for G protein-coupled receptors. Nucleic Acids Res 44: D356–D364. https://doi.org/10.1093/nar/gkv1178
22. Bauer MR, Ibrahim TM, Vogel SM, Boeckler FM (2013) Evaluation and optimization of virtual screening workflows with DEKOIS 2.0--a public library of challenging docking benchmark sets. J Chem Inf Model 53:1447–1462. https://doi.org/10.1021/ci400115b
23. Huang N, Shoichet BK, Irwin JJ (2006) Benchmarking sets for molecular docking. J Med Chem 49:6789–6801. https://doi.org/10.1021/jm0608356
24. Mysinger MM, Carchia M, Irwin JJ, Shoichet BK (2012) Directory of useful decoys, enhanced (DUD-E): better ligands and decoys for better benchmarking. J Med Chem 55:6582–6594. https://doi.org/10.1021/jm300687e
25. Bento AP, Gaulton A, Hersey A et al (2014) The ChEMBL bioactivity database: an update. Nucleic Acids Res 42:D1083–D1090. https://doi.org/10.1093/nar/gkt1031
26. Liu T, Lin Y, Wen X et al (2007) BindingDB: a web-accessible database of experimentally determined protein–ligand binding affinities. Nucleic Acids Res 35:D198–D201. https://doi.org/10.1093/nar/gkl999
27. Southan C, Sharman JL, Benson HE et al (2016) The IUPHAR/BPS guide to PHARMACOLOGY in 2016: towards curated quantitative interactions between 1300 protein targets and 6000 ligands. Nucleic Acids Res 44:D1054–D1068. https://doi.org/10.1093/nar/gkv1037

28. Sali A, Blundell TL (1993) Comparative protein modelling by satisfaction of spatial restraints. J Mol Biol 234:779–815. https://doi.org/10.1006/jmbi.1993.1626
29. Sievers F, Wilm A, Dineen D et al (2011) Fast, scalable generation of high-quality protein multiple sequence alignments using Clustal omega. Mol Syst Biol 7:539. https://doi.org/10.1038/msb.2011.75
30. Hu Y, Furtmann N, Gütschow M, Bajorath J (2012) Systematic identification and classification of three-dimensional activity cliffs. J Chem Inf Model 52:1490–1498. https://doi.org/10.1021/ci300158v
31. Bender A, Glen RC (2005) A discussion of measures of enrichment in virtual screening: comparing the information content of descriptors with increasing levels of sophistication. J Chem Inf Model 45:1369–1375. https://doi.org/10.1021/ci0500177
32. Lätti S, Niinivehmas S, Pentikäinen OT (2016) Rocker: open source, easy-to-use tool for AUC and enrichment calculations and ROC visualization. J Chem 8:45. https://doi.org/10.1186/s13321-016-0158-y

Chapter 10

Single Step Determination of Unlabeled Compound Kinetics Using a Competition Association Binding Method Employing Time-Resolved FRET

David A. Sykes and Steven J. Charlton

Abstract

The competition association binding method allows the characterization of the kinetics of unlabeled compounds and the calculation of receptor-drug affinity (K_d). The K_d value is defined as the ratio of the dissociation constant (or k_{off}) of the receptor-bound ligand to its association rate constant (or k_{on}) for a system at equilibrium. Traditionally, competition association binding experiments have been carried out using radiometric detection methods with limited assay throughput. Here we describe a novel method for the determination of unlabeled compound kinetics using the technique of time-resolved fluorescence resonance energy transfer (TR-FRET) performed at physiological temperature and sodium ion concentration. Based on a traditional screening format (10-point curves), up to 28 compounds can be tested on a single 384-well plate by this method.

Key words Time-resolved fluorescence resonance energy transfer, Competition association binding kinetics, Fluorescent ligand, Terbium cryptate, SNAP-tagged GPCR, Association rate, Dissociation rate

1 Introduction

The competition association binding approach first described by Motulsky and Mahan [1] involves the use of a previously characterized tracer to determine the kinetics of unlabeled compounds. Until recently quantifying the competition between unlabeled compounds and tracer, traditionally a radioligand, has been achieved mainly using filtration binding assays [2–4], although scintillation proximity assays have also been described [5]. More recently, a higher-throughput, whole cell nonradioactive method has been published that utilizes time-resolved fluorescence resonance energy transfer (TR-FRET) between terbium-labeled receptor and fluorescently labeled ligand [6], although in this instance the authors needed to modify the competition association binding

Thomas Mavromoustakos and Tahsin F. Kellici (eds.), *Rational Drug Design: Methods and Protocols*, Methods in Molecular Biology, vol. 1824, https://doi.org/10.1007/978-1-4939-8630-9_10, © Springer Science+Business Media, LLC, part of Springer Nature 2018

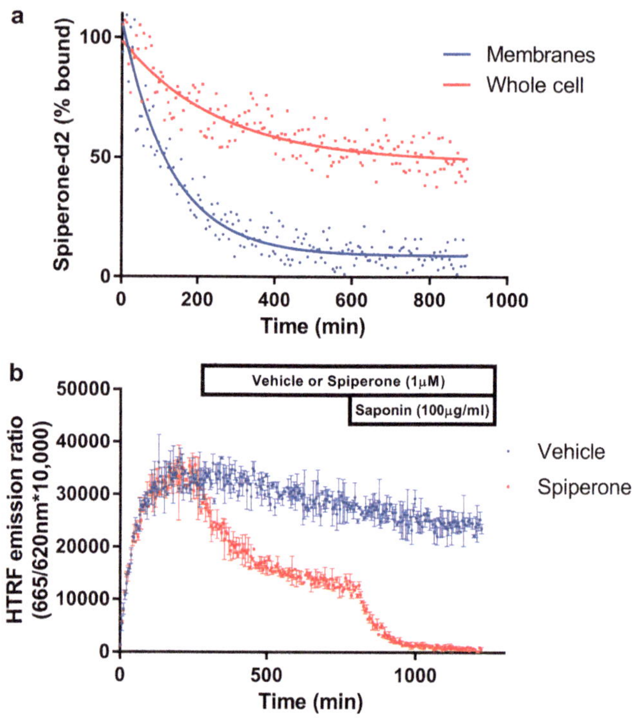

Fig. 1 (**a**) Spiperone-red dissociation from membranes and whole cells following addition of an excess of spiperone and (**b**) spiperone-red dissociation from whole cells treated with saponin in the presence or absence of an excess of spiperone

equation to account for signal drift which they attributed to photobleaching.

Here we describe the TR-FRET methodology employed in our laboratory. Rather than using whole cells, we have preferred to utilize membrane preparations [4, 7, 8]. This is because whole cells represent an additional compartment into which tracer and competitor ligands may partition, therefore complicating interpretation of kinetic data. This problem of differential partitioning is perhaps best highlighted by the incomplete reversal of spiperone-red binding from the dopamine D_2 receptor expressed in whole cells following addition of a vast excess of competitor (Fig. 1a). This incomplete reversal of binding (with trapped tracer likely bound to intracellular receptors) can be overcome by adding a cell-permeabilizing agent such as saponin (Fig. 1b), demonstrating that the membrane of whole cells is a barrier to free diffusion of the competing compound. This figure also suggests that the changes in specific binding observed over time may be attributed to loss of receptors rather than depletion of ligand since levels do not return back to their peak on addition of saponin. The Motulsky-Mahan competition association model is based on the laws of mass action [1, 9], and its accuracy relies on unhindered competition between the tracer and the unlabeled ligand.

Traditionally the first step in the competition association approach involves the accurate quantification of the tracer association and dissociation rates (or on- and off-rates). This is achieved by monitoring the association of binding of increasing concentrations of the tracer and then fitting the data directly to a global association equation or through linear transformation of the observed rate of association where the slope of the resulting line is equal to the on-rate and the Y-intercept is equal to the off-rate [4]. The second step involves the direct competition between a fixed concentration of the tracer and increasing concentrations of the unlabeled competitor. Using the plate map described in Subheading 3.7, we effectively combine both steps on a single 384-well plate (96 wells in total), characterizing 7 compounds at 10 different concentrations. Practically we use this plate map on 4 quadrants, allowing up to 28 compounds to be tested per plate.

We have recently used this method to determine the association and dissociation rates and equilibrium affinities of a series of dopamine D_2 receptor agonists [10] and antagonists [11].

2 Materials

Prepare all solutions using ultra-high purity water and analytical grade reagents. Prepare all reagents at room temperature, and store as indicated.

2.1 Labeling Receptors with Terbium Cryptate

1. Prepare 1× concentrated Tag-lite labeling medium: Add 10 mL of LABMED (5× concentrated from Cisbio Bioassays (Bagnols-sur-Cèze, France)) to a 50 mL tube. Add 40mL of water making a 1× concentrated LABMED solution (50 mL). Mix and store at 4 °C.
2. To 20 mL of Tag-lite labeling medium, add 20 μL of 100 μM SNAP-Lumi4-Tb (Cat. No. SSNPTBC from Cisbio Bioassays (Bagnols-sur-Cèze, France)) dissolved in DMSO (100 nM final concentration). Mix and store at −20 °C.
3. Cell wash buffer: D-PBS (Cat. No. D8537 Sigma-Aldrich) store at room temperature.
4. Cell culture media: DMEM:F12 (Cat. No. D6421 Sigma-Aldrich) supplemented with 2 mM glutamine and 10% fetal calf serum (Gibco). Store at 4 °C.
5. Hank's-based cell dissociation buffer is obtained from GIBCO (Gibco™ 13,150,016).

2.2 Membrane Preparation

1. Membrane preparation buffer: 10 mM HEPES, 10 mM EDTA, pH 7.4. Dissolve 2.38 g HEPES and 3.80 g of disodium EDTA in 1 L of water, and adjust pH to 7.4 with 3 N HCl. This solution can be made and kept at 4 °C until day of experiment (store up to 1 week).

2. Membrane storage buffer: 10 mM HEPES, 0.1 mM EDTA, pH 7.4. Dissolve 2.38 g HEPES and 0.038 g of disodium EDTA in 1 L of water, and adjust pH to 7.4 with 3 N NaOH. This solution can be made and kept at 4 °C until day of experiment (store for up to 1 week).
3. Polytron tissue homogenizer (e.g., Werke, Ultra-Turrax).
4. 25 mL centrifuge tubes (Universals) and bench top centrifuge (e.g., Sigma 3–16 10270).
5. Ultracentrifuge tubes and ultracentrifuge (e.g., Beckman Ultracentrifuge).
6. 1 mL syringe and 0.5 gauge needles.
7. Protein assay: e.g., bicinchoninic acid assay kit for protein determination (BCA1 Sigma-Aldrich).

2.3 Fluorescent and Unlabeled Ligand Characterization Studies

1. PPHT derivative labeled with a red fluorescent probe (PPHT-red) is obtained from Cisbio Bioassays (Bagnols-sur-Cèze, France).
2. Pluronic acid F127 (Cat. No. P2443 purchased from Sigma-Aldrich): 20% pluronic acid F127 solution in DMSO. Dissolve 0.2 g pluronic acid F127 in 1 mL of DMSO. Store at room temperature (*see* **Note 1**).
3. Assay buffer: 20 mM HEPES containing 100 mM NaCl, 6 mM $MgCl_2$, 1 mM EGTA, 1 mM EDTA, 0.02% pluronic acid and 1% DMSO. Weigh each buffer component, and then add 800 mL of water to a 1 L measuring cylinder. Add each buffer component and mix, adjusting the pH with 3 N sodium hydroxide. Make up to 1 L with water, filter (*see* **Note 2**) and transfer to a 1 L Duran. Store at 4 °C. Add 0.02% pluronic acid (10 μL per 10 mL) and 1% DMSO (90 μL per 10 mL—*see* **Note 3**) fresh on the day of experiment.
4. Alternative assay buffers can be substituted (*see* **Note 4**).
5. GppNHp (Cat. No. G0635 from Sigma-Aldrich) solution: GppNHp is dissolved in water to a stock concentration of 20 mM. Store at −20 °C.
6. Temperature-controlled hot box.
7. White 384-well Optiplates (Cat. No. 6007290 purchased from PerkinElmer, Beaconsfield, UK) or equivalent microplate suitable for use with BMGs Pherastar FS (or equivalent plate reader—*see* **Note 5**).
8. 384-well compatible multichannel pipettors (8 or 12 channel) and reagent reservoirs (e.g., Matrix).
9. Integra Viaflo 384 and 384 tips (Cat. No. 6463).
10. Optical plate sealers (*see* **Note 6**) e.g., Whatman UniSeal™ (Cat. No. 7704-0009).

3 Methods

3.1 Terbium Labeling of SNAP-Tagged D_{2L} Cells

1. Cell culture medium is aspirated from the T150 cm^2 flasks containing confluent adherent CHO-D_{2L} cells.
2. Cells are washed 2× with 10 mL of D-PBS (GIBCO Carlsbad, CA) and then 1× with 10 mL of Tag-lite labeling medium (i.e., 1× concentrated LABMED, from Cisbio Bioassays, Bagnols-sur-Cèze, France).
3. 10 mL of Tag-lite labeling medium containing 100 nM of SNAP-Lumi4-Tb is added to the flask and incubated for 1 h at 37 °C under 5% CO_2.
4. Cells are washed 2× in D-PBS to remove the excess of SNAP-Lumi4-Tb.
5. Cells are then detached using 5 mL of enzyme-free Hank's-based cell dissociation buffer (GIBCO) and collected in a 25 mL Universal containing 5 mL of DMEM:F12 supplemented with 2 mM glutamine and 10% fetal calf serum (*see* **Note 7**).
6. Cells are pelleted by centrifugation (5 min at 1500 rpm), and the pellets were frozen and stored at −80 °C.

3.2 Membrane Preparation of Terbium Labeled D_{2L} Cells

To prepare membranes homogenization steps are conducted at 4 °C (to avoid receptor degradation).

1. 20 mL per t150-cm^2 flask of membrane preparation buffer (10 mM HEPES and 10 mM EDTA, pH 7.4) is added to the pellet previously thawed and placed on ice.
2. The pellet is resuspended and then homogenized using an electrical homogenizer Ultra-Turrax (Ika-Werk GmbH & Co. KG, Staufen, Germany) (position 6, 4 × 5 s bursts).
3. The resulting cell homogenate is centrifuged at 48,000 × *g* at 4 °C (Beckman Avanti J-251 Ultracentrifuge; Beckman Coulter, Fullerton, CA) for 30 min.
4. The supernatant is discarded, and the pellet is resuspended in 20 mL of membrane preparation buffer (10 mM HEPES and 10 mM EDTA, pH 7.4), and then re-homogenized and centrifuged as described above.
5. The supernatant is discarded, and the pellet is suspended in ice-cold membrane storage buffer (10 mM HEPES and 0.1 mM EDTA, pH 7.4), at a concentration of 5–10 mg/mL.
6. Protein concentration is determined using the bicinchoninic acid assay kit (Sigma-Aldrich), BSA as a standard and aliquots maintained at −80 °C until required.

7. Prior to their use, the frozen membranes are thawed, and the membranes are suspended in the assay buffer at a membrane concentration of 0.1 mg/mL.

3.3 Tracer Characterization Through Saturation Binding

Prepare serial dilutions of the fluorescent ligand at 4× final concentration.

1. Prepare a 200 nM stock solution of F-PPHT by adding 1 μL of 20 μM PPHT-red to 99 μL of assay buffer in a 0.5 mL Eppendorf.
2. Add 50 μL of assay buffer using a multichannel pipettor to 11 × 0.5 mL Eppendorf tubes used to prepare serial dilutions of the fluorescent ligand.
3. Serially dilute the stock PPHT-red 1–2 by adding 50 μL from the stock solution to 50 μL of assay buffer in a second Eppendorf using a suitable pipette (to yield fluorescent ligand concentrations four times the final assay concentration). Mix by pipetting up and down, and then continue the serial dilution using the remaining 10 Eppendorfs (*see* **Note 8**).

Perform the binding assay in a final volume of 40 μL per well (*see* **Note 9**) in a white 384-well Optiplate (assay plate). Add the following components to the assay plate to measure total and nonspecific binding (NSB).

1. Add 10 μL of assay buffer to wells in rows A–D (1–12) of a 384-well Optiplate using a multichannel pipettor.
2. Add 10 μL of assay buffer to wells in rows A–B (1–12) using a multichannel pipettor.
3. Add 10 μL of unlabeled 40 μM haloperidol (used to define NSB; 10 μM final) to wells in rows C–D (1–12), using a multichannel pipettor.
4. Transfer 10 μL of each of the 4× PPHT-red fluorescent ligand serial dilutions (**step 3**) to its corresponding well on the assay plate Fig. 2.
5. Cover the plate with an optical plate seal to prevent evaporation.
6. Measure the fluorescent intensity of the sample prior to the addition of tissue, and construct a standard curve (ligand concentration versus fluorescent intensity—*see* **Note 10**).
7. Thaw a frozen membrane sample (*see* **Note 11**), and dilute the membranes in assay buffer (0.6 mL required) in a 1.5 mL polypropylene Eppendorf tube to a final concentration of 100 μg/mL. Add GppNHp (400 μM directly to the membranes, 100 μM final concentration—*see* **Note 12**), and heat the membranes to 37 °C.

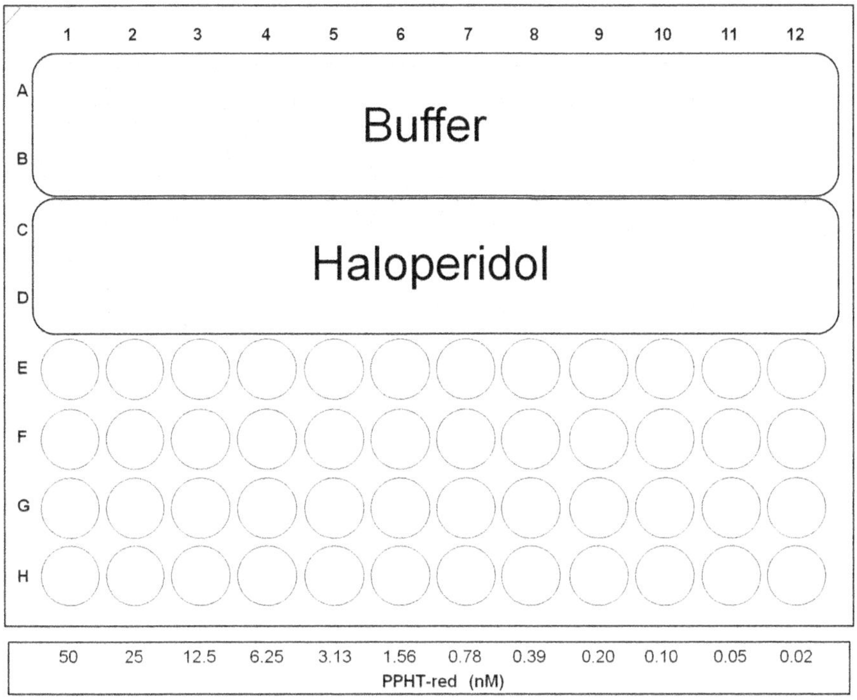

Key: PPHT-red various concentrations; Buffer defines total binding; haloperidol (10μM) defines non-specific binding

Fig. 2 Plate map saturation binding of PPHT-red

8. Place the assay plate in the temperature-controlled plate reader, and heat to 37 °C (*see* **Note 13**). Add 10 μL of this membrane stock to rows A to D using a multichannel pipettor (or using the Integra Viaflo) (i.e., 1 μg of membrane per well; *see* **Note 14**).
9. Immediately transfer the plate to the plate reader, and use a stop clock to determine the time from the addition of membranes to first read on the plate reader (e.g., Pherastar FS; *see* **Notes 15** and **16**).

3.4 Saturation Binding Data Analysis

Saturation binding of radioligands traditionally allows the calculation of two key parameters receptor tracer affinity (or K_d) expressed as concentration and the maximal number of binding sites (or B_{max}) expressed in terms of the number of moles of receptor per milligram of protein. One minor drawback of TR-FRET is that the detection of tracer binding is dependent on the level of terbium bound to the receptor, but since the true efficiency of labeling is unknown, it is not possible to calculate a true B_{max}. Receptor tracer affinity can be calculated in two ways from saturation binding data.

Specific binding is calculated by subtracting nonspecific binding (NSB) from total binding, and a saturation binding curve (or binding isotherm) is created by plotting the specific binding

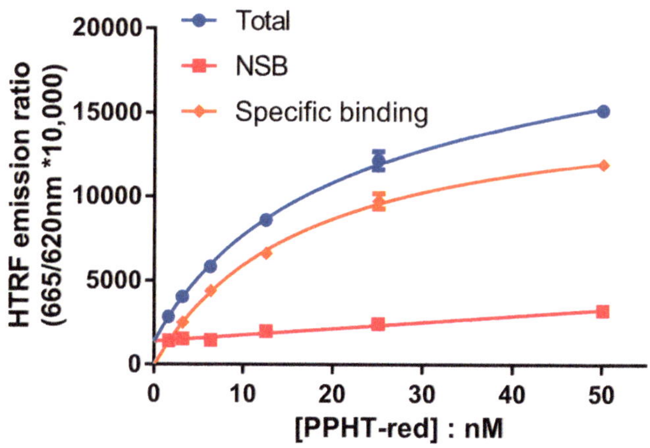

Fig. 3 PPHT-red saturation binding curve

(or bound) versus the concentration of tracer added (or free tracer). Data from a typical saturation curve showing the binding of PPHT-red to membranes prepared from CHO-D_{2L} cells are shown in Fig. 3. In this example only the concentrations of PPHT-red which made a significant contribution to specific binding are shown.

NSB is conventionally described by a linear function, and specific binding to a single site should begin to saturate at highest tracer concentrations employed. Specific binding is displayed by applying the Hill-Langmuir equation that describes a hyperbolic relationship as follows:

$$\Upsilon = \frac{[B_{\max}][X]}{[X] + K_{\mathrm{d}}} \tag{1}$$

where the $B_{\max}$ = maximum TR-FRET signal and K_{d} denotes the tracer equilibrium dissociation constant.

The equation for nonspecific binding reveals a straight line:

$$\Upsilon = \mathrm{NS}\tilde{n}X \tag{2}$$

Therefore, the equation for the total binding curve represents both specific binding together with NSB:

$$\Upsilon = \frac{[B_{\max}][X]}{[X] + K_{\mathrm{d}}} + \mathrm{NS}[X] \tag{3}$$

Data can also be globally fitted to determine specific binding using the raw saturation binding data. Thus by fitting total and NSB together, there is no need to subtract one data set from another to determine specific binding. Outlined below is the GraphPad Prism 7 equation syntax for global fitting of saturation binding data:

```
Nonspecific = NS*X
Specific = Bmax*X/(KD+X)
<A> Y = Specific + Nonspecific
<B> = Nonspecific
```

Where total binding is input into column A and the nonspecific binding into column B, with the parameter NS shared between both data sets.

3.5 Determining the Dissociation Rate of the Fluorescent Ligand from the Receptor

The dissociation rate of the fluorescent ligand can be obtained directly by adding an excess of unlabeled competitor to the various concentrations of fluorescent tracer preassociated in the saturation binding assay described above. An example procedure is described for dissociation of PPHT-red from the dopamine D_{2L} receptor.

1. Preassociate PPHT-red with the D_{2L} receptor as described above. Once fully associated establish a baseline TR-FRET read, and then pause the reader.
2. Remove the plate from the reader, and peel back the optical seal. Add 2 μL of 20× haloperidol (200 μM) to the reaction mixture, start the stop clock, mix and reseal, and then return to the plate reader [*see* **Note 17**. If binding is truly reversible then, the TR-FRET ratio should reach the level of the pre-existing NSBs (in rows C and D)].
3. Use a stop clock to determine the time from the addition of haloperidol to first read on the plate reader (e.g., Pherastar FS; *see* **Note 15**).

3.6 Dissociation Rate (k_{off}) Data Analysis

Dissociation binding experiments measure the "off-rate" of the tracer dissociating from the receptor. It is particularly important to demonstrate that specific binding of the fluorescent ligand is truly reversible.

To experimentally determine the k_{off}, a single concentration of PPHT-red is incubated with CHO-D_{2L} cell membranes until equilibrium is attained, at which point a saturating concentration ($\geq$1000 × K_i) of haloperidol (10 μM), a competitive receptor antagonist, is added to initiate dissociation of PPHT-red.

Data from a typical dissociation experiment are shown in Fig. 4. The results are shown as the mean total PPHT-red bound (TR-FRET emission ratio 665 nm/620 nm * 10,000) plotted against time (Fig. 4). Ideally initial k_{off} determinations should be conducted over a wide range of time points at regular intervals with a minimal cycle time (e.g., 5 s), as the time frame over which the tracer dissociates may be unknown. If the whole curve is not accurately defined, then it will affect the accuracy of the k_{off} determined.

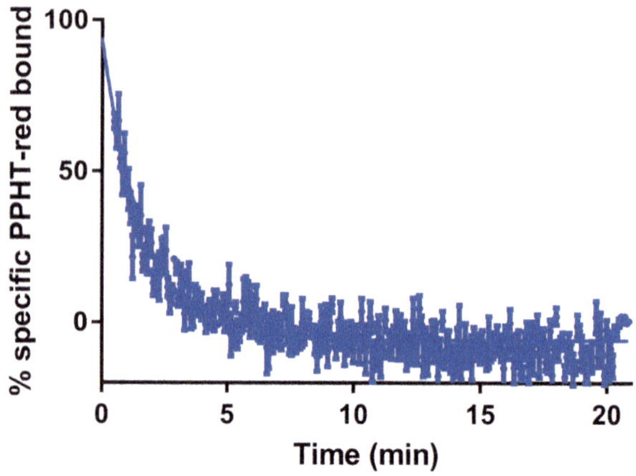

Fig. 4 PPHT-red dissociation from CHO-D_{2L} membranes

If binding is to a single receptor species, then dissociation data can be fit into a one-phase exponential decay function using Prism 7.0 (GraphPad):

$$\text{Total binding} = \text{NS} + (\text{Total} - \text{NS}) * e^{-k_{\text{off}} * t} \tag{4}$$

where total binding and nonspecific binding (NS) are expressed as (TR-FRET emission ratio 665 nm/620 nm * 10,000). Time (t) is usually expressed in minutes. The $t_{1/2}$ value obtained is transformed into a k_{off} rate using Eq. 5:

$$k_{\text{off}} = {}^{0.693}\!/_{t_{1/2}} \tag{5}$$

The dissociation rate constant (k_{off}) is expressed in units of inverse time, usually min^{-1}. More commonly, the half-life for dissociation, which equals $\ln(2)/k_{\text{off}}$ or $0.6931/k_{\text{off}}$, is calculated. In one half-life, half the tracer will have dissociated from the receptor. In this example, PPHT-red dissociation is monophasic with a half-time of dissociation ($t_{1/2}$) of 1.37 min (Fig. 4). When these values are applied to Eq. 5, they yield a k_{off} of 0.50 min^{-1}. The k_{off} value calculated from this experiment should be equivalent to the k_{off} value calculated from the kinetic association rate experiment (*see* Fig. 6).

3.7 Determining Tracer and Unlabeled Compound Kinetics (Combined Single Step or Separate)

Prepare serial dilutions of the fluorescent ligand at 4× final concentration

1. Prepare a 200 nM stock solution of PPHT-red by adding 2 μL of 20 μM PPHT-red to 198 μL of assay buffer in a 0.5 mL Eppendorf.
2. Add 100 μL of assay buffer using a multichannel pipettor to 5 × 0.5 mL Eppendorf tubes used to prepare serial dilutions of the fluorescent ligand.

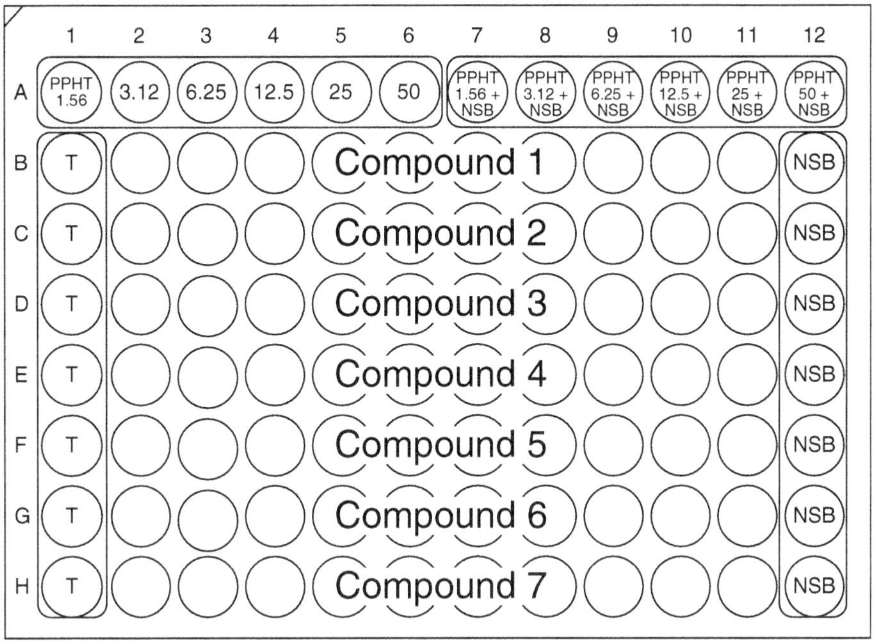

Key: Total = total binding (absence of competitor); Compound = D_2 ligands at various concentrations based on estimated K_i; NSB = haloperidol (10μM) defines non-specific binding

Fig. 5 Plate map competition association assay

3. Serially dilute the stock PPHT-red 1–2 by adding 100 μL from the stock solution to 100 μL of assay buffer in a second Eppendorf using a multichannel pipettor (to yield fluorescent ligand concentrations four times the final assay concentration). Mix by pipetting up and down, and then continue the serial dilution using the remaining four Eppendorfs (*see* **Note 8**).

Perform the binding assay in a final volume of 40 μL per well in a white 384-well Optiplate (assay plate).

Add the following components to the assay plate to measure total and nonspecific binding (NSB) allowing the calculation of specific binding.

1. Add 10 μL of assay buffer to wells in rows A to H (1–12) of a 384-well Optiplate using a multichannel pipettor (*see* Plate Map Fig. 5).
2. Add 10 μL of assay buffer to wells in row A (1–6) and row B to H (1) using a multichannel pipettor.
3. Add 10 μL of unlabeled 40 μM haloperidol (used to define NSB; 10 μM final) to wells in rows A (6–12) and row B to H (12), using a multichannel pipettor.
4. Transfer 10 μL of each of the 4× fluorescent ligand serial dilutions (**step 3**) to its corresponding well on the assay plate.

5. Prepare 10-point serial dilution 1–3 of test compounds in a 96-well PP plate (diluting from right to left), and then transfer using an expandable Matrix pipette 10 μL of each of the 4× test compound serial dilutions to its corresponding well on the assay plate (*see* Plate Map Fig. 5).
6. Prepare a 50 nM stock concentration of 4× fluorescent ligand in assay buffer (950 μL), final assay concentration 12.5 nM, and add to rows B–H (1–12).
7. Cover the plate with an optical plate seal to prevent evaporation.
8. Measure the fluorescent intensity of the sample prior to the addition of tissue, and construct a standard curve (ligand concentration versus fluorescent intensity—*see* **Note 10**).
9. Thaw a frozen membrane sample (*see* **Note 11**), and dilute the membranes in assay buffer (1.2 mL required) in a 1.5 mL polypropylene Eppendorf tube to a final concentration of 100 μg/mL. Add GppNHp (400 μM directly to the membranes, 100 μM final concentration), and heat the membranes to 37 °C.
10. Place the assay plate in the temperature-controlled plate reader, and heat to 37 °C (*see* **Note 13**). Add 10 μL of this membrane stock to rows A to H using a multichannel pipettor (or using the Integra Viaflo) (i.e., 1 μg of membrane per well; *see* **Note 14**).
11. Immediately transfer the plate to the plate reader, and use a stop clock to determine the time from the addition of membranes to first read on the plate reader (e.g., Pherastar FS; *see* **Note 15**).

3.8 Association Rate (k_{on}) Determination Data Analysis

The observed association rate of a ligand is dependent upon its concentration, k_{on} and k_{off} values. By constructing a family of association curves using a range of tracer concentrations, it is possible to calculate the k_{on} and k_{off} values by simultaneously fitting all curves to generate global estimates for the rate parameters, as described in Method 1 below:

Method 1: *Global fitting*. The equation below taken from for GraphPad Prism 7 allows global fitting of kinetic association data with tracer concentration entered as the column title for each data set.

$$k_{ob} = [\text{Tracer}]^{*} k_{on} + k_{off}$$

$$Y = Y_{max}{}^{*}(1 - \exp(-1^{*} K_{ob}{}^{*} X))$$

For example, PPHT-red curves fitted in this manor are shown in Fig. 6; using this method, a k_{on} of 2.98×10^7 M^{-1} min^{-1} and a k_{off} value of 0.52 min^{-1} are obtained. These same parameters can

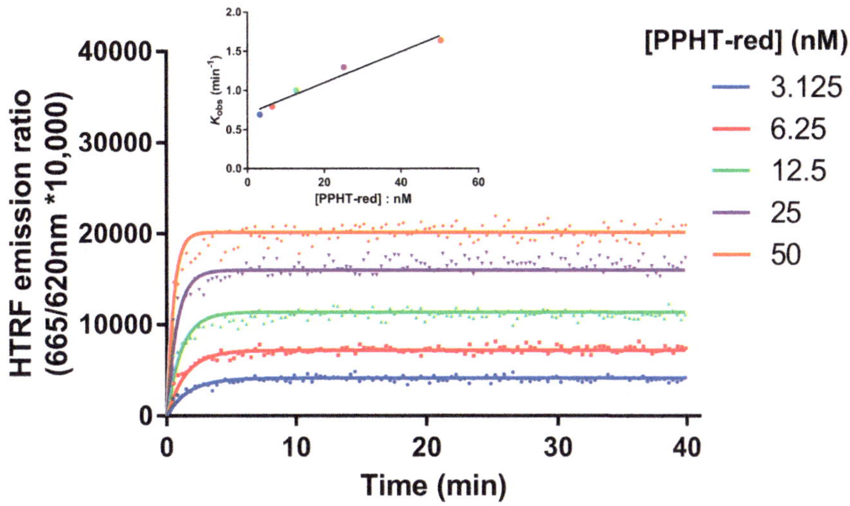

Fig. 6 PPHT-red association to membranes containing the dopamine D_{2L} receptor

be used to calculate a kinetically derived K_d value ($K_d = k_{off}/k_{on}$) at the D_{2L} receptor. The kinetically derived K_d calculated should be the same as that derived from a saturation binding studies. In this example, the kinetically derived K_d calculated by global kinetic fitting (17.4 nM) was in good agreement with the value obtained from PPHT-red saturation experiments (17 nM).

Method 2: Linear plot of k_{ob} *versus tracer concentration.* If PPHT-red binding follows a simple law of mass action model, k_{ob} should increase in a linear manner as a function of tracer concentration. The slope of the line should equate to the association rate, and extrapolation of the plot to $y = 0$ should yield the dissociation rate [4, 12]. In this example, when k_{ob} values were plotted against tracer concentration (Fig. 6 inset), the data yielded a straight line, consistent with PPHT-red binding to a single site. Values obtained from this plot were $1.98 \times 10^7\ M^{-1}\ min^{-1}$ and $0.7\ min^{-1}$ for k_{on} and k_{off}, respectively.

3.9 Competition Association Binding Data Analysis: Calculation of Unlabeled Compound Kinetics

Competition association binding data are displayed in Fig. 7 A and B, for dopamine and aripiprazole, respectively in competition with the tracer PPHT-red for binding to the human D_{2L} receptor. Data are plotted as specifically bound tracer versus time. Each unlabeled ligand is assayed at ten different concentrations. Data are obtained using a range of concentrations of dopamine, which has a faster dissociation rate than the tracer PPHT-red and aripiprazole which is slower to dissociate than the tracer (*see* **Note 18**).

Association and dissociation rates for unlabeled antagonists are calculated by globally fitting the data in Prism 7.0 to the equations

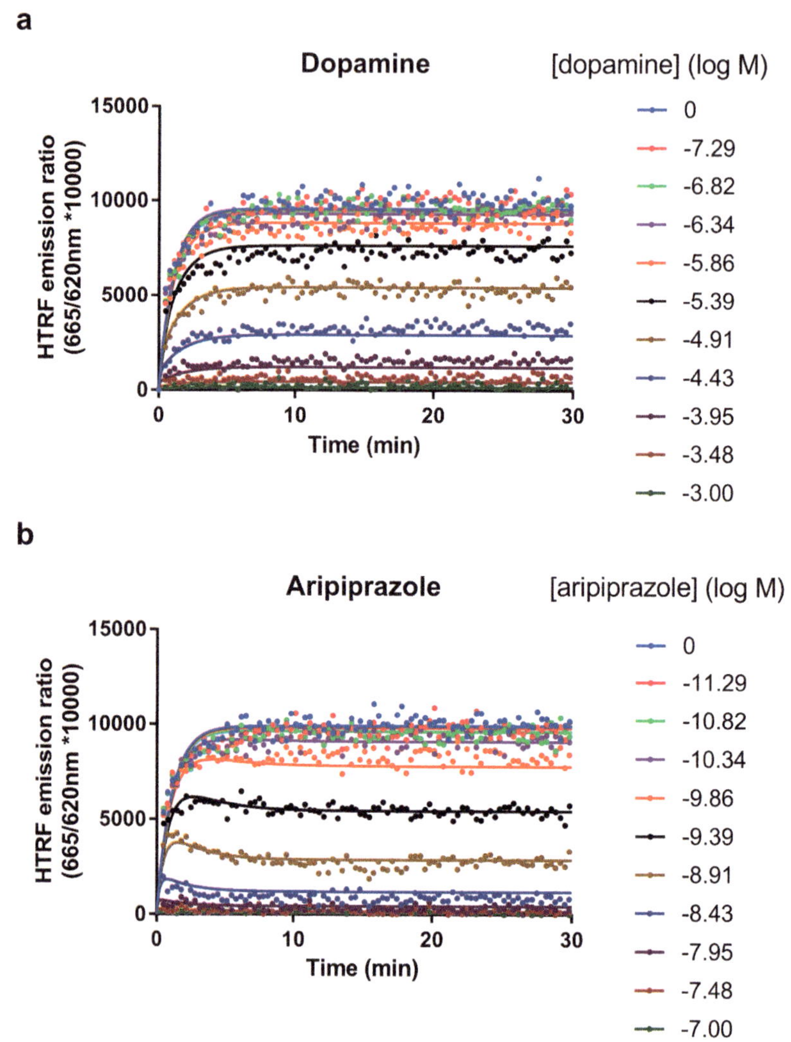

Fig. 7 PPHT-red competition association binding kinetics

described by Motulsky and Mahan [1] (see below), with all parameters fixed apart from $k3$, $k4$, and B_{max} [10].

```
KA = K1*L*1E-9 + k2
KB = K3*I*1e-9 + K4
S = SQRT((KA-KB)^2+4*K1*K3*L*I*1e-18)
KF = 0.5 * (Ka + KB + S)
KS = 0.5 * (KA + KB - S)
DIFF = KF - KS
Q = Bmax*K1*L*1e-9/DIFF
Y = Q*(k4*DIFF/(KF*KS)+((K4-Kf)/KF)*exp(-KF*X)-((K4-KS)/KS)
*exp(-KS*X))
```

where X = time (min), Y = specific binding (TR-FRET emission ratio 665 nm/620 nm * 10,000), $k1 = k_{on}$ tracer (PPHT-red), $k2 = k_{off}$ tracer (PPHT-red), L = concentration of tracer (PPHT-red) used (nM), and I = concentration unlabeled antagonist/agonist (nM).

Fixing the parameters above allows calculation of the following: B_{max} = total binding (TR-FRET emission ratio 665 nm/620 nm * 10,000), $k3$ = association rate of unlabeled ligand (M^{-1} min^{-1}), and $k4$ = dissociation rate of unlabeled ligand (min^{-1}).

The values of k_{on} and k_{off} obtained from the competition association analysis of dopamine and aripiprazole competition data are shown in Fig. 7. Kinetically derived K_d values (k_{off}/k_{on}) for the unlabeled competitors were in good agreement with the K_i values obtained at equilibrium (i.e., kinetic reads at 60 min read) in competition association binding experiments.

3.10 K_i Determination from Competition Association Binding Experiments

Competition association binding data obtained at the point of equilibrium may be fitted to a sigmoidal curve (variable slope *n*H) using a four parameter logistic equation using Prism 7.0 (GraphPad):

$$\Upsilon = \text{Bottom} + (\text{Top} - \text{Bottom})/\left(1 + 10^{(X - \log EC_{50})\tilde{n}n_H}\right) \quad (6)$$

where Bottom is the Υ value at the bottom plateau, Top is the Υ value at the top plateau, *n*H is the slope factor, and EC_{50} (or IC_{50}) is the X value when the response is midway between Bottom and Top. IC_{50} values obtained by fitting the data using Prism 7.0 from the inhibition curves are converted to K_i values using the method of Cheng and Prusoff [13]. The K_i value is calculated from the IC_{50} value according to the relationship $K_i = IC_{50}/[1 + (F/K_d)]$, where F is the concentration of tracer and K_d is the affinity of the tracer for the receptor. This is also known as the Cheng-Prusoff correction [13]. Typical competition association binding displacement data are shown in Fig. 8 from an experiment in which the D_2 agonists inhibited the binding of PPHT-red ($F = 12.5$ nM, $K_d = 17$ nM) to human D_{2L} receptors transfected into CHO cells.

4 Notes

1. 20% pluronic acid F127 solution in DMSO has a tendency to solidify at temperatures below 20–22 °C. Therefore it is recommended that solutions are warmed and mixed prior to pipetting.
2. It is recommended that assay buffers are filtered prior to use to remove any particulates.

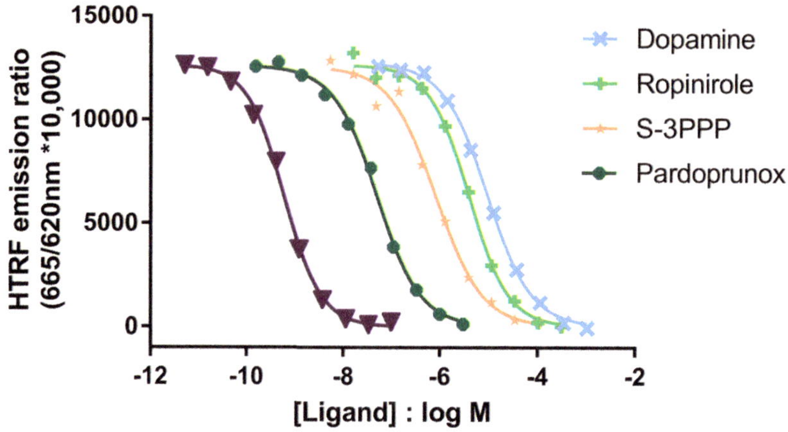

Fig. 8 Equilibrium competition binding

3. Pluronic acid is made up in DMSO; therefore any additional DMSO added should account for this.
4. Alternative assay buffers can be substituted to those detailed in the protocol, e.g., HBSS/HEPES buffer: Use 1× HBSS (137 mM NaCl, 5.4 mM KCl, 0.25 mM Na_2HPO_4, 0.44 mM KH_2PO_4, 1.3 mM $CaCl_2$, and 1.0 mM $MgSO_4$) with 5 mM HEPES. 1× HBSS and 1 M HEPES solutions were procured from Life Technologies (Carlsbad, California, USA) or those with salts removed.
5. Alternative plate readers are available, but speed and assay sensitivity are important considerations, and the use of alternative instruments may compromise assay quality.
6. Non-optical plate sealers will prevent evaporation but also prevent accurate TR-FRET measurements.
7. If cells are difficult to detach, then alternatively they can be scrapped into cell dissociation media and then the remaining protocol steps followed.
8. Ideally a range of fluorescent ligand concentrations should be employed 5–30-fold above and below the anticipated K_d.
9. Total assay volume is dependent upon the affinity of the ligand and the concentration of the receptor. Specific binding should equal less than 10% of the total fluorescent ligand added. Significant tracer depletion can be overcome by increasing the amount of fluorescent ligand added, either by increasing concentration or through an increase in reaction volume or alternatively reducing the amount of tissue or a combination of these methods [14].
10. Unlike radiometric assays it is not possible to accurately determine the concentration of fluorescent ligand added; however it

is possible to measure the relative levels of compound added to the assay plate by taking a fluorescent intensity read prior to the addition of tissue. This serves two purposes. Firstly, it allows you to check for inconsistencies in fluorescent ligand addition, and secondly it also checks whether the unlabeled competitor compound has any effect on the fluorescent ligand intensity in solution, as any compound-related reductions in fluorescent ligand intensity (e.g., due to quenching) will lead to artificial reductions in the resulting TR-FRET signal.

11. In order to thoroughly resuspend membranes, it is important to pass the membranes through a fine-gauge needle using a 1 mL syringe.
12. GTP can be substituted for GppNHp in certain circumstances. The addition of GTP or GppNHp converts high-affinity binding sites into low-affinity binding sites by uncoupling receptor from the cognate G proteins.
13. Assay plates and binding reactions must be preheated to the desired assay temperature.
14. Membrane concentrations (or alternatively laser/lamp flashes on BMG' Pherastar Fs) may need to be adjusted in order to observe a more stable TR-FRET signal. A 620 nm (red) or 520 nm (green) emission value in the range of 1000 should produce a good signal to noise ratio.
15. Offline additions mean that, following the addition of membranes or drugs, a timer must be used to monitor the first read time following insertion into the reader and subsequent timing adjusted to reflect this delay.
16. Saturation binding experiments can be performed as an end-point read in which case a kinetic read is not necessary, however some pre-knowledge of the kinetics of the tracer is useful when selecting concentrations of the fluorescent ligand to be employed in the competition association binding assay.
17. Another important internal check is to perform the direct determination of the dissociation rate (k_{off}) of the fluorescent tracer from the receptor of interest. This serves two purposes; it proves that the tracer of interest is fully reversible from the receptor (i.e., law of mass of action obeyed) and that the indirectly determined dissociation rate of the tracer is correct. If binding is truly reversible, then the TR-FRET ratio should reach the level of the pre-existing NSB ratios.
18. For more slowly associating compounds, higher concentrations of unlabeled ligand may need to be employed to obtain suitable resolution of PPHT-red inhibition of binding within the experimental timeframe.

Acknowledgments

Catherine Wark (BMG Labtech Ltd.) for expert technical assistance and BMG for personal sponsorship of David Sykes. Nicolas Pierre, Louise Affleck, Thomas Roux and François Degorce from CisBio Bioassays for their continuing support. Rob Lane from the Monash Institute for Pharmaceutical Sciences for supplying the dopamine D_2 agonists used in the competition association binding studies.

References

1. Motulsky HJ, Mahan LC (1984) The kinetics of competitive radioligand binding predicted by the law of mass action. Mol Pharmacol 25 (1):1–9
2. Dowling MR, Charlton SJ (2006) Quantifying the association and dissociation rates of unlabelled antagonists at the muscarinic M3 receptor. Br J Pharmacol 148(7):927–937. https://doi.org/10.1038/sj.bjp.0706819
3. Sykes DA, Dowling MR, Charlton SJ (2009) Exploring the mechanism of agonist efficacy: a relationship between efficacy and agonist dissociation rate at the muscarinic M3 receptor. Mol Pharmacol 76(3):543–551. https://doi.org/10.1124/mol.108.054452
4. Sykes DA, Dowling MR, Charlton SJ (2010) Measuring receptor target coverage: a radioligand competition binding protocol for assessing the association and dissociation rates of unlabeled compounds. In: Current protocols in pharmacology. John Wiley & Sons, Inc. https://doi.org/10.1002/0471141755.ph0914s50
5. Xia L, de Vries H, AP IJ et al (2016) Scintillation proximity assay (SPA) as a new approach to determine a ligand's kinetic profile. A case in point for the adenosine A1 receptor. Purinergic Signal 12(1):115–126. https://doi.org/10.1007/s11302-015-9485-0
6. Schiele F, Ayaz P, Fernández-Montalván A (2015) A universal homogeneous assay for high-throughput determination of binding kinetics. Anal Biochem 468:42–49. https://doi.org/10.1016/j.ab.2014.09.007
7. Sykes DA, Parry C, Reilly J et al (2014) Observed drug-receptor association rates are governed by membrane affinity: the importance of establishing "micro-pharmacokinetic/pharmacodynamic relationships" at the beta2-adrenoceptor. Mol Pharmacol 85 (4):608–617. https://doi.org/10.1124/mol.113.090209
8. Sykes DA, Bradley ME, Riddy DM et al (2016) Fevipiprant (QAW039), a slowly dissociating CRTh2 antagonist with the potential for improved clinical efficacy. Mol Pharmacol 89 (5):593–605. https://doi.org/10.1124/mol.115.101832
9. Motulsky HJ, Mahan LC, Ansel PA (1985) Radioligand, agonists and membrane receptors on intact cells: data analysis in a bind. Trends Pharmacol Sci 6:317–319. https://doi.org/10.1016/0165-6147(85)90149-x
10. Klein Herenbrink C, Sykes DA, Donthamsetti P et al (2016) The role of kinetic context in apparent biased agonism at GPCRs. Nat Commun 7:10842. https://doi.org/10.1038/ncomms10842
11. Sykes DA, Moore H, Stott L et al (2017) Extrapyramidal side effects of antipsychotics are linked to their association kinetics at dopamine D2 receptors. Nat Commun 8(1):763. https://doi.org/10.1038/s41467-017-00716-z
12. Motulsky H, Christopoulos A (2004) Fitting models to biological data using linear and nonlinear regression: a practical guide to curve fitting. Oxford University Press, Oxford, New York
13. Cheng Y, Prusoff WH (1973) Relationship between the inhibition constant (K1) and the concentration of inhibitor which causes 50 per cent inhibition (I50) of an enzymatic reaction. Biochem Pharmacol 22(23):3099–3108
14. Carter CM, Leighton-Davies JR, Charlton SJ (2007) Miniaturized receptor binding assays: complications arising from ligand depletion. J Biomol Screen 12(2):255–266. https://doi.org/10.1177/1087057106297788

Chapter 11

Dynamic Undocking: A Novel Method for Structure-Based Drug Discovery

Maciej Majewski, Sergio Ruiz-Carmona, and Xavier Barril

Abstract

Computer-aided methods have been broadly used in pharmaceutical research to identify potential ligands and design effective therapeutics. Most of the approaches rely on the binding affinity prediction and approximate thermodynamic properties of the system. Our alternative approach focuses on structural stability, provided by native protein–ligand interactions, in particular hydrogen bonds. Based on this idea, we designed new fast computational method, called dynamic undocking (DUck), that evaluates stability by calculating the work necessary to break the most important native contact in a ligand-receptor complex. This property is effective in distinguishing true ligands from decoys and is orthogonal to currently existing docking methods, thus making it exceptionally useful in virtual screening. Here, we present a protocol suitable for DUck's application in drug design strategy, as well as notes that will help to solve common problems addressed by users.

Key words Drug discovery, Molecular docking, Molecular dynamics, Structure-based drug design, Virtual screening, Hydrogen bonds, Structural stability

1 Introduction

There is a continuous need for new methods that increase the efficacy and efficiency of rational drug design. Structure-based approaches aim to predict the binding free energy of protein–ligand complexes, but this is an elusive property that is extremely difficult to calculate in a rigorous manner. As a result, commonly used tools apply various layers of approximations, and the resulting estimates carry a large, and often unknown, absolute error. Recently, we have postulated that protein–ligand complexes could be evaluated, not only by their binding free energy but also by their ability to form a precise and stable binding mode. Structural stability is relatively easy to compute, as one can start with the bound state, introduce minor perturbations, and measure the resistance that the system opposes to that change.

Thomas Mavromoustakos and Tahsin F. Kellici (eds.), *Rational Drug Design: Methods and Protocols*, Methods in Molecular Biology, vol. 1824, https://doi.org/10.1007/978-1-4939-8630-9_11, © Springer Science+Business Media, LLC, part of Springer Nature 2018

In this book chapter, we describe a particular computational approach, termed dynamic undocking (DUck) [1], that we have implemented to assess the robustness of protein–ligand interactions. DUck is fast and automatic and, thus, amenable to high-throughput applications. The method is very effective in distinguishing active from inactive compounds and is virtually free from false negatives. At the same time, it is orthogonal to existing approaches as they focus on fundamentally different properties. In this introduction, we will present the conceptual basis for DUck and summarize the most important results validating the method. Then we will present and discuss all the methodological details involved in the practical application of DUck.

1.1 Structural Stability and Binding

In target-based drug design, K_D is the parameter that defines efficacy. The thermodynamic equilibrium constant (or other parameters that are easier to determine experimentally—IC_{50}, AC_{50}, K_I—and are used as proxy) informs about the potency of a ligand for its macromolecular target and is the main parameter under optimization. Not surprisingly, structure-based drug design has always focused on predicting K_D (or mathematical transformations of the same, such as ΔG_{BIND}) in order to guide and accelerate the discovery of new bioactive molecules. Inevitably, this involves a comparison of the bound (protein–ligand complex in solution) and unbound states (independently solvated entities). These states are difficult to characterize, and their comparison leads to an accumulation of errors. In spite of the economic and intellectual incentives in solving this problem, accurate solutions are—at best—impractical, and common methods offer very qualitative estimates [2].

We propose to consider a different property of protein–ligand complexes, which is not related to a thermodynamic constant but appears to be ubiquitous. Most protein–ligand complexes are structurally robust (i.e., they have a single binding site that is preserved under dynamic conditions). This implies that active ligands—irrespective of their ΔG_{BIND}—must present a deep and narrow free energy minimum around the bound state (Fig. 1). As this is a local magnitude, it would be relatively straightforward to predict, simply starting from the bound state and measuring the resistance that the ligand opposes to small perturbations. Note, however, that (1) structural stability is not an essential condition for binding (consider, i.e., the case of a lipid inside a bilayer), but—empirically—most protein–ligand complexes form robust complexes, and (2) a priori, structural stability should not correlate with any thermodynamic constant (K_D, k_{off}).

1.2 Hydrogen Bonds as Structural Anchors

The calculation of structural stability could be realized in many different ways. Here we postulate that hydrogen bonds are privileged anchoring motifs and decide to monitor specifically this

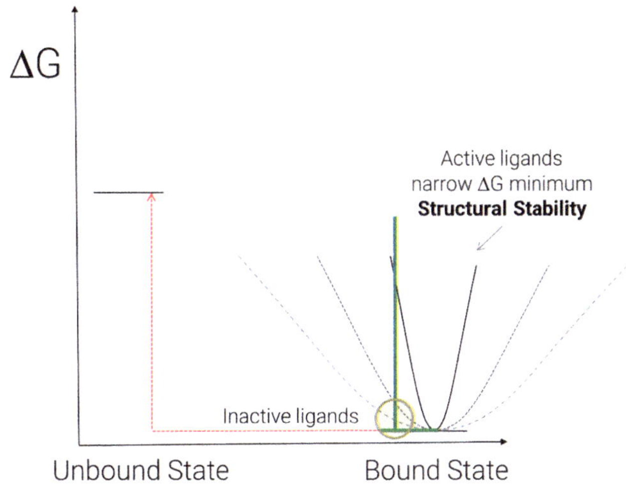

Fig. 1 Graphical representation of the quasi-bound state (green lines and circle) in relation to bound and unbound states

type of interactions. The choice is based on the fact that hydrogen bonds have very strict geometric requirements (maximal fluctuation ~0.5 Å). Additionally, we have observed that protein–ligand complexes can form water-shielded hydrogen bonds, which create steep barriers to dissociation [3]. Hydrogen bonds are an essential feature of most protein–ligand complexes, including fragment-sized ligands [4], and most well-studied binding sites present a polar interaction point that is fulfilled by all known ligands. In the initial implementation of the method, we have decided to consider only the single most important hydrogen bond, as defined by a pharmacophore analysis of known ligands. In the future, we will investigate the use of multiple hydrogen bonds and also other types of molecular interactions. The designated hydrogen bond is then pulled from 2.5 Å to 5.0 Å, which covers the whole range from a very strong hydrogen bond to a water-mediated interaction. In order to exclude effects that are unrelated to the hydrogen bond under investigation, we use a small portion of the receptor. The judicious definition of this subsystem is essential, as it must preserve the local environment that modulates the rupture of the hydrogen bond while removing interactions that may preclude displacement by unrelated mechanisms (e.g., steric blockage). Simulating only a subset of the system offers the additional advantages of simplifying the dissociation pathway and speeding up the calculations, which scale linearly with the number of particles. Having defined the system and the scope of the simulation, we have designed a computational protocol to realize it.

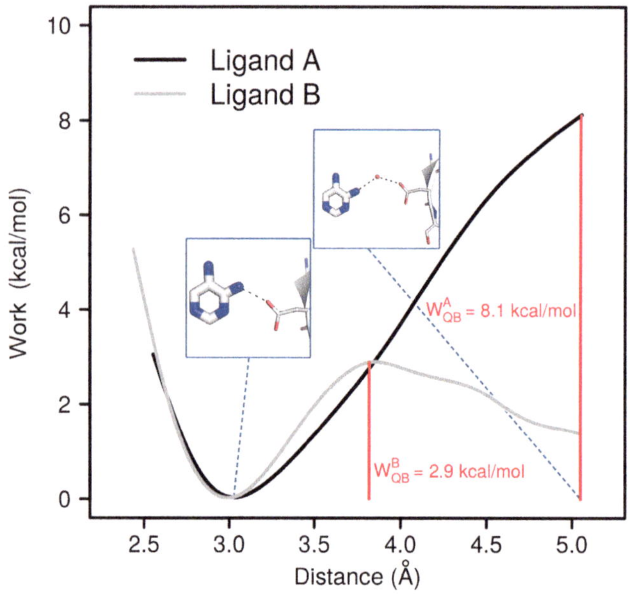

Fig. 2 Representative work profiles obtained from DUck simulations for a strong (black) and a weak (gray) ligand. The QB state is defined as the point with the highest energy relative to the ideal hydrogen-bond geometry

1.3 Dynamic Undocking and the Quasi-Bound State

Dynamic undocking per se is a particular type of steered molecular dynamics (SMD) simulation, where we force the rupture of an intermolecular hydrogen bond formed between a predefined interaction point in the receptor and a complementary atom in the ligand. The distance between the said two atoms is the reaction coordinate, and steering is carried out at constant velocity, monitoring the force (and thus the work) needed to proceed at each point along the reaction coordinate. Then, we define the quasi-bound state as the point where work reaches a maximum (Fig. 2). The work needed to reach the quasi-bound state (W_{QB}) is used as a measure of structural stability. If our hypothesis is correct, potent ligands must present relatively large W_{QB} values, while weak ligands or inactive molecules should oppose little resistance to dissociation. Initial experiments were devised to test the hypothesis and to identify a relationship between W_{QB} and binding that could be used in virtual screening applications.

1.4 Hypothesis Validation

Figure 3 shows the distribution of W_{QB} values observed for a set [5] of strong CDK2 binders ($IC_{50} < 1$ μM), weak CDK2 binders ($IC_{50} > 1$ μM), and decoys (i.e., molecules that have similar properties and can dock to CDK2 but have no reported activity against this protein). Strikingly, all strong binders present high W_{QB} (>5 kcal/mol) values, while the vast majority of decoys present no or very low W_{QB} values (<3 kcal/mol). Weak binders present larger dispersion on the low end of the distribution but must also

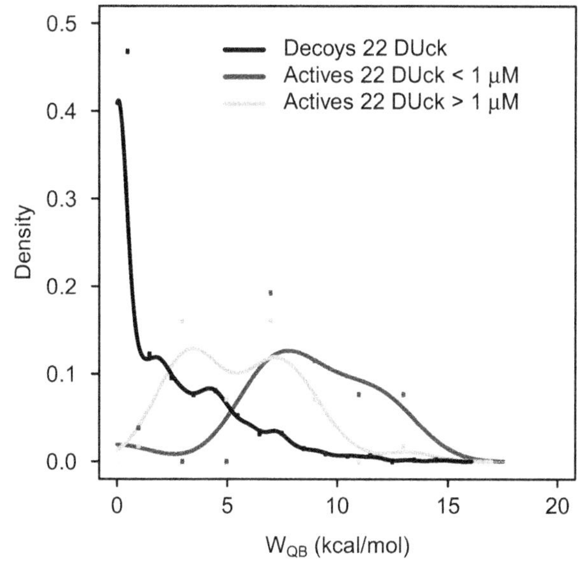

Fig. 3 Distribution of W_{QB} values of potent CDK2 ligands (IC50 $<$ 1 μM, dark gray), weak CDK2 ligands (IC50 $>$ 1 μM, light gray), and non-binding decoys (black). Points indicate population values from which the smooth lines are extrapolated

offer strong resistance to dissociation. This result is a strong indication that, as we hypothesized, true ligands form hydrogen bonds that make the protein–ligand complex structurally robust. It also indicates that this property can be used to separate active compounds from inactive ones. In consequence W_{QB} can be used in virtual screening applications. This is shown in the ROC curves plotted in Fig. 4. Here we considered one member of each of the following protein families: kinases (CDK2), GPCRs (adenosine A2A receptor), and proteases (trypsin). As shown, a selection based on this metric produces a clear enrichment in true active compounds (curves well above the diagonal). It is important to appreciate that W_{QB} offers a completely new, yet complementary, perspective on binding. While existing methods, such as docking score, try to capture the overall complementarity between two molecules in their bound state, DUck evaluates the resistance that a particular interaction opposes to geometrical perturbation. It is not surprising then that both parameters are uncorrelated (Fig. 5). Using both methods together increases the effectiveness of virtual screening over each individual method. DUck has also proven its worth in prospective validation, confirming that it can multiply the efficacy of docking-based virtual screening by detecting many of the false positives that this method produces, without introducing any false negatives [1].

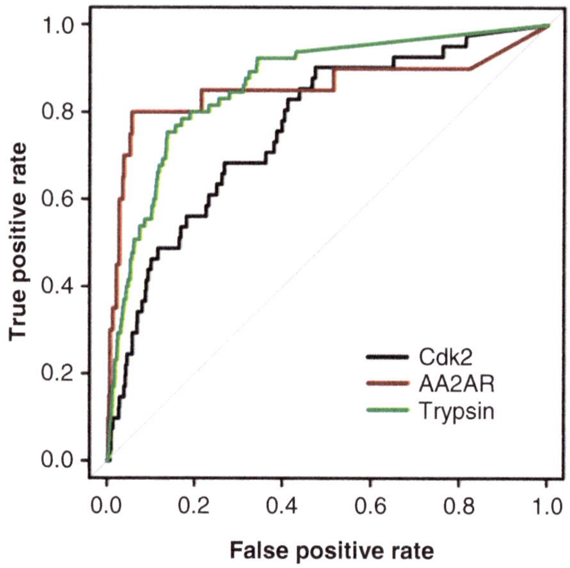

Fig. 4 ROC curves for the CDK2 (black), AA2AR (red), and trypsin (green) sets from the directory of useful decoys. The plotted results correspond to two DUck runs per ligand

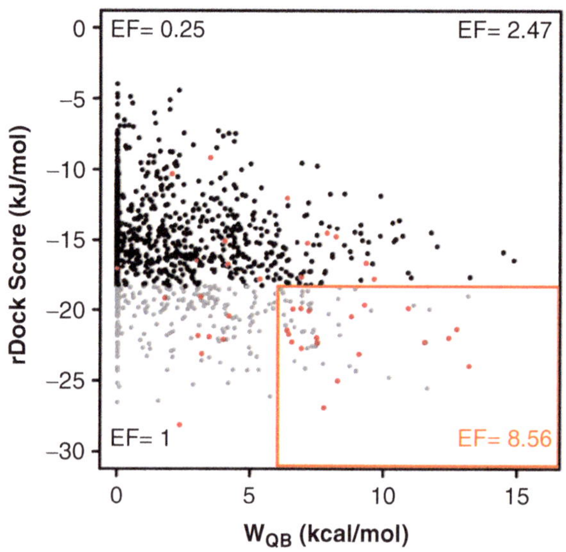

Fig. 5 Docking score (rDock) versus W_{QB} values for active (red) and inactive (black or gray) compounds in the CDK2 retrospective virtual screening dataset. The quadrant in orange highlights the area that corresponds to the top 25% docking score and top 25% W_{QB} values in which the optimal enrichment factors (EFs) are achieved

In the following sections, you will find a detailed explanation about how to prepare and run dynamic undocking. A step-by-step guide will walk you through the whole process, and a final section of "Notes" will help you in case any issues or errors arise.

2 Materials

1. Molecular Operating Environment (MOE) [6]. Download MOE (versions 2015, 2016, and above). License is required. Open MOE installer, and follow the instructions.
2. Molecular dynamics package (AMBER) [7]. Download Amber and AmberTools (version 16) from their website (http://ambermd.org/), and follow the installation instructions for your platform. AmberTools is free, but you will need a license for running Amber. Make sure AmberTools is installed locally and their binaries are visible (adapt $PATH variable if needed) so MOE can run them.
3. PyMOL [8]. Download the PyMOL molecular viewer at http://www.pymol.org/. Click on "Download." On the next page, fill out the information according to your status. Follow the instructions to download and install PyMOL.
4. R [9]. Download R software from https://cran.r-project.org/ for your platform. Follow the instructions, and make sure that R and Rscript binaries are visible during production stage.
5. DUck scripts. Download the public DUck scripts from https://github.com/CBDD/duck. Make sure $MOE_SVL_LOAD variable is declared and pointing to the DUck scripts directory (MOE2015). Make sure all scripts are located in $HOME/moefiles/svl directory (MOE2016 and newer).
6. Hardware: a computer workstation with Linux or MAC OS for DUck preparations; a computational cluster with Linux-based OS for parallelization, and GPUs for MD simulations (DUck is compatible with SGE and SLURM queuing systems).

3 Methods

3.1 Dynamic Undocking

Dynamic undocking is a particular type of molecular dynamics (MD). As such, the system must get parameters from an existing molecular mechanics force field (protein) or must be parameterized according to a compatible protocol (ligands). The protein–ligand complex must also be solvated and treated as a periodic system. Ultimately, running the dynamic undocking is just a matter of creating certain files that contain the parameters describing the system (topology file); the initial atomic positions (coordinate files); the parameters that control execution of the MD software (input files); and, finally, the sequence of commands that establish how, where, and in which order the various simulations and analysis scripts will be executed (execution files). Preparation of these files could be done in different ways, and the expert user may choose to adopt their own protocols. Equally, most MD software packages have the capability of running steered MD and could be used to carry out DUck. However, here we will describe the current protocols developed in our group. They have the advantage of being automatic and computationally efficient, but they rely on commercial software (MOE and AMBER). We are currently working to provide an open-source solution, which will follow a similar workflow to the one described herein.

3.2 Ligand Preparation

For running the dynamic undocking, we first need a collection of small molecules, or ligands, which will be subjected to the simulation. In order to correctly create this collection, the following steps should be carried out:

1. Starting from a file with all ligand structures (we use the MDL SD file format (sdf)), open it with MOE, and save it as an mdb (molecular database) file. The structure of the ligands should already be in the binding site, either from a crystallographic structure or from a binding mode predicted by docking (*see* **Note 1**).
2. All the ligands must have a well-defined protonation and tautomeric state, as parameterization and DUck simulations will use the ligands as provided by the user (*see* **Note 2**). Also, hydrogen atoms must be explicit for all molecules: to add them to all the ligands with MOE, click on Compute > Molecule > Wash. Unmark all the options, and set the Hydrogens value to Add Explicit, and name the destination field "mol" (*see* **Note 3**).

3.3 Identification of H-Bond

Dynamic undocking relies on the presence of a key interaction, specifically a hydrogen bond, which is considered fundamental for binding. Almost all protein–ligand complexes form at least one hydrogen bond. On the other hand, most systems form more than one hydrogen bond, and each of them could potentially be used as the key interaction point for DUck simulations. In practice, we use a single hydrogen bond formed between the ligand and a particular atom on the protein side. Depending on the existing data, different approaches can be used in order to identify the key interaction.

3.3.1 Case A: Multiple Protein–Ligand Complexes Are Known

1. Align the protein structures to obtain a 3D superimposition of the ligands. Then a pharmacophore can be elucidated. There are plenty of options (free and licensed software such as Maestro [10] or MOE) that allow the user to identify a

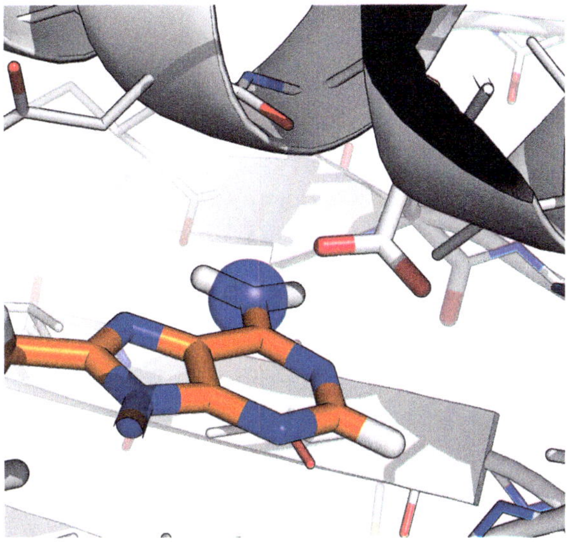

Fig. 6 An example of a complex with a single key interaction

pharmacophore for a specific protein from a given set of known binders (and non-binders).

2. From this pharmacophore identification, hydrogen bonds are detected and applied for DUck simulations, as detailed in Subheading 3.5.
3. The cases where only 1 hydrogen bond is identified, DUck will only be run for this key interaction (Fig. 6). On the other hand, there might be protein–ligand complexes with more than one hydrogen bond (Fig. 7). In this case, if there is not any additional information to identify which of these hydrogen bonds should be selected, independent DUck simulations for each of these interactions should be carried out (*see* **Note 4**).

3.3.2 Case B: Novel Binding Sites

If a pharmacophore definition can't be obtained due to a lack of known protein–ligand complexes, other approaches should be followed in order to identify possible key interaction points:

1. The structure can provide valuable hints, as the interaction will usually occupy a central position in the binding site. Further, the polar group in the protein will likely display the characteristics of an almost buried polar atom (low SASA, convex local surface curvature) and generally corresponds to a low mobility area.
2. Empirical data, especially the effect of point mutations on substrate recognition, may also be useful. On enzymes, the residues that are important for ligand recognition are often the ones that define the most important interaction with the inhibitors.

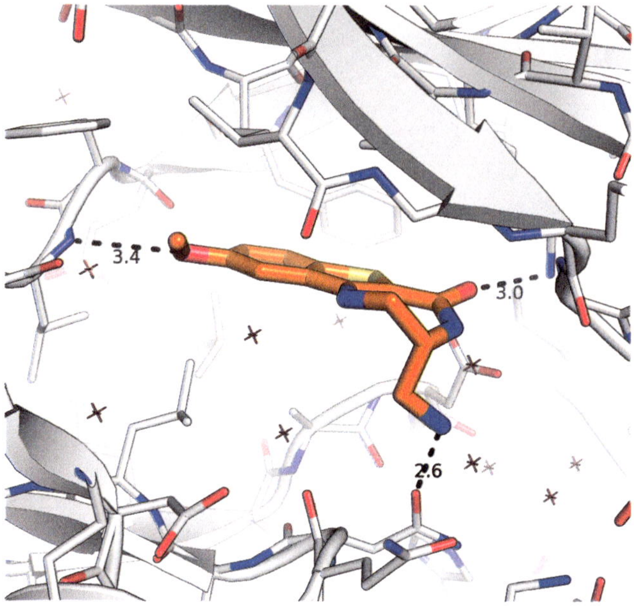

Fig. 7 An example of a complex with multiple hydrogen bonds

3. Computational methods that identify binding hot spots can be used to select a candidate interaction point. We find MDmix (MD simulations with mixed cosolvents) very useful to prioritize interaction points based on the relative strength of their binding hot spots. Other methods exist, but it's out of the scope of this book chapter to list or compare the alternatives, so we recommend the user to look to the bibliography for more details on the technique [11, 12].

3.4 Chunk Creation

One of the most important steps in system preparation is chunk selection. "Chunk" is a minimal subset of residues that preserve the local environment around the key hydrogen bond (Fig. 8).

Selection of residues is essential for the accurate result of dynamic undocking; thus very careful visual inspection is required (*see* **Note 5**). Excess residues will slow down calculation and can potentially block the ligand from leaving the pocket, resulting in very high W_{QB} values that do not reflect the strength of the hydrogen bond. An incomplete structure will result in artificially high solvent exposure, which will render the hydrogen bond more labile and cause to underestimate W_{QB} value. The following steps describe chunk preparation process:

1. If dynamic undocking was preceded by docking, it is best to use the same protonated structure. In any other case, e.g., X-ray structure, the protein structure must be prepared by protonation with a standard protocol implemented in MOE software or other protonation methods. Essential water molecules for complex stability must be identified and preserved in the

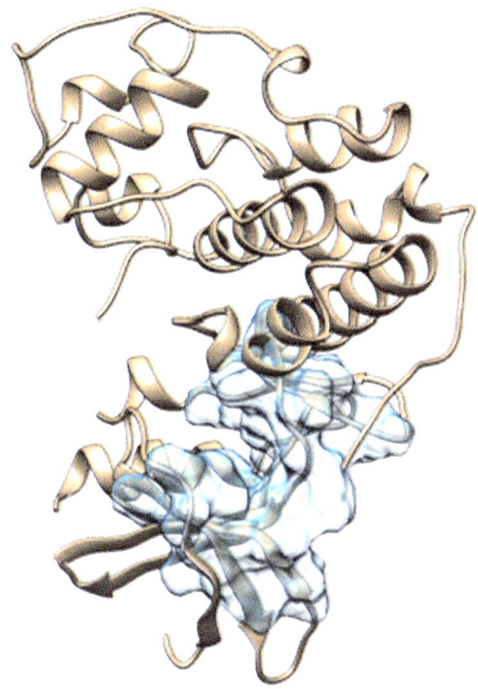

Fig. 8 Chunk of protein, constructed from pocket residues, compared to whole protein structure

structure (*see* **Note 6**). The rest of water molecules, ions, and other ligands must be removed from the system.

2. Initially, chunk is created by selecting residues within 6 Å of the atom of reference. To complete the base selection further, visual inspection is needed. Additional residues must be added, based on following rules:
   (a) Residues important for protein–ligand interaction.
   (b) Residues blocking the channels in the structure, preventing solvent molecules from accessing the key H-bond through holes created when carving the chunk out of the protein matrix.
   (c) Residues connecting parts of the chunk, if sequence gap between two selected parts of the protein is less than three residues.
   (d) Preserve interstitial water molecules that may be essential for complex stability.
3. Unselected residues are eliminated. Typically, this causes polypeptide chains to split into separate chains. To prevent charged ends and unnatural electrostatic forces, chains must be capped with acetyl and N-methyl groups.
4. Final structure has to be saved in MOE format, with names of residues adjusted to AMBER force field (*see* **Note 7**).

3.5 Simulation Preparation

In this step that has to be run in MOE, the system and simulation parameter files are generated automatically by a MOE SVL script. Before proceeding further, make sure that the MOE format file with the prepared chunk and the mdb file with ligand/poses library are located in the same directory.

1. First, the chunk structure has to be opened in MOE, and the atom defining the key protein–ligand hydrogen bond has to be selected.
2. The duck.svl script must be loaded in MOE (from $MOE_SVL_LOAD directory in MOE2015 and previous versions, for newer versions see details in **Note 8**). It opens a window with parameters for the simulation (Fig. 9).
   (a) "load additional params"—field is useful in cases of structures of ligands with metal ions (Zn^{2+}, Ca^{2+}, or Mn^{2+}), since the force field parameters for metal ions are not included in the standard force field.
   (b) The other variable is a queue system that will be used for the simulation, either SGE or SLURM. However, it is also possible to run calculations on local UNIX. Appropriate *.sh files are created when the box is marked.

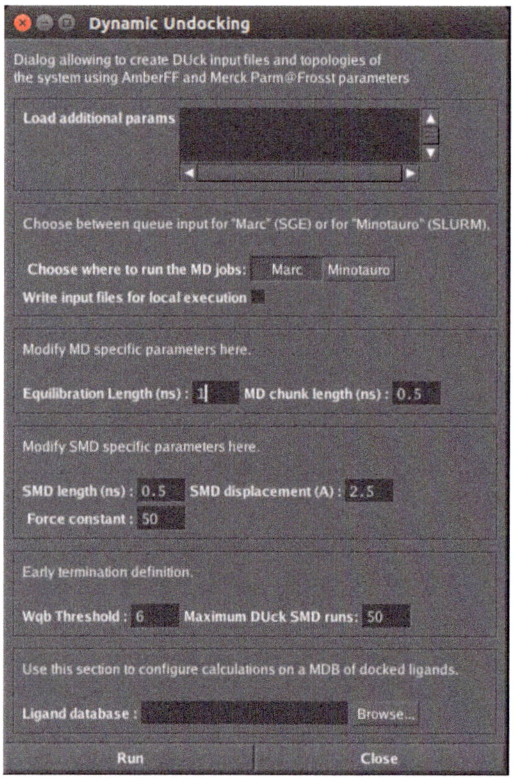

Fig. 9 Duck.svl graphical window in MOE

(c) In the next section, MD parameters can be modified:
   - "Equilibration Length" (default 1 ns).
   - "MD chunk length" (default 0.5 ns)—length of free MD between consecutive SMD simulations in order to generate different starting points for SMD.

(d) In the next section, SMD parameters can be modified:
   - "SMD length" (default 0.5 ns)—length of each SMD step.
   - "SMD displacement" (default 2.5 Å)—the distance that the ligand is going to be displaced, starting at the distance of 2.5 Å from reference atom in ligand, finishing at 5 Å by default.
   - "Force constant" (default 50 kcal/mol Å^2)—force constant of the spring that is pulling the ligand out of the pocket.

(e) In the "Early termination definition" section, following actions can be done:
   - "W_{QB} threshold" (default 6 kcal/mol)—establishes threshold of work value, below which calculations will be terminated. Optimal value depends on the system and set of ligands. For most cases, the threshold 6 kcal/mol is sufficient. If, for your system, known ligands bind with weak forces, a lower W_{QB} threshold may be necessary (*see* **Note 9**).
   - "Max DUck SMD runs" (default 50)—sets the maximum number of calculations (*see* **Note 10**).

(f) In the last section, the ligand database must be selected. Ligands have to be in the binding site, as mentioned in previous sections.

3. Executed script performs the following steps:
   (a) Calculates AM1-BCC charges [13] for all the ligands (*see* **Note 11**).
   (b) Assigns Parm@Frosst [14], atom types, and nonbonded parameters to the ligands.
   (c) Identifies the atom of each ligand that makes the hydrogen bond with the protein's reference atom (based on the distance).
   (d) Writes input and execution files to carry out the MD simulations with AMBER.
   (e) Calls AMBER's tleap to generate valid topology and coordinate files for each individual receptor–ligand complex (*see* **Note 12**).

4. The script creates a series of files that will perform the dynamic undocking, which can be later transferred to a server. For the protein, AMBER force field 99SB is used. Each system is placed in a cuboid box spanning at least 18 Å more than the furthest atom in each direction. The box is then filled with TIP3P water molecules to create periodic boundary conditions. When needed, Na^+ or Cl^- are added to force the neutrality of the whole system. As an output, the duck.svl script creates series of files:
   (a) submit_duck_smd_gpu.csh – calls *.q files in subdirectories and submits SMDs to the queue system.
   (b) getWqbValues.R – R script that calculates the value of W_{QB}. More details are given in "Result Analysis" section.
   (c) The rest of the files are collected in LIG_target_* folders, separated for every ligand:
      - duck_template_gpu.q and duck_template_gpu_325K.q—submit the SMD to queue system.
      - equil.q, md*.q—equilibration file submits a job with equilibration of the system to the server queue; the md*q files submit jobs that perform the SMDs (both in 300 K and 325 K), preceded by 0.5 ns of unbiased molecular dynamics, to increase the sampling.
      - 1_min.in, 2_eq.in, 3_eq_200.in, 3_eq_250.in, 3_eq_300.in, 4a_eq.in, 4b_eq.in—AMBER input files for the equilibration stage.
      - md.in—AMBER input files containing the parameters for the MD stage.
      - duck.in and duck_325K.in—AMBER input files with parameters for the SMD stage at 300 K and 325 K, respectively. The different temperature is simply used to ensure that both SMDs follow different trajectories even though they start from the same restart file.
      - dist_md.rst—file needed for MD simulations. It includes the indexes of the atoms that form the defined hydrogen bond and the parameters of restraints applied to ligand during MD.
      - dist_duck.rst—file needed for SMD simulations. It includes the indexes of the atoms that form the defined hydrogen bond and the initial and final distance between key atom in the receptor and end of the string that applies the force to the ligand during the SMD.
      - lib/—directory that gathers the files with coordinates and topology of the solvated system in the simulation box that will be used as input for the simulation.

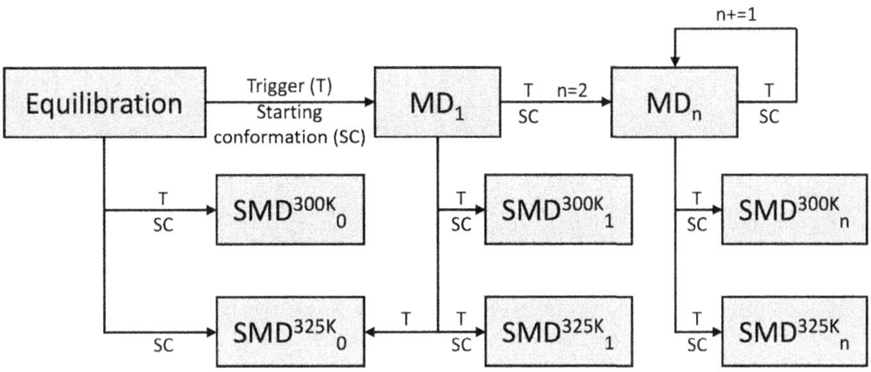

Fig. 10 Scheme of the DUck workflow

3.6 Production Stage

In the production stage, a series of MD and SMD simulations using AMBER are performed for every ligand in the library. All files required for proper execution are generated in previous stage, and they are located in LIG_target_* folders (Fig. 10).

The process is comprised by different parts:

1. First, the system is equilibrated in the following steps:
   (a) Energy minimization for 1000 cycles.
   (b) Assignment of random velocities at 100 K and gradual warming to 300 K for 400 ps in the NVT ensemble.
   (c) Equilibration of the system for 1 ns in the NPT ensemble (1 atm, 300 K).
2. Equilibration stage produces:
   (a) *.rst—restart files for the next step of calculations.
   (b) *.out—standard AMBER output files.
   (c) equil.q.e equil.q.o—files helping identifying process and errors in the simulation.
3. Equilibration stage is followed by a series of MDs and SMDs with conditions as follows:
   (a) At all stages, harmonic restraints with a force constant of 1 kcal/mol Å^2 are placed on all non-hydrogen atoms of the receptor to prevent structural changes.
   (b) Spontaneous rupture of the key hydrogen bond during non-steered simulations is prevented with a gradual restraint for distances beyond 3 Å (parabolic with $k = 1$ kcal/mol, Å^2 between 3 Å and 4 Å, and linear with $k = 10$ kcal/mol Å^2 beyond 4 Å).
   (c) All equilibration and simulation steps were run using Langevin thermostat with a collision frequency of 4 ps^{-1}, and the cutoff for nonbonded interactions was set to 12 Å.
   (d) Bonds involving hydrogen are constrained using SHAKE.

4. The first step of SMD is executed in 300 K. The SMD lasts 500 ps, during which time the distance between the atoms forming the key hydrogen bond is steered, by default, from 2.5 Å to 5.0 Å (this distance, however, can be changed in the parameters, as explained in Subheading 3.5), with constant velocity of 5 Å/ns and spring constant of 50 kcal/mol Å^2. Once the first SMD is completed, W_{QB} is evaluated, which can trigger the continuation of the process or stop the simulation altogether if W_{QB} is lower than the predefined threshold. Thus, running the first SMD only at one temperature saves calculation time. Results of SMD are gathered in DUCK_* folder:
   (a) duck.dat—file with four columns (*see* **Note 13**):
      - Distance between reference atom in chunk and place where the additional potential is applied.
      - Distance between key atom in chunk and equivalent atom in ligand.
      - Value of force applied to ligand.
      - Value of work.
   (b) duck_*.q.e duck_*.q.o—files that help the identifying process and errors in the simulation.
5. The first step of MD follows the trajectory generated by equilibration stage in the previous step.
6. The MD stage produces:
   (a) *.rst—restart files for the next step of calculations.
   (b) *.out—standard AMBER output files.
   (c) md.q.e md.q.o—files helping identifying process and errors in the simulation.
7. The first MD triggers the first SMD in 325 K and two new SMDs in both temperatures. The first SMD in higher temperature starts from the same restart file as the first SMD in 300 K (**step 4**). The two subsequent SMDs follow the trajectory generated by first MD and proceed at different temperatures (300 K and 325 K) to ensure different trajectories.
8. To generate diverse starting points for SMD trajectories, we perform 0.5 ns of unbiased MD simulation, and repeat the process as many times as set in the SVL window (e.g., 50 steps of unbiased MD simulations are needed to execute 100 SMD trajectories). Fifty is enough repetitions to satisfactory evaluate W_{QB} value. To decrease time of calculation for virtual screening, 5 SMDs runs are recommended.
   (a) Before and after performing every DUck step, getWqbValues.R script calculates the W_{QB} value, and if it is greater than established threshold, md{n + 1}.q will be submitted.

Jobs must be submitted to server queue manager.

(a) SLURM queue system:

- $ sbatch equil.q.

(b) SGE queue system:

- $ qsub equil.q.

3.7 Analysis

Once the production stage is finished, the work necessary to reach the quasi-bound state can be calculated:

1. In the simulation preparation stage, the script for calculating the W_{QB} is created and stored in the main folder of the DUck project. To run it, enter the desired folder, and run it as Rscript ../getWqbValues.R that will return the W_{QB} value on standard output. It will read the output from all completed SMDs that have finished, and return the lowest value of all W_{QB} values calculated for each replica.
2. To visualize the results, the same script can be called with the flag "plot" that will generate a summary plot, "wqb_plot.png" (Fig. 11), and a file, "wqb_final.txt," with the calculated W_{QB} in the first and only line (8.29 for the example in Fig. 11).
3. This script can be called at any time, so it might happen that some SMD simulations are still running or they have finished earlier than they should. These and other types of errors are taken into account by the script. More details on how these errors are managed are provided in **Note 14**.

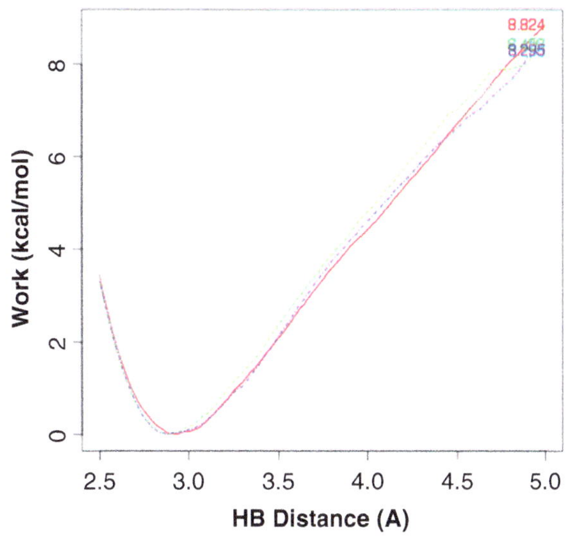

Fig. 11 Example of summary plot of W_{QB} obtained by running Rscript ../ getWqbValues.R plot

4 Notes

1. Dynamic undocking needs a starting pose of the ligand in the binding site. This starting pose can be obtained from a crystallographic structure, ideally, but also from binding mode prediction programs such as docking. In the latter case, the user needs to be sure that the starting pose is representative of true pose; otherwise dynamic undocking calculations might be wrong.
2. Having the correct protonation and tautomeric states is something that has been widely discussed in the past years. For docked poses, the different stereoisomers should be generated prior to running docking, i.e., with programs like Schrödinger's ligprep or Chemaxon suite. On the other hand, most of the ligands that come from crystallographic structures of the PDB are correct. However, some of them have incorrectly assigned topologies, or the tautomeric state is not well defined. Double checking the structure by digging in the publication could avoid problems in the following stages.
3. After washing the molecules to add the explicit hydrogen atoms, be sure that the field is called mol. Dynamic undocking will use the "mol" field to prepare the simulations and parametrize the ligands. If no "mol" field is found, the first field with "molecule" format will be used.

   In order to avoid problems regarding this issue, it is strongly recommended to change the field name of the unwashed molecule to "mol_unwashed," for example, and then save the washed molecules in a field named "mol."
4. One common problem in the identification of the key hydrogen bond is the case where more than one hydrogen bond could be selected. In ref. 1, there is a specific example addressing this issue: a ligand had three different hydrogen bonds, and it turned out that the one used for the rest of the ligands in the dataset was not the key interaction point for this ligand. After running two more DUck simulations with the other possibilities, the key interaction was identified. The suggested approach when the user happens to be in such scenario is to run independent runs for each of the possible hydrogen bonds and select the one with higher W_{QB}.
5. In case of multiple interaction points (hydrogen bonds) are selected, individual chunks of protein must be created for each key atom separately.
6. Water molecules can have a big influence on complex stability. Some water molecules mediate interactions between ligand and protein. It is worth inspecting the structure more closely and preserving important water molecules. For example, in

complexes of Hsp90, water molecules are crucial in mediating interactions between protein and ligand.

7. If the structure of the chunk contains ASH residue, duck.svl will crash during tleap system preparation stage. Crash is caused by different namings of residues in MOE and AMBER. To fix the problem, remove HD2 hydrogen from the structure, and run duck.svl script on modified system.
8. Preparation process described in the chapter is adjusted to MOE2015. In MOE2016, developer changed the way that environmental variables are handled. In the new version of MOE, copy the svl files /scripts and /tleap to the $HOME/moefiles/svl directory, and run svl as described in the chapter.
9. If structures of protein with ligands are available, the best way to estimate W_{QB} threshold value is to run DUck for the known complexes. Use exhaustive sampling (20–50 SMDs).
10. 50 SMD runs are recommended for precise estimation of W_{QB} value. For accurate estimation, 20 runs is enough. For virtual screening purposes, 5–7 runs with threshold-based early termination are recommended.
11. SVL script might crash during calculation of AM1-BCC charges for the ligand. If so, the script will not create systems for invalid ligands, leaving a gap in LIG_target_* folders numbering. The easiest way to avoid the problem is calculating partial charges in MOE. Load *.mdb file with ligand/pose library, and calculate partial charges (Compute > Molecule > Partial charges…) with "AM1-BCC" selected in the "Method" field. If charges are calculated for all of ligands without problem, SVL script should run smoothly. Otherwise, discard or fix the problematic ligands. Sometimes crash is caused by the initial 3D geometry (e.g., internal clash), and slight changes of atomic positions (e.g., bond rotation) can fix the issue.
12. Another problem with system preparation might be caused by tleap. In case system cannot be created, the following error will be displayed:

    Error, tleap did not manage to build the system.
    There might be a couple of reasons for such error:

    (a) tleap cannot be run from the terminal. Make sure that AmberTools is properly installed and can be executed in the terminal. Loading appropriate module might be necessary.
    (b) If the chunk contains ASH residue. For solution look at **Note 7**.
    (c) Wrong force field file pointed in SVL script. For new version of AmberTools (16), FF file is named leaprc.

ff99Bild; however for older versions, this file may be in oldFF directory. In this case to fix the error, editing duck.svl script is required.

$ sed 's/leaprc\.ff99Bild/oldFF\/leaprc\.ff99Bild/' duck.svl > tmp.
$ mv tmp duck.svl

13. Checking duck.dat is the best way to ensure that the step of the simulation is completed. With the default parameters, this file should be exactly 5000 lines long. If something went wrong during the simulation, e.g., the server crashed, for some of the ligands, this file will be shorter.
14. The script to calculate the W_{QB} can be run at any point of the DUck simulation. This can lead to error where some SMD simulations are not over or have been abruptly terminated, which is of particular importance when the script is used to decide whether more steps of MD + SMD simulations need to be carried or not.

A correctly finished SMD simulation will have a duck.dat file similar to:

2.50000	2.92018	−42.01769	0.00000
2.50050	2.78965	−28.91455	−0.01097
2.50100	2.55078	−4.97794	−0.02026
2.50150	2.71974	−21.82384	−0.02933
2.50200	2.63421	−13.22120	−0.03907
[...]			
4.99700	5.02624	−2.92401	0.30579
4.99750	5.09999	−10.24863	0.30125
4.99800	4.98177	1.62251	0.30058
4.99850	5.00014	−0.16448	0.29868
4.99900	5.06074	−6.17372	0.29649
4.99950	5.04282	−4.33195	0.29338

where 2.5 and 5.0 are the defined starting and final point of the hydrogen bond distance. The script will check that the final line is actually the defined final point (±0.001 A); otherwise it will return a W_{QB} of 100.

References

1. Ruiz-Carmona S, Schmidtke P, Luque FJ et al (2017) Dynamic undocking and the quasi-bound state as tools for drug discovery. Nat Chem 9(3):201–206. https://doi.org/10.1038/nchem.2660
2. Chodera JD, Mobley DL, Shirts MR et al (2011) Alchemical free energy methods for drug discovery : progress and challenges. Curr Opin Struct Biol 21(2):150–160. https://doi.org/10.1016/j.sbi.2011.01.011
3. Schmidtke P, Luque FJ, Murray JB, Barril X (2011) Shielded hydrogen bonds as structural determinants of binding kinetics: application in drug design. J Am Chem Soc 133 (46):18903–18910. https://doi.org/10.1021/ja207494u
4. Ferenczy GG, Keseru GM (2012) Thermodynamics of fragment binding. J Chem Inf Model 52(4):1039–1045. https://doi.org/10.1021/ci200608b
5. Huang N, Shoichet BK, Irwin JJ (2006) Benchmarking sets for molecular docking. J Med Chem 49(23):6789–6801. https://doi.org/10.1021/jm0608356
6. Molecular Operating Environment (MOE), 2013.08 (2016) Chemical Computing Group Inc., 1010 Sherbooke St. West, Suite #910, Montreal, QC, Canada, H3A 2R7
7. Case DA et al (2016) Amber 16. University of California, San Francisco
8. DeLano WL (2014) The PyMOL Molecular Graphics System, Version 1.8. Schrödinger LLC. http://www.pymol.org. https://doi.org/10.1038/hr.2014.17
9. R Core Team (2017) R: a language and environment for statistical computing. R Foundation for Statistical Computing, Vienna, Austria https://www.R-project.org/
10. Schrödinger Release 2017-3: Maestro, Schrödinger, LLC, New York, NY, 2017
11. Seco J, Luque FJ, Barril X (2009) Binding site detection and druggability index from first principles. J Med Chem 52(8):2363–2371. https://doi.org/10.1021/jm801385d
12. Álvarez-García D, Barril X (2014) Molecular simulations with solvent competition quantify water displaceability and provide accurate interaction maps of protein binding sites. J Med Chem 57(20):8530–8539. https://doi.org/10.1021/jm5010418
13. Jakalian A, Jack DB, Bayly CI (2002) Fast, efficient generation of high-quality atomic charges. AM1-BCC model: II. Parameterization and validation. J Comp Chem 23(16):1623–1641. https://doi.org/10.1002/jcc.10128
14. Bayly CI, McKay D, Truchon J-F (2011) An Informal AMBER Small Molecule Force Field: parm@Frosst. Computational Chemistry Ltd.

Chapter 12

The Impact of Lipophilicity in Drug Discovery: Rapid Measurements by Means of Reversed-Phase HPLC

Constantinos Giaginis, Fotios Tsopelas, and Anna Tsantili-Kakoulidou

Abstract

Lipophilicity constitutes a vital physicochemical property in drug design as it is connected with pharmacodynamic and pharmacokinetic properties as well as toxicological aspects of candidate drugs. Traditional partitioning experiments to determine *n*-octanol-water coefficients are laborious and time-consuming, while they cannot be reliably performed for highly lipophilic or compounds undergoing degradation. Alternatively, lipophilicity of candidate drugs can be accurately and reproducibly determined using reversed-phase liquid chromatography. In this chapter, the details of protocols for lipophilicity assessment using reversed-phase HPLC, under conditions which provide the best simulation of *n*-octanol-water partition coefficients, are described.

Key words Lipophilicity, *n*-Octanol-water partition coefficient, Reversed-phase HPLC, Extrapolated retention factors, *n*-Octanol as mobile phase additive

1 Introduction

Lipophilicity, expressed by the logarithm of *n*-octanol-water partition coefficient log*P* or distribution coefficient log*D*, if ionized molecular species are present, constitutes a physicochemical property of paramount importance in the design of new drug molecules, influencing both pharmacokinetic and pharmacodynamic behavior as well as toxicological aspects [1–4]. The importance of lipid solubility in biological activity has been demonstrated already at the dawn of the twentieth century, when Meyer [5] and Overton [6] independently reported the correlation of narcosis with oil-water partition coefficients. However, research on lipophilicity was systematically investigated by the pioneer team of C. Hansch, T. Fujita, and A. Leo, who associated this property both with the probability of a drug to access its site of action and its hydrophobic binding to macromolecules. The same authors introduced *n*-octanol-water as the reference system to construct an empirical scale for partition coefficients [7, 8]. They defined log*P* as the logarithm of

Thomas Mavromoustakos and Tahsin F. Kellici (eds.), *Rational Drug Design: Methods and Protocols*, Methods in Molecular Biology, vol. 1824, https://doi.org/10.1007/978-1-4939-8630-9_12, © Springer Science+Business Media, LLC, part of Springer Nature 2018

the concentration of the neutral species of the compound in the partition solvent (*n*-octanol) to the concentration of the same species in water, keeping into consideration that the compound exists in monomeric species (Eq. 1).

$$\log P = \log\,[\text{neutral species}]_{\text{oct}} \backslash [\text{neutral species}]_{\text{water}} \quad (1)$$

Lipophilicity changes as a function of pH for ionizable compounds. The log*D* value denotes the lipophilicity at a given pH and corresponds to the logarithm of the concentration ratio of all electrical (monomeric) species in the organic and aqueous phase (Eq. 2).

$$\log D = \log\,[\text{all species}]_{\text{oct}}/[\text{all species}]_{\text{water}} \quad (2)$$

For a solute with a single ionizable group, log*D* is the outcome of the partition coefficient of the neutral species P^{N} plus the partition coefficient of the ionized species P^{I}, each multiplied by the fraction *f* present in the mixture (Eq. 3).

$$\log D_{\text{pH}} = \log\,(f_{\text{N}} \cdot P^{\text{N}} + f_{\text{I}} \cdot P^{\text{I}}) \quad (3)$$

If the p*K*a of a monofunctional solute is known, log*P* and log*D* can be interconverted according to Eq. 4, provided that only the neutral species partition into the organic solvent.

$$\log P = \log D + \log\left[10^{\pm(\text{pH}-\text{p}K\text{a})}\right] \quad (4)$$

where positive sign counts for acids and negative for bases.

However, in the case of a high degree of ionization, charged species, accompanied by a counterion, may contribute to the "true" log*D* value as ion pairs, which are able to partition into *n*-octanol, while they may also partition into the saturation water present in wet *n*-octanol [9, 10].

For solutes with more ionizable groups, more complex equations are used for the interconversion, taking into account all p*K*as. In the case of ampholytes, log*P* can be calculated from log*D* and p*K*a only if acidic p*K*a is higher than basic p*K*a (ordinary ampholytes). For ampholytes forming zwitterionic species, maximum log*D* ($\log D_{\text{max}}$) at isoelectric point is considered, since no "true" log*P* value exists. The particular behavior of zwitterionic drugs may have implications in their pharmacokinetic behavior [11].

1.1 Lipophilicity in Drug Action

Lipophilicity is essential for drug accessibility to the site of action, as it influences permeability through membranes. Membrane permeability may follow parabolic or bilinear relationships with log*P* or log*D*, and optimum log*P* (log*Po*) or log*D* (log*Do*) values have been defined for penetration through certain biological barriers [4, 12–14]. Characteristically, for blood-brain barrier penetration, the crucial biological barrier for CNS action, an optimum lipophilicity around 2, is considered. Sigmoidal relationships between permeability and log*D* have also been reported [15, 16].

On the other hand, hydrophobic binding usually correlates linearly with log*P*. Hydrophobic binding is considered as an indirect non-specific "bond." It is the result of the displacement of water molecules from the nonpolar surfaces to interact between them, thus leading to an increase in entropy [17, 18]. High lipophilicity of drug molecules favors hydrophobic binding and may increase affinity to the target receptor. It should be noted that in binding studies, lipophilicity is expressed by log*P* of the neutral species, even in the case of ionizable compounds.

There is however strong evidence that high lipophilicity is associated with undesired drug features. It is generally considered that very lipophilic compounds are "preferred" targets for biotransformation, thus leading to extensive and unpredictable metabolism. High plasma protein binding, influencing drug efficacy and drug safety and often responsible for drug-drug interactions, is also observed for highly lipophilic compounds, as well as promiscuous binding to off-targets or accumulation to tissues [19–21].

Hansch et al. were the first to outline such problems, and in a paper published in 1987, they formulated the concept of minimum hydrophobicity. According to this concept, research should focus on compounds with no more lipophilicity than that required for their biological action (permeability and affinity [12]. Ten years later, upper limits for log*P* values were proposed by Lipinski et al. who included lipophilicity (as clog*P*) in the well-known rule of 5 (RoF) [22]. RoF was the first rule of "thumb," formulated as an alert or filter for oral bioavailability. Ro5 influenced the perception of medicinal chemists regarding drug physicochemical properties and chemical space exploration. It was soon followed by other "metrics," identifying additional properties to define the drug-like space [23–26]. In most of these metrics, lipophilicity (expressed as log*P* or log*D*) keeps its central role often coupled to molecular weight. The term "molecular obesity" as an unfavorable molecular feature refers to the big size and high lipophilicity and is expressed by ligand efficiency (LE) and ligand lipophilicity efficiency (LLE) which normalize affinity to the number of heavy atoms and to log*P*, respectively [27, 28].

1.2 Advantages of Chromatographic Techniques in Lipophilicity Assessment

In light of the above discussion, it is evident that rapid knowledge of log*P* is essential in early drug discovery phases, and research efforts to develop high-throughput experimental techniques or to establish reliable calculation methods are well justified. Predictions of log*P* are valuable for compound library screening, filtering, and preselection of molecules, and many relevant softwares are available [29]. However the complex nature of lipophilicity as the outcome of inter- and intramolecular interactions is far from being precisely encoded in the various algorithms, and the reliability of the available software depends on the chemical structure and the inherent conception of the method [29, 30], while it cannot always follow the advances in synthetic chemistry. It should be noted that, considering the equations correlating the observed log*P* values to those predicted by the calculation systems, an error of about 0.8 log unit is tolerated, according to the two times the standard deviation criterion. Thus, for new chemotypes, synthesized as potential drug candidates, calculated log*P* values may be misleading in modeling their biological activity or in estimating their permeability potential [31].

In this aspect, there is a vital need for accurate measurements in the laboratory, while new experimental log*P* values provide feedback for updating existing software. Different experimental protocols for log*P* or log*D* determination have been reported in literature. The classical shaking flask method for direct partitioning experiments is tedious and time-consuming, not suitable for degradable compounds, less amenable to automation, while it presents limitations concerning the log*P* (or log*D*) range which can be reliably measured [32, 33]. The dual-phase potentiometric titration suitable for ionizable drugs, on the other hand, requires special equipment, not always available in an analytical laboratory [34].

Chromatographic techniques and in particular reversed-phase HPLC offer a friendly alternative for lipophilicity assessment, since it is well known that under suitable conditions, retention factors simulate octanol-water partition coefficients [35–37]. The practical advantages of chromatographic techniques such as speed, accuracy, repeatability, broader dynamic range (especially to high lipophilicity areas), high automatization ability, insensitivity to impurities/degradation products, and reduced sample handling/sample sizes [35–37] justify the considerable research interest devoted to the investigation of HPLC-based lipophilicity, compared to traditional octanol-water partitioning and the common factors underlying the two processes [37–39]. Retention factors, either isocratic log*k* or extrapolated to 100% aqueous phase $\log k_w$, correlate with log*P* according to Collander-type equations.

$$\log P = a \log k (\text{or} \log k_w) + b \tag{5}$$

A problem that had to be faced early enough in lipophilicity assessment by HPLC is the silanophilic effect, e.g., interactions with remaining free silanol groups of the reversed-phase C18-silanized columns, which may interfere to the partition mechanism [36, 37]. Such interactions can be reduced by the selection of suitable stationary and mobile phases.

The most widely used stationary phases are C18-silanized silica gel columns, either end-capped (BDS column) or polar-embedded (ABZ^+, Discovery RP-Amide C16, Discovery BioWide Pore C-18 column). In end-capped columns, free silanol groups react with small alkyls in a second silanization process. On the other hand, polar-embedded columns contain an amide functional group which provides electrostatic shielding to the silanol sites, while a high degree of orientation of the alkyl chains is achieved [40]. Polar end-capped Aquasil column has also been suggested for hydrophilic compounds [41].

Mobile phases usually consist of methanol as organic modifier at different proportions and morpholine propanesulfonic acid (MOPS) or phosphate buffer as the aqueous component. Methanol has the advantage to disturb less the structure of water, while it provides H-bond sensitivity to the stationary phase by creating a monolayer on it [36]. Addition of small amounts of hydrophobic amines (usually *n*-decylamine) is a common practice in order to further suppress silanophilic interactions [36–38].

Equations of type (5) can be used as calibration equations to calculate $\log P$ of unknown compounds. If isocratic $\log k$ values are used, it is recommended to construct more than one calibration equation at different proportions of organic modifier and to calculate the mean $\log P$ values [42], since a lipophilicity inversion can occur with varying percentage of organic modifier. Extrapolated $\log k_{\mathrm{w}}$ values are determined considering the linear part of the $\log k/\varphi$ relationship according to Eq. 6.

$$\log k = -S\,\varphi + \log k_{\mathrm{w}} \tag{6}$$

where φ is the fraction of organic modifier.

Alternative chromatographic measure for lipophilicity assessment is the chromatographic hydrophobicity index (CHI), which corresponds to the fraction of organic modifier φo which produces equal distribution ($\log k = 0$) of the compounds between stationary and mobile phase [43, 44]. The organic modifier fraction φo, as the quotient of the slope to the intercept of Eq. 6, exhibits good correlation with $\log P$ [45], whereas it has been shown that it correlates with the gradient retention times. Thus, CHI indices can be determined by a fast gradient method and can be projected to $\log D$ (CHI$\log D$) via a calibration equation, constructed with measured octanol-water $\log D$ values of standard compounds [44, 45]. For CHI determination, acetonitrile is used as organic modifier and ammonium acetate as buffer. Such conditions do not take into account the effect of silanophilic interactions, while acetonitrile does not deliver any polar functionalities to the stationary phase [36]. Thus, CHI indices perform better in the case of the neutral state of compounds [43]. Moreover they cannot be applied for hydrophilic compounds where the presence of organic modifier produces very rapid elution.

Other authors and our group orient research efforts to the standardization of the chromatographic conditions for most appropriate $\log k_{\mathrm{w}}$ retention factors as $\log P$ or $\log D$ surrogates and to the establishment of a relevant calibration equation for general use [46–49]. This goal has been practically achieved for neutral and basic compounds, as well as for acidic compounds in their neutral state or at relatively low ionization. In such cases 1:1 correlations are obtained, with a and b in Eq. 5 close to 1 and 0, respectively, indicating homoenergetics between retention mechanism and n-octanol-water partitioning. In those reports, a crucial common factor for better simulation of $\log k_w$ with $\log P$ (or $\log D$) is the presence of small amounts of n-octanol as mobile phase additive, which render an "octanol-like character" to the stationary phase. The influence of n-octanol on retention decreases with increasing lipophilicity, and for compounds with $\log P > 2$, its effect is negligible [49].

For basic and neutral drugs, the $\mathrm{E}\log D$ approach suggests as standard chromatographic conditions the use of ABZ^+ column and mobile phases consisting of mixtures of methanol/MOPS, pH 7.4, with the addition of small amounts of n-decylamine and n-octanol [46]. Retention factors of $\log k_w$ are obtained upon extrapolation of only three isocratic $\log k$ values, depending on lipophilicity range. The high-quality calibration Eq. ($R = 0.982$, $s = 0.309$), obtained using a training set of 90 drugs, has a slope close to unity ($a = 1.13$) and a small intercept ($b = 0.21$). The approach achieves an average determination time < 20 min with reproducibility and good accuracy in most cases. However, the use of only three fractions of organic modifier may not always be appropriate, since it does not guarantee that measurements fall within the linear range of the $\log k/\varphi$ relationship.

We have proposed an analogous procedure using a BDS column and the same mobile phase conditions, but at least five isocratic $\log k$ values, carefully selected in the range $-0.5 < \log k < 1.1$, so as to belong to the linear part of the $\log k/\varphi$ relationship [48]. Under these conditions the high-quality calibration equation obtained for 64 drugs corresponds to a true 1:1 correlation (Eq. 7). Thus, practically $\log k_w$ values do not differ from $\log P$ or $\log D$, in most cases being below the error tolerated by the calculation systems.

$$\log D_{7.4} = 1.03(\pm 0.03) \log k_w + 0.14(\pm 0.07)$$
$$n = 64 \; r = 0.966 \; s = 0.288 \qquad (7)$$

In a further step, we extended our research to account for acidic and ampholytic compounds. For pH 2.5 a 1:1 correlation was obtained using a BDS column and methanol/MOPS mixtures, upon saturation of the buffer with n-octanol and no further addition of n-octanol in the volume of methanol (Eq. 8) [41, 49].

$$\log D_{2.5} = 1.02(\pm 0.03) \log k_w + 0.05(\pm 0.07)$$
$$n = 43 \; r = 0.966 \; s = 0.311 \qquad (8)$$

Analogous but slightly inferior results were obtained using a ABZ^+ column under the same mobile phase conditions [41].

For pH 7.4, the addition of 0.25% n-octanol in the volume of methanol proved necessary. However, it was not possible to obtain a general calibration equation, and the data set should be divided into weak acid and strong acid subsets. Strong acids were considered as those fully ionized at pH 7.4. For weak acids a high significant 1:1 correlation was obtained (Eq. 9).

$$\log D_{7.4} = 1.04(\pm 0.05)\log k_{\mathrm{w}} + 0.09(\pm 0.09)$$
$$n = 22 \; r = 0.966 \; s = 0.338 \qquad (9)$$

For strong acids a good calibration equation was also obtained, however with a slope lower than unity and a large negative intercept, indicating a strong affinity of anions to the silica-based stationary phase, although not absolutely systematic (Eq. 10).

$$\log D_{7.4} = 0.85(\pm 0.04)\log k_{\mathrm{w}} - 0.91(\pm 0.08)$$
$$n = 21 \; r = 0.952 \; s = 0.266 \qquad (10)$$

In the next section, the details of the above described protocols for lipophilicity assessment of basic/neutral (training set I) and acidic ampholytic (training set II) compounds are described.

2 Materials

1. The data set including 40 basic and 24 neutral drugs is described in ref. 48.
2. The data set including 40 acidic and 5 ampholytic drugs is described in ref. 49.

Morpholine propanesulfonic acid (MOPS) and *n*-decylamine were analytical grade. N-octanol was extra pure. Water was deionized and further purified by means of a Milli-Q Plus water purification system, Millipore Ltd.

2.1 Chromatographic Conditions

An HPLC isocratic pumping system (GBC Model 1126 pump) and a Rheodyne Model 7725i GBC injector with a 20 μl loop, coupled to a UV-Vis detector, are used. The detector operates at appropriate wavelength (220, 254, 268 nm) depending on the drugs analyzed. Data acquisition is performed using WinChrom chromatography software package version 2.1 implemented in the chromatographic system (*see* **Note 1**).

The stationary phase is a Hypersil BDS C18 Column (250 × 4.6 mm i.d., 5 μm particle size, pore volume 0.67 cc/g) (*see* **Note 2**).

The mobile phase consists of different mixtures of methanol/20 mM MOPS, in the range 10–75%, depending on compound lipophilicity (*see* **Note 3**). The pH is adjusted to 7.4 or 2.5 by 1 M NaOH or concentrated phosphoric acid, respectively. MOPS is previously saturated with *n*-octanol (*see* **Note 4**).

The following additives are used:

1. For basic and neutral drugs, buffer at pH 7.4 was used: *n*-decylamine 0.15% v/v in respect to the total volume of the mobile phase + *n*-octanol 0.25% in respect to the volume of methanol.
2. For acidic compounds in their neutral state (pH 2.5): *n*-octanol present in saturated MOPS was used with no further addition. For ionized acidic compounds, pH 7.4 was used: *n*-octanol 0.25% in respect to the volume of methanol.

3 Methods

After equilibration of stationary/mobile phase (*see* **Note 5**), retention times *tr* are measured at least from three separate injections and converted to the logarithm of retention factors via Eq. 11

$$\log k = \log \frac{tr - to}{to} \tag{11}$$

t_o being the retention time of methanol.

The eluent flow rate was 1 mL/min. All measurements were performed at room temperature.

Retention factors corresponding to 100% water ($\log k_w$) are derived from the linear part of the $\log k/\varphi$ relationship, using at least five isocratic $\log k$ values (*see* **Note 6**) according to Eq. 6 (*see* **Note 7**).

3.1 Calculation of logP and logD7.4

1. The $\log k_w$ values of neutral and basic compounds are fitted to Eq. 7, reported in ref. 48, in order to calculate $\log P$ or $\log D_{7.4}$, respectively. However since differences between $\log P$ and $\log k_w$ values are very small (1:1 correlation), the latter can also be used as such.
2. The $\log k_w$ values of acidic drugs are fitted to Eq. 8, reported in ref. 49 to calculate $\log P$ (*see* **Note 8**).

To calculate $\log D_{7.4}$, Eq. 9 reported in ref. 49 is used for partially ionized acidic drugs, or $\log k_w$ can be used as such (1:1 correlation). Equation 10 also reported in ref. 49 is used to calculate $\log D_{7.4}$ for strongly ionized drugs (*see* **Note 9**).

4 Notes

1. Any other HPLC instrumentation can be used.
2. ABZ^+ column, a Discovery RP-Amide or a Discovery BioWide Pore C-18 column can also be used.
3. It is recommended before experiment to estimate compound lipophilicity using a calculation system. Estimation of

lipophilicity enables to choose the percentage of methanol to start with. For lipophilic compounds ($\log P > 2$), one can start with 50% methanol; for less lipophilic compounds, initial methanol percentage can be 30%.

4. Saturation is achieved by gently shaking the buffer with a small volume of *n*-octanol, leaving it overnight and separating the aqueous phase.
5. Equilibration may need more time due to the presence of *n*-octanol in the mobile phase. A very good washing of the HPLC system is required before a new mobile phase is used and at the end of the experiments.
6. For highly lipophilic compounds, where high percentages of methanol are used, extrapolation can be performed with four or even three $\log k$ values, provided that the correlation coefficient is high enough. For less lipophilic compound, linearity should always be checked.
7. If the entire organic modifier range is considered, the relationship between retention factors and the fraction of the organic modifier φ follows the Schoenmakers' solubility parameter model expressed by Eq. 12 [50].

$$\log k = A\varphi + B\varphi^2 + E\sqrt{\varphi} + \log k_{\mathrm{w}} \qquad (12)$$

The $B\varphi^2$ term accounts for the curvature (concave) at higher organic modifier concentrations partly attributed to silanophilic interactions, while $E\sqrt{\varphi}$ accounts for a curvature (concave or convex) observed at water-rich mobile phases ($\varphi < 20\%$) due to stationary phase solvation problems.

Extrapolation is performed using linear regression analysis using the linear part of Eq. 12, which corresponds to Eq. 6.

8. Zwitterionic compounds should be considered with caution. Retention factors of zwitterionic thiazolidinediones (pioglitazone and rosiglitazone) included in data set II did not show linearity at any proportion of organic modifier, and extrapolated retention factors could not be obtained at pH 2.5. In this pH the basic function is protonated and may interact with the silanols via hydrogen bond interactions.
9. Despite the high affinity of organic anions for silica-based stationary phases, very hydrophilic anionic drugs may elute with the dead time even at 100% aqueous phase. This is a limitation of the HPLC technique, which cannot be used in those cases.

References

1. Hansch C, Leo A (eds) (1995) Exploring QSAR: fundamentals and applications in chemistry and biology. American Chemical Society, Washington, D.C.

2. Testa B, Crivori P, Reist M, Carrupt P-A (2000) The influence of lipophilicity on the pharmacokinetic behavior of drugs: concepts and examples. Perspect Drug Discov 17:179–211. https://doi.org/10.1023/A:1008741731244
3. Arnott JA, Planey SL (2012) The influence of lipophilicity in drug discovery and design. Expert Opin Drug Discov 7(10):863–875. https://doi.org/10.1517/17460441.2012.714363
4. Tsopelas F, Giaginis C, Tsantili-Kakoulidou A (2017) Lipophilicity and biomimetic properties to support drug discovery. Expert Opin Drug Discov 12(9):885–896. https://doi.org/10.1080/17460441.2017.1344210
5. Meyer H (1899) Zur Theorie der Alkoholnarkose. Arch Exp Pathol Pharmakol 42:109–118. https://doi.org/10.1007/BF01834480
6. Overton E (1901) Studien uber die narkose zugleich ein beitrag zur allgemeinen pharmakologie. Gustav Fischer, Jena
7. Hansch C, Fujita T (1964) ρ-σ-π analysis. A method for the correlation of biological activity and chemical structure. J Am Chem Soc 86:1616–1626. https://doi.org/10.1021/ja01062a035
8. Leo A, Hansch C, Elkins D (1971) Partition coefficients and their uses. Chem Rev 71:525–616. https://doi.org/10.1021/cr60274a001
9. Avdeef A (2003) Absorption and drug development. Solubility, permeability and charge state. Wiley, Hoboken, NJ. https://doi.org/10.1002/047145026X
10. Tsantili-Kakoulidou A, Piperaki S, Panderi I et al (1997) Prediction of distribution coefficients from structure. The influence of ion pair formation as reflected in experimental and calculated values. QSAR Comb Sci 16(4):315–316. https://doi.org/10.1002/qsar.19970160407
11. Pagliara A, Carrupt P-A, Caron G et al (1997) Lipophilicity profiles of Ampholytes. Chem Rev 97(8):3385–3400. https://doi.org/10.1021/cr9601019
12. Hansch C, Bjorkroth JP, Leo A (1987) Hydrophobicity and central nervous system agents: on the principle of minimal hydrophobicity in drug design. J Pharm Sci 76(9):663–687. https://doi.org/10.1002/jps.2600760902
13. Kubinyi H (1979) Lipophilicity and biological activity. Drug transport and drug distribution in model systems and in biological systems. Arzneimittelforschung 29(8):1067–1080
14. Dearden JC (1990) Molecular structure and drug transport. In: Ramsden CA, Hansch C, Sammer PG, Taylor JB (eds) Comprehensive medicinal chemistry. The rational design, mechanistic study & therapeutic applications of chemical compounds, vol 4. Pergamon, Oxford, pp 375–411
15. G C, Alsenz J, van de Waterbeemd H, Folkers G (1998) Estimation of permeability by passive diffusion through Caco-2 cell monolayers using the drugs' lipophilicity and molecular weight. Eur J Pharm Sci 6(4):317–324. https://doi.org/10.1016/S0928-0987(97)10019-7
16. Camenisch G, Folkers G, van de Waterbeemd H (1998) Shapes of membrane permeability-lipophilicity curves: extension of theoretical models with an aqueous pore pathway. Eur J Pharm Sci 6(4):321–329. https://doi.org/10.1016/S0928-0987(98)00033-5
17. Snyder PW, Mecinović J, Moustakas DT et al (2011) Mechanism of the hydrophobic effect in the biomolecular recognition of arylsulfonamides by carbonic anhydrase. Proc Natl Acad Sci U S A 108:17889–17894. https://doi.org/10.1073/pnas.1114107108
18. Freire E (2004) Isothermal titration calorimetry: controlling binding forces in lead optimization. Drug Discov Today Technol 1:295–299. https://doi.org/10.1016/j.ddtec.2004.11.016
19. Smith DA, van de Waterbeemd H (1999) Pharmacokinetics and metabolism in early drug discovery. Curr Opin Chem Biol 4:373–378. https://doi.org/10.1016/S1367-5931(99)80056-8
20. Rowley M, Kulagowski JJ, Watt AP et al (1997) Effect of plasma protein binding on in vivo activity and brain penetration of glycine/NMDA receptor antagonists. J Med Chem 40:4053–4068. https://doi.org/10.1021/jm970417o
21. Lambrinidis G, Vallianatou T, Tsantili-Kakoulidou A (2015) In vitro, in silico and integrated strategies for the estimation of plasma protein binding. A review. Adv Drug Deliv Rev 86:27–45. https://doi.org/10.1016/j.addr.2015.03.011
22. Lipinski CA, Lombardo F, Dominy BW, Feeney PJ (2001) Experimental and computational approaches to estimate solubility and permeability in drug discovery and development settings. Adv Drug Deliv Rev 23:3–25. https://doi.org/10.1016/S0169-409X(00)00129-0
23. Veber DF, Johnson SR, Cheng HY et al (2002) Molecular properties that influence the oral bioavailability of drug candidates. J Med

Chem 45:2615–2623. https://doi.org/10.1021/jm020017n

24. Congreve M, Carr R, Murray C, Jhoti H (2003) A 'rule of three' for fragment-based lead discovery? Drug Discov Today 8:876–877. https://doi.org/10.1016/S1359-6446(03)02831-9
25. Gleeson MP (2008) Generation of a set of simple, interpretable ADMET rules of thumb. J Med Chem 51:817–834. https://doi.org/10.1021/jm701122q
26. Vallianatou T, Giaginis C, Tsantili-Kakoulidou A (2015) The impact of physicochemical and molecular properties in drug design: navigation in the "drug-like" chemical space. Adv Exp Med Biol 822:187–194. https://doi.org/10.1007/978-3-319-08927-0_21
27. Keseru GM, Makara GM (2009) The influence of lead discovery strategies on the properties of drug candidates. Nat Rev Drug Discov 8 (3):203–212. https://doi.org/10.1038/nrd2796
28. Ferenczy GG, Keseru GM (2015) The impact of binding thermodynamics on medicinal chemistry optimizations. Future Med Chem 7 (10):1285–1303. https://doi.org/10.4155/fmc.15.63
29. Mannhold R, Poda GI, Ostermann C, Tetko IV (2009) Calculation of molecular Lipophilicity: state-of-the-art and comparison of log P methods on more than 96,000 compounds. J Pharm Sci 98(3):861–893. https://doi.org/10.1002/jps.21494
30. Testa B, Carrupt PA, Gaillard P, Tsai RS (1996) Intramolecular interactions encoded in lipophilicity: their nature and significance. In: Pliska V, Testa B, van de Waterbeemd H (eds) Lipophilicity in drug action and toxicology. VCH, Weinheim, pp 49–71. https://doi.org/10.1002/9783527614998.ch4
31. Chrysanthakopoulos M, Koletsou A, Nicolaou I et al (2009) Lipophilicity studies on pyrrolylacetic acid derivatives. Experimental versus predicted logP values in relationship with aldose reductase inhibitory activity. QSAR Comb Sci 28:551–560. https://doi.org/10.1002/qsar.200860138
32. Hersey A, Hill AP, Hyde RM, Livingstone DJ (1989) Principles of method selection in partition studies. Quant Struct Act Relat 8:288–296. https://doi.org/10.1002/qsar.19890080405
33. Sangster J (1997) Octanol-water partition coefficients: fundamentals and physical chemistry. John Wiley & Sons, Inc., New York
34. Avdeef A (1993) pH-metric logP. 2. Refinement of partition coefficients and ionization constants of Multiprotic substances. J Pharm Sci 82:183–190. https://doi.org/10.1002/jps.2600820214
35. Dorsey JG, Khaledi MG (1993) Hydrophobicity estimations by reversed-phase liquid chromatography. Implications for biological partitioning processes. J Chromatogr A 656:485–499. https://doi.org/10.1016/0021-9673(93)80815-P
36. Bechalany A, Tsantili-Kakoulidou A, El Tayar N, Testa B (1991) Measurement of lipophilicity indices by reversed-phase high-performance liquid chromatography: comparison of two stationary phases and various eluents. J Chromatogr 541:221–229. https://doi.org/10.1016/S0021-9673(01)95994-1
37. Giaginis C, Tsantili-Kakoulidou A (2008) Current state of the art in HPLC methodology for lipophilicity assessment of basic drugs. A review. J Liq Chromatogr Relat Technol 31 (1):79–96. https://doi.org/10.1080/10826070701665626
38. Van de Waterbeemd H, Kansy M, Wagner B, Fischer H (1996) Lipophilicity measurement by high performance liquid chromatography (RP-HPLC). In: Pilska V, Testa B, Van de Waterbeemd H (eds) Lipophilicity in drug action and toxicology. VCH, Weinheim, p 73. https://doi.org/10.1002/9783527614998.ch5
39. Vrakas D, Panderi I, Hadjipavlou-Litina D, Tsantili-Kakoulidou A (2005) Investigation of the relationships between logP and various chromatographic indices for a series of substituted coumarins. Evaluation of their similarity/dissimilarity using multivariate statistics. Quant Struct Act Relat 24:254–269. https://doi.org/10.1002/qsar.200430898
40. Pagliara A, Khamis E, Trinh A et al (1995) Structural properties governing retention mechanisms on RP-HPLC stationary phases used for lipophilicity measurements. J Liq Chromatogr 18(9):1721–1745. https://doi.org/10.1080/10826079508010002
41. Giaginis C, Theocharis S, Tsantili-Kakoulidou A (2013) Octanol/water partitioning simulation by RP-HPLC for structurally diverse acidic drugs: comparison of three columns in the presence and absence of *n*-octanol as the mobile phase additive. J Sep Sci 36:3830–3836. https://doi.org/10.1002/jssc.201300711
42. Tsantili-Kakoulidou A, Antoniadou-Vyza A (1989) Determination of the partition coefficients of adamantyl derivatives by reversed phase TLC and HPLC. Prog Clin Biol Res 291:71–74
43. Valko K, Bevan C, Reynolds D (1997) Chromatographic hydrophobicity index by fast-gradient RPHPLC: a high-throughput

alternative to log P/log D. Anal Chem 69:2022–2029. https://doi.org/10.1021/ac961242d
44. Valko K (2004) Application of high-performance liquid chromatography based measurements of lipophilicity to model biological distribution. J Chromatogr A 1037:299–310. https://doi.org/10.1016/j.chroma.2003.10.084
45. Valko K, Slegel P (1993) New chromatographic hydrophobicity index (φ0) based on the slope and the intercept of the log k_ versus organic phase concentration plot. J Chromatogr A 631:49–61. https://doi.org/10.1016/0021-9673(93)80506-4
46. Lombardo F, Shalaeva MY, Tupper KA, Gao F (2001) ElogDoct: a tool for Lipophilicity determination in drug discovery. 2. Basic and neutral compounds. J Med Chem 44(15):2490–2497. https://doi.org/10.1021/jm0100990
47. Liu X, Tanaka H, Yamauchi A et al (2005) Determination of lipophilicity by reversed-phase high-performance liquid chromatography: influence of 1-octanol in the mobile phase. J Chromatogr A 1091:51–59. https://doi.org/10.1016/j.chroma.2005.07.029
48. Giaginis C, Theocharis S, Tsantili-Kakoulidou A (2006) Contribution to the standardization of the chromatographic conditions for the lipophilicity assessment of neutral and basic drugs. Anal Chim Acta 573:311–318. https://doi.org/10.1016/j.aca.2006.03.074
49. Giaginis C, Theocharis S, Tsantili-Kakoulidou A (2007) Octanol/water partitioning simulation by reversed phase HPLC for structurally diverse acidic drugs: effect of octanol as mobile phase additive. J Chromatogr A 1166:116–125. https://doi.org/10.1016/j.chroma.2007.08.004
50. Schoenmakers PJ, Billiet HAH, de Galan L (1979) Influence of organic modifiers on the retention behaviour in reversed-phase liquid chromatography and its consequences for gradient elution. J Chromatogr 185:179–195. https://doi.org/10.1016/S0021-9673(00)85604-6

Chapter 13

Exploring Polypharmacology in Drug Design

Patricia Saenz-Méndez and Leif A. Eriksson

Abstract

Nowadays it is widely accepted that one compound can be able to hit several targets at once. This "magic shotgun" approach for drug development properly describes the mechanism of biomolecular recognition. The need to take into account the polypharmacology in structure-based drug design has led to the development of several computational tools. Here we present a computational protocol to identify promising compounds against several biological targets, a protocol known as inverse docking.

Key words Multi-target docking, Inverse docking, Selectivity, Polypharmacology, Docking score normalization, Target-fishing experiments

1 Introduction

Until recently, the paradigm of drug discovery has been the design of selective compounds, following the original idea of Paul Ehrlich of a "magic bullet," i.e., drugs that go directly to their predetermined biological target [1–3]. However, this one target-centric picture is a simplification of reality, while the idea of drugs acting on multiple targets is more appropriate. Therefore, the so-called magic shotguns or silver bullets appear to better represent the reality [4]. Polypharmacology or pharmacological promiscuity has emerged as a valuable concept in drug discovery [5]. Most drug candidates do not reach the market [6, 7], with high attrition rates of bioactive compounds being the major and more expensive reason for it. Late-stage drug attrition (frequently caused by toxicity) is highly costly and must be reduced by assessing hits and leads at key points in the drug discovery pipeline. This assessment has to be performed as early as possible to reduce the cost associated to a possible failure. Besides the evident problems with nonselective drugs producing undesirable side effects, polypharmacology may also be favorable, for instance, in treatment of complex diseases, such as cancer or psychosis [8–10]. Polypharmacology is also desirable in the treatment of infectious diseases: if the drug hits several

Thomas Mavromoustakos and Tahsin F. Kellici (eds.), *Rational Drug Design: Methods and Protocols*, Methods in Molecular Biology, vol. 1824, https://doi.org/10.1007/978-1-4939-8630-9_13, © Springer Science+Business Media, LLC, part of Springer Nature 2018

bacterial targets, it is more difficult for the bacteria to develop resistance [10]. Finally, considering that almost all drugs have off-target interactions, drug repurposing, i.e., utilizing a side effect for another indication, is an economic way to make a drug candidate reach the market [11]. Thus, by exploiting the polypharmacological properties of small molecules, it is possible to focus on the drug discovery process considerably.

In a single-target drug design project, high-throughput virtual screening (HTVS) is a straightforward methodology for identifying hits, but it is not sufficient when multiple targets are considered simultaneously. Thus, a multi-target approach has to be designed in order to address polypharmacology. Aiming to find the "magic shotgun" targeting multiple receptors at once, inverse docking techniques has to be employed. Inverse docking was first described by Chen and Zhi in 2001 [12] and is employed to find the best target (from a library of receptor structures) for a specific ligand. This allows to predict the bioactivity and secondary effects of a potential new drug, as well as to reposition old drugs [13–18].

In this chapter, we present a standard detailed protocol to perform the inverse docking of several potential inhibitors in the binding site of a small library of bacterial adenosine 5′-diphosphate-ribosylating toxins encoded by three pathogens, i.e., *Pseudomonas aeruginosa* (exotoxin A, ETA), *Corynebacterium diphtheria* (diphtheria toxin, DT), and *Vibrio cholera* (cholix toxin, CT). Our inverse docking approach was successfully applied for identifying selective and multi-target inhibitors of bacterial toxins, aiming toward the design of antibiotics active against resistant pathogens [18]. However, this protocol can be extrapolated to any other system. We:

1. Prepared the receptors using the University of California San Francisco (UCSF) Chimera [19].
2. Selected and prepared the ligands.
3. Optimized the docking parameters, such as the size of the box used.
4. Ran docking rounds employing UCSF DOCK (version 6.7) [20, 21].
5. Normalized the inverse docking scores aiming to remove any possible bias originating from the different internal energy of the receptors (Fig. 1).

2 Materials

To implement the inverse docking calculation procedure, it is necessary to have access to a copy of University of California San Francisco (UCSF) Dock [20, 21] and UCSF Chimera [19].

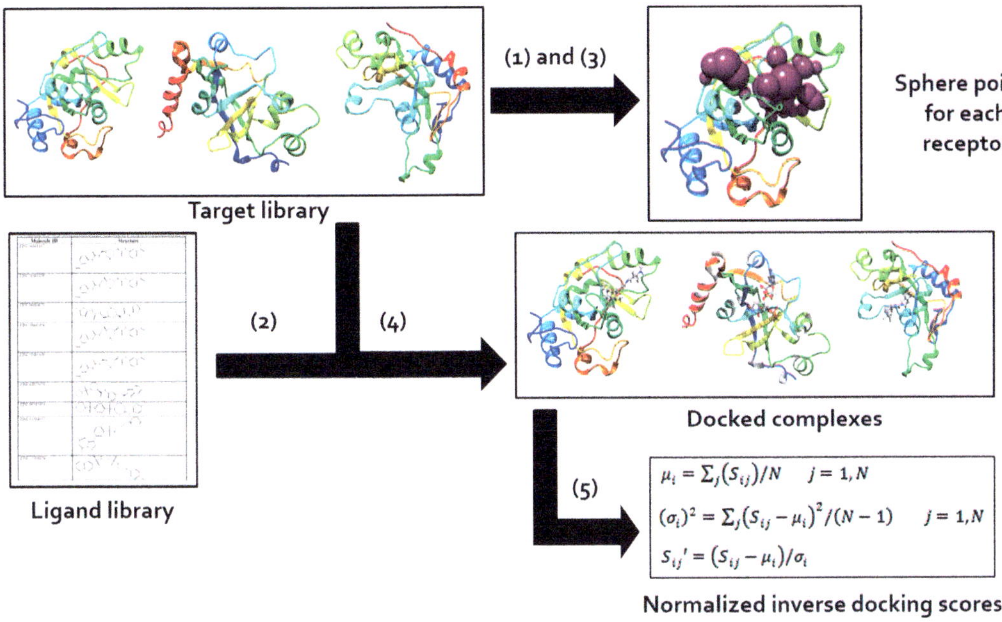

Fig. 1 Flowchart showing the inverse docking protocol described in this chapter [1]. Preparation of receptors, [2] selection and preparation of ligands, [3] optimization of docking parameters, [4] independent docking of each ligand against all receptors, and [5] normalization of inverse docking scores and prediction of the best receptor for each ligand

3 Methods

In this section, we describe the four main steps involved in our inverse docking protocol. When necessary, some variants and further details are described in Subheading 4.

3.1 Protein Preparation

1. Download the crystal structures of the proteins of interest from the Protein Data Bank [22]. In this case, the protein crystallographic coordinates of ETA (PDB id 1AER [23]), DT (PDB id 1DTP [24]), and CT (PDB id 2Q6M [25]) were retrieved. However, these methodologies can be transferable to any system, as mentioned in Subheading 1.
2. Structure preparation was performed using UCSF Chimera [19]. Several steps must be carried out aiming to obtain all different files needed to perform the molecular docking rounds. To this end, open the corresponding pdb file in Chimera. If the crystal structure contains a ligand, the user must select and delete the ligand and then use the Dock Prep tool to prepare the receptor (Tools > Structure Editing > Dock Prep). Once the structure is prepared, it must be saved as mol2 file (*receptor_charged.mol2*). An additional file (*receptor_unprotonated.pdb*) must be generated by deleting all hydrogen atoms. For details and different options, *see* **Note 1**.

3.2 Selection and Preparation of Ligands

The preparation of ligands depends on the origin of the structures. If the ligand is obtained from a crystal structure, then the user must select and delete everything except the ligand from the crystal structure complex. Then, hydrogen atoms must be added (Tools > Structure Editing > AddH). The Chimera Add Charge tool can be employed to calculate charges based on AM1-BCC calculations [26, 27], using *antechamber* and by properly setting the net charge [28]. Antechamber recognizes the atom and bond types, generates the topology file, and adds missing force field parameters for most organic molecules. If the ligand is obtained from a ZINC database [29], the charges are already present, and the user can accept those charges or calculate them as mentioned above. Finally, save the prepared ligand as mol2 file (*ligand_charged.mol2*).

3.3 Optimization of Docking Parameters

1. Generation of the molecular surface of the receptor using the DMS tool included in Chimera [30]. To this end, open the file *receptor_unprotonated.pdb*, create the surface (Actions > Surface > Show), and finally save the dms file containing the surface information (Tools > Structure Editing > Write DMS), e.g., *receptor.dms.*
2. Generation and selection of spheres corresponding to the binding site. This set of overlapping spheres is created in order to represent the topology of the surface [31]. Thus, spheres making a "negative image" of the binding site surface are generated using the "sphgen" program accessory to DOCK, within some radius. The overlapping spheres are used during the docking rounds to generate the orientations of the ligands within the active site. Thus, a low number of spheres (small radius) may neglect some representative binding poses, and an artificially large search space (large radius or high number of spheres) may generate irrelevant binding poses. Therefore, selecting the correct number/size of spheres is of utmost importance. To this end, the user must first generate the spheres file, employing the command line program **sphgen**. Then, the docking site must be defined by selecting spheres within some radius of a desired location, usually around a co-crystallized ligand in the original pdb file, employing the **sphere_selector** command of DOCK (*see* **Note 2**).
3. Generation of a box around the active site using the command

   showbox < box.in

   where *box.in* is the input file containing the required information (*see* **Note 3**). The file *receptor_box.pdb* is then created.
4. Generation of the energy scoring grid file using the grid program included in DOCK. To this end, the following command line must be executed:

   grid -i grid.in -o receptor_grid.out.

The file *grid.in* contains the parameters for the calculation. Several files are then generated, as follows: first *receptor_grid.out* (or simply *grid.out* if a different name is not specified), which summarizes the parameters employed and the grid generated. Two additional files are created, named *grid.nrg* and *grid.bmp*. The nrg file contains the energy calculation scores, and the bmp file includes the size, position and grid spacing, and bump calculations (i.e., if there are any overlaps with receptor atoms). Details about the input file are included in **Notes 4** and **5**.

3.4 Molecular Docking

At this point, the user has several options, rigid ligand docking, flexible ligand docking, and induced fit (Amber scoring in DOCK), being ordered from the lowest to the highest accuracy and computational cost of the calculation. The first one implies that both the ligand and the receptor are fixed. In the second case, the ligand is considered flexible and capable of structurally rearranging within the receptor. Finally, induced fit treats both the receptor and the ligand as flexible, allowing structural rearrangements while calculating scoring. In this example, we employed rigid docking running the command line dock6 -i rigid.in -o rigid.out.The file *rigid.in* contains the input parameters, while the output file contains a list of the parameters employed during the docking calculation, any error messages and summary information of the best scoring pose. A mol2 file, *rigid_ranked.mol2*, contains the geometric coordinates and a summary of the interaction energy of the best pose. If the ligand file is a database of several ligands (such as a ZINC database), the *rigid_ranked.mol2* file will contain the best pose for every ligand included in the database.To summarize, the files needed for running DOCK are the following: *grid.nrg* and *grid.bmp*, for energy scoring, *selected_spheres.sph* for placing the ligand within the binding site, and the *ligand_charged.mol2* file. Details about the input file are included in **Note 5**.

3.5 Normalization of Docking Scores

The success of normal virtual screening relies on the accurate prediction of interactions between several ligands and a target receptor. However, the prediction of the best receptor for a particular ligand represents a particularly challenging task. Scoring functions implemented in docking protocols (rigid, flexible, and induced fit) are designed to find the best ligand for a particular receptor (normal docking), but they cannot be employed to find the best receptor from a panel of targets for a particular ligand (inverse docking). Different receptors usually do not share the same binding pocket shape or internal energy (due to different protein size and composition). In order to properly account for this effect, a normalization protocol must be implemented.

In this example the multiple active site correction (MASC) [32] is employed as follows:

$$\mu_i = \sum_j (S_{ij})/N \quad j = 1, N$$
$$(\sigma_i)^2 = \sum_j (S_{ij} - \mu_i)^2/(N-1) \quad j = 1, N \qquad (1)$$
$$S_{ij}' = (S_{ij} - \mu_i)/\sigma_i$$

where S_{ij} is the original calculated docking score for the *i*th compound and the *j*th pocket (in kcal mol^{-1}) and S_{ij}' is the normalized score for the compound i in the active site and *j*, μ_i, and σ_I are the average and standard deviations of the scores for compound *i* across all pockets *j*, respectively. The MASC score includes relevant information in the sign of the normalized score, i.e., if the MASC score is negative, the binding interaction between the ligand and that particular receptor is better than the average among all receptors. Results obtained by following the protocol described in this chapter were reported in a recent work [18]. Further details regarding score normalization are included in **Note 6**.

4 Notes

1. The user can choose several options during the preparation of the receptor, such as delete solvent, add hydrogens, and add charges. In particular, the user can select the method for protonating histidine residues: based on the residue name (HIS/HID/HIE/HIP), individually chosen, or determined by the method, i.e., the employed method will determine the protonation state, and the hydrogen bonding network will be optimized. Charges for standard amino acids are calculated using AMBER ff14SB [33]. When saving the unprotonated receptor as pdb file, the user must select the box "Use untransformed coordinates" in the Save As dialog box.
2. To run the sphgen command line, the dms file created before is needed as input, and the following line must be executed:

   sphgen –i receptor.dms –o receptor.sph
   where the input and output file are the dms and sph files, respectively. Then, to select the spheres within a defined radius around the ligand, the syntax of the sphere_selector program included in dock is:
   sphere_selector receptor.sph ligand_charged.mol2 8.0
   This line implies that the user selects all spheres within 8.0 Å RMSD from every atom of the ligand and always generates a file named *selected_spheres.sph*. The resulting spheres can be visualized in Chimera by opening the *receptor_charged.mol2* file and then opening the *selected_spheres.sph* file (Fig. 2).
3. Showbox is the program defining the size and location of the box that will be employed to create the docking grid. The command requires an input file, for instance, named as *box.in*, including the following lines (explained as comments after #) (Table 1):

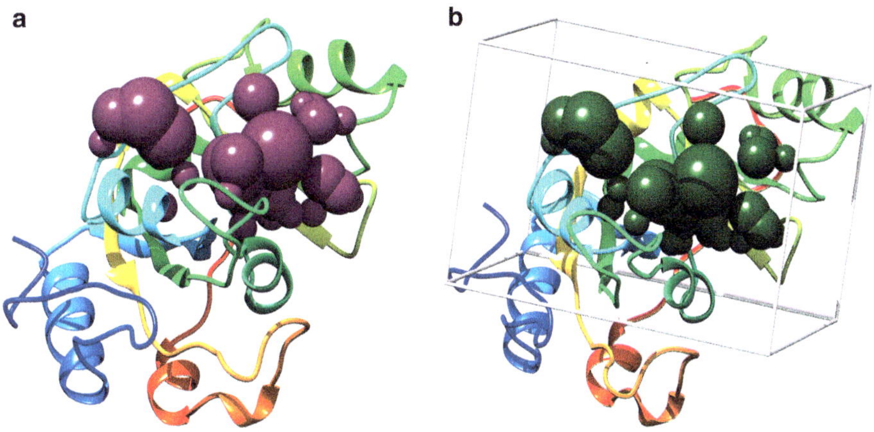

Fig. 2 (**a**) Selected spheres corresponding to 8 Å are represented in magenta. (**b**) Box generated around the ligand, including selected spheres in green

Table 1
Example of input file for defining the size and the location of the box

Y	# YES, generate the box
8.0	# Size of desired box in Å
selected_spheres. sph	# Selected spheres file. When located in another # folder, the path must be included
1	# Cluster number
receptor_box.pdb	# Output file

Since the output file is a pdb file, the box can be visualized in Chimera (*see* Fig. 2b).

4. An example of the input file required for the generation of the grid, together with an explanation of the lines included, is shown below in Table 2.

   compute_grids: compute scoring grid (YES/NO).

   grid_spacing: distance between grid points along each axis in Å (float number).

   output_molecule: writes the coordinates of the receptor into a new file (YES/NO).

   contact_score: define if constructing a contact grid (YES/NO). Default is no.

   energy_score: define if computing energy score (YES/NO).

   energy_cutoff_distance: define the maximum distance between atoms for the energy contribution to be included.

   atom_model: atom model **u** implies a united atom model (i.e., hydrogen atoms are included in the united atom and the

Table 2
Example of input file for the generation of the grid

compute_grids	Yes
grid_spacing	0.3
output_molecule	No
contact_score	No
energy_score	Yes
energy_cutoff_distance	9999
atom_model	a
attractive_exponent	6
repulsive_exponent	12
distance_dielectric	Yes
dielectric_factor	4
bump_filter	Yes
bump_overlap	0.75
receptor_file	receptor_charged.mol2
box_file	receptor_box.pdb
vdw_definition_file	/location-of-dock/parameters/vdw_AMBER_parm99.defn
score_grid_prefix	grid

partial charge of a particular hydrogen transferred to the corresponding heavy atom where it is attached), while model **a** means an all-atom model where hydrogen atoms are treated independently.

attractive_exponent: exponent of the attractive van der Waals term in the Lennard-Jones potential.

repulsive_exponent: exponent of the repulsive van der Waals term in the Lennard-Jones potential.

distance_dielectric: define if the dielectric depends linearly on the distance (YES/NO).

dielectric_factor: represents the coefficient of the dielectric (user defined).

bump_filter: determines if the user wants to screen orientation for clashes before scoring and minimizing (YES/NO).

bump_overlap: represents the amount of van der Waals overlap allowed, and it is a float number between 0 and 1, being 0 complete overlap allowed and 1 no overlap allowed. If two atoms are closer than the bump overlap definition, then the position is defined as a bump.

receptor_file: receptor file (mol2 file) including the partial charges and atom types, i.e., prepared receptor file as discussed before.

box_file: box file (pdb file) is the file containing the box generated with the showbox program.

vdw_definition_file: van der Waals parameters file, including the path where DOCK is installed.

score_grid_prefix: prefix for the name of grid files (user defined). File extensions are included automatically.

5. The generation and selection of spheres, box, and grid will define the accuracy of the docking studies [34]. The goal for molecular docking is to predict the correct binding pose and affinity. Therefore, the user must study the effect of the size of the grid, usually by docking known ligands with available crystal structures for the corresponding complexes. Those docking parameters (i.e., box size) allowing the best reproduction of experimental results must be selected to perform docking experiments aiming to predict binding poses and energies.

   An example of the input file required for running a rigid docking experiment, together with an explanation of the lines included, is shown below in Table 3.

   ligand_atom_file: ligand input filename.

   limit_max_ligands: define if there is a limit in the number of ligands to be read from the ligand atom file (YES/NO).

   skip_molecule: skip some molecules at the beginning of the library of ligands (YES/NO).

   read_mol_solvation: define if the atomic desolvation information is read from the ligand file.

   calculate_rmsd: perform an RMSD calculation between the final pose and the initial structure (YES/NO).

   orient_ligand: orient ligand to spheres (YES/NO).

   automated_matching: defines if performing automated or manual matching (YES for automated, NO for manual).

   receptor_site_file: file containing the receptor spheres calculated.

   max_orientations: maximum number of orientations tried during posing (user defined).

   critical_points: use critical points sphere labeling to define orientations to particular spheres (YES/NO).

   chemical_matching: use chemical coloring of spheres to match chemical labels on ligand atoms (YES/NO).

Table 3
Example of input file for running a rigid docking experiment

ligand_atom_file	ligand_charged.mol2
limit_max_ligands	No
skip_molecule	No
read_mol_solvation	No
calculate_rmsd	No
orient_ligand	Yes
automated_matching	Yes
receptor_site_file	selected_spheres.sph
max_orientations	500
critical_points	No
chemical_matching	No
use_ligand_spheres	No
use_internal_energy	Yes
internal_energy_rep_exp	12
flexible_ligand	No
bump_filter	No
score_molecules	Yes
contact_score_primary	No
contact_score_secondary	No
grid_score_primary	Yes
grid_score_secondary	No
grid_score_rep_rad_scale	1
grid_score_vdw_scale	1
grid_score_grid_prefix	Grid
multigrid_score_secondary	No
dock3.5_score_secondary	No
continuous_score_secondary	No
gbsa_zou_score_secondary	No
gbsa_hawkins_score_secondary	No
SASA_descriptor_score_secondary	No
amber_score_secondary	No
minimize_ligand	Yes

(continued)

Table 3 (continued)

simplex_max_iterations	500
simplex_max_cycles	1
simplex_score_converge	0.1
simplex_cycle_converge	1
simplex_trans_step	1
simplex_rot_step	0.1
simplex_tors_step	10
simplex_random_seed	0
atom_model	All
vdw_defn_file	/location-of-dock/parameters/vdw_AMBER_parm99.defn
flex_defn_file	/location-of-dock/parameters/flex.defn
flex_drive_file	/location-of-dock/parameters/flex_drive.tbl
ligand_outfile_prefix	Rigid
write_orientations	No
num_scored_conformers	1
rank_ligands	Yes
max_ranked_ligands	10,000

use_ligand_spheres: this option allows for using a sphere file representing ligand heavy atoms during posing (YES/NO).

use_internal_energy: use van der Waals internal energy for minimization (YES/NO).

internal_energy_rep_exp: repulsive van der Waals exponent in the Lennard-Jones potential.

flexible_ligand: defines if the docking protocol is rigid (NO) or flexible (YES).

bump_filter: determines if the user wants to screen orientation for clashes before scoring and minimizing (YES/NO).

score_molecules: defines if using a scoring function (YES/NO).

contact_score_primary: defines if performing contact scoring as the primary scoring function (YES/NO).

contact_score_secondary: defines if performing contact scoring as the secondary scoring function (YES/NO).

grid_score_primary: defines if performing a grid-based scoring as the primary scoring function (YES/NO).

grid_score_secondary: defines if performing a grid-based scoring as the secondary scoring function (YES/NO).

grid_score_rep_rad_scale: scalar multiplier of the van der Waals radius for the repulsive term of the Lennard-Jones potential (user defined).

grid_score_vdw_scale: scalar multiplier of the van der Waals energy (user defined).

grid_score_grid_prefix: prefix of the grid nrg file.

multigrid_score_secondary: defines if performing a multigrid score as the secondary scoring function (YES/NO).

dock3.5_score_secondary: defines if performing dock3.5 scoring as the secondary scoring function (YES/NO).

continuous_score_secondary: defines if performing continuous scoring as the secondary scoring function (YES/NO).

gbsa_zou_score_secondary: defines if performing Zou GB/SA scoring as the secondary scoring function (YES/NO).

gbsa_hawkins_score_secondary: defines if performing Hawkings-Cramer-Thrular GB/SA scoring as the secondary scoring function (YES/NO).

SASA_descriptor_score_secondary: defines if performing SASA score as the secondary scoring function (YES/NO).

amber_score_secondary: defines if performing AMBER scoring as the secondary scoring function (YES/NO).

minimize_ligand: performs score optimization (YES/NO).

simplex_max_iterations: maximum number of minimization iterations (user defined).

simplex_max_cycles: maximum number of minimization cycles (user defined).

simplex_score_converge: end cycles when the energy converge to the specified cutoff (user defined).

simplex_cycle_converge: exit minimization when cycles converge to the specified cutoff (user defined).

simplex_trans_step: defines the initial translation step size.

simplex_rot_step: defines the initial rotation step size.

simplex_tor_step: defines the initial torsion angle step size.

simplex_random_seed: initial seed for random number generator.

atom_model: choice between all atoms (all) and united atoms (united) models.

vdw_def_file: van der Waals parameters file, including the path where DOCK is installed.

flex_def_file: conformational search parameters file, including the path where DOCK is installed.

flex_drive_file: conformational search parameters file, including the path where DOCK is installed.

ligand_outfile_prefix: the prefix that all output files will have (user defined).

write_orientations: defines if writing all anchor orientations (YES/NO).

num_scored_conformers: defines the number of conformations scored for each ligand (user defined).

rank_ligands: defines if enabling a ligand top scoring list (YES/NO). If yes, these selected top poses are included in the *rigid_ ranked.mol2* file.

max_ranked_ligands: maximum number of ranked ligands included in the *rigid_ ranked.mol2* file (user defined).

The file containing all ranked ligands will get the prefix specified by the user as "ligand_outfile" and the suffix "_ranked. mol2," i.e., in this example will be named as *rigid_ ranked. mol2.*

6. Other normalization protocols are available, such as the normalization proposed by Lauro et al. [35, 36]. In this approach, the normalized score is calculated using Eq. 2:

$$V = V_0/[(M_L + M_R)/2] \quad (2)$$

where V is the normalized score for each ligand on each receptor, V_0 is the docking score obtained as described in this protocol through docking calculations, M_L is the average binding energy of each ligand on different receptors, and M_R is the average binding energy of each receptor on different ligands. The higher the V, the more promising is the interaction between a ligand and particular target. This correction is dependent not only on the panel of targets but also on the ligands selected, as M_L is the average binding energy of each ligand. This means that different results can be obtained if a different set of ligands is included and is considered as a pitfall of this approach.

Acknowledgments

This work has been supported by the People Program (Marie Curie Actions) of the European Union's Seventh Framework Program (FP7/2007–2013) under REA grant agreement N° 608746. We gratefully acknowledge funding from the Swedish Research Council and the Faculty of Science at the University of Gothenburg. We also acknowledge the generous allocation of computer time at the C3SE supercomputing center via a grant from the Swedish National Infrastructure for Computing (SNIC).

References

1. Ehrlich P (1878) Beiträge zur theorie und praxis der histologischen färbung. Leipzig University, Leipzig
2. Ehrlich P (1897) Die wertbemessung des diphterieheilserums und deren theoretische grundlagen. Klinisches Jahrbuch 6:299–326
3. Strebhardt K, Ullrich A (2008) Paul Ehrlich's magic bullet concept: 100 years of progress. Nat Rev Cancer 8:473–480
4. Medina-Franco JL, Giulianotti MA, Welmaker GS et al (2013) Shifting from the single to the multitarget paradigm in drug discovery. Drug Discov Today 18(9–10):495–501. https://doi.org/10.1016/j.drudis.2013.01.008
5. AbdulHameed MDM, Chaudhury S, Singh N et al (2012) Exploring Polypharmacology using a ROCS-based target fishing approach. J Chem Inf Model 52(2):492–505. https://doi.org/10.1021/ci2003544
6. Hay M, Thomas DW, Craighead JL et al (2014) Clinical development success rates for investigational drugs. Nature Biotechnol 32:40–51
7. Waring MJ, Arrowsmith J, Leach AR et al (2015) An analysis of the attrition of drug candidates from four major pharmaceutical companies. Nat Rev Drug Discov 14 (7):475–486. https://doi.org/10.1038/nrd4609
8. Zimmermann GR, Lehar J, Keith CT (2007) Multi-target therapeutics: when the whole is greater than the sum of the parts. Drug Discov Today 12(1–2):34–42. https://doi.org/10.1016/j.drudis.2006.11.008
9. Roth BL, Sheffler DJ, Kroeze WK (2004) Magic shotguns versus magic bullets: selectively non-selective drugs for mood disorders and schizophrenia. Nat Rev Drug Discov 3:353–359
10. Peters J-U (2013) Polypharmacology – Foe or friend? J Med Chem 56(22):8955–8971. https://doi.org/10.1021/jm400856t
11. Ye H, Liu Q, Wei J (2014) Construction of drug network based on side effects and its application for drug repositioning. PLoS One 9(2):e87864. https://doi.org/10.1371/journal.pone.0087864.t001
12. Chen YZ, Zhi DG (2001) Ligand–protein inverse docking and its potential use in the computer search of protein targets of a small molecule. Proteins 43:217–226
13. Zahler S, Tietze S, Totzke F et al (2007) Inverse in silico screening for identification of kinase inhibitor targets. Chem Biol 14 (11):1207–1214. https://doi.org/10.1016/j.chembiol.2007.10.010
14. Grinter SZ, Liang Y, Huang SY et al (2011) An inverse docking approach for identifying new potential anti-cancer targets. J Mol Graph Model 29(6):795–799. https://doi.org/10.1016/j.jmgm.2011.01.002
15. Xie L, Xie L, Bourne PE (2011) Structure-based systems biology for analyzing off-target binding. Curr Opin Struct Biol 21 (2):189–199. https://doi.org/10.1016/j.sbi.2011.01.004
16. Wang W, Zhou X, He W et al (2012) The interprotein scoring noises in glide docking scores. Proteins 80(1):169–183. https://doi.org/10.1002/prot.23173
17. Eric S, Ke S, Barata T et al (2012) Target fishing and docking studies of the novel derivatives of aryl-aminopyridines with potential anticancer activity. Bioorg Med Chem 20 (17):5220–5228. https://doi.org/10.1016/j.bmc.2012.06.051
18. Saenz-Méndez P, Eriksson M, Eriksson LA (2017) Ligand selectivity between the ADP-Ribosylating toxins: an inverse-docking study for multitarget drug discovery. ACS Omega 2(4):1710–1719. https://doi.org/10.1021/acsomega.7b00010
19. Pettersen EF, Goddard TD, Huang CC et al (2004) UCSF chimera—a visualization system for exploratory research and analysis. J Comput Chem 25(13):1605–1612
20. DOCK 6.7 (2015) University of California San Francisco. http://dock.compbio.ucsf.edu/
21. Lang PT, Brozell SR, Mukherjee S et al (2009) DOCK 6: combining techniques to model RNA-small molecule complexes. RNA 15 (6):1219–1230. https://doi.org/10.1261/rna.1563609

22. Protein Data Bank. http://www.rcsb.org/pdb/home/home.do
23. Li M, Dyda F, Benhar I et al (1996) Crystal structure of the catalytic domain of *Pseudomonas* exotoxin a complexed with a nicotinamide adenine dinucleotide analog: implications for the activation process and for ADP ribosylation. Proc Natl Acad Sci U S A 93:6902–6906
24. Weiss MS, Blanke SR, Collier RJ et al (1995) Structure of the isolated catalytic domain of diphtheria toxin. Biochemistry 34:773–781
25. Jorgensen R, Purdy AE, Fieldhouse RJ et al (2008) Cholix toxin, a novel ADP-ribosylating factor from vibrio cholerae. J Biol Chem 283(16):10671–10678. https://doi.org/10.1074/jbc.M710008200
26. Jakalian A, Bush BL, Jack DB et al (2000) Fast, efficient generation of high-quality atomic charges. AM1-BCC model: I. Method. J Comput Chem 21(2):132–146
27. Jakalian A, Jack DB, Bayly CI (2002) Fast, efficient generation of high-quality atomic charges. AM1-BCC model: II. Parameterization and validation. J Comput Chem 23(16):1623–1641. https://doi.org/10.1002/jcc.10128
28. Wang J, Wang W, Kollman PA et al (2006) Automatic atom type and bond type perception in molecular mechanical calculations. J Mol Graph Mod 25(2):247–260. https://doi.org/10.1016/j.jmgm.2005.12.005
29. Irwin JJ, Sterling T, Mysinger MM et al (2012) ZINC: a free tool to discover chemistry for biology. J Chem Inf Model 52(7):1757–1768
30. Richards FM (1977) Areas, volumes, packing, and protein structure. Ann Rev Biophys Bioeng 6:151–176
31. Kuntz ID, Blaney JM, Oatley SJ et al (1982) A geometric approach to macromolecule-ligand interactions. J Mol Biol 161:269–288
32. Vigers GPA, Rizzi JP (2004) Multiple active site corrections for docking and virtual screening. J Med Chem 47:80–89
33. Maier JA, Martinez C, Kasavajhala K et al (2015) ff14SB: improving the accuracy of protein side chain and backbone parameters from ff99SB. J Chem Theory Comput 11 (8):3696–3713. https://doi.org/10.1021/acs.jctc.5b00255
34. Feinstein WP, Brylinski M (2015) Calculating an optimal box size for ligand docking and virtual screening against experimental and predicted binding pockets. J Cheminform 7 (1):1–10. https://doi.org/10.1186/s13321-015-0067-5
35. Lauro G, Romano A, Riccio R et al (2011) Inverse virtual screening of antitumor targets: pilot study on a small database of natural bioactive compounds. J Nat Prod 74 (6):1401–1407. https://doi.org/10.1021/np100935s
36. Lauro G, Masullo M, Piacente S et al (2012) Inverse virtual screening allows the discovery of the biological activity of natural compounds. Bioorg Med Chem 20(11):3596–3602. https://doi.org/10.1016/j.bmc.2012.03.072

Chapter 14

Development of Nuclear Receptor Modulators

Simone Schierle and Daniel Merk

Abstract

With 49 members identified thus far, the superfamily of nuclear receptors offers a large number of targets to be pharmacologically exploited. Some nuclear receptors already look back to a successful history as drug targets, while others still lack any identified ligand. The development of small molecules targeting nuclear receptor is a challenging task and has to consider not only high affinity binding but also aspects as the nuclear localization of the target protein or transactivation efficacy. In this chapter, we summarize characteristics of nuclear receptors as target family, strategies of hit and lead identification, and the variety of methods for in vitro characterization of nuclear receptor modulators. A detailed method chapter describes an example optimization of a nuclear receptor modulator as well as hybrid reporter gene assays as a very flexible method of choice for in vitro characterization. Thereby, the chapter provides an introduction to nuclear receptor ligand development.

Key words Nuclear receptors, Transactivation assay, Reporter gene assay, Farnesoid X receptor, Medicinal chemistry, Drug discovery

1 Introduction to Nuclear Receptors

Nuclear receptors are looking back to a long successful history as drug targets and have been addressed by drug discovery over decades. However, although some nuclear receptors are exploited very successfully in pharmacotherapy, for the bigger part of the nuclear receptor superfamily, no ligands—not to mention drugs—have been identified. In view of the widespread roles and physiological importance of nuclear receptors, this target family holds great potential for drug discovery in numerous disease complexes.

1.1 The Nuclear Receptor Superfamily

The nuclear receptor superfamily is composed of 49 proteins identified thus far, of which 24 possess a known ligand, while no modulator has been identified for the remaining 25, yet. The receptors for which a ligand remains to be discovered are termed orphan nuclear receptors. Nuclear receptors can be classified either by sequence identity resulting in seven families (NR0–NR6) or by four distinct dimerization characteristics. Steroid receptors usually

Thomas Mavromoustakos and Tahsin F. Kellici (eds.), *Rational Drug Design: Methods and Protocols*, Methods in Molecular Biology, vol. 1824, https://doi.org/10.1007/978-1-4939-8630-9_14, © Springer Science+Business Media, LLC, part of Springer Nature 2018

form homodimers, while the so-called RXR heterodimers exhibit most of their functions as heterodimer with the retinoid X receptors (RXRα, RXRβ, RXRγ). This class contains most nuclear receptors that are already used or at least evaluated as drug target including the peroxisome proliferator-activated receptors (PPARα, PPARβ/δ, PPARγ), the retinoic acid receptors (RARα, RARβ, RARγ), the liver X receptors (LXRα, LXRβ), the thyroid hormone receptors (TRα, TRβ), and the farnesoid X receptor (FXR). An important characteristic of these RXR heterodimers is that most of them are permissive and can be activated by agonists of either partner receptor. Only few, e.g., the RAR-RXR heterodimers, require an agonist of both receptors for activation.

Nuclear receptors translate ligand signals to changes in gene expression and thereby act as ligand-activated transcription factors. Most of them share a common architecture and are composed of five to six domains. The N-terminal region is poorly conserved and often unstructured. In some nuclear receptors, it mediates ligand-independent activation. It is followed by the DNA-binding domain (DBD) containing two zinc finger motifs that mediate binding to specific nuclear receptor response elements (RE) on the DNA. The DBD is connected via a flexible hinge region to the ligand-binding domain (LBD) that recognizes specific ligands and undergoes conformational changes upon ligand binding leading to activation or inhibition of target gene transcription. The LBD interacts with co-regulatory proteins including coactivators and corepressors that govern the activity of the complex toward gene transcription. Some nuclear receptors, e.g., the neuron-derived orphan receptor 1 (NOR-1), also seem to possess intrinsic transactivation activity and do not require a ligand to be activated. However, these receptors have not been extensively studied, yet, and it is not clear to which extent their activity can be regulated by modulators. The LBD also contains surfaces for dimer formation with other nuclear receptors. At the C-terminal end, the ligand-dependent activation function is located [1–7].

1.2 Nuclear Receptors as Targets

Modulation of nuclear receptors by small molecules can be achieved in different manners resulting in activation of the transcription factor and gene transcription or in stabilization of the nuclear receptor's inactive state with inhibition of gene expression. In absence of an agonist, the LBD usually has higher affinity to corepressors and upon agonist binding undergoes conformational changes that shift the equilibrium to release of corepressors and recruitment of coactivators. For this purpose, agonist binding leads to recruitment of the terminal ligand-dependent activation function to the core LBD forming a new surface for coactivator binding. Nuclear receptor agonists can possess different transactivation efficiency and exist as full agonists and partial agonists. Recently, gene-selective modulators are getting increasingly into focus, but there are few successful examples of gene-selective nuclear receptor modulation.

An antagonist binds to the same ligand-binding pocket as an agonist but does not form interactions with the LBD that lead to recruitment of the ligand-dependent activation function. It competes with (endogenous) agonists and does not induce gene transcription. Inverse agonists by forming different interactions with the LBD prevent recruitment of the ligand-dependent activation function and thereby stabilize the inactive state of the nuclear receptor shifting the equilibrium toward interaction with corepressors. The discrimination of antagonist and inverse agonist can be difficult since many nuclear receptors lack intrinsic activities but require an agonist for activation whose activity is competed by antagonist and inverse agonist. Great interest is also dedicated to allosteric modulation of nuclear receptors. However, few small-molecule allosteric nuclear receptor modulators have been reported thus far.

Nuclear receptors constitute intracellular targets, and therefore, synthetic modulators must be able to reach the cytosol and nucleus to be active. Small molecules can pass the barrier of the cell membrane by various mechanisms including passive diffusion and active uptake by cellular transporters. This aspect should be considered in the design and development of nuclear receptor targeting compounds.

2 Hit/Lead Identification

Many nuclear receptors share a large and lipophilic ligand-binding site that usually can accommodate various different ligands. Still, nuclear receptors precisely distinguish their respective endogenous ligands mainly through a specific shape and angle on one hand and a certain region for potent polar contacts on the other hand. The farnesoid X receptor, for example, is activated by bile acids that comprise a steroidal scaffold. Steroid hormones, in contrast, do not activate FXR (Fig. 1) [8]. The receptor distinguishes steroidal bile acids from other steroids by forming a potent neutralizing interaction with the carboxylic acid of its endogenous ligands via two arginine residues and by accommodating the specific shape of bile acids that comprise a cis configuration at the A/B ring connection. These prerequisites, especially regions for potent polar contacts in the widely lipophilic nuclear receptor ligand-binding site should be considered in lead structure finding and in modulator optimization.

Hit and lead identification for nuclear receptor modulator development can, of course, be achieved by screening approaches using a suitable in vitro test system (described in Subheading 5.2). For a favorable hit rate, either a suitable focused library or a computer-assisted approach should be selected. Focused screening libraries are available for several classes of compounds, and a

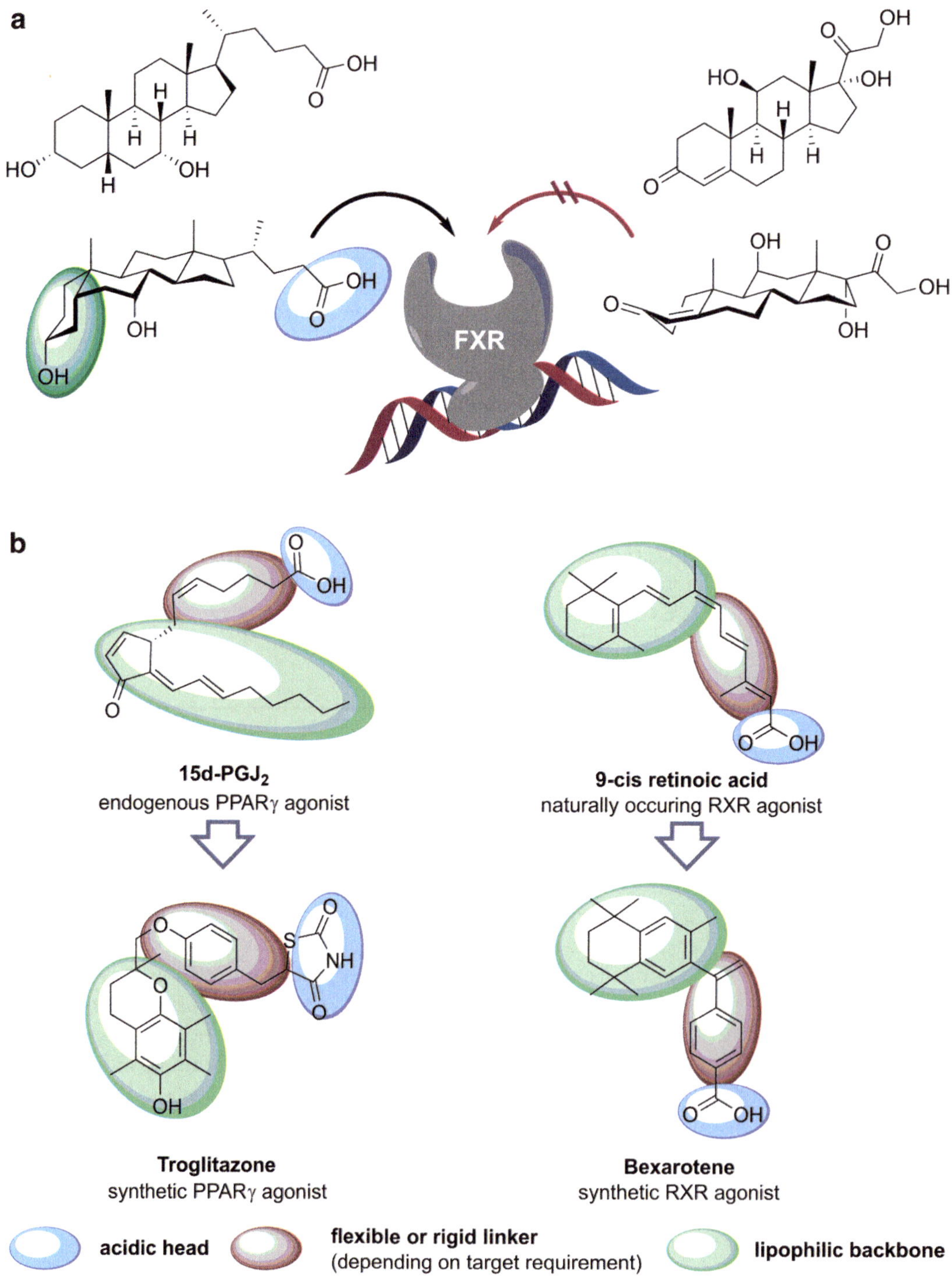

Fig. 1 (**a**) Shape and electrostatics are important in nuclear receptor ligand discrimination. (**b**) Natural and synthetic ligands of PPARγ (15d-PGJ2 and troglitazone) as well as RXR (9-*cis* retinoic acid and bexarotene) share shape and polarity. The synthetic ligands are fatty acid mimetics and can be divided in acidic head group, geometry-governing linker region, and lipophilic backbone as molecular building blocks

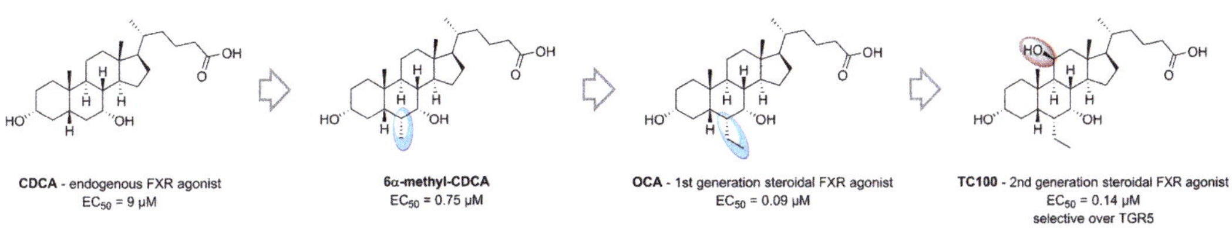

Fig. 2 Successful optimization of the natural FXR ligand CDCA to highly potent (investigational) drugs

suitable selection should be oriented at the endogenous ligand or other known modulators of the receptor in question. Peroxisome proliferator-activated receptors or retinoid X receptors that are physiologically activated by fatty acid metabolites prefer an acidic function in their ligands (although also non-acidic modulators have been reported) and except for the binding region of this acidic residue comprise very lipophilic ligand-binding sites. Therefore, PPAR or RXR ligands are fatty acid mimetics, and focused libraries containing this compound class will likely provide a higher hit rate than neutral compounds (Fig. 1) [9].

Computer-assisted approaches to nuclear receptor modulator development have been very successful, particularly as supportive approach in hit identification. However, several studies have shown that the binding sites of most nuclear receptors are very flexible and accommodate to various scaffolds. Therefore, ligand-based screening approaches seem superior to structure-based methods. If a structure-based method is required, for example, to study ligand interactions by docking, only the use of co-crystallized structures with very similar ligands will provide robust results.

As alternative to screening-derived structures, also the natural ligand can serve as valuable starting point for nuclear receptor modulator development. The discovery of obeticholic acid and other steroidal FXR agonists (Fig. 2), for example, has shown that highly potent nuclear receptor targeting drugs can be derived from the endogenous agonist. Obeticholic acid (OCA) was discovered by systematic exploration of the natural scaffold with chenodeoxycholic acid (CDCA) derivatives carrying an additional methyl residue in various positions. Thereby, 6α-methyl-CDCA was identified as more potent on FXR than CDCA. Subsequently, the 6α-position was further investigated with alternative substituents of which the ethyl chain of OCA turned out as most favored. Using the support of a co-crystallized structure of the FXR-LBD in complex with CDCA, OCA was further investigated to enhance potency and selectivity over the membrane bile acid receptor TGR5. The FXR ligand-binding site revealed a small pocket near C11 of CDCA that could be exploited by β-oriented hydroxy group which remarkably enhanced selectivity over TGR5 [10–12].

3 Test Systems

In general, there are two common approaches to evaluate modulation of nuclear receptors by small molecules in vitro. First, several methods are available to observe coactivator recruitment to the purified recombinant ligand-binding domain of a nuclear receptor in the presence of an agonist. They rely on the interaction between the LBD and a coactivator peptide that can be detected by fluorescence resonance energy transfer (FRET), the alpha screen technology, or simple fluorescence polarization. Each of these methods requires that at least one of the interaction partners—nuclear receptor LBD or coactivator peptide—is labeled. Coactivator recruitment assays provide the advantage that they detect a specific interaction between a small molecule and the ligand-binding domain of a nuclear receptor without unspecific effects from cellular background. Moreover, coactivator recruitment allows an estimation of a test compound's transactivation efficacy which ought to be correlated to the efficacy of coactivator recruitment. However, coactivator recruitment assays ignore a crucial aspect of nuclear receptor modulator development, namely, the nuclear localization of the target and the cellular background. A potent inducer of coactivator recruitment can be totally inactive at a cellular background if it fails to access the site inside the cell where the target is located or if it is inactivated by the cell [13].

This crucial information can in contrast be retrieved from reporter gene assays, the second widespread method to characterize nuclear receptor modulators in vitro. They rely on the physiological ability of a nuclear receptor to govern the expression of a target gene. By genetic engineering, a construct is generated that codes for a reporter gene whose expression rate can easily be detected under the control of a promoter/response element which is specific for the nuclear receptor to be studied. Two types of such transactivation assays exist for nuclear receptors. The more physiological setting employs the full human nuclear receptor and its response element to govern reporter gene expression. Such full-length assays constitute the least artificial in vitro test systems for the characterization of nuclear receptor modulators as they reproduce the cellular background with nuclear target localization as well as the entire human nuclear receptor protein as monomer, homodimer, or heterodimer bound to a natural response element. However, as such full-length assays are based on the full nuclear receptor, also alternative transactivation mechanisms can occur, and, therefore, full-length assays often provide rather small signal-to-noise ratios and are less robust than hybrid systems [13].

The more artificial transactivation assay system is based on hybrid receptors composed of the human nuclear receptor ligand-binding domain and the DNA-binding domain of the yeast receptor Gal4. Such hybrid transactivation assays require a plasmid construct coding for the hybrid receptor and a reporter construct with the reporter gene under the control of a specific response element for the Gal4 DNA-binding domain. Though more artificial, such hybrid transactivation assays provide several advantages when used for screening in the process of nuclear receptor modulator development [13].

As reporter genes, luciferases (firefly, renilla) and ß-galactosidase are most common. Newer systems also successfully used fluorescent proteins making the assay significantly less expensive. In addition, a robust reporter gene assay should implicitly be equipped with a constitutively expressed control gene to monitor transfection efficiency and test compound toxicity. Otherwise, false positive hits might be retrieved, especially in antagonistic testing [13].

In summary, cellular reporter gene assays provide most information as test systems in nuclear receptor modulator development as they not only reveal the activity of test compounds on the nuclear receptor in question but also have a cellular background. This ensures that only substances are identified as active which are able to penetrate the barrier of the cell membrane and reach the cellular compartment where they are expected to be active. Additionally, test systems equipped with a control gene also give a hint on the toxicity of test compounds. Among the reporter gene assay types, hybrid receptor systems though artificial are the more specific approach to characterize test compound activity on one particular nuclear receptor. Additionally, the Gal4 system is very robust and provides favorable signal-to-noise ratios. It is also very flexible and can be established for many human nuclear receptors. As nuclear receptor modulator test system of choice, an example Gal4 hybrid reporter gene assay is described in detail in the method chapter [13].

4 Materials

For a typical Gal4 hybrid reporter gene assay, the following materials are required:

1. A plasmid encoding the Gal4-DBD-hNR-LBD hybrid receptor. It is generated by inserting the DNA sequence of the desired human nuclear receptor ligand-binding domain and hinge region obtained from cDNA amplification into the multiple cloning sites of the commercially available vector pFA-CMV. The resulting construct codes for the required hybrid receptor which is constitutively expressed under the CMV promoter. Example constructs for 15 hybrid receptors can be found in [14].
2. pFR-Luc or a comparable reporter vector with Gal4 response element as reporter gene construct.

3. pRL-SV40 or a similar constitutively expressed reporter gene construct for normalization and toxicity control.
4. HEK293T cells (or an alternative cell line that can be easily transfected and cultured in serum-free medium).
5. Light microscope.
6. Clear 96-well plates.
7. Cell culture media: DMEM high glucose supplemented with 10% FCS, sodium pyruvate (1 mM), penicillin (100 U/mL), and streptomycin (100 μg/mL), unsupplemented Opti-MEM and Opti-MEM supplemented with penicillin (100 U/mL) and streptomycin (100 μg/mL) (*see* **Note 1**).
8. Trypsin/EDTA solution (TE), trypan blue solution (0.5% solution in 0.9% NaCl solution), and a cell counter or counting chamber for cell seeding.
9. Lipofectamine® LTX for transfection.
10. Dual-Glo® Luciferase Assay system, opaque 96-well plates and a plate reader for luminescence measurement.
11. Standard cell culture consumables (reaction tubes, culture flasks, etc.).
12. Reference agonist for the respective nuclear receptor as positive control, test compounds, and DMSO.

5 Methods

5.1 Exemplified Optimization of a Nuclear Receptor Modulator

There is no general strategy of compound optimization, but a systematic approach for the exploration of a lead compound usually is a good start. Additionally, some demands to compounds should not be neglected when targeting nuclear receptors. In this chapter, we describe a successful optimization of a nuclear receptor modulator as example and discuss the strategy and considerations in the optimization process.

1. A FXR modulator development started with a ligand- and structure-based virtual screening approach using self-organizing maps which retrieved the moderately potent FXR ligand **A** as lead structure (Fig. 3) [15]. Ligand **A** comprised the typical structure of fatty acid mimetics and seemed suitable to target FXR which is endogenously activated by bile acids. (Furthermore, **A** was identified in a reporter gene assay and, therefore, was obviously able to reach the nucleus as prerequisite to nuclear receptor modulation. Inspection of the molecular structure of **A** indicated that the lipophilic backbone as typical structural element of nuclear receptor targeting fatty acid mimetics was rather small. Hence, this moiety was addressed as initial optimization step. Among several larger and more lipophilic residues

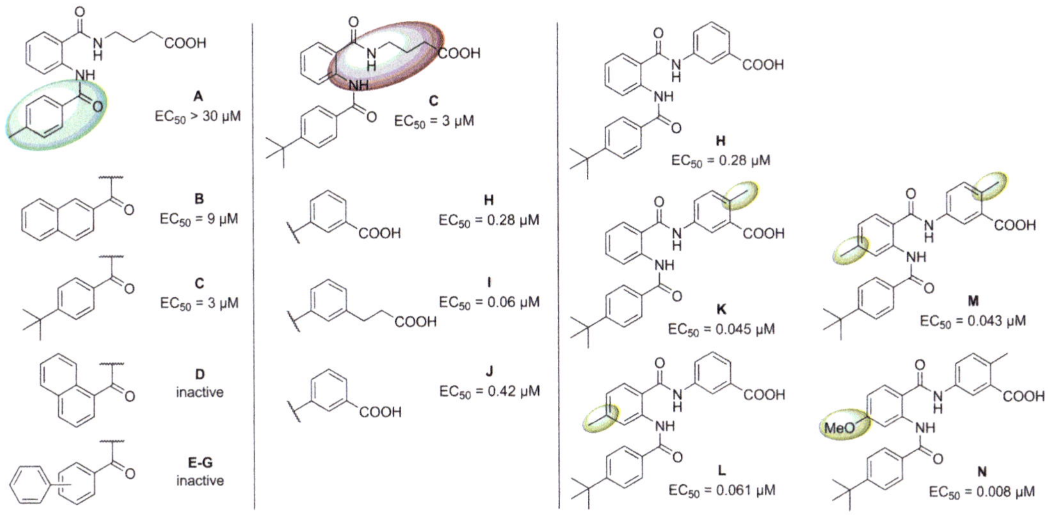

Fig. 3 Key compounds of an exemplified nuclear receptor modulator development

than the original 4-methylbenzamide in **A**, the 2-naphthamide (**B**) and the 4-tert-butylbenzamide (**C**) turned out as most favorable. As expected, enlargement of the lipophilic backbone generated a marked improvement in potency but as exemplified by the inactivity of 1-naphthamide derivative **D** and all biphenyls **E–G** (*see* Fig. 3), also the geometry of this region can play a major role.)

2. The next optimization step addressed the linker region of the compound class that mediates positioning of the acidic head and the lipophilic backbone regions. Exploration of the linker's structure activity relationship started with chain length variations, but no alternative chain length produced any improvement. Subsequently, the geometry of the linker was studied by inverting each amide bond which in both cases leads to inactivity. Also methylation of the amide nitrogen atoms was not tolerated indicating that the amide bonds either formed polar contacts to the target or intramolecular H-bonds that significantly contributed to a favorable geometry [16].
3. Compared to the rigid scaffold of the bile acids as natural FXR ligands, the linker region of **A–C** seemed rather flexible. Thus, aminobenzoic acids, aminomethylbenzoic acids, aminophenylacetic acids, and aminophenylpropionic acids were evaluated as more rigid linkers [16, 17] (*see* **Note 2**).
4. After linker optimization, the essential acidic head was studied by bioisosteric replacement. This strategy has already been very successful in nuclear receptor modulator development, for example, in the glitazones that contain a thiazolidinedione as carboxylic acid bioisostere which significantly contributes to their potency and selectivity [9, 16–18] (*see* **Note 3**).

5. Lipophilic backbone and linker optimization that were accompanied by larger structural changes had already remarkably improved the potency. For further activity enhancement, smaller changes were addressed [17] (*see* **Note 4**).

This example depicts a successful systematic approach to nuclear receptor modulator development. Starting with a screening hit that comprised moderate activity, larger scaffold changes were investigated for potency improvement. By targeted structural variations, the amide bonds were identified as essential moieties enabling a favorable geometry and were then conserved throughout the SAR exploration. After optimizing the scaffold and its geometry with major structural changes, additional space in the binding site for further substituents was evaluated by introducing methyl in every free position. This strategy revealed two suitable positions to further expand the compounds for improvements in potency. Thus identified substituent vectors were then combined and further explored with alternative residues replacing the methyl groups which led to identification of a methoxy group as further optimized residue.

Compound optimization in a systematic approach should always introduce only one structural change at a time, and activity should always be determined in the same test system to obtain comparable data. In brief, the exemplified successful optimization strategy can be summarized in few key steps:

1. Exploration of the lipophilic backbone with several large lipophilic moieties that covered various geometries for optimally filling the hydrophobic part of the nuclear receptor ligand-binding site.
2. Inspection of the linker length and geometry to position the acidic head and lipophilic backbone in suitable distance and angle.
3. Bioisosteric replacement of the acidic head group considering favorable interaction with the target but also suitable properties/p*K*a to reach the site of action in the nucleus.
4. Systematic evaluation of unexplored space in the ligand-binding site by separate introduction of a methyl group in every free position of the ligand.
5. Deep investigation of identified positions for further substitution in every position in which the methyl group was at least tolerated without loss of activity by replacing methyl with trifluoromethyl, halogens, methoxy, trifluoromethoxy, hydroxy, amino, etc. Potentially also larger groups such as phenyl, etc. should be studied.
6. Another promising approach that was, however, not explored in the example would be heterocyclic replacement of aromatic

residues to improve solubility by introducing more dipolmoment and to potentially identify unexplored polar contacts with the target from additional heteroatoms.

A nuclear receptor modulator development should also consider the following points:

(a) The activity of the hit/lead structure on the receptor to be targeted should be confirmed with a robust test system and at best be confirmed by an independent alternative method. For example, activity from a cellular reporter gene assay or a cell-free coactivator recruitment assay combined with binding affinity to the recombinant nuclear receptor LBD determined by isothermal titration calorimetry would be a reliable start.

(b) A nuclear receptor modulator has to reach the nucleus to be active. Therefore, it is of no use to optimize a compound for high potency in a cell-free test system if it will not get through the cell membrane to the site of action. If a modulator development is conducted with a cell-free assay, alternative methods to confirm cellular availability should be included.

(c) Due to high similarity in the architecture of nuclear receptors and similar ligand-binding sites, nuclear receptor modulators are prone to possess poor selectivity. Therefore, the activity of a compound class on related receptors should be studied early in modulator development, and measures to obtain the desired selectivity profile should be taken before the potency on the desired target is excessively optimized.

(d) The high lipophilicity of the ligand-binding sites in many nuclear receptors naturally leads to rather lipophilic ligands. Therefore, the development of nuclear receptor modulators with favorable solubility is an additional challenge, but drug-like properties such as acceptable solubility and log P should also be evaluated and addressed early in development. Classical strategies such as heterocyclic replacement can improve solubility to a certain extent, and sometimes avoiding an extensively flat geometry can be of considerable benefit.

5.2 Gal4 Hybrid Reporter Gene Assay

The detailed procedure of a typical Gal4 assay is described below. It takes 3 days, with an average of 2–3 h/day (depending on the number of 96-well plates used).

5.2.1 0 h: Seeding Cells

- Have HEK293T cells with approx. 80% confluence ready.
- Trypsinate cells, transfer cell suspension to a 50 mL tube, and count cell number per mL.
- Centrifuge and resuspend cells in fresh cell culture medium.
- Seed cells in 96-well plates with 30,000 cells and 100 μL volume per well (cell density 300,000 cells/mL).
- Keep cells in the incubator at 37 °C and 5% CO_2.

5.2.2 24 h: Transfection

- Preparations (note: the following procedure including plasmid and reagent amounts as well as incubation times are an example and are subject to changes and optimization for some hybrid receptor constructs, alternative cell lines, or other plate sizes):
  - Prepare plasmid mixture according to the following specifications:

    Final volume: 15.1 μL/well in Opti-MEM without supplements.

    pFA-CMV-hybrid receptor construct: 12–50 ng/well.

    pFR-Luc: 100 ng/well.

    pRL-SV40: 2 ng/well.
  - Prepare lipofectamine reagent mixtures:

    0.12 μL/well PLUS reagent + 1.88 μL/well Opti-MEM without supplements.

    0.20 μL/well LTX reagent reagent + 2.70 μL/well Opti-MEM without supplements.
  - Change culture medium on the 96-well plates to Opti-MEM without supplements (100 μL/well).
- Transfection procedure:
  - Add 2.0 μL/well PLUS reagent mix to plasmid mix, incubate 5 min.
  - Add 2.9 μL/well LTX reagent mix to plasmid mix, incubate 25 min.
  - Transfer the plasmid/reagent mixture to the 96-well plate (20 μL/well).
- Incubate cells for 4.5–5.0 h.

5.2.3 29 h: Incubation with Test Compounds

- Preparations:
  - Prepare stock solutions (100 mM) of the test compounds in DMSO. If solubility at 100 mM is insufficient, reduce concentration.
  - Prepare a master dilution (100 μM) of each test compound by adding 1 μL of the stock solution to 1 mL Opti-MEM with supplements.
  - Prepare dilution series for each test compound in Opti-MEM with supplements containing 0.1% DMSO.
  - For antagonistic testing, use Opti-MEM with supplements and DMSO additionally containing a fixed concentration (e.g., 1 μM) of the reference agonist for the dilution series.
- Incubation:
  - Remove medium/transfection mix from the 96-well plates, and replace it with the dilutions of the test compounds (50 μL/well).

- Do not remove medium from more than 12 wells at a time.
- Test each compound concentration in triplicates (or at least in duplicates).
- Include at least one negative (Opti-MEM with supplements containing 0.1% DMSO) and one positive control (reference agonist for the receptor that is tested at a sound concentration, 1 μM usually works well) on each 96-well plate.
- Validate actives by repeating a single concentration measurement without transfecting the hybrid receptor construct.

- Incubate the cells in the incubator for 14–16 h.

5.2.4 43 h: Luminescence Measurement

- Preparations:
  - Thaw Dual-Glo firefly substrate mix (2.5 mL/96-well plate).
  - Dilute Dual-Glo firefly substrate mix 1:1 with Opti-MEM without supplements.
  - Prepare DualGlo stop&glo renilla substrate mix (2.5 mL/96-well plate) according to manufacturer's procedure.
- Remove medium/incubation mix from 96-well plates, and add 50 μL dilutes Dual-Glo firefly substrate mix to each well (do not execute more than 48 wells at a time).
- Incubate for 10 min at room temperature.
- Transfer lysed cells to an opaque 96-well plate.
- Measure (firefly) luminescence (1000 ms integration time, no specific wavelength) in a plate reader immediately (not later than 60 after lysis).
- After firefly luminescence measurement, add 25 μL DualGlo stop&glo mix to every well.
- Incubate for 10 min.
- Measure (renilla) luminescence (1000 ms integration time, no specific wavelength) in a plate reader immediately.

5.2.5 Data Analysis

- Data analysis for individual assays:
  - Use Microsoft Excel or a similar software to calculate relative light units (RLUs), fold activation, and relative activation by performing the following operations for each well:

$$\text{RLU} = \frac{\text{luminescence} \quad (\text{firefly})}{\text{luminescence} \quad (\text{renilla})} * 1000$$

$$\text{fold-activation} = \frac{\text{RLU} \ (\text{testcompound})}{\text{RLU} \ (\text{negativecontrol})}$$

$$\text{relative activation} = \frac{\text{fold-activation} \ (\text{testcompound})}{\text{fold-activation} \ (\text{positivecontrol})} * 100$$

  - The selection between RLU, fold activation, and relative activation for compound characterization has to be made according to the demands. In general, relative activation gives the most stable results, while RLUs usually have high inter-assay variance.

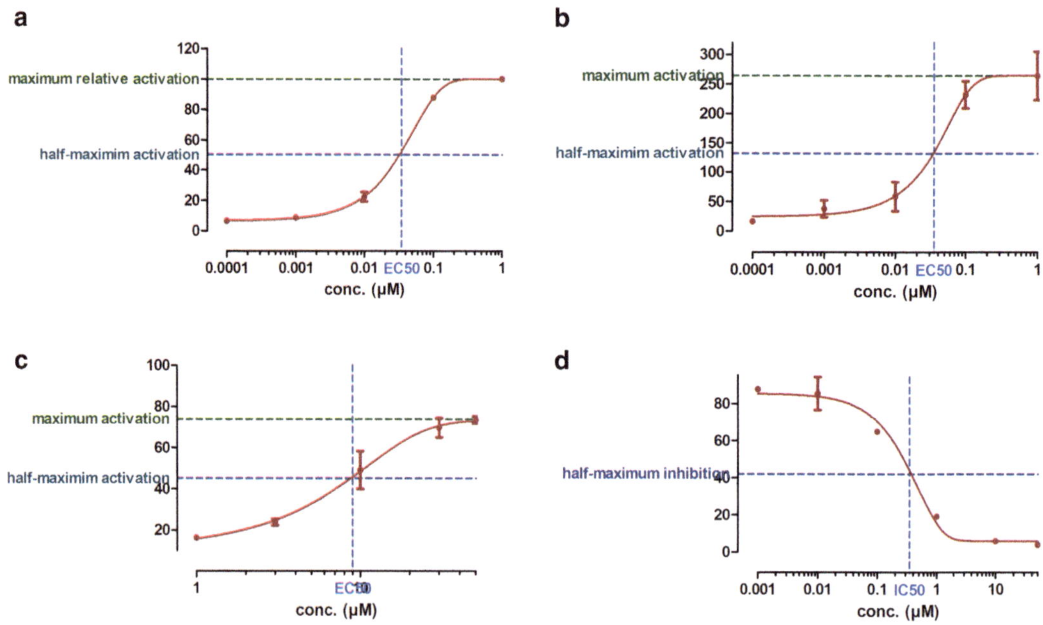

Fig. 4 Example of dose–response curves: (**a**) Activity of the RAR reference agonist retinoic acid on RARγ with maximum relative activation. (**b**) The same data analyzed by fold activation gives a very similar curve but with significantly higher variance for each single point. (**c**) Activity of the endogenous FXR agonist CDCA analyzed by relative activation compared to the reference agonist GW4064: the maximum relative activation of CDCA is lower than of the synthetic reference agonist and does not reach 100%. (**d**) Typical antagonistic dose–response curve of a synthetic FXR antagonist in presence of a fixed concentration of the reference agonist analyzed with relative activation

- Data analysis for compound characterization (Fig. 4):
  - The potency of a test compound, expressed as its EC_{50} or IC_{50} value, can be determined from a sigmoidal dose–response curve.
  - To obtain such sigmoidal curve, determine RLU, fold activation, or relative activation for a concentration range that contains concentrations where the compound is inactive and concentrations in the saturation of maximum activity.
  - Plot concentration (*x*-axis, logarithmic) vs. RLU, fold activation, or relative activation.
  - Calculate EC_{50} or IC_{50} value using *SigmaPlot* (Systat Software) or *GraphPad Prism* (GraphPad Software) with four-parameter logistic regression.

5.3 Concluding Remarks

Nuclear receptors are expected to gain increasing relevance as pharmaceutical targets as they regulate innumerable physiological and pathophysiological processes. The development of small molecules that activate or antagonize this class of receptors is a challenging though promising approach to new drugs. One major challenge beyond simple optimization of potency often rests in achieving the required selectivity within a subfamily of related nuclear receptors that accommodate the same chemotype of ligands. Additionally, the large number of genes that is induced or repressed by each nuclear receptor also holds a potential for considerable side effects, and modulator development must consider this risk. Therefore, the future of nuclear receptor targeting drugs might especially lie in tissue or even target gene-selective modulators.

6 Notes

1. If not clearly indicated otherwise, DMEM with supplements is used.
2. Among these, 3-aminophenylbenzoic acid **H** and 3-aminophenylpropionic acid **I** remarkably enhanced the potency. The fact that 3-aminophenylacetic acid **J** did not exhibit a potency between **H** and **I** depicts the importance of optimal positioning of the acidic function. Virtual inspection of the binding modes of **H**–**J** suggested that the benzoic acid (**H**) forms favorable interactions with a water molecule coordinated by the basic arginine residues at the polar end of the FXR ligand-binding site. Phenylpropionic acid **I** displaces the water molecule and directly forms polar contacts with the arginine residue, whereas phenylacetic acid **J** has the wrong geometry for both kinds of interaction (*see* Fig. 3). It is too long for water-mediated interactions but also does not reach the arginines for direct contacts [16, 17].
3. Additionally, carboxylic acids can be a weak spot in a compound's metabolic conversion, and bioisosteres can markedly enhance their half-life. Bioisosteric replacement should ensure that the interactions of the moiety to be replaced with the target protein can also be formed by the bioisoster. In this particular example, a group able to carry a negative charge and to participate as H-bond acceptor for the neutralizing interaction with FXR's arginines was required. However, acidity should also not exceed a p*K*a of approx. 3 to ensure cell penetration and bioavailability [9]. Based on these considerations, bioisosteres such as a tetrazole were evaluated but significantly reduced the potency and were not suitable [16–18].
4. To identify positions that would tolerate additional substituents, first a methyl group was introduced in every free position of the scaffold. The lipophilic backbone had been studied like this earlier in the optimization and, therefore, was neglected. Thereby, two positions where the methyl group enhanced potency were identified (**K**, **L**) and further explored with halogens as well as methoxy and trifluoromethoxy groups as alternative residues. No further activity increase was achieved in ortho position of the carboxylic acid, and also combination of

both methyl substituents in one compound (**M**) was not superior. However, replacement of the 4-methyl group at the central aromatic ring by methoxy (**N**) produced the desired further optimization.

References

1. Aranda A, Pascual A (2001) Nuclear hormone receptors and gene expression. Physiol Rev 81 (3):1269–1304
2. Germain P, Chambon P, Eichele G et al (2006) International Union of Pharmacology. LX. Retinoic acid receptors. Pharmacol Rev 58(4):712–725
3. Evans RM, Mangelsdorf DJ (2014) Nuclear receptors, RXR, and the big bang. Cell 157 (1):255–266. https://doi.org/10.1016/j.cell.2014.03.012
4. Germain P, Chambon P, Eichele G et al (2006) International Union of Pharmacology. LXIII. Retinoid X receptors. Pharmacol Rev 58 (4):760–772. https://doi.org/10.1124/pr.58.4.7
5. de Lera AR, Bourguet W, Altucci L, Gronemeyer H (2007) Design of Selective Nuclear Receptor Modulators: RAR and RXR as a case study. Nat Rev Drug Discov 6(10):811–820. https://doi.org/10.1038/nrd2398
6. Nuclear Receptors Nomenclature Committee (1999) A unified nomenclature system for the nuclear receptor superfamily. Cell 97 (2):161–163. https://doi.org/10.1016/S0092-8674(00)80726-6
7. Germain P, Staels B, Dacquet C et al (2006) Overview of nomenclature of nuclear receptors. Pharmacol Rev 58(4):685–704. https://doi.org/10.1124/pr.58.4.2
8. Merk D, Steinhilber D, Schubert-Zsilavecz M (2012) Medicinal chemistry of Farnesoid X receptor ligands: from agonists and antagonists to modulators. Future Med Chem 4 (8):1015–1036. https://doi.org/10.4155/fmc.12.47
9. Proschak E, Heitel P, Kalinowsky L, Merk D (2017) Opportunities and challenges for fatty acid Mimetics in drug discovery. J Med Chem 60(13):5235–5266. https://doi.org/10.1021/acs.jmedchem.6b01287
10. Pellicciari R, Passeri D, De Franco F et al (2016) Discovery of 3α,7α,11β-Trihydroxy-6α-ethyl-5β-Cholan-24-Oic acid (TC-100), a novel bile acid as potent and highly selective FXR agonist for Enterohepatic disorders. J Med Chem 59(19):9201–9214. https://doi.org/10.1021/acs.jmedchem.6b01126
11. Costantino G, Macchiarulo A, Entrena-Guadix A et al (2003) Binding mode of 6ECDCA, a potent bile acid agonist of the Farnesoid X receptor (FXR). Bioorg Med Chem Lett 13 (11):1865–1868. https://doi.org/10.1016/S0960-894X(03)00281-6
12. Pellicciari R, Fiorucci S, Camaioni E et al (2002) 6α-ethyl-Chenodeoxycholic acid (6-ECDCA), a potent and selective FXR agonist endowed with Anticholestatic activity. J Med Chem 45(17):3569–3572. https://doi.org/10.1021/jm025529g
13. Merk D, Steinhilber D, Schubert-Zsilavecz M (2014) Characterizing ligands for Farnesoid X receptor-available in vitro test Systems for Farnesoid X Receptor Modulator Development. Expert Opin Drug Discov 9(1):27–37. https://doi.org/10.1517/17460441.2014.860129
14. Flesch D, Cheung S-Y, Schmidt J et al (2017) Non-acidic Farnesoid X receptor modulators. J Med Chem 60(16):7199–7205. https://doi.org/10.1021/acs.jmedchem.7b00903
15. Achenbach J, Gabler M, Steri R et al (2013) Identification of novel Farnesoid X receptor modulators using a combined ligand- and structure-based virtual screening. MedChemComm 4(6):920. https://doi.org/10.1039/C3MD00049D
16. Merk D, Gabler M, Gomez RC et al (2014) Anthranilic acid derivatives as novel ligands for Farnesoid X receptor (FXR). Bioorg Med Chem 22(8):2447–2460. https://doi.org/10.1016/j.bmc.2014.02.053
17. Merk D, Lamers C, Ahmad K et al (2014) Extending the structure-activity relationship of anthranilic acid derivatives as Farnesoid X receptor modulators: development of a highly potent partial Farnesoid X receptor agonist. J Med Chem 57(19):8035–8055. https://doi.org/10.1021/jm500937v
18. Merk D, Lamers C, Weber J et al (2015) Anthranilic acid derivatives as nuclear receptor modulators—development of novel PPAR selective and dual PPAR/FXR ligands. Bioorg Med Chem 23(3):499–514. https://doi.org/10.1016/j.bmc.2014.12.013

Chapter 15

In Silico Screening of Compound Libraries Using a Consensus of Orthogonal Methodologies

Vassilios Myrianthopoulos, George Lambrinidis, and Emmanuel Mikros

Abstract

A number of diverse approaches for efficient screening of compound collections in silico are nowadays available, each with their own methodological background, successes and limitations. Implementation of such virtual screening methods has enabled an impressive acceleration in the search toward the most biologically relevant regions of chemical space and has greatly facilitated the discovery of novel biologically active molecules. It is noteworthy that the range of principles on which the available virtual screening methodologies are based is wide enough for several of these methods to be considered as orthogonal to a good extent. We hereby propose a simple and extensible protocol aiming at integrating the diverse information derived by such virtual screening methods in a consensus manner that can achieve an improvement of the hit rate obtained by individual use of those methods. The protocol can be performed in its basic version as described in this work, but it can also be extended manually by integrating a number of different screening tools and their case-specific variations to further increase the performance of virtual screening in prioritizing the most promising compounds for in vitro evaluations.

Key words Structure-based screening, Ligand-based screening, Docking-scoring, Similarity search, Sampling optimization, Frequency-based ranking, Linear integration, NCI/DTP repository

1 Introduction

Drug discovery is a laborious and lengthy process estimated to reach a total mean cost of $2500 million (2013 data) spread over a sequence of phases lasting more than 10 years for each new approved entity [1]. In the last decades, the preclinical stages of the drug discovery pipeline have been considerably shortened [1] by successful implementation of a variety of state-of the-art technologies. Among these, innovative cheminformatics and bioinformatics methods nowadays play a prominent role in all steps of early-stage drug discovery and preclinical development, such as target identification and validation, primary hit identification, hit-to-lead optimization and rational drug design [2, 3]. Of utmost importance in the discovery of new and promising drug candidates are the

Thomas Mavromoustakos and Tahsin F. Kellici (eds.), *Rational Drug Design: Methods and Protocols*, Methods in Molecular Biology, vol. 1824, https://doi.org/10.1007/978-1-4939-8630-9_15, © Springer Science+Business Media, LLC, part of Springer Nature 2018

various computational algorithms used for predicting the likelihood of small molecules to interact in a therapeutically relevant fashion with a given biological target in silico [4]. Such predictions are enabled by a diverse set of procedures collectively characterized as virtual screening (VS) [5].

The array of currently available VS methodologies comprises an integral part of most drug discovery campaigns and their contribution in facilitating increased hit rates is indisputable. In parallel to VS evolution, the accessible chemical space has also increased in the last decade by a number of public compound libraries such as PubChem [6], ChEMBL [7], ZINC [8], or commercial like Enamine, Chembridge, Sellekchem, ChemDiv, Maybridge, and many others along with a wide array of smaller focused libraries facilitating drug repurposing (e.g., LOPAC® or Drug Repurposing Hub [9]). Furthermore, advances in genetic engineering, X-ray crystallography, and NMR spectroscopy enabled the successful realization of a series of structural genomics projects that deliver a continuously increasing number of experimental structures for emerging drug targets.

VS can be based both on the structure and physicochemical characteristics of the small molecules (ligand/pharmacophore-based approach) [10] and on the simulation of their interaction with the target protein by docking-scoring calculations (structure-based approach) [11]. Pharmacophore perception is a key concept in medicinal chemistry and its empirical modeling through extensive synthetic efforts for establishing extensive structure–activity relationships used to characterize traditional drug discovery. The corresponding computational tools provide a comprehensive description of important pharmacophore features such as hydrogen-bond donors/acceptors, charged or polarizable groups or atoms, hydrophobicity, molecular surface and shape, dipole moment and others. Additional pharmacophore features can be derived by mapping the binding region of the drug target in case the protein structure is known. Assuming that target recognition is mainly driven by such factors, integration of these features with biological activity data can derive statistical models that can be used to screen compound libraries for bioactive molecules. Several software for pharmacophore modeling and similarity screening exist such as CATALYST [12], PHASE [13], LIGANDSCOUT [14], GALAHAD [15], GASP [16], and ROCS [17].

On the other hand, structure-based VS is based on accurate prediction of the protein–ligand complex geometry (docking) [18] and the corresponding change in free energy (scoring) [19]. Sampling of ligand orientation within the binding domain of the target is mainly based on stochastic search techniques such as Monte Carlo and genetic or fragment-based algorithms [20, 21]. Evaluation of each binding pose is carried out by force-field, empirical, or knowledge-based scoring functions leading to rank ordering the different docked poses for each ligand [22]. Docking-scoring tools include both open access and commercial algorithms such as DOCK [23], AutoDock [24] and AutoDock Vina [25], Glide [26], GOLD [27], and rDOCK [28].

Real-life applications have shown the limitations of the different approaches, while pitfalls have been recognized and thoroughly described with the aim to assist the efficiency of the VS procedures [29]. A significant approximation is that the majority of existing software considers only ligand flexibility, in order to reduce computational time. Different techniques have been proposed to address the protein flexibility issue, among them the use of protein ensembles derived from MD simulations [30, 31]. More importantly, the existing scoring functions deal with the entropic term of the interaction only implicitly. New approaches that take into account the displacement of water molecules located within the protein-binding cavity could address, at least partly, the entropic penalties related to protein–ligand interaction [32].

The detailed and systematic assessment of VS performance is a research topic of key importance for promoting rational use of the available algorithms. High-quality preassembled sets of known active compounds (training sets) or structurally related inactives (decoy sets) such as the DUD-E (Database of Useful Decoys—Enhanced) are available to assist validation of VS campaigns on a case-by-case basis [33]. Moreover, a number of benchmarking tests have been carried out to evaluate performance of the most popular docking-scoring software [34–36].

The majority of benchmarks have highlighted VS method limitations in terms of their overall success toward qualitative prediction of binding geometry but at the same time of moderate, to poor in many cases, performance over quantitative reproduction of experimental binding affinity [37]. Moreover, to advance evolution of computer-aided drug discovery, community-wide, blinded prediction assessment challenges have been organized such as CSAR [38] or D3R (https://drugdesigndata.org). In a recent (2016) D3R challenge, the pose prediction median RMSD varied from 1 up to 7 Å, while free energy prediction RMSE varied from 0.7 up to 5.0 kcal/mol.

It is unquestionable though that VS can indeed facilitate enrichment of compound collections and lead to a systematic reduction in the need for actual in vitro experiments that can reach up to three orders of magnitude compared to randomized HTS [39]. Moreover, VS has been proposed as a successful tool to avoid HTS artifacts and provide a more rational approach to hit discovery [40]. Toward this objective, benchmarking studies moreover suggest that the performance of VS endeavors can be considerably advanced by integrating a range of diverse VS algorithms in a consensus fashion [34, 41]. On the other hand, many studies underline the need of any VS-derived dataset to be treated with a critical thought and always in comparison with experimental data [42] for securing confidence of all stages of research in which such a tool is involved.

Aiming at suggesting a versatile VS workflow with its main emphasis being on rational implementation of all methods involved and, moreover, on optimal time and cost efficiency, we hereby describe an expansible consensus protocol for in silico screening of compound collections and prioritization of the most promising molecules for subsequent in vitro evaluations. Applications of this approach have been already reported [43, 44]. The basic version presented here comprises a combination of one ligand-based (three-dimensional similarity screening) and one structure-based method (docking-scoring calculations), but it is accompanied by a thorough discussion on the different sampling methods and algorithms that can be manually integrated for further enhancement of the basic protocol (*see* **Notes 1–3**). Finally, to address the need of users with less experience to validate the error-free implementation of the two individual screening tools utilized in the basic protocol, we provide a small focused tutorial section (*see* **Notes 4** and **5**).

2 Materials

1. Protein structures and protein–ligand complexes are obtained from the Protein Data Bank (PDB) [45] (www.rcsb.org), which is a worldwide repository of information about the 3D structures of large biological molecules.
2. The NCI/DTP repository, a collection of approximately 260,000 drug-like small molecules available on demand (https://cactus.nci.nih.gov/download/nci/), is also provided as a virtual database in .sdf format.
3. Software and tools:
   (a) Maestro software (Schrödinger Inc., http://www.schrodinger.com), a molecular visualization program, free of charge for all academic users.
   (b) Protein preparation wizard (Schrödinger Inc., http://www.schrodinger.com), implemented on Maestro software (commercially available).
   (c) LigPrep workflow (Schrödinger Inc., http://www.schrodinger.com), implemented in Maestro software (commercially available).
   (d) Glide software (Schrödinger Inc., http://www.schrodinger.com), implemented in Maestro software (commercially available).
   (e) ROCS software and vROCS graphical user interface (Openeye Inc., http://www.eyesopen.com), a commercial program providing free academic license usage.

(f) Omega software (Openeye Inc., http://www.eyesopen.com), a commercial program providing free academic license usage.

(g) VIDA software (Openeye Inc.), a commercial molecular visualization program providing academic license usage.

3 Methods

3.1 Compound Collection Preparation and Enumeration

Each database of small molecules needs to be prepared prior to its use for virtual screening calculations. Most databases provide 2D structures in .smi (SMILES) or .sdf format which need to be converted into 3D structures with correct protonation states, tautomerism and enumeration of possible stereoisomers whenever such information is missing from the original database. In our case the entries of the NCI/DTP repository are provided as 3D structures in .sdf format and it will be prepared, enumerated and finally energy-minimized using the LigPrep tool as implemented in Maestro software, but other programs can be used for the same purpose as well.

1. Download the "NCI_Open_2012-05-01.sdf.gz" file of the NCI/DTP repository to your computer.
2. Open the LigPrep workflow (Applications → LigPrep).
3. On "Use structure from," choose "File," and on "File name," select "Browse," and find the file downloaded in **step 1**.
4. In "Ionization" select "Generate possible states at target pH: 7.0 ± 2.0" option, and in "Using" select "Epik."
5. Check that "Desalt" and "Generate tautomers" options are selected.
6. On "Stereoisomers" choose "Retain specified chiralities (vary other chiral centers)".
7. On "Generate low energy ring conformations," set a value of "1".
8. Select .mae (maestro) as output file format and press "Run". After completion of the calculation, a .mae file containing the enumerated NCI/DTP compound collection ready to be used for docking will be created in the working directory. Meanwhile the resulted collection will be incorporated to the current project and selected (marked as yellow on the project table).
9. Convert the selected collection to .sdf ("File" → "Export") and select the .sdf format from the dropdown list in the "Export" window.
10. Perform a conformer enumeration for the prepared NCI/DTP collection by using Omega software. Open a terminal inside the directory where the LigPrep output file is saved, type

"omega2 –in [filename.sdf]" where "filename.sdf" is the file exported on **step 10**, and press Enter. The calculation creates a file named [filename.oeb.gz] which contains 200-member ensembles for each of the molecules contained in the collection and can be used for similarity screening using ROCS.

3.2 Structure-Based Screening Using a Docking-Scoring Method

In this step, the workflow of performing a docking-based ranking of the NCI/DTP compounds is described. In this approach, an appropriately selected crystal structure of the target protein (*see* **Notes 2** and **5**) will be used to create grids necessary for performing rigid docking calculations, then docking will be undertaken, scoring of the NCI/DTP molecules will be performed and finally a list of the screened molecules will be created. In this list, the molecules are ranked based on their predicted affinity for the protein. Ranking is based on their docking score, where a more negative value corresponds to a higher binding affinity for the given protein.

3.2.1 Protein Preparation

1. Download the crystal structure of the protein, which will be used for docking calculations from the PDB.
2. Open the Maestro software.
3. From "Project" menu select "Change Directory," and create a new directory where all calculations will be further stored. Open the .pdb file downloaded in the previous step ("File" → "Import structures").
4. Press the "PrepWiz" button and the "Protein Preparation Wizard" appears. At the "Job prefix" field, define an appropriate name. Then, at the "Import and Process" tab, press the "Preprocess" button.
5. At the tab "Refine," select "Sample water orientations," then use "PROPKA for pH 7.0," and press "Optimize."
6. Finally proceed to "Restrained minimization" using the default "Converge heavy atoms to RMSD," set the value of "0.3 Å" for RMSD, select the "OPLS3" force field, and press the "Minimize" button. The software will run small restrained minimizations to eliminate crystallographic strain. Hydrogen atoms are always fully optimized. Heavy atoms are restrained so the resulting structure will not exceed the RMSD value set from starting coordinates.
7. The created protein structure is ready for docking-scoring calculations.

3.2.2 Creation of Protein Grid Files

1. Select from the "Entry List" the resulting protein from Subheading 3.2.1, **step 5**.
2. From "Applications" choose "Glide" and "Receptor Grid Generation." The Receptor Grid Generation panel opens.

3. At the “Receptor” tab, check “Pick to identify the ligand,” and left click on any atom of ligand on the workspace. The ligand will be excluded from receptor grid generation. Everything not defined as “ligand” will be treated as part of the protein. Set the “Van der Waals radius scaling” value at “1.0”.
4. At the “Site” tab, the “Center” section defines the center of mass for the enclosing grid box. Since the crystal structure contains a ligand, the “Center” is defined as the “Centroid of workspace ligand” (selected in the “Receptor” tab). The “Size” option refers to the size of ligands allowed to be docked. If you press the “Advanced Settings” button, you can observe the size of this box. The diameter midpoint of each ligand must remain within this green box.
5. At the “Rotatable Groups” tab, all residues inside the grid box containing hydroxyl or thiol groups are shown. The user can allow rotation of one or more residues based on the structural knowledge of the protein. For this protocol no rotation will be chosen.
6. Provide an appropriate job name and press “Run.” A folder containing a .zip archive of the grid files of the protein will be generated in the working directory.

3.2.3 Docking-Scoring Calculations

1. From “Application” menu choose “Glide” → “Ligand Docking.”
2. On the “Receptor grid” tab, select the .zip file of grid created in Subheading 3.2.2, **step 6**.
3. On the “Ligands” tab at the “Use ligands from” option, choose “File,” and select the output file of LigPrep ligand preparation created in Subheading 3.1, **step 9**.
4. On the “Settings” tab, choose at the “Precision” option the SP (standard precision) level.
5. On “Ligand sampling” choose “Flexible” so all single bonds are free to be rotated in docking calculations.
6. On “Job name” write an appropriate job name and press “Run.” A folder with the files containing the results of docking calculation will be created in the working directory. The “[filename]_pv.mae” file contains a list of the ligands ranked on the basis of their predicted binding affinity for the target protein (*see* **Notes 6** and 7).

3.3 Ligand-Based Screening Using a Three-Dimensional Similarity Method

In this step the workflow of performing a similarity-based screen of the NCI/DTP molecules against the structure of a molecule that is active against the specified protein target is described. In this approach, the bioactive conformation of the known active will be extracted from a crystal structure of the active in complex with the given protein. Then, the algorithm will perform a rapid overlay between the structure of the known active and the structure of each of the NCI/DTP molecules and it will afford a list of scores based on the three-dimensional similarity for each comparison, with high resemblance in terms of shape and pharmacophore sites indicated by a high similarity score.

1. Select the crystal structure, which contains the bioactive conformation of the known active molecule ligand that will be used as a three-dimensional template for screening.
2. Download and open the corresponding .pdb file using Maestro ("File" → "Import structures"). Delete all atoms that do not belong to the specific ligand ("Quick select" → "Ligand", "Invert", "Edit" → "Delete atoms"). Correct bond order and add explicit hydrogens to the ligand ("Edit" → "3D builder"). If more than one ligand molecules appear, manually delete the remaining atoms so that you keep only one copy of the ligand. Save the ligand structure in .pdb format ("File" → "Export structures").
3. Open the vROCS software interface.
4. Select "Perform a simple ROCS run." In the "Inputs" menu, define a name for the run, select the "Implicit Mills-Dean" color force field, and use the "Query" option to open the . pdb file of the three-dimensional ligand structure as it was saved in the previous step. Use the "Database" option to select the preprocessed .oeb.gz file of the NCI/DTP repository from Subheading 3.1, **step 11**.
5. In the "Input and output" section of the "Options" menu, select the working directory in which all files will be saved. Set a value of 5000 as the number of best hits to be saved. The value should be between 10^3 and 10^4 depending on the size of the screened collection so that a reasonable percentage of top ranked molecules is included in the derived list (in this case, approximately 2% of the NCI repository).
6. Select a prefix for the run files to be saved, and in the "Rank by" option, choose "Tanimoto Combo" as the scoring method to rank the screened ligands.
7. In the "Shape and color" section, make sure that only the "Inertial" option in "Start type" and the "Color optimize," "Full optimization," and "3D view" options are ticked.

8. Choose the "Run" option at the lower part of the screen. Wait until the screening percentage reaches 100% and the screening output is displayed on the lower part of the screen as a spreadsheet.

3.4 Consensus Ranking

In this step, the integration of the resulting lists created by each of the utilized screening methods will be performed. Each method produces a ranked list that will be introduced to a spreadsheet for determining the frequency of appearance for each compound of those that are included in the individual lists. Compounds that are identified as promising by more than one method will be highlighted by a higher frequency (*see* **Note 8**).

1. Export the results of each individual screening experiment from Subheadings 3.2 and 3.3 as a comma delimited .csv file. Use either the Maestro environment for results obtained by Glide ("Window" → "Project table" → "Table" → "Export" → "Spreadsheet") or Vida for results obtained by ROCS ("File" → "Export" → "Spreadsheet").
2. Open each .csv file separately in Microsoft Excel ("Data" → "Get external data" → "From text/csv"). Make sure that the data are sorted on the basis of the specific score selected to rank the molecules in each screening experiment (e.g., the "docking score" column in Glide and the "ROCS_TanimotoCombo" column in ROCS). Then, create the ranked list by deleting all columns except from the one that includes the identifiers of the screened molecules (e.g., the "NSC number" column for the NCI/DTP repository compounds), *see* also **Note 9**.
3. Specify a cutoff for choosing the percentage of top-ranked molecules that will be included in the consensus analysis and discard all elements of the list that are below this cutoff, if any. We suggest the use of a cutoff value that retains about 10^3–10^4 top ranked entries (in this case 5000 entries, or about top 2% of the NCI repository).
4. Open a new Excel spreadsheet (consensus spreadsheet), and collect all ranked and preprocessed lists from the previous two steps in adjacent columns of the consensus spreadsheet. The columns at this step can be increased depending on the sampling enhancement strategy selected, in accordance with **Notes 1** and **2**.
5. Save the consensus spreadsheet as an .xlsx file. To this point each different screening experiment performed so far should be represented by exactly one column in the consensus spreadsheet ('Ranks Spreadsheet' or Spreadsheet 1), in a table of dimensions N (rows, maximum number of ligands ranked) times M (columns, number of different screens performed).

In case a smaller number of ligands are ranked by one or more of the utilized screens, fill the empty cells that appear at the end of the corresponding lists with "0" manually.

6. Define a separate table of the same dimensions ('Frequencies Spreadsheet' or Spreadsheet 2) adjacent to the former by introducing at the upper left cell of the new table the following function: {COUNTIF($C1$R1:$C2$R2;C1R1)}, and use Ctrl+Shift+Enter to enter the specific function as an array. In that syntax, C1 is the column, and R1 is the row of the upper left element of Spreadsheet 1, C2 is the column, and R2 is the row of the lower right not empty element of Spreadsheet 1 (e.g., A2 and D9 in a table of 4 columns × 9 rows starting at A1 and including headers in the first row), and C1R1 is the first element of the array (e.g., cell A2).
7. Copy and paste the formula over all cells comprising Spreadsheet 2. The result is a table of frequencies for each of the elements appearing in Spreadsheet 1, which are the molecules that advanced beyond a defined threshold in the individual screens. The identifiers of molecules appearing with high scores in more than one of the orthogonal screening calculations will afford high frequencies, on the basis of which the selection for experimental evaluations can be performed in accordance with the experimental screening capacities available each time.

4 Notes

1. The key concept of the present consensus ranking protocol is combined utilization of an array of virtual screening methods characterized by high orthogonality and their linear integration. For each molecule of the screened collection, its capacity to rank high in one or more of the screening techniques is quantified as the frequency of its appearance in a top-ranked position in the lists derived by screening. This approach provides a highly affordable way to exploit information contained in each screening method to its extreme by facilitating identification of those compounds that are independently identified as promising by distinct algorithms based on orthogonal principles. In this sense any screening method can be integrated into the present basic protocol, provided that it demonstrates a degree of orthogonality with respect to the rest of methods applied. For optimal results, in addition to the combination of one three-dimensional similarity method and one based on docking-scoring calculations as discussed in the abovementioned basic protocol, we suggest the use of one fingerprint-based, two-dimensional similarity method (e.g., Canvas, Schrodinger Inc.) and one pharmacophore-based method (e.g., LigandScout, Inte:Ligand Inc.).

2. An issue of major importance for successful implementation of the protocol is the sampling level used for each method involved in consensus ranking. Sampling can be adjusted by different parameters characteristic for each screening method with diverse impact on time efficiency. In Glide such parameters are the precision level (SP or XP), the VdW scaling factor of ligand atoms and the scoring function, in ROCS the similarity scoring method (Tanimoto or Tversky and their variations) and the different weighting of selected pharmacophore atoms of the query. However, it should be emphasized that the higher degree of sampling achieved, the more confident the resulting consensus ranking output is expected to be. It should be noted that sampling can be increased in a stepwise manner, such as that described in **Note** 7, to ensure the optimal speed-accuracy trade-off. We suggest the use of the following series of screens for achieving a good speed-accuracy compromise toward sampling optimization with respect to the basic consensus protocol:

   (a) In structure-based screening, we utilize at least two distinct crystal structure templates (same protein isoform and organism, different co-crystallized ligand but similar mode of binding, e.g., structures of two different type I ATP-competitive inhibitors complexed with the same protein kinase). We then prepare the structures as in Subheading 3.2.1, and we create two different grids as described in Subheading 3.2.2 for each protein structure (a total of four grids) by adjusting the scaling factor of protein atoms van der Waals radii at either 80% or 100% of nominal value ("Applications" → "Glide" → "Receptor grid generation" → tab "Receptor" "Van der Waals radius scaling" → " Scaling factor"). We proceed with individual docking calculations at the SP accuracy level with each of the four grids, as described in Subheading 3.2.3.

   (b) In ligand-based screening, we select and extract structures of four to ten different known active molecules, if available. We prepare them individually as described in Subheading 3.3, **steps 1** and **2,** and we perform an equal number of similarity screens, as described in Subheading 3.3, **step 4**. The more diverse the known actives are in terms of structure, the higher sampling efficacy is achieved. To have a measure of structural diversity, we can use the matrix of Tanimoto distances for all available actives and select those with the lowest scores. The Tanimoto distance can be determined using software like Canvas ("File" → "New project," "File" → "Import," import all structures as .sdf files; then "Applications" → "Binary fingerprints," select an appropriate fingerprint-like

MOLPRINT2D by "Fingerprint type: MOLPRINT2D," "create;" and then "Similarity distance matrix" → "Create from fingerprints," select fingerprint column and then "Create").

3. A critical issue related to sampling efficacy is selection of water molecules that are regarded as important for ligand binding and thus should be taken into account in screening calculations. Those water molecules are either crystallographically determined and show a conserved interaction motif in several crystal structures of the same or a related protein, or they are predicted with high confidence using solvation mapping algorithms like SZMAP (Openeye Inc.). Concerning structure-based screening, such critical water molecules can be incorporated in calculations first by being retained and not deleted in the protein preparation stage (Subheading 3.2.1) and then by including them as atoms that constitute a part of the protein in the stage of creating the corresponding grids (Subheading 3.2.2). Concerning ligand-based and pharmacophore screening, they can be incorporated by creating a pseudomolecule that is comprised by merging the atoms of the actual ligand query with those of water molecules as they appear in the complex of the corresponding ligand with its protein target. No definition of bonds between the ligand and waters is necessary for creating the structure file of a pseudo query molecule, the structure of which can then be imported in ROCS to perform similarity screening as it is described in Subheading 3.3, **step 3**. We strongly suggest considering different screening calculation sets performed both with and without the critical water molecules, in systems where their contribution to binding is inconclusive.

4. As a tutorial we use the structure of Estrogen Receptor alpha (ERα) in complex with diethylstilbestrol (DES) (PDB id: 3ERD) [46]. This specific crystal structure of ERα adopts an agonist conformation where the ligand-binding domain (LBD) is narrow compared to the antagonist conformation in order to accommodate bulkier molecules such as 4-hydroxytamoxifene. One can find in PDB more than 300 structures with different ligands bound to ER. In our case, the 3ERD structure is a dimer with two symmetrical ERα monomers in complex with a coactivator.

   (a) Open the 3ERD.pdb file in Maestro. On the ligand molecule, there are no multiple bonds because the PDB file contains only data about connectivity of atoms and not multiplicity of bonds. On the "Entry List," right click on entry titled "3ERD," and select "Split by Chain," and four separate entries will be created. The A and B chains are the ER protein monomers, while chains C and D are the co-crystallized coactivators. Select and include the entry "3ERD_chainA" in workspace.

(b) Start the Protein preparation wizard as described in Subheading 3.2.1 to prepare a correct protein structure. This procedure will add hydrogen to all atoms, assign bond orders, and create zero-order bonds for metals (if any) and disulfide bonds based on the distance between cysteine residues. Finally all water molecules beyond 5.0 Å from the protein will be deleted. This step will also optimize the hydrogen-bonding network by calculating the protonation states of residues at given pH from a p*K*a prediction by PROPKA (http://propka.org/) as implemented in Maestro software. Additionally, the orientation of Asn, Gln, and His side chains will be optimized in order to achieve the maximum number of H-bonds with surrounding residues. After completion of this step, some histidine residues are labeled "His," "Hie," or "Hip" based on their protonation state and site. In the case of ER, this step is very crucial since His524 needs to be protonated in nitrogen Nε instead of Nδ, in order to create a hydrogen network between the hydroxyl group of DES, the side chain of His524, and the backbone carbonyl group of Glu419.

(c) Another important decision in ER preparation stage is treatment of crystallographic water molecules. The occurrence of water molecules inside a protein-binding pocket may be crucial for ligand recognition. In our case, we have already shown that the crystallographic water molecules between the ligand and the side chains of residues Arg394 and Glu353 are fundamental for binding [47].

(d) After protein preparation in Subheading 3.2.1, the user should visually inspect the resulting structure for errors, especially with respect to protonation. For example in the final structure by ER in complex with 4-hydroxytamoxifene, the nitrogen of the ligand is neutral although, based on literature, this atom is well known to be protonated and forming a salt bridge with Asp351. In this instance, the user must manually add a positive charge to the nitrogen atom by using the "Increment formal charge" button (yellow thunder with "+" symbol on "Built" toolbar) and finally add a hydrogen atom on the nitrogen by using the "Add H+" icon.

(e) When the grid files of ER (3ERD) are created as compressed .zip files as described in Subheading 3.2.2 and the ligand database is fully prepared as described in Subheading 3.1, we proceed to the final step of docking simulations as described in Subheading 3.2.3. At the end of the ligand preparation stage, in our case, the prepared NCI/DTP repository database contains 644,589 entries and is ready for virtual screening.

(f) Once the docking calculation is completed, the results are imported to the current project. Click on "Import" icon. Select on the left "Working Directory," and double-click on the folder having the job name from Subheading 3.2.1, **step 3**. Double-click on file having the "job name" with the extension "pv.maegz." The receptor is the first entry which is "fixed" (you can see the lock icon next to "Title"), and the user can include each ligand to examine the binding mode together with the interactions formed. All ligands are sorted so that the first entry has the lowest GlideScore. In our case the top ligand "10,839" has a docking score of −12.64 kcal/mol. This compound is an analogue of DES, while Estradiol is ranked 14th with docking score −10.98 kcal/mol, and DES is ranked 116th with docking score −10.45 kcal/mol. Those values are not directly comparable to experimental values, but the rank can be used for further selection of molecules for in vitro experiments. While the protein and a ligand are included in the workspace, click the "Lig. Int." button to see in 2D the ligand interaction diagram, which visualizes all interactions between the protein and ligand.

(g) To perform a ROCS calculation using DES as a known active, extract, correct the bond order and add hydrogens to the ligand of 3ERD structure as described in Subheading 3.3, **step 2**. Then, perform a similarity screen as described in Subheading 3.3, **steps 4–7**. DES is ranked on top (NSC Id 3070) as this is our query molecule.

(h) After the user is familiar enough with the basic screening procedure, they can try to download the ER decoy set for DUD-E database (http://dude.docking.org/targets/esr1/decoys_final.sdf.gz) and check if the known agonists afford a higher glide score compared to the decoys in the final ranking.

5. Selection of the appropriate crystal structure is critical and is exclusively dependent on the objective of the screening effort. Many protein target classes show a high potential of adopting different conformations as a result of their activation state or their role as signal transduction factors. In the ER case, the utilized crystal structure has the agonist conformation, and the binding pocket adopts a topology for accommodating molecules such as estradiol or diethylstilbestrol. Bulkier molecules such as raloxifen or 4-hydroxytamoxifen, which are known

antagonists, are automatically excluded from virtual screening since they cannot fit inside the agonist conformation of the ligand-binding domain. The user needs to perform the same workflow using an antagonist conformation of ER such as 3ERT in complex with 4-hydroxytamoxifene in case screening aims at the recovery of antagonists.

6. When running Glide software, the user can define the number of subjobs based on the number of available PC or cluster CPUs. In Subheading 3.2.3, **step** 7, next to "Job name," click on the "Gear" icon, select job settings, and on the "Separate job into:" box give the number of processors to use. Glide software can run in parallel by separating the ligands to be docked and at the end combines results to give one final output file.
7. When performing virtual screening on large databases, in Subheading 3.2.3, **step 5,** it is suggested to use the "high-throughput virtual screening (HTVS)" precision mode. This procedure will screen the database at high speed and then the top 10–20% of the top-ranked compounds can be subsequently re-docked by implementing the Glide SP standard precision for more accurate scoring.
8. A small number of 3–5 molecules appearing at the top of the individual lists derived by each screening approach utilized are considered as potential hits and are advanced to experimental screening regardless of their consensus frequency. Those structures are potentially false-negative results with respect to consensus, and it is safe to consider them as good candidates on the basis of the corresponding method that singularly identified them as such.
9. The preservation of a comprehensive identifier for each molecule that is included in the screened collection (e.g., the "NSC" or "CID" identifiers of NCI repository) should be secured throughout the calculations and checked periodically, as in many instances this highly important information might be lost along the course of read/write steps along the various calculations, especially in the enumeration and preparation stages.

References

1. DiMasi JA, Grabowski HG, Hansen RW (2016) Innovation in the pharmaceutical industry: new estimates of R&D costs. J Health Econ 47:20–33. https://doi.org/10.1016/j.jhealeco.2016.01.012
2. Bleicher KH, Böhm H-J, Müller K et al (2003) A guide to drug discovery: hit and lead generation: beyond high-throughput screening. Nat Rev Drug Discov 2(5):369–378. https://doi.org/10.1038/nrd1086
3. Hughes J, Rees S, Kalindjian S et al (2011) Principles of early drug discovery: principles of early drug discovery. Br J Pharmacol 162 (6):1239–1249. https://doi.org/10.1111/j.1476-5381.2010.01127.x

4. Zhang W (ed) (2016) Computer-aided drug discovery. Springer, New York, NY. https://doi.org/10.1007/978-1-4939-3521-5
5. Shoichet BK (2004) Virtual screening of chemical libraries. Nature 432:862–865. https://doi.org/10.1038/nature03197
6. Li Q, Cheng T, Wang Y et al (2010) PubChem as a public resource for drug discovery. Drug Discov Today 15(23-24):1052–1057. https://doi.org/10.1016/j.drudis.2010.10.003
7. Gaulton A, Bellis LJ, Bento AP et al (2012) ChEMBL: a large-scale bioactivity database for drug discovery. Nucleic Acids Res 40: D1100–D1107. https://doi.org/10.1093/nar/gkr777
8. Irwin JJ, Shoichet BK (2005) ZINC--a free database of commercially available compounds for virtual screening. J Chem Inf Model 45 (1):177–182. https://doi.org/10.1021/ci049714+
9. Ma D-L, Chan DS-H, Leung C-H (2013) Drug repositioning by structure-based virtual screening. Chem Soc Rev 42:2130. https://doi.org/10.1039/c2cs35357a
10. Langer T (2010) Pharmacophores in drug research. Mol Inform 29(6-7):470–475. https://doi.org/10.1002/minf.201000022
11. Rognan D (2010) Structure-based approaches to target fishing and ligand profiling. Mol Inform 29(3):176–187. https://doi.org/10.1002/minf.200900081
12. Hecker EA, Duraiswami C, Andrea TA et al (2002) Use of Catalyst Pharmacophore models for screening of large combinatorial libraries. J Chem Inf Comput Sci 42(5):1204–1211. https://doi.org/10.1021/ci020368a
13. Dixon SL, Smondyrev AM, Rao SN (2006) PHASE: a novel approach to Pharmacophore Modeling and 3D database searching. Chem Biol Drug Des 67(5):370–372. https://doi.org/10.1111/j.1747-0285.2006.00384.x
14. Wolber G, Dornhofer AA, Langer T (2007) Efficient overlay of small organic molecules using 3D pharmacophores. J Comput Aided Mol Des 20(12):773–788. https://doi.org/10.1007/s10822-006-9078-7
15. Richmond NJ, Abrams CA, Wolohan PRN et al (2006) GALAHAD: 1. Pharmacophore identification by hypermolecular alignment of ligands in 3D. J Comput Aided Mol Des 20 (9):567–587. https://doi.org/10.1007/s10822-006-9082-y
16. Schneidman-Duhovny D, Dror O, Inbar Y et al (2008) PharmaGist: a webserver for ligand-based pharmacophore detection. Nucleic Acids Res 36:W223–W228. https://doi.org/10.1093/nar/gkn187
17. Hawkins PCD, Skillman AG, Nicholls A (2007) Comparison of shape-matching and docking as virtual screening tools. J Med Chem 50(1):74–82. https://doi.org/10.1021/jm0603365
18. Irwin JJ, Shoichet BK (2016) Docking screens for novel ligands conferring new biology: Miniperspective. J Med Chem 59(9):4103–4120. https://doi.org/10.1021/acs.jmedchem.5b02008
19. Lavecchia A, Di Giovanni C (2013) Virtual screening strategies in drug discovery: a critical review. Curr Med Chem 20(23):2839–2860. https://doi.org/10.2174/09298673113209990001
20. Dias R, de Azevedo WF (2008) Molecular docking algorithms. Curr Drug Targets 9 (12):1040–1047. https://doi.org/10.2174/138945008786949432
21. Kontoyianni M, McClellan LM, Sokol GS (2004) Evaluation of docking performance: comparative data on docking algorithms. J Med Chem 47(3):558–565. https://doi.org/10.1021/jm0302997
22. Huang S-Y, Grinter SZ, Zou X (2010) Scoring functions and their evaluation methods for protein-ligand docking: recent advances and future directions. Phys Chem Chem Phys PCCP 12(40):12899–12908. https://doi.org/10.1039/c0cp00151a
23. Ewing TJ, Makino S, Skillman AG et al (2001) DOCK 4.0: search strategies for automated molecular docking of flexible molecule databases. J Comput Aided Mol Des 15 (5):411–428. https://doi.org/10.1023/A:1011115820450
24. Morris GM, Goodsell DS, Halliday RS et al (1998) Automated docking using a Lamarckian genetic algorithm and an empirical binding free energy function. J Comput Chem 19 (14):1639–1662. https://doi.org/10.1002/(SICI)1096-987X(19981115)19:14<1639::AID-JCC10>3.0.CO;2-B
25. Trott O, Olson AJ (2010) AutoDock Vina: improving the speed and accuracy of docking with a new scoring function, efficient optimization, and multithreading. J Comput Chem 31 (2):455–461. https://doi.org/10.1002/jcc.21334
26. Wu G, Robertson DH, Brooks CL et al (2003) Detailed analysis of grid-based molecular docking: a case study of CDOCKER-A CHARMm-based MD docking algorithm. J Comput Chem 24(13):1549–1562. https://doi.org/10.1002/jcc.10306
27. Jones G, Willett P, Glen RC et al (1997) Development and validation of a genetic algorithm

for flexible docking. J Mol Biol 267 (3):727–748. https://doi.org/10.1006/jmbi.1996.0897

28. Ruiz-Carmona S, Alvarez-Garcia D, Foloppe N et al (2014) rDock: a fast, versatile and open source program for docking ligands to proteins and nucleic acids. PLoS Comput Biol 10(4): e1003571. https://doi.org/10.1371/journal.pcbi.1003571
29. Scior T, Bender A, Tresadern G et al (2012) Recognizing pitfalls in virtual screening: a critical review. J Chem Inf Model 52(4):867–881. https://doi.org/10.1021/ci200528d
30. Waszkowycz B, Clark DE, Gancia E (2011) Outstanding challenges in protein-ligand docking and structure-based virtual screening. Wiley Interdiscip Rev Comput Mol Sci 1 (2):229–259. https://doi.org/10.1002/wcms.18
31. Lam PC-H, Abagyan R, Totrov M (2017) Ligand-biased ensemble receptor docking (LigBEnD): a hybrid ligand/receptor structure-based approach. J Comput Aided Mol Des. https://doi.org/10.1007/s10822-017-0058-x
32. Spyrakis F, Ahmed MH, Bayden AS et al (2017) The roles of water in the protein matrix: a largely untapped resource for drug discovery. J Med Chem 60(16):6781–6827. https://doi.org/10.1021/acs.jmedchem.7b00057
33. Lagarde N, Zagury J-F, Montes M (2015) Benchmarking data sets for the evaluation of virtual ligand screening methods: review and perspectives. J Chem Inf Model 55 (7):1297–1307. https://doi.org/10.1021/acs.jcim.5b00090
34. Plewczynski D, Łaźniewski M, Augustyniak R et al (2011) Can we trust docking results? Evaluation of seven commonly used programs on PDBbind database. J Comput Chem 32 (4):742–755. https://doi.org/10.1002/jcc.21643
35. Wang Z, Sun H, Yao X et al (2016) Comprehensive evaluation of ten docking programs on a diverse set of protein-ligand complexes: the prediction accuracy of sampling power and scoring power. Phys Chem Chem Phys PCCP 18:12964–12975. https://doi.org/10.1039/C6CP01555G
36. Chaput L, Martinez-Sanz J, Saettel N et al (2016) Benchmark of four popular virtual screening programs: construction of the active/decoy dataset remains a major determinant of measured performance. J Cheminform 8:56. https://doi.org/10.1186/s13321-016-0167-x
37. Warren GL, Andrews CW, Capelli A-M et al (2006) A critical assessment of docking programs and scoring functions. J Med Chem 49 (20):5912–5931. https://doi.org/10.1021/jm050362n
38. Carlson HA, Smith RD, Damm-Ganamet KL et al (2016) CSAR 2014: a benchmark exercise using unpublished data from Pharma. J Chem Inf Model 56(6):1063–1077. https://doi.org/10.1021/acs.jcim.5b00523
39. Polgár T, Baki A, Szendrei GI et al (2005) Comparative virtual and experimental high-throughput screening for glycogen synthase kinase-3beta inhibitors. J Med Chem 48 (25):7946–7959. https://doi.org/10.1021/jm050504d
40. Ferreira RS, Simeonov A, Jadhav A et al (2010) Complementarity between a docking and a high-throughput screen in discovering new Cruzain inhibitors. J Med Chem 53 (13):4891–4905. https://doi.org/10.1021/jm100488w
41. Spitzer R, Jain AN (2012) Surflex-Dock: docking benchmarks and real-world application. J Comput Aided Mol Des 26(6):687–699. https://doi.org/10.1007/s10822-011-9533-y
42. Cross JB, Thompson DC, Rai BK et al (2009) Comparison of several molecular docking programs: pose prediction and virtual screening accuracy. J Chem Inf Model 49 (6):1455–1474. https://doi.org/10.1021/ci900056c
43. Myrianthopoulos V, Gaboriaud-Kolar N, Tallant C et al (2016) Discovery and optimization of a selective ligand for the switch/sucrose nonfermenting-related Bromodomains of Polybromo Protein-1 by the use of virtual screening and hydration analysis. J Med Chem 59(19):8787–8803. https://doi.org/10.1021/acs.jmedchem.6b00355
44. Myrianthopoulos V, Cartron PF, Liutkevičiūtė Z et al (2016) Tandem virtual screening targeting the SRA domain of UHRF1 identifies a novel chemical tool modulating DNA methylation. Eur J Med Chem 114:390–396. https://doi.org/10.1016/j.ejmech.2016.02.043
45. Berman HM, Westbrook J, Feng Z et al (2000) The Protein Data Bank. Nucleic Acids Res 28 (1):235–242. https://doi.org/10.1093/nar/28.1.235
46. Shiau AK, Barstad D, Loria PM et al (1998) The structural basis of Estrogen receptor/Coactivator recognition and the antagonism of this interaction by Tamoxifen. Cell 95 (7):927–937. https://doi.org/10.1016/S0092-8674(00)81717-1
47. Lambrinidis G, Halabalaki M, Katsanou ES et al (2006) The estrogen receptor and polyphenols: molecular simulation studies of their interactions, a review. Environ Chem Lett 4 (3):159–174. https://doi.org/10.1007/s10311-006-0065-y

Chapter 16

Insights in Organometallic Synthesis of Various Adamantane Derivatives with Sigma Receptor-Binding Affinity and Antiproliferative/Anticancer Activity

Ioannis Papanastasiou

Abstract

Organometallic reactions, such as those involving Grignard and organocadmium reagents, are very useful but require prudent laboratory skills. In many papers related to the medicinal chemistry of adamantane derivatives with sigma receptor (σR)-binding affinity and antiproliferative/anticancer activity, organometallics play a crucial role in the synthetic pathways. In this work, the experimental procedures utilizing Grignard and organocadmium reagents are presented in detail, because these techniques are not analyzed and are important in the rational drug design.

Key words Adamantane derivatives, Sigma receptor, Organocadmium reaction, Grignard reaction

1 Introduction

Adamantane is a lipophilic symmetrical hydrocarbon that has become a target for many drugs in clinical trial practice, due to improving or providing "drug-like" properties to pharmacophore moieties [1, 2]. Quite recently, sigma receptor (σR) ligands have been used as radiolabeled and fluorescent molecular probes, biomarkers, and remedial agents in the diagnosis or treatment of various types of cancer [3–5]. Many adamantane derivatives display σR-binding affinity not related to antiproliferative or anticancer activity [6–10]. However, the following adamantane phenylalkylamines **I**, **II,** and **III**, illustrated in Fig. 1, exhibit σR-binding affinity in combination with antiproliferative and anticancer activity [11–17].

The aforementioned adamantane adducts possess the structural requirements for σR-binding affinity [18] (Fig. 1). In the first adamantane scaffold **I**, benzene ring A is attached to the first piperazine nitrogen via a chain of three atoms (N, 2C), and in template **II**, the benzene rings are linked to an amine nitrogen atom via a spacer of one, two, and three methylene carbons. The

Thomas Mavromoustakos and Tahsin F. Kellici (eds.), *Rational Drug Design: Methods and Protocols*, Methods in Molecular Biology, vol. 1824, https://doi.org/10.1007/978-1-4939-8630-9_16, © Springer Science+Business Media, LLC, part of Springer Nature 2018

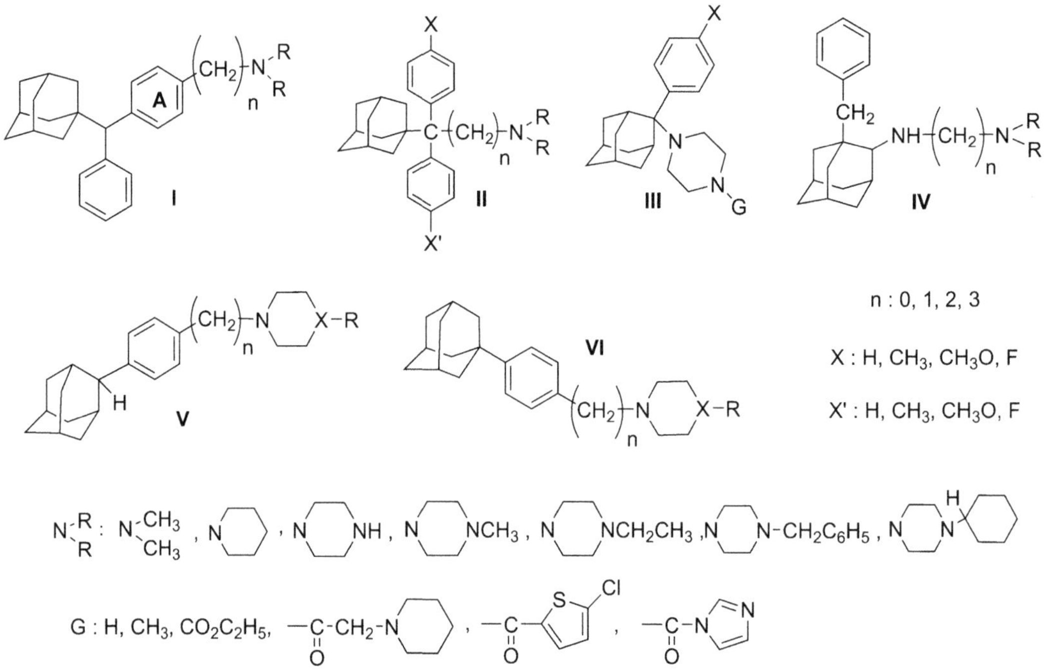

Fig. 1 Adamantane derivatives with σR-binding affinity and antiproliferative or anticancer activity

substitution of the adamantane moiety has changed in 1-(2-aryl-2-adamantyl)piperazine derivatives **III**. All the above adamantane derivatives have a significant binding affinity for the σ1R and σ2R at a low nanomolecular range. Their antiproliferative activity against numerous cancer cell lines (colon, prostate, breast, ovarian, central nervous system, leukemia, pancreas, liver) was significant. These results in conjunction with their affinity for site 2 of the Na^+ channels imply that the adamantane phenylalkylamines **I, II,** and **III** have the pharmacological profile of mixed σ1/σ2R ligands. The phenylalkylamine analogues of general types **IV** [19], **V** [20], and **VI** [21] have been designed as σR ligands and share structural similarities in their scaffold with compounds **I** and **II**. These adamantane derivatives **IV, V,** and **VI** are reported for their antiproliferative activity, but their binding affinities have not been yet investigated (Fig. 1).

Herein, we report the crucial steps of organometallic reactions with Grignard and organocadmium reagents, in different synthetic pathways of the aforementioned adamantane derivatives.

2 Materials

2.1 Organocadmium Reagents

1. Magnesium turnings: The magnesium turnings should look shiny or silver. If they look black, a magnesium oxide coat is formed on the metal surface, and they are reluctant to react.

2. Cadmium chloride: Cadmium chloride is very hydroscopic and should be dried in an oven at 110 °C for 1 h before use.
3. Anhydrous solvents, diethyl ether, and benzene: Commercially available dry solvents are maintained in the presence of powder of calcium hydride and under an argon atmosphere.
4. 1-Adamantyl carbonyl chloride: 1-Adamantylcarbonyl chloride is prepared by heating of 1-adamantanecarboxylic acid at 60–65 °C with freshly distilled thionyl chloride for 45 min. Upon completion of the reaction, the excess of unreacted thionyl chloride is removed azeotropically in vacuo with the aid of dry benzene. Thionyl chloride is prepared by distillation in the presence of quinoline.

2.2 Grignard Reagents

1. Magnesium turnings: the magnesium turnings should look shiny or silver. If they look black, a magnesium oxide coat is formed on the metal surface, and they are reluctant to form Grignard reagents.
2. Anhydrous solvents, diethyl ether, or tetrahydrofuran: the solvent of the Grignard should be scrupulous dry without water traces. The presence of moisture destroys the Grignard reagent, once it is formed (*see* **Note 1**). The solvent should be freshly distilled and stored in sealed flask under an argon atmosphere. Powder of calcium hydride should be added into the solvent beaker to maintain the dryness of the solvent.
3. Other reagents: 2-Adamantanone, 1-adamantylphenyl ketone, 4-bromo-α-phenyl-α-(1-adamantyl)methyl-benzene, *p*-dibromobenzene, *p*-bromotoluene, and *p*-allylbromobenzene should be also dry without any trace of moisture.

3 Methods

3.1 Organocadmium Reaction

1-Adamantylphenyl ketone is prepared either by reacting diphenylcadmium with 1-adamantanecarbonyl chloride in boiled benzene or by reacting phenyllithium with 1-adamantanecarboxylic acid in di-*n*-butylether at −80 °C. The in situ transmetallation, the exchange between phenylmagnesium bromide and cadmium chloride, as a more difficult experimental procedure, is presented in detail in Fig. 2 [22, 23].

3.1.1 Preparation of Organocadmium Reaction

1. Set up a three-necked round-bottom flask, fitted with a pressure-equalizing dropping funnel, a condenser in the middle, and a glass stopper, which will be replaced by a distillation head connected with a side condenser adapted to a receiving flask. A calcium chloride drying tube is attached to the condenser in the middle, and an argon line is attached to the dropping funnel.

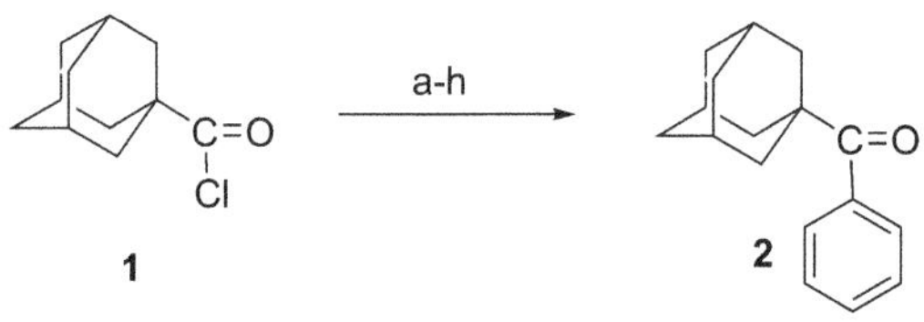

Fig. 2 *Reagents and conditions*: (**a**) Mg turnings; (**b**) bromobenzene/Et_2O; (**c**) $CdCl_2$ at 0 °C; reflux, 90 min; (**d**) dry benzene/Et_2O, reflux, 2 h; (**e**) **1** in dry benzene, gentle reflux, 1 h; (**f**) H_2SO_4 20% at 0 °C; (**g**) NaOH 10%, reflux, 2 h; (**h**) distillation

2. Add a stirrer and Mg turnings into the round-bottom flask, and grease all the ground-glass joints to ensure an airtight seal.
3. Heat and dry the apparatus without cooling water in the condensers, with flame, until there is no cloudiness of moisture in the glassware. Let the apparatus cool down under argon atmosphere (*see* **Note 2**).
4. Add dropwise the solution of bromobenzene in dry diethyl ether into the round-bottom flask with the Mg turnings under stirring. Upon completion of the addition, add cadmium chloride in small portions under chilled water bath. Reflux the reaction mixture in a hot water bath for 1 h (*see* **Note 3**).
5. Add a distillation head connected with a side condenser adapted to a receiving flask to distill diethyl ether. Add dry benzene to the reaction mixture to replace the distilled diethyl ether, and remove the side condenser (*see* **Note 4**) [24].
6. Add a solution of 1-adamantanecarbonyl chloride in dry benzene, and heat the reaction mixture in a gentle reflux.
7. Keep efficient stirring throughout the whole reaction time (*see* **Note 5**).

3.1.2 Treatment of the Organocadmium Reaction

1. Set an ice bath under the reaction mixture, and quench the reaction with an aqueous solution of H_2SO_4 (20%).
2. Evaporate the organic phase in vacuo, and treat the residue with an aqueous solution of NaOH (10%). Reflux the reaction mixture for 2 h (*see* **Note 6**).
3. Extract the reaction mixture with diethyl ether, wash the organic phase with brine, dry it over Na_2SO_4, and evaporate. The residue should be distilled in vacuo.

3.2 Grignard Reactions

The Grignard reactions involved in the studied synthetic pathways are depicted in Fig. 3.

3.2.1 Preparation of Grignard Reaction

1. Set up a three-necked round-bottom flask, fitted with a condenser, a pressure-equalizing dropping funnel, and a rubber septum. A calcium chloride drying tube is attached to the condenser, and an argon line is attached to the dropping funnel.

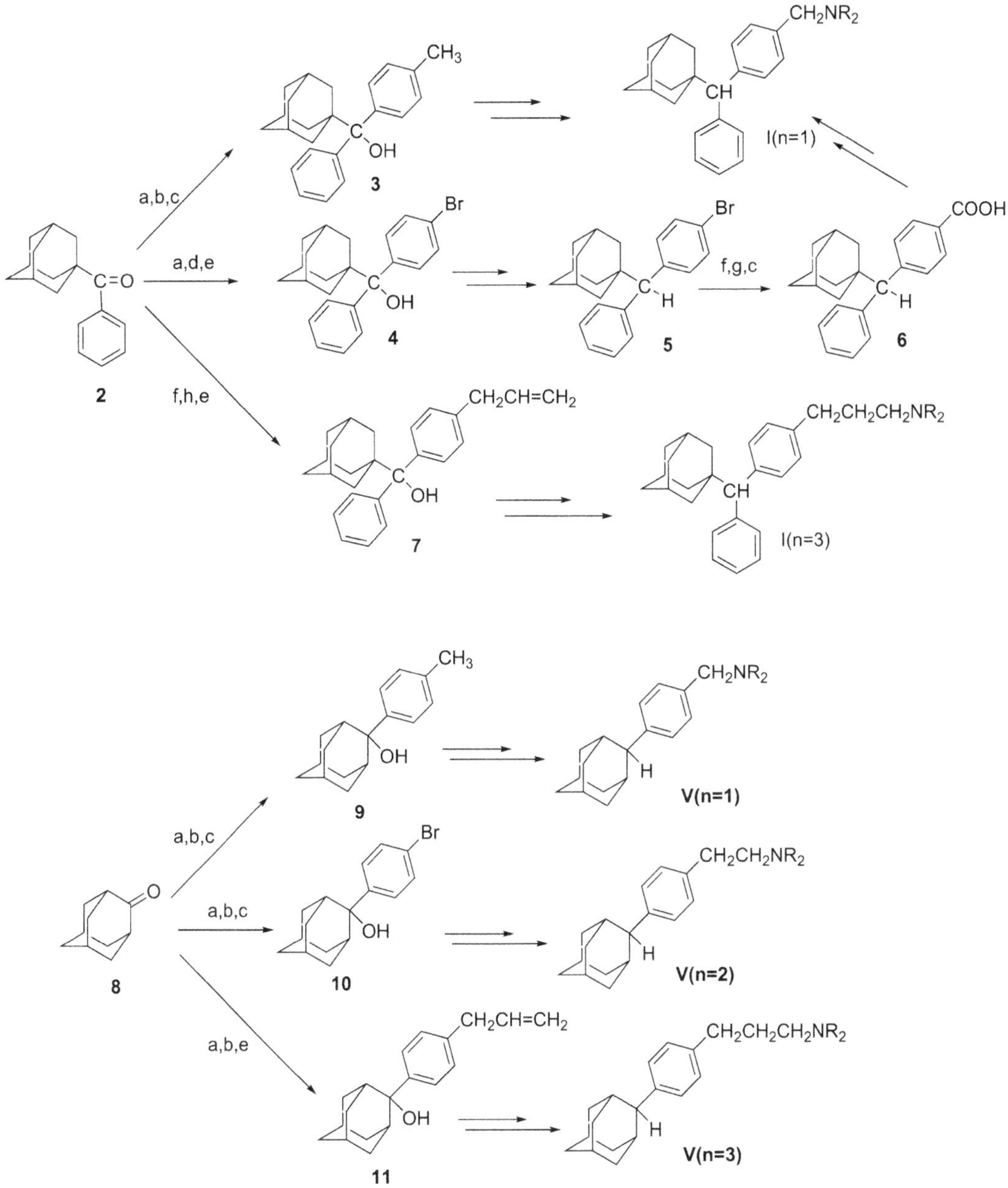

Fig. 3 *Reagents and conditions*: (*a*) Mg turnings; (*b*) *p*-tolyl bromide/Et_2O (in case of 1-adamantylphenyl ketone: reflux, 2 h, in case of 2-adamantanone: rt., 3 h); (*c*) HCl 10% at 0 °C; (*d*) *p*-dibromobenzene/Et_2O, reflux, 2 h; (*e*) sat. sol. NH_4Cl at 0 °C; (*f*) Mg turnings/THF; (*g*) dry CO_2 gas, 3 h; (*h*) *p*-allylphenyl bromide/THF

2. Add a stirrer, Mg turnings, and a few crystals of iodine or copper (I) iodine into the round-bottom flask (*see* **Note 7**), and grease all the ground-glass joints to ensure an airtight seal.

3. Heat and dry the apparatus without cooling water in the condenser, with flame until the glassware turns purple from iodine vapors. Let the apparatus cool down under argon atmosphere.
4. Prepare a hot water bath to initiate the reaction and an ice bath in case the reaction becomes too vigorous (*see* **Note 8**).
5. Add a few ml of the halide solution into the round-bottom flask up to the point to cover the surface of Mg turnings, and turn on the stirring (*see* **Note 9**). At the same time, set the hot water bath under the flask.
6. Do not add all the alkyl halide at once, because you will not be able to cool the reaction fast enough to control it. Add the halide solution in a way to maintain a gentle boiling.
7. Maintain a steady gentle reflux. Remove the hot bath, and check if boiling continues. If there is no reaction, add a few drops of 1,2-dibromoethane, and renew the hot bath under the reaction mixture.
8. Do not let the Grignard reagent solvent free by no means. Grignard reagents explode when they are hot without solvent.
9. The red-purple color of the reaction mixture should have disappeared and become transparent gray. By that time, only a few Mg remnants should have been unconsumed, and the solvent should not boil anymore. These signs indicate the formation of the Grignard reagent.
10. The addition of the carbonyl derivative should be slow and steady, as well (*see* **Note 10**).

3.2.2 The Hydrolysis of the Grignard Reaction

1. Set an ice bath under the reaction mixture, and quench the reaction with an aqueous solution of HCl (10%) or a saturated solution of NH_4Cl (*see* **Note 11**). A white precipitate should be formed.
2. Separate the aqueous layer, and extract with diethyl ether. Wash the combined organics with brine and saturated solution of Na_2CO_3 (10%), dry them over Na_2SO_4, and concentrate in vacuo.

4 Notes

1. Water consumes and wastes the Grignard reagent once formed and complicates the preparation, since the produced Mg(OH) X can coat the surface of the metal and prevents further the proceeding of the organometallic reaction:

$$RMgX + H_2O \rightarrow RH + Mg(OH)X$$

2. Organocadmium compounds are sensitive to air, light, and moisture.

3. Once the Grignard reagent has been formed in ether, it is allowed to react with solid cadmium chloride at the boiling temperature. The time required for this reaction varies, probably because of the variation in particle size of the cadmium chloride.
4. Acid chlorides react with diethyl ether in the presence of anhydrous magnesium halide:

$$RCOCl + (C_2H_5)_2O \rightarrow RCO_2C_2H_5 + C_2H_5Cl$$

5. The organometallic reactions are heterogeneous, and the metallic halides produced during the reaction precipitate and form heavy sludge. Failure of efficient stirring at any time of the reaction decreases the yield significantly.
6. There is unreacted 1-adamantanecarbonyl chloride which is saponified with NaOH.
7. Iodine reacts with the magnesium to form the very reactive magnesium iodide (MgI_2).
8. If the reaction boils so vigorously that the reflux condenser cannot condense all the ether vapor, you have to slow down the reaction by cooling it in an ice water bath. Do not slow the reaction down too much, because you will have to start it again.
9. The stirring should prevent crust buildup.
10. The reaction of the Grignard reagent with the carbonyl functional group is extremely exothermic.
11. The alkoxide product of the Grignard reaction is hydrolyzed to the tertiary alcohol. The acidic pH makes the magnesium ions soluble, while the alkaline pH promotes the formation of gelatinous precipitate of magnesia $Mg(OH)_2$.

References

1. Wanka L, Iqbal K, Schreiner PR (2013) The lipophilic bullet hits the targets: medicinal chemistry of adamantane derivatives. Chem Rev 113(5):3516–3604. https://doi.org/10.1021/cr100264t
2. Spilovsk K, Zemek F, Korabecny J et al (2016) Adamantane – a lead structure for drugs in clinical practice. Curr Med Chem 23 (29):3245–3266. https://doi.org/10.2174/0929867323666160525114026
3. Narayanan S, Bhat R, Mesangeau C et al (2010) Early development of sigma-receptor ligands. Fut Med Chem 3(1):79–94. https://doi.org/10.4155/fmc.10.279
4. Akhtar MJ, Ahamed M, Alhadlaq HA et al (2014) Targeted anticancer therapy: overexpressed receptors and nanotechnology. Clin Chim Acta 436:78–92
5. Van Waarde A, Rybczynska AA, Ramakrishnan NK et al (2015) Potential applications for sigma receptor ligands in cancer diagnosis and therapy. Biochim Biophys Acta 1848 (10):2703–2714. https://doi.org/10.1016/j.bbamem.2014.08.022
6. Kornhuber J, Schoppmeyer K, Riederer P (1993) Affinity of 1-amino- adamantanes for the binding site in post-mortem human frontal cortex. Neurosci Lett 163(2):129–131. https://doi.org/10.1016/0304-3940(93)90362-O
7. Ronsisvalle G, Marrazzo A, Prezzavento O et al (2000) Substituted 1-phenyl-2-cyclopropylmethylamines with high affinity and selectivity for sigma sites. Bioorg Med Chem 8 (6):1503–1513. https://doi.org/10.1016/S0968-0896(00)00072-9

8. Bourrie B, Bribes E, De Nys N et al (2002) SSR125329A, a high affinity sigma receptor ligand with potent anti-inflammatory properties. Eur J Pharmacol 456:123–131. https://doi.org/10.1016/S0014-2999(02)02646-8
9. Bucolo C, Marrazzo A, Ronsisvalle S et al (2006) A novel adamantane derivative attenuates retinal ischemia–reperfusion damage in the rat retina through σ1 receptors. Eur J Pharmacol 536:200–203. https://doi.org/10.1016/j.ejphar.2006.02.026
10. Banister SD, Yoo DT, Wern Chua S et al (2011) N-Arylalkyl-2-azaadamantanes as cage-expanded polycarbocyclic sigma (σ) receptor ligands. Bioorg Med Chem Lett 21:5289–5292. https://doi.org/10.1016/j.bmcl.2011.07.028
11. Riganas S, Papanastasiou I, Foscolos GB et al (2012) New adamantane phenylalkylamines with σ-receptor binding affinity and anticancer activity, associated with putative antagonism of neuropathic pain. J Med Chem 55:10241–10261. https://doi.org/10.1021/jm3013008
12. Riganas S, Papanastasiou I, Foscolos GB et al (2012) Synthesis, σ1, σ2-receptors binding affinity and antiproliferative action of new C1-substituted adamantanes. Bioorg Med Chem 20:3323–3331. https://doi.org/10.1016/j.bmc.2012.03.038
13. Riganas S, Papanastasiou I, Foscolos GB et al (2012) New adamantane derivatives with sigma affinity and antiproliferative activity. Med Chem 8:569–586. https://doi.org/10.2174/157340612801216201
14. Fytas C, Zoidis G, Tsotinis A et al (2015) Novel 1-(2-aryl-2-adamantyl)piperazine derivatives with antiproliferative activity. Eur J Med Chem 93:281–290. https://doi.org/10.1016/j.ejmech.2015.02.021
15. Fytas G, Kolocouris N, Foscolos GB, Pouli N (1989) Aminoethers de quelques aryladamantanols. Chimika Chronika New Ser 18:47–57
16. Liu KT, Sheu HC (1991) Solvolysis of 2-aryl-2-chloroadamantanes. A new Y scale benzylic chlorides. J Org Chem 56(9):3021–3025. https://doi.org/10.1021/jo00009a018
17. Georgiadis M-O, Karoutzou O, Foscolos A-S, Papanastasiou I (2017) Sigma receptor (σR) ligands with antiproliferative and anticancer activity. Molecules 22(9):1408. https://doi.org/10.3390/molecules22091408
18. De Costa BR, He X (1994) Structure–activity relationships and evolution of σ receptor ligands. In: Itzhak Y (ed) Sigma receptors. Academic Press, London, pp 45–111
19. Papanastasiou I, Tsotinis A, Kolocouris N et al (2014) New aminoadamantane derivatives with antiproliferative activity. Med Chem Res 23:1966–1975. https://doi.org/10.1007/s00044-013-0798-7
20. Papanastasiou I, Riganas S, Foscolos GB et al (2015) Synthesis and cytotoxicity of 4-(2-Adamantyl)phenylalkylamines. Lett Org Chem 12(5):319–323. https://doi.org/10.2174/1570178612051505092024 19
21. Koperniku A, Foscolos A-S, Papanastasiou I et al (2016) 4-(1-Adamantyl)phenyl alkylamines with potential anti- proliferative activity. Lett Org Chem 13(3):171–176. https://doi.org/10.2174/1570178613666160104233856
22. Papaconstantinou-Garoufalias S, Foscolos GB, Costakis E (1984) Adamantane analogs of diphenhydramine. Chim Chron, *New series*, 13:225–237
23. Stetter H, Rauscher E (1960) Uber verbindungen mit urotropin-struktur XVII. Zur kenntnis der adamantan-carbosäure-(I). Chem Ber 93(5):1161–1166. https://doi.org/10.1002/cber.19600930527
24. Cason J (1947) The use of organocadmium reagents for the preparation of ketones. Chem Rev 40(1):15–32. https://doi.org/10.1021/cr60125a002

Chapter 17

Supervised Molecular Dynamics (SuMD) Approaches in Drug Design

Davide Sabbadin, Veronica Salmaso, Mattia Sturlese, and Stefano Moro

Abstract

Supervised MD (SuMD) is a computational method that enables the exploration of ligand–receptor recognition pathway in a reduced timescale. The performance speedup is due to the incorporation of a tabu-like supervision algorithm on the ligand–receptor approaching distance into a classic molecular dynamics (MD) simulation. SuMD enables the investigation of ligand–receptor binding events independently from the starting position, chemical structure of the ligand (small molecules or peptides), and also from its receptor-binding affinity. The application of SuMD highlights an appreciable capability of the technique to reproduce the crystallographic structures of several ligand–protein complexes and can provide high-quality protein–ligand models of for which yet experimental confirmation of binding mode is not available.

Key words Ligand–protein binding, Peptide–protein binding, Recognition pathway, Molecular dynamics, Supervised molecular dynamics, Meta-binding site

1 Introduction

The increasing number of structural information released daily in the Protein Data Bank (www.rcsb.org) [1] provides high-quality models that enable atomistic level of detailed understanding of protein–ligand interactions at the final stage of the mutual recognition process. This information is a key enabler for structure-based drug design (SBDD). Such structures are also a valuable starting point for computer-aided biophysical investigations, for example, using molecular dynamics (MD) simulations. In this context of steady increase of structural-biology input over time [2], the computer-aided investigation of ligand–protein recognition events enabled computational chemists to draw a parallelism between experimental observations and the atomistic-level description of the in silico simulated system.

As an example, in late 2011, long μs timescale unbiased molecular dynamics (MD) simulations of co-crystallized ligand placed at

Thomas Mavromoustakos and Tahsin F. Kellici (eds.), *Rational Drug Design: Methods and Protocols*, Methods in Molecular Biology, vol. 1824, https://doi.org/10.1007/978-1-4939-8630-9_17,

an arbitrary position (away from the binding site) of membrane-embedded *pseudo-apo* β adrenergic receptor were performed. This pioneering simulation demonstrated that drug molecules can spontaneously associate with G protein-coupled receptors [3]. The incorporation of the receptor protein in a membrane-like environment and explicit water molecules, solvation shell, in fact, enabled to describe the phenomena at an unprecedented atomistic level of detail and paved a way to establish a rigorous link between simulated and measurable macroscopic properties. In particular, (a) the qualitative convergence of the binding mode determined by molecular dynamics with the spectroscopically determined one (X-ray spectroscopy) and (b) agreement of ligand-binding thermodynamic calculations with macroscopically measurable free-energy of binding represented a milestone in computational drug discovery [4, 5].

It was the first proof of concept demonstrating that long μs timescale MD simulations possessed the intrinsic advantage of reproducing the spectroscopically determined binding conformation, which represents a solid starting point for SBD [6]. However, such simulations were (and are to date) extremely time-consuming and require high-end hardware.

Supervised molecular dynamics (SuMD) addresses this shortcoming by enabling the complete ligand–protein recognition process to be elucidated, using unbiased all-atom molecular dynamics, in a reduced timescale—up to three orders of magnitude compared to classical MD (Fig. 1) [7]. A tabu-like algorithm supervises the ligand–receptor distance over the course of the simulation. The algorithm performs a supervision on the ligand position during the simulation.

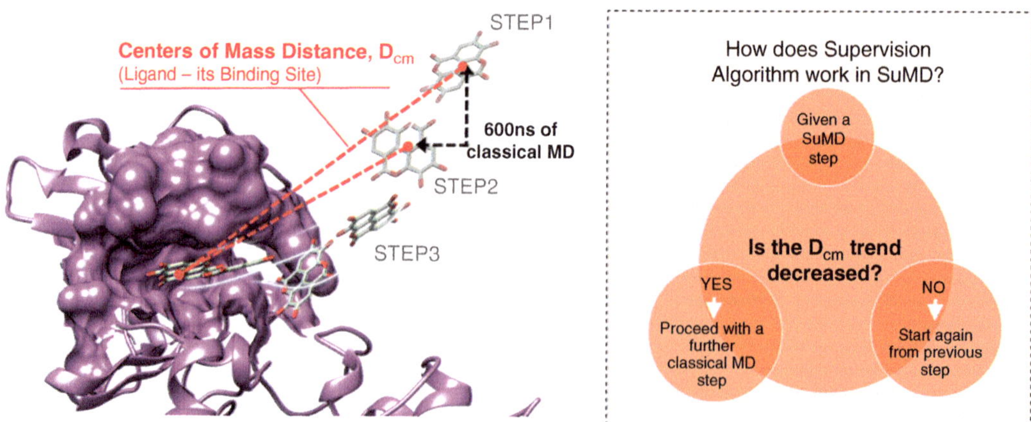

Fig. 1 A schematic representation of the supervised molecular dynamics (SuMD). The supervision algorithm using ellagic acid recognition process to human casein kinase 2 (CK2) is given as an example

When the ligand is drifting away from the receptor (i.e., ligand–receptor distance—named Dcm—increases over a simulation step of 600 ns), the simulation is restarted from the initial set of coordinates, and random velocities, drawn from the Boltzmann distribution, are reassigned (Fig. 1). This has the effect of causing the restarted simulation to explore a different region of configuration space while maintaining sampling from the correct NVT ensemble. The tabu-like supervision algorithm is repeatedly applied until the ligand–receptor distance is less than a threshold defined by the user. Generally this threshold is reached when centroids of the mass of ligand and the protein vestibule, the region that anticipates the orthosteric binding pocket cavity, match. No energetic bias is introduced to the MD simulation.

1.1 Key Aspects of SuMD: Performance on Graphical Processing Units (GPUs) and Case Study History

After placing the ligand far away from the binding pocket, SuMD simulations enable to reproduce the X-ray-determined bound conformation in hundreds of nanoseconds [7, 8]. On average an explicitly solvated class A GPCR model, embedded in a lipid environment, constitutes a system for MD simulation of the size of approximately 60,000–100,000 atoms in a cubic simulation box, using periodic boundary conditions (PBCs). A recent commodity single NVIDIA GPU card can deliver about 100 ns/day (on a 100,000 atoms system), thus enabling to probe ligand–protein recognition events with excellent throughput even on moderate-sized GPU clusters.

SuMD studies carried on the hA_{2A} adenosine receptor (AR) have proved the ability to retrospectively reproduce the crystallographic binding conformation of three strong binders such as ZM 241385 ($pK_D = 9.18$—Fig. 2) [9], T4G ($pK_D = 8.9$), and T4E ($pK_D = 9.6$) [10] and a weaker binder such as caffeine

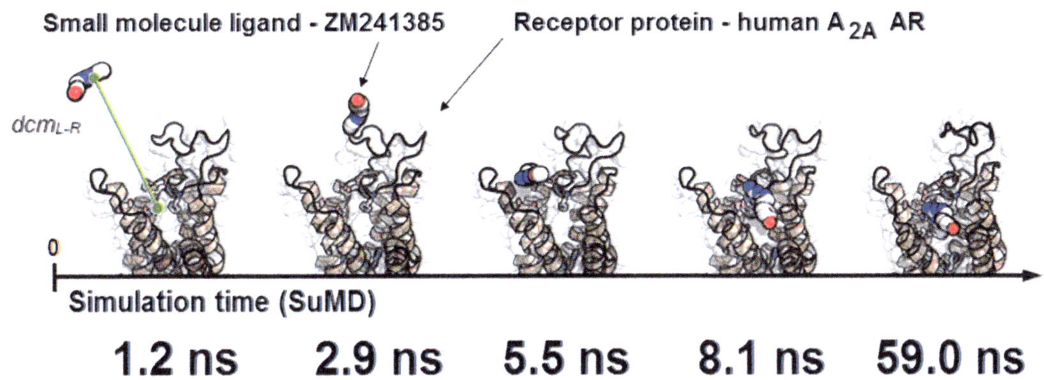

Fig. 2 Binding event of human adenosine A2A receptor antagonist ZM241385 to its receptor protein. Supervised MD simulation was applied to accelerate the recognition process. Qualitative convergence of the binding mode determined by molecular dynamics with the spectroscopically determined one (X-ray spectroscopy—PDB ID: 3EML) was reached in less than 100 ns

($pK_D = 5.31 \pm 0.44$) [11]. According to these performances, it is reasonable to assume that the endpoint of a SuMD simulation can provide high-quality models of novel ligands bound to AR and other GPCRs for which experimental confirmation of binding mode is not yet available (Fig. 2).

SuMD was also used to study protein–ligand recognition mechanism of globular and membrane proteins not belonging to the GPCR superfamily. Six different case studies were considered: (a) the human casein kinase 2 (CK2) in complex with ellagic acid, (b) the P1-1 isoform of glutathione S-transferase (GSTP1-1) in complex with sulfasalazine (2-hydroxy-(5-{[4-(2-pyridinylamino) sulfonyl]phenyl}azo) benzoic acid, SASP), (c) the human peroxiredoxin 5 (PRDX5) in complex with a benzen-1,2-diol, and (d) the human serum albumin (HSA) in complex with (*S*)-naproxen (for more applications of SuMD, *see* **Note 1**). Considering the membrane proteins, we selected the leucine transporter (LeuT) from *Aquifex aeolicus* in complex with (*S*)-fluoxetine [8]. Also in these cases, one of the key aspects to underline is the remarkable reduction of the computational time needed to reproduce with high confidence the X-ray-determined ligand-binding conformation in comparison to classical MD (unsupervised) simulations. The computation time is in the range from few hours to tens of hours (per ligand–protein complex) for the presented case studies using a single NVIDIA GPU graphic card (for performance issues *see* **Note 2**).

SuMD has also been used to explore protein–peptide recognition pathways (pepSuMD) [12]. In particular, to evaluate the performance and robustness of pepSuMD, three well-renowned complexes were selected, among a subset of characterized protein–-protein interaction (PPI) targets [13], specifically, two of them containing natural peptides (Bcl-X_L/BAD and MDM2/p53) [14, 15] and one containing a stapled peptidomimetic (MDM2/SAH-p53-8; Fig. 3) [16]. The preliminary results are very encouraging. In fact, pepSuMD methodology allows the simulation of the entire process of protein–peptide recognition (from the unbound to the bound state) in a shortened timescale with an appreciable capability to reproduce the crystallographic structures of the native complexes.

SuMD simulations enable the identification of a variety of metastable intermediate ligand-bound states that anticipate the ligand recognition at the orthosteric site. Due to the positional bias introduced by the application of the supervision algorithm, the binding events that anticipate the X-ray bound conformation might help in forming novel hypotheses and challenge current knowledge on the pharmacological properties of known ligands to their putative receptor. With the aim to stimulate otherwise neglected discussion on the matter, we applied and discussed the simulation outcome to interpret some other aspects of ligand-GPCR recognition which are yet less explored in the scientific literature. These include the differential binding profile of the

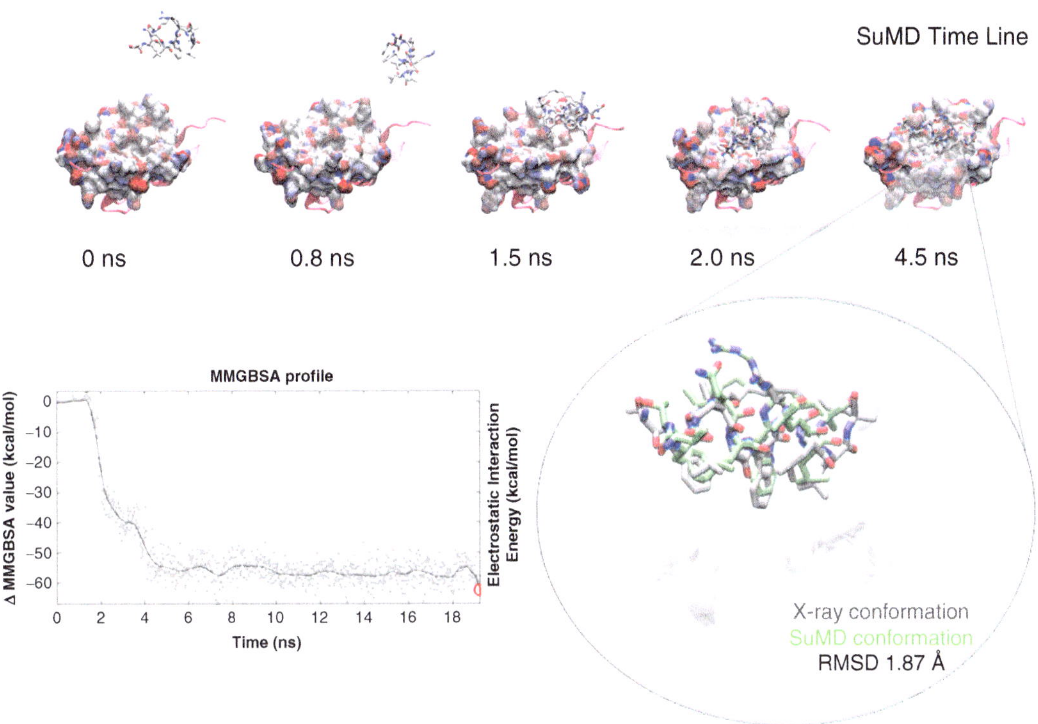

Fig. 3 Snapshots of the binding process of SAH-p53-8 cyclic peptide to MDM2 protein. The peptide reaches a conformation close to the experimental X-ray one (PDB ID: 3V3B) in 4.5 ns. It is important to note that 4.5 ns do not consider the unproductive simulation time that was discarded due to the applied supervision algorithm. From that moment, the peptide–protein interaction energy (calculated using MM-GBSA approximation) highlights a low-energy state which corresponds with the X-ray bound protein–protein complex

natural agonist adenosine and inosine at the hA_{2A} AR [17] and a mechanistic view on the positive allosteric modulation mediated by LUF6000 toward the human A_3 adenosine receptor (hA_3 AR) which corroborates the available experimental data.

In 2014 in the original SuMD paper, a challenging statement to the state-of-the-art knowledge was made by us [7]. We hypothesized the possible dual-binding mode that caffeine could adopt at the hA_{2A} AR orthosteric site. This was subsequently proven to be true by X-ray crystallography [18].

We, therefore, encourage the scientific community to adopt such tool to stimulate hypothesis creation and design appropriate "wet lab" experiments to challenge and shed more light on the observed insights gained from the simulated system.

2 Materials

SuMD is a command line tool written in python, tcl, and bash that operates the supervision of MD trajectories according to the algorithm that has been previously described. The program exploits visual molecular dynamics (VMD) and Gnuplot functionalities [19]. In its current implementation, SuMD is interfaced with the ACEMD [20] engine and supports AMBER and CHARMM force fields [21–26]. An implementation of SuMD for GROMACS has been reported to be developed in the Filipek Molecular Modeling group [27].

3 Methods

1. At the beginning of the simulation, the SuMD algorithm detects the atoms that identify the ligand and the target binding site, to define the distance between their mass centers $Dcm_{(L\text{-}R)}$ that will be monitored.
2. Then, a series of 600 ps classical MD simulations are performed (suMD step). The SuMD step has been empirically set up to guarantee a significant translation of the center of mass of the ligand during this short time of conventional MD simulation. After each simulation, five $Dcm_{(L\text{-}R)}$ distance points are collected at regular intervals of 150 ps.
3. Using these points, the slope value (m) is derived by a linear fitting. As previously described, if the resulting slope m is negative or below the user-selected threshold (i.e., the distance $Dcm_{(L\text{-}R)}$ is decreasing), the next simulation step starts from the last set of coordinates produced; otherwise, the simulation is restarted by randomly assigning the atomic velocities. To avoid problematic starting geometries (i.e., geometries prone to lead to dead-end pathway), in the first simulation step, SuMD supervises the distance $Dcm_{(L\text{-}R)}$ with a maximum threshold of 31 failed attempts (preliminary run). If this threshold is reached, SuMD callbacks a randomization process on the set of coordinates supplied by the user, which consists of a classical 600 ps MD simulation.
4. During the following steps, the simulations are perpetuated under the supervision rules. In particular, the first time a slope value below the threshold is recorded, the program enters the so-called SuMD Run. When the distance $Dcm_{(L\text{-}R)}$ drops below 5 Å, the supervision is disabled, and the simulation proceeds through a classical MD simulation.
5. At the end of the simulation, only the production steps are saved, numbered in chronological order, and stored in a separate directory. The output is then analyzed (*see* **Note 3**).

4 Notes

1. *On the applicability domain of supervised molecular dynamics simulations*: In the lead optimization phase of small molecule, bioactive linear, or cyclic peptides, intrinsic potency to the target protein is a singular challenge whose success needs to be balanced with the improvement of pharmacokinetic (PK) properties. Therefore providing solid structure-based working hypotheses to guide compound optimization, in fact, allows chemists to introduce targeted modifications to the lead compound in order to improve ADME properties with minimum impact on intrinsic potency to the relevant target.

   Providing such a high-quality model may be a challenge per se since the protein–ligand recognition energy landscape is a complex ensemble of transitioning events that happen on the surface of the receptive protein. Prior the final stage of the binding event which triggers the initiation of signaling cascade, the ligand may be recognized in a distant region from the orthosteric binding pocket [3]. As described by Buch et al. [4], the binding events which may chronologically anticipate the orthosteric site sit on higher-energy potential wells in comparison to the ligand-bound X-ray-determined low-energy state. Long μs timescale MD simulations enable the ligand to fully explore the receptive protein surface and overcome small energy barriers that it may encounter when approaching the receptor. The trade-off for the very high computational cost of such long simulations is offset by the high-value outcome which consists in reproducing the spectroscopically determined binding conformation without adding any bias to the system. In such simulations, a lot of unproductive simulation time is spent by the ligand to wobble around bulk solvent which solvates the system. In addition, the possibility to identify pockets located in the proximity of the orthosteric site can be exploited in the design of bitopic ligands [28].

   In SuMD a supervision algorithm is applied regularly at a checkpoint time (Δtck). This enables to avoid running simulations when the ligand is carried away from the protein surface by the turbulent movement of bulk solvent.

   For $\Delta tck \rightarrow +\infty$, no supervision algorithm is applied throughout the entire simulation, and there is no distinction to classical molecular dynamics. In case of a defined Δtck of, i.e., 0.6 ns, there is a great increase in the probability of ligand–receptor binding events to occur in a shorter period of simulation time which leads to a speedup (three orders of magnitude) in obtaining an X-ray like ligand–protein bound conformation.

   Ligand–receptor models obtained through the employment of SuMD alone can, therefore, be obtained in desktop computing solutions equipped with GPU computing equipment at a fraction of a cluster cost.

2. *Performance breakthrough comes to a potential downside*: In SuMD, ligand conformational exploration while approaching the receptor is limited to the timeframe of the set checkpoint time (Δtck). The longer the checkpoint time, the less the performance speedup. On the contrary, the shorter the checkpoint time, the greater the probability of the ligand to be trapped in high-energy potential well which may be an allosteric-binding pocket, a flexible loop region, or the vestibule of the binding pocket.

Looking for extreme performances may be potentially dangerous when the objective of the SuMD simulation is to provide a reasonable hypothesis of the final stage of ligand recognition. Adenosine A2A receptor-binding site location is in spatial proximity to the extracellular surface, and the binding pocket vestibule is solvated by bulk-like water molecules (Fig. 4) [29]. Supervised molecular dynamics simulations of small molecule agonists and antagonists can reproduce an X-ray binding

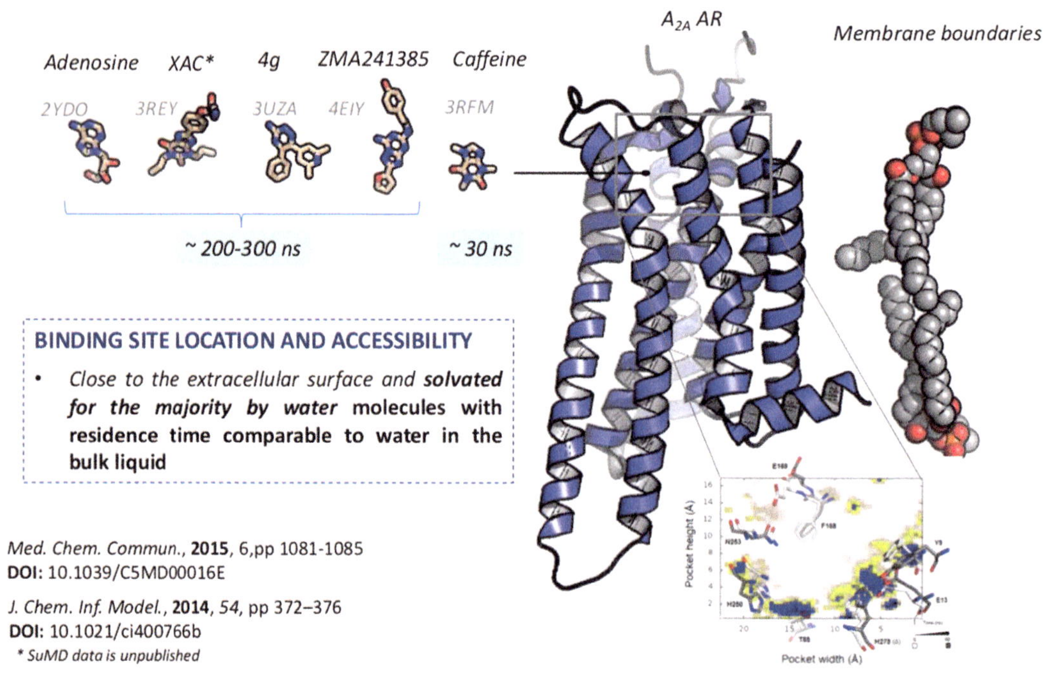

Fig. 4 In SuMD, ligand conformational exploration, while approaching the receptor, is limited to the timeframe of the Δtck. Reproducing the X-ray binding pose or providing a high-quality ligand–receptor model for a compound of unknown binding conformation can be successful in a short simulation time span (~200 ns) when the receptor proteins possess a binding pocket which is close to the extracellular surface and vestibule of the binding pocket can be easily desolvated by the incoming ligand. Adenosine A2A receptor is an example of a protein which has these characteristics and is suitable for high-performance-oriented SuMD simulations. SuMD settings: Δtck of 0.2 ns [7]

pose in about 30–200 ns [7]. This is considerably a short time-scale, and the performance improvement does not compromise the quality of the output.

On the other hand, P2Y12 receptor possesses a more complex binding pocket structure and dynamics [30]. Residues E273 and K174, which constitute the binding pocket vestibule, form a salt bridge. This feature enables to form an effective trap for ligand molecules that transit toward the orthosteric site. Performance speedups by lowering the checkpoint time (Δtck) should not be sought in this case. Using a Δtck of 0.2 ns does not lead to convergent-binding poses after running long μs supervised simulations. This is clearly an indication that a longer checkpoint time (up to 1 ns) should be used. Performance speedups, in comparison to classical MD, will be therefore less pronounced (Fig. 5).

3. *Avoiding blind acceptance of a SuMD simulation output*: As for molecular docking, inspection of the output is needed to avoid the blind acceptance of a solution that might be simply wrong due to artifacts of molecular mechanics (MM) [31] in sampling

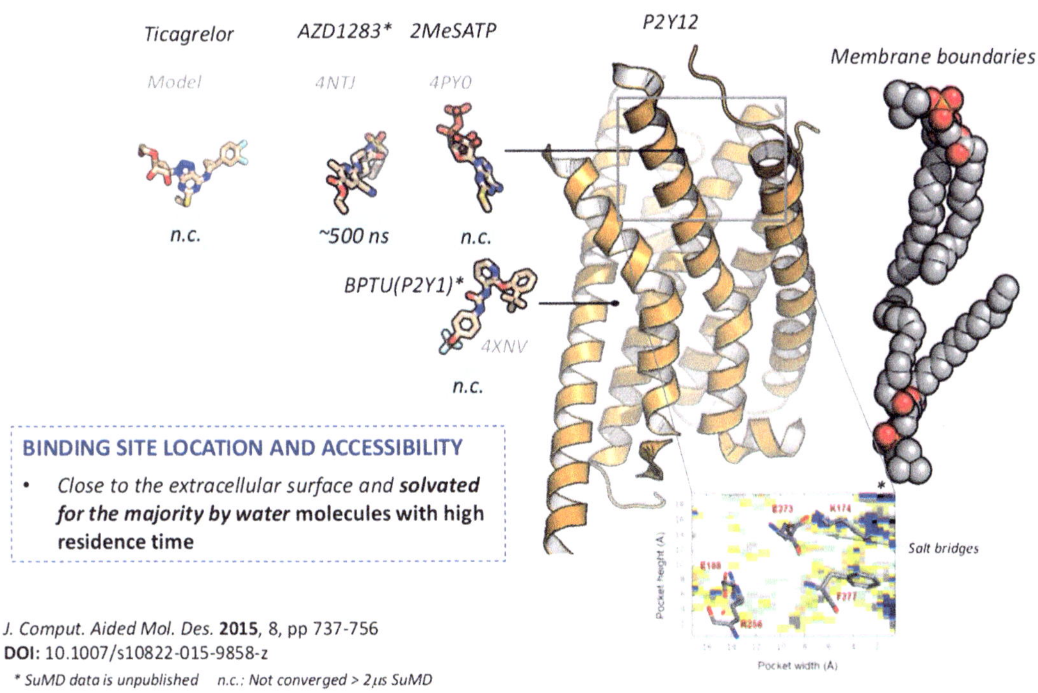

Fig. 5 Reproducing the X-ray binding pose or providing a high-quality ligand–receptor model for a compound of unknown binding conformation to P_2Y_{12} receptor has proven to be unsuccessful in a long simulation time span (~2 μs) and relatively short checkpoint time (Δtck = 0.2 ns). The P_2Y_{12} receptor proteins possess a binding pocket which is in the spatial vicinity of the extracellular surface, but the vestibule of the binding pocket cannot be easily desolvated by the incoming ligand. Such receptor is an example of a protein which has these characteristics and is not suitable for high-performance-oriented SuMD simulations

and scoring favorable ligand and protein conformational and contact preferences. Questioning the model in the output of a supervised molecular dynamics simulation is important to appreciate the usability of the technique in an industrial or academic environment. First, it is important to ensure that system preparation and MD equilibration guarantee the stereochemical quality of a protein structure and that the membrane-calculated biophysical parameters are in agreement with experimentally determined ones. Secondly, it is necessary to be aware of the caveats in the treatment of ligand conformational flexibility by judging conformational and contact preferences of both amino acid side chains and bound ligand.

Querying small molecule conformation and atom-contact preferences from structural databases [32, 33], such as the Cambridge Structural Database (CSD) [34] and the Protein Data Bank (www.rcsb.org) [1], is a complementary analysis that enables to question, with scientific rigor, the output of a supervised MD simulation. This analysis should regularly be carried out with the final aim to build solid hypotheses of protein–ligand interaction and drive the creative thinking process in medicinal chemistry [35].

References

1. Berman HM, Westbrook J, Feng Z et al (2000) The protein data bank. Nucleic Acids Res 28 (1):235–242. https://doi.org/10.1093/nar/28.1.235
2. Cooke RM, Brown AJH, Marshall FH, Mason JS (2015) Structures of G protein-coupled receptors reveal new opportunities for drug discovery. Drug Discov Today 20 (11):1355–1364. https://doi.org/10.1016/j.drudis.2015.08.003
3. Dror RO, Pan AC, Arlow DH et al (2011) Pathway and mechanism of drug binding to G-protein-coupled receptors. Proc Natl Acad Sci U S A 108(32):13118–13123. https://doi.org/10.1073/pnas.1104614108
4. Buch I, Giorgino T, De Fabritiis G (2011) Complete reconstruction of an enzyme-inhibitor binding process by molecular dynamics simulations. Proc Natl Acad Sci U S A 108 (25):10184–10189. https://doi.org/10.1073/pnas.1103547108
5. Ferruz N, Harvey MJ, Mestres J, De Fabritiis G (2015) Insights from fragment hit binding assays by molecular simulations. J Chem Inf Model 55(10):2200–2205. https://doi.org/10.1021/acs.jcim.5b00453
6. Kuhn B, Guba W, Hert J et al (2016) A real-world perspective on molecular design. J Med Chem 59(9):4087–4102. https://doi.org/10.1021/acs.jmedchem.5b01875
7. Sabbadin D, Moro S (2014) Supervised molecular dynamics (SuMD) as a helpful tool to depict GPCR-ligand recognition pathway in a nanosecond time scale. J Chem Inf Model 54 (2):372–376. https://doi.org/10.1021/ci400766b
8. Cuzzolin A, Sturlese M, Deganutti G et al (2016) Deciphering the complexity of ligand-protein recognition pathways using supervised molecular dynamics (SuMD) simulations. J Chem Inf Model 56(4):687–705. https://doi.org/10.1021/acs.jcim.5b00702
9. Jaakola V-P, Griffith MT, Hanson MA et al (2008) The 2.6 angstrom crystal structure of a human A2A adenosine receptor bound to an antagonist. Science 322(5905):1211–1217. https://doi.org/10.1126/science.1164772
10. Congreve M, Andrews SP, Doré AS et al (2012) Discovery of 1,2,4-triazine derivatives as adenosine A(2A) antagonists using structure based drug design. J Med Chem 55 (5):1898–1903. https://doi.org/10.1021/jm201376w
11. Doré AS, Robertson N, Errey JC et al (2011) Structure of the adenosine A(2A) receptor in complex with ZM241385 and the xanthines

XAC and caffeine. Structure 19 (9):1283–1293. https://doi.org/10.1016/j.str.2011.06.014
12. Salmaso V, Sturlese M, Cuzzolin A, Moro S (2017) Exploring protein–peptide recognition pathways using a supervised molecular dynamics approach. Structure 25(4):655–662.e2. https://doi.org/10.1016/j.str.2017.02.009
13. Scott DE, Bayly AR, Abell C, Skidmore J (2016) Small molecules, big targets: drug discovery faces the protein–protein interaction challenge. Nat Rev Drug Discov 15 (8):533–550. https://doi.org/10.1038/nrd.2016.29
14. Kussie PH, Gorina S, Marechal V et al (1996) Structure of the MDM2 oncoprotein bound to the p53 tumor suppressor transactivation domain. Science 274(5289):948–953. https://doi.org/10.1126/science.274.5289.948
15. Petros AM, Nettesheim DG, Wang Y et al (2000) Rationale for Bcl-xL/bad peptide complex formation from structure, mutagenesis, and biophysical studies. Protein Sci 9 (12):2528–2534. https://doi.org/10.1110/ps.9.12.2528
16. Baek S, Kutchukian PS, Verdine GL et al (2012) Structure of the stapled p53 peptide bound to Mdm2. J Am Chem Soc 134 (1):103–106. https://doi.org/10.1021/ja2090367
17. Deganutti G, Welihinda A, Moro S (2017) Comparison of the human A2A adenosine receptor recognition by adenosine and Inosine: new insight from supervised molecular dynamics simulations. ChemMedChem 12 (16):1319–1326. https://doi.org/10.1002/cmdc.201700200
18. Cheng RKY, Segala E, Robertson N et al (2017) Structures of human A1 and A2A adenosine receptors with Xanthines reveal determinants of selectivity. Structure 25 (8):1275–1285.e4. https://doi.org/10.1016/j.str.2017.06.012
19. Williams T, Kelley C Gnuplot 4.5: an interactive plotting program, version 4.5; http://gnuplot.info (Accessed October 2015)
20. Harvey MJ, Giupponi G, Fabritiis GD (2009) ACEMD: accelerating biomolecular dynamics in the microsecond time scale. J Chem Theory Comput 5(6):1632–1639. https://doi.org/10.1021/ct9000685
21. Case DA, Babin V, Berryman JT et al (2014) AMBER 14
22. Wang J, Wolf RM, Caldwell JW, Kollman PA, Case DA (2004) Development and testing of a general amber force field. J Comput Chem 25 (9):1157–1174. https://doi.org/10.1002/jcc.20035
23. MacKerell AD, Bashford D, Bellott M et al (1998) All-atom empirical potential for molecular modeling and dynamics studies of proteins. J Phys Chem B 102(18):3586–3616. https://doi.org/10.1021/jp973084f
24. MacKerell AD, Banavali N, Foloppe N (2000) Development and current status of the CHARMM force field for nucleic acids. Biopolymers 56(4):257–265. https://doi.org/10.1002/1097-0282(2000)56:4<257::AID-BIP10029>3.0.CO;2-W
25. Vanommeslaeghe K, MacKerell AD (2012) Automation of the CHARMM general force field (CGenFF) I: bond perception and atom typing. J Chem Inf Model 52(12):3144–3154. https://doi.org/10.1021/ci300363c
26. Vanommeslaeghe K, Raman EP, MacKerell AD (2012) Automation of the CHARMM general force field (CGenFF) II: assignment of bonded parameters and partial atomic charges. J Chem Inf Model 52(12):3155–3168. https://doi.org/10.1021/ci3003649
27. Jakowiecki J, Filipek S (2016) Hydrophobic ligand entry and exit pathways of the CB1 cannabinoid receptor. J Chem Inf Model 56 (12):2457–2466. https://doi.org/10.1021/acs.jcim.6b00499
28. Fronik P, Gaiser BI, Sejer Pedersen D (2017) Bitopic ligands and metastable binding sites: opportunities for G protein-coupled receptor (GPCR) medicinal chemistry. J Med Chem 60 (10):4126–4134. https://doi.org/10.1021/acs.jmedchem.6b01601
29. Sabbadin D, Ciancetta A, Moro S (2014) Perturbation of fluid dynamics properties of water molecules during G protein-coupled receptor-ligand recognition: the human A2A adenosine receptor as a key study. J Chem Inf Model 54 (10):2846–2855. https://doi.org/10.1021/ci500397y
30. Paoletta S, Sabbadin D, von Kügelgen I et al (2015) Modeling ligand recognition at the P2Y12 receptor in light of X-ray structural information. J Comput Aided Mol Des 29 (8):737–756. https://doi.org/10.1007/s10822-015-9858-z
31. Lipkowitz K (1995) Abuses of molecular mechanics: pitfalls to avoid. J Chem Educ 72 (12):1070. https://doi.org/10.1021/ed072p1070
32. Brameld KA, Kuhn B, Reuter DC, Stahl M (2008) Small molecule conformational preferences derived from crystal structure data. A medicinal chemistry focused analysis. J Chem

Inf Model 48(1):1–24. https://doi.org/10.1021/ci7002494

33. Lovell SC, Word JM, Richardson JS, Richardson DC (2000) The penultimate rotamer library. Proteins 40(3):389–408. https://doi.org/10.1002/1097-0134(20000815)40:3<389::AID-PROT50>3.0.CO;2-2
34. Allen FH (2002) The Cambridge structural database: a quarter of a million crystal structures and rising. Acta Crystallogr B 58:380–388
35. Stahl M, Baier S (2015) How many molecules does it take to tell a story? Case studies, language, and an epistemic view of medicinal chemistry. ChemMedChem 10(6):949–956. https://doi.org/10.1002/cmdc.201500091

Chapter 18

Lead Identification Through the Synergistic Action of Biomolecular NMR and In Silico Methodologies

Konstantinos D. Marousis, Aikaterini C. Tsika, Maria Birkou, Minos-Timotheos Matsoukas, and Georgios A. Spyroulias

Abstract

The combination of virtual screening with biomolecular NMR can be a powerful approach in the first steps toward drug discovery. Here, we describe how computational methodologies to screen large databases readily available for testing small molecules, in synergy with NMR techniques focused on protein–ligand interactions, can be used in the early lead compound identification process against a protein drug target.

Key words NMR, Structural biology, SAR, Virtual screening, Pharmacophore modeling

1 Introduction

Structure–activity relationship methods using nuclear magnetic resonance (NMR) [1] in combination with computational virtual screening schemes [2] are often applied in the process of identifying and characterizing lead compounds. The main advantage in the study of protein–ligand interactions is the elucidation of the interaction dynamics at the atomic level even if low affinity binders are identified [3]. Several methodologies can be applied in the elucidation of protein–protein interface identification [4] and the exploration of molecular determinants of protein–ligand binding [5]. Libraries of small molecules can be easily evaluated applying protein- and ligand-based NMR experiments [6, 7]. Here, we attempt to cover, in a comprehensive way, the process of identifying the binding interface of a protein, targeting this interface through virtual screening and evaluating the binding of selected compounds via NMR [8–10].

Konstantinos D. Marousis and Aikaterini C. Tsika contributed equally to this work.

Thomas Mavromoustakos and Tahsin F. Kellici (eds.), *Rational Drug Design: Methods and Protocols*, Methods in Molecular Biology, vol. 1824, https://doi.org/10.1007/978-1-4939-8630-9_18, © Springer Science+Business Media, LLC, part of Springer Nature 2018

1.1 Protein–Protein Interaction Using NMR

Proteins have many miscellaneous biological functions which are intimately linked with the formation of a complex with another macromolecule or a small ligand. The binding effect is elicited by conformational changes of various properties which can affect the overall conformation of the protein complex [11]. Thus, the plasticity of the protein scaffold during the binding process can affect positively or negatively [12–14] the interaction of the complex in such a way that cellular processes can be regulated or controlled [15]. Chemical shift difference (CSD) analysis is the most ordinary procedure to investigate the interaction of a protein–protein complex and can spotlight a big variety of bimolecular responses [16]. In this case NMR titration experiments and CSD analysis of protein–protein interaction protocol are described, as well as a typical procedure for the estimation of the dissociation constant (K_d) in some of the exchange regimes on the NMR timescale [17].

1.2 Virtual Screening

There are many computational methods and software packages for target identification, target selection, and computer-aided drug design using docking, pharmacophore, or other methods [18]. Pharmacophore modeling has been used in the past in several successful virtual screening studies to identify novel compounds against protein targets of pharmaceutical interest [19, 20]. However, not many web services exist that support structure-based virtual screening [21]. The mostly used ones are typically batch-processing services of existing molecule libraries, where jobs may be submitted and the results can be gathered after hours or days. A relatively new pharmacophore-based web service, Pharmit, allows both pharmacophore and molecular shape searching, in addition to ligand energy minimization, which enables the ranking of compounds given that a molecular target is available [22]. It can be used for fast-searching of already defined or user-defined libraries and can deliver results within seconds. In this case, NMR structural data of a protein of interest can be used for a virtual screening of molecules, as well as provide with specific protein–ligand interactions to optimize an initial pharmacophore model for enhanced hit selection.

1.3 Protein–Ligand Interactions Through NMR

Saturation transfer difference (STD) is an approach that it is used in order to screen small molecules against a specific target [23]. Small compounds having small differences in certain moieties can be evaluated via this technique and simultaneously can be performed under competitive conditions. Identification of the important binding moieties is characterized as ligand mapping [24]. The high sensitivity along with low non-labeled protein concentration and K_d determination listed as the main advantage of this methodology. STD is based on the nuclear Overhauser effect allowing the observation of the resonances of the bound ligand protons. Thus, relying on the "on resonance" and "off resonance" experiment, one can obtain a spectrum containing only the signal of the protein and ligand which are exhibiting saturation, i.e., involved in the binding [25].

Additionally, the chemical shift mapping method can be applied to identify the ligand-binding pocket in order to ensure that the specific crevice is targeted, as well as to evaluate the binding strength of the interaction that takes place [1, 26]. This method requires the protein (target molecule) to be in a ^{15}N-labeled form. Usually, the ^{15}N-labeled protein is titrated by the small molecule (binder), and in case that this molecule interacts with the protein, differences in the chemical shifts of the NH amide groups are observed. These chemical shift changes may differ in nature or in extent, and they are monitored by ^{1}H–^{15}N 2D HSQC experiments. The nature of the chemical shift changes depends on the binding affinity and the binding kinetics of the binder [17]. The binding constant of the small molecule can also be determined, using a function that correlates the NH chemical shift changes as a function of the molecular ratio of the protein target and the binder [27].

The above methods can provide valuable information about the binding of the ligand but cannot provide quantitative information about the binding orientation of the ligand and the binder-protein contacts. Therefore, for the structural determination of protein–ligand complex via NMR spectroscopy, the identification of the intermolecular NOEs that define the ligand's orientation is required. The filtered-edited NOESY experiment was developed to provide such kind of information for the structure-based drug design, since the results reveal the bond "network" between protein and ligand atoms [28, 29]. The technique is useful even without the assignment of the complex via the standard method and sparse assignment of resonances belonging to the protein and binder groups may be adequate to extract NOE-based structural constraints. Complexes characterized by $K_d < 100$ nM are ideal for this type of study. However, there are some examples in which the technique was applied efficiently in much weaker binding events [30]. The critical step is the ^{1}H assignment of the small molecules. Initially, the ligand assignment, through its intramolecular NOEs, can be achieved since only the ^{12}C-attached protons at the edited-edited TOCSY and NOESY spectrum are observed. Consecutively, intermolecular NOEs due to the bond between the ^{1}H and ^{1}H ^{13}C can be obtained from the filtered-edited NOESY spectrum containing these specific NOE peaks.

Therefore, what is described below is the experimental protocols applied in the preparation of protein samples in appropriate form (labeled in ^{15}N and/or $^{13}C/^{15}N$ form) and the application of NMR experiments in order to obtain data that can be exploited in experimental or computational drug design efforts.

2 Materials

2.1 Protein Production

2.1.1 Protein Expression

1. BL21(DE3) (Stratagene) or Rosetta™2 (DE3) Singles™ (Novagen).
2. Luria-Bertani (LB) medium: 1L H2), 10g/L NaCl, 10g/L Tryptone, 5g/L Yeast Extract, Autoclave.
3. M9 medium: 1L H_20 6.8 g Na_2HPO_4, 3 g KH_2PO_4, 0.5 g NaCl. Autoclave. Add 4 g glucose or ^{13}C-glucose, 1 g $^{15}NH_4Cl$ or $^{14}NH_4SO_4$, 0.3 mL/L $CaCl_2$ (from 1 M stock), 1 mL/L $MgSO_4$ (from 1 M stock), 2 mL/L solution Q (8 mL HCl, 184 mg $CaCl_2$ 2 H_2O, 64 mg H_3BO_3, 18 mg $CoCl_2$ $6H_2O$, 4 mg $CuCl_2$ $2H_2O$, 340 mg $ZnCl_2$, 605 mg Na_2oMO_4 $2H_2O$, 40 mg $MnCl_2$ $4H_2O$, IL H_2O), 2 mL/L thiamin and biotin (from 0.5 mg/mL stock), 1 mL/L BioExpress® (CIL).
4. Ampicillin 1 mL/L (100mg/ml stock) and/or chloramphenicol 1 mL/L (34mg/ml stock).
5. Isopropyl-β-D-galactopyranoside, IPTG (1 M stock).

2.1.2 Protein Purification

Affinity Chromatography Purification

His-Tagged Protein Purification

1. 5 mL HisTrap HP column (GE Healthcare).
2. Binding Buffer: 10 mM imidazole, 20 mM Na_2HPO_4, 0.5 M NaCl, pH 8.0 Elution Buffer: 400 mM imidazole, 20 mM Na_2HPO_4, 0.5 M NaCl, pH 8.0.

GST-Tagged Protein Purification

1. 5 mL GSTrap FF column (GE Healthcare).
2. Wash buffer: phosphate-buffered saline, PBS, pH 7.4 ± 0.2 GST. Elution buffer: 50 mM Tris–HCl, 10 mM reduced glutathione, pH 8.0.

Size-Exclusion Chromatography Purification

1. Elution buffer: According to the optimal protein stability (*see* **Note 1**).
2. Amicon® Ultra 15 mL centrifugal filters (Merck).
3. AKTA purifier (GE Healthcare).
4. Superose® 12 10/300 GL (GE Healthcare).

NMR Sample Preparation

1. 10% deuterium oxide (D_2O).
2. 2 μL 2,2-dimethyl-2-silapentane-5-sulfonate (DSS).
3. 1 μL NaN_3 (from 1 M stock).
4. 50 mm NMR tubes.

All stock solutions were filter-sterilized.

2.2 NMR Experiments

The NMR sample conditions and experimental parameters described below refer to measurements acquired in a Bruker 700 MHz Avance III HD magnet equipped with a triple-resonance TCI CryoProbe. All Pulse sequences used and mentioned below are standard pulse programs included in the Bruker library. All measurements are carried out at 25 °C, and the data are acquired and processed with the TopSpin 3.5 software.

2.2.1 Titration Experiments

For the analysis of the interaction between a protein and a ligand or another protein, a series of titration experiments is required. There is a big variety of NMR pulse sequences inside the Bruker library that can be used depending on the size and stability of the labeled protein. One has to choose between the typical ^{15}N-HSQC, the TROSY (transverse relaxation-optimized spectroscopy) version, and the fast-acquisition ^{15}N-HSQC pulse program (the so-called "sofast" version of HSQC experiments). These ^{15}N-HSQC experiments are experiments that can provide the ^{1}H–^{15}N correlation of a protein, and these resonances are the fingerprint of each polypeptide, since they are diagnostic for the folding, the oligomerization, and the dynamics of each protein target (*see* Fig. 1—HSQC of folded and unfolded protein). The most common pulse programs are hsqcetfpgpsi2, trosyf3gpph19, and fhsqcf3gpph. The acquisition parameters depend on the size and the concentration of the protein. In the protocol described below, the trosyf3gpph19 pulse program is used, and a protein concentration of ~0.3 mM is considered. The basic acquisition and processing parameters for the above pulse programs are illustrated in Tables 1–3.

2.2.2 Saturation Transfer Difference (STD)

1. Purified protein (unlabeled) as mentioned previously, concentrated at the selected buffer (the solution of the NMR sample should always contain a deuterated solvent; for aqueous water solution, this is D_2O in 5–10% v/v).
2. Ligand stock solutions for each of the compounds should be in much higher concentration than the protein solution. This stock will be diluted into the protein solution; therefore mixtures of P(protein)–L(ligand) should have a ligand excess of 50–100-fold higher than the protein concentration. Thus, stock solutions about 5 mM should be used (the same buffer as the protein-containing buffer should be prepared, given that it is permitted by the solubility of the compounds).
3. The NMR pulse program used for such an analysis is stddiffgp19.3 and zgesgp for the reference spectra, both stored inside the Bruker pulse program library. The basic experimental conditions are illustrated in Table 4.

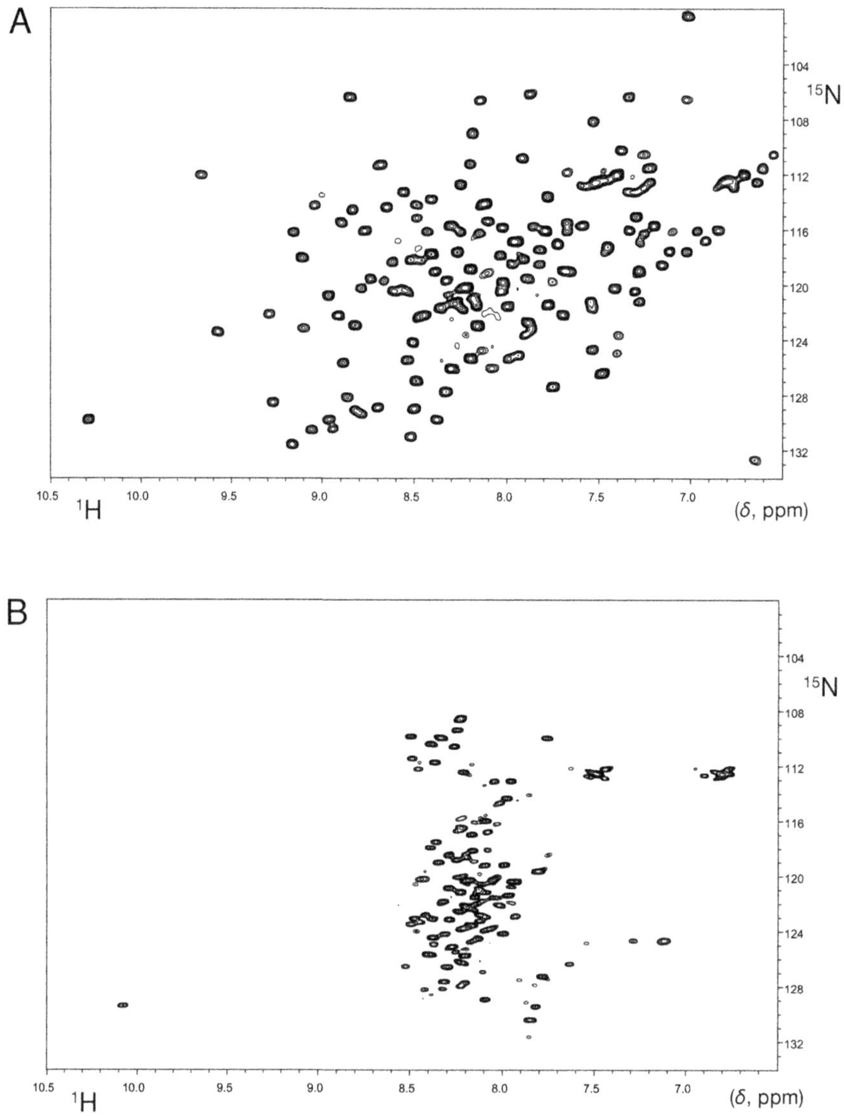

Fig. 1 ^{15}N-HSQC spectra of a ~150 amino acid polypeptide. The signal dispersion is characteristic for a well-folded protein (**a**), while the absence of any secondary or tertiary structure elements results to the accumulation of ^{1}H–^{15}N signals in the region of around 8.0–8.5 ppm, typical for structureless polypeptides (**b**)

2.2.3 Protein–Ligand Interaction Studies Through Chemical Shift Mapping

1. Purified protein (^{15}N labeling) as mentioned previously is diluted in the selected buffer (D_2O is used in 5–10% v/v) up to a final concentration >0.2 mM.
2. Ligand stock solutions of ten molar excess (in the same buffer used for the protein) in such concentrations so the final total volume of each sample containing protein and titrated ligand does not exceed 50 μL (this ensures that the protein solution will not be extremely diluted at the end of the titration and that signal disappearance during the titrations is due to the interaction and not the decrease of the signal intensity).

Table 1
Basic experimental parameters for trosyf3gpph19

^{15}N–^{1}H Trosy HSQC		
Pulse program	**trosyf3gpph19**	
Acquisition parameters		
Dimension	F1(^{15}N)	F2(^{1}H)
Time domain (TD)	256	1024
Spectral width (SW)	40 ppm	14 ppm
O1p	120 ppm	4.7 ppm
Number of scans (NS)	4	
Relaxation delay (D1)	1 sec	
Time	20 min 13 s	
Processing parameters		
Size of real Spect (SI)	2048	2048
Line broadening (LB)	0.3	0.3
Window Func (WDW)	QSINE	QSINE
Sine bell shift (SSB)	2	2

Table 2
Basic experimental parameters for hsqcetfpgpsi2

^{15}N–^{1}H HSQC		
Pulse program	**hsqcetfpgpsi2**	
Acquisition parameters		
Dimension	F1(^{15}N)	F2(^{1}H)
Time domain (TD)	256	2048
Spectral width (SW)	40 ppm	14 ppm
O1p	120 ppm	4.7 ppm
Number of scans (NS)	4	
Relaxation delay (D1)	1 sec	
Time	19 min 55 sec	
Processing parameters		
Size of real Spect (SI)	1024	2048
Line broadening (LB)	0.3	0.3
Window Func (WDW)	QSINE	QSINE
Sine bell shift (SSB)	2	2

2.2.4 X-Filtered-X-Edited

An important aspect of determining a protein–ligand complex is the investigation of any intermolecular NOE signal. For $^{13}C/^{15}N$ isotope-labeled proteins and non-labeled ligand complexes, a series of filtered-edited experiments can be used to identify and measure such NOE signals [31]. There are three useful types of experiments: filtered-edited NOESY, edited-edited NOESY, and TOCSY (*see* **Note 2**).

Table 3
Basic experimental parameters for fhsqf3gpph

^{15}N–^{1}H fast HSQC		
Pulse program	**fhsqcf3gpph**	
Acquisition parameters		
Dimension	F1(^{15}N)	F2(^{1}H)
Time domain (TD)	256	2048
Spectral width (SW)	40 ppm	14 ppm
O1p	120 ppm	4.7 ppm
Number of scans (NS)	4	
Relaxation delay (D1)	1 s	
Time	19 min 41 s	
Processing parameters		
Size of real Spect (SI)	2048	2048
Line broadening (LB)	0.3	0.3
Window Func (WDW)	QSINC	QSINC
Sine bell shift (SSB)	2	2

Table 4
Basic experimental parameters for stddiffgp19.3 and zgesgp

STD-NMR		
Pulse program	**stddiffgp19.3**	**zgesgp**
Acquisition parameters		
Dimension	F2(^{1}H)	F1(^{1}H)
Time domain (TD)	16,000	2048
Spectral width (SW)	16 ppm	16 ppm
O1p	4.7 ppm	4.7 ppm
Number of scans (NS)	128	128
Relaxation delay (D1)	4 s	2.5 s
Time	25 min 43 s	5 min 55 s
Processing parameters		
Size of real Spect (SI)	32,000	4096
Line broadening (LB)	0.3	3.0
Window Func (WDW)	EM	QSINE
Sine bell shift (SSB)	2	2

1. Protein sample: Purified protein (^{15}N and ^{13}C labeling) as mentioned previously concentrated at the selected buffer (the solution has to contain a deuterated solvent; usually D_2O is used) up to a final concentration of 500 μM. The final protein–ligand ratio will be determined by the binding affinity. For a strong interaction, a ratio about 1:2 is sufficient.

Table 5
Basic experimental parameters for noesyhsqcf3gpwgx13d

Filtered-edited NOESY			
Pulse program	**noesyhsqcf3gpwgx13d**		
Acquisition parameters			
Dimension	F1(^{1}H)	F2(^{13}C)	F3(^{1}H)
Time domain (TD)	256	1	2048
Spectral width (SW)	14 ppm	140 ppm	14
O1p	4.7 ppm	70 ppm	4.7 ppm
Number of scans (NS)	512		
Relaxation delay (D1)	1 s		
Time	1d 22 h 52 min 20 s		
Processing parameters			
Size of real Spect (SI)	2048	N/A	2048
Line broadening (LB)	0.1	N/A	0
Window Func (WDW)	QSINE	N/A	QSINE
Sine bell shift (SSB)	2	N/A	2

Table 6
Basic experimental parameters for noesygpphwgxf.2

Edited-edited NOESY		
Pulse program	**noesygpphwgxf.2**	
Acquisition parameters		
Dimension	F1(^{1}H)	F2(^{1}H)
Time domain (TD)	640	2048
Spectral width (SW)	14 ppm	14 ppm
O1p	4.7 ppm	4.7 ppm
Number of scans (NS)	256	
Relaxation delay (D1)	1 s	
Time	2d 11 h 22 min 51 s	
Processing parameters		
Size of real Spect (SI)	1024	1024
Line broadening (LB)	1	0.3
Window Func (WDW)	QSINE	QSINE
Sine bell shift (SSB)	2	2

2. The pulse sequences for these experiments are the following: noesyhsqcf3gpwgx13d, noesygpphwgxf.2 (edited-edited NOESY), and dipsi2gpphwgxf (edited-edited TOCSY). The basic experimental and processing parameters for these experiments are shown in Tables 5–7, respectively.

Table 7
Basic experimental parameters for dipsi2gpphwgxf

Edited-edited TOCSY		
Pulse program	**dipsi2gpphwgxf**	
Acquisition parameters		
Dimension	F1(^{1}H)	F2(^{1}H)
Time domain (TD)	640	2048
Spectral width (SW)	14 ppm	14 ppm
O1p	4.7 ppm	4.7 ppm
Number of scans (NS)	256	
Relaxation delay (D1)	1 s	
Time	2d 8 h 59 min 3 s	
Processing parameters		
Size of real Spect (SI)	1024	1024
Line broadening (LB)	1	0
Window Func (WDW)	QSINE	QSINE
Sine bell shift (SSB)	2	2

2.3 Computational Methods

1. The three-dimensional (3D) small-molecule web database of MolPort can be used in such circumstances, providing with chemical information a wide range of already synthesized purchasable organic compounds. MolPort has a web platform which contains approximately seven million unique and in stock compounds (as of September 2017). These compounds are sold by 18 synthetic chemistry companies, such as Enamine (~1.6 M), ChemDiv (~1 M), Vitas-M (~1.2 M), Chembridge (~0.9 M), and others, which have deposited their compound database information into MolPort.
2. For the pharmacophore virtual screening process, Pharmit [22] is a web-based interactive environment for the fast screening of large compound databases, enhanced with molecular shape and energy minimization methods.

3 Methods

3.1 Protein Expression-Purification-Production

1. Transform cells with the plasmid carrying the gene of interest.
2. Pick a colony from the plate and inoculate a 10–15 mL culture of LB medium, at 37 °C overnight (o/n).
3. Add the pre-culture in 1 L of sterile M9 medium. Incubate the culture in a shaking incubator (200–220 rounds per minute, rpm) at 37 °C until it reaches an optical density (OD_{600}) of ~0.6.
4. Add IPTG to induce expression, and continue incubating for the appropriate time.

5. Harvest cells by centrifugation at 5400 × *g* for 10 min at 4 °C.
6. Lyse the cell suspension. Sonicate on ice for 2:30 min using 2:30 min off mode.
7. Purify the protein of interest with affinity chromatography.
8. If necessary, cleave the tag with the appropriate protease.
9. Increase the purity of the protein with size-exclusion chromatography.
10. Concentrate the protein using Amicon Ultra 15 mL.
11. Transfer protein to 50 mm NMR tube.

3.2 Protein–Protein Interactions with NMR Spectroscopy

3.2.1 Mapping the Interaction Interface

For the analysis and identification of the interaction between two macromolecules with NMR, two titration experiments should be performed: one with the first protein ^{15}N labeled and the other unlabeled and the reverse one with the second one labeled and the first one unlabeled. For both of the cases, a typical protocol is described below:

1. Record a reference 2D ^{1}H–^{15}N HSQC spectrum of the ^{15}N-labeled protein. Sample concentration typically ranges from 0.1 to 0.3 mM.
2. Add unlabeled protein sample using a concentration stock about ten times the concentration of the labeled protein sample.
3. Record a 2D ^{1}H–^{15}N HSQC spectrum of the mixture with exactly the same experimental parameters as in **step 1**.
4. Repeat **steps 2–3** until the final mixture reach saturation. The unlabeled protein is added incrementally with typical ratios of 1:0.1, 1:0.25, 1:0.5, 1:0.75, 1:1, 1:2, and 1:5 until no new spectral changes are observed.
5. Analyze all the spectra with any assignment software (CARA [32], TopSpin, NMRPipe [33], etc.), and measure the chemical shift difference (CSD) from the reference spectrum to the saturated state using Eq. 1 [34].

$$\Delta\delta_{\mathrm{ppm}} = \sqrt{(\Delta\delta_{\mathrm{HN}})^2 + \left(\frac{\Delta\delta_{\mathrm{N}}}{5}\right)^2} \quad (1)$$

6. Plot the CSD against the residue number to a column bar graph.
7. Calculate the standard deviation of the CSD values (if the protein has flexible or unstructured segments, use the residues that belong to the rigid body). Use this value as threshold for the CSD plot [16].

8. Residues with CSD values significant higher than the threshold are highlighted and used to map the interaction interface of the binding.

In order to identify the interaction interface of the second protein, the reverse titration experiment should be performed. Follow the procedure described above, but this time with the second protein ^{15}N labeled, and observe the CSD in this macromolecule.

3.2.2 Determining the Dissociation Constant

With all the data collected from the titration experiments, it is possible to determine the dissociation constant (K_d) of the interaction. This analysis is ideally suited for protein interactions with K_d ranging from ~2 μM to ~1 mM, thus leading to a fast exchange regime on the NMR timescale. In order to determine unambiguously the K_d value, protein concentration must be in a similar magnitude to the K_d.

1. The initial protein concentration $[P_0]$ should be $\sim 0.5 \times K_d$.
2. The maximum concentration of the titrant should be $\sim 10 \times [P_0]$.
3. Follow the procedure described in section above to measure the CSD for every residue from each step of the titration.
4. Plot the CSD against the titrant concentration for each of the interacting residues.
5. Perform a nonlinear fitting for each graph with Eq. 2:

$$[\Delta\delta_{\mathrm{obs}}] = \frac{\Delta\delta_{\mathrm{max}}}{2[P_{\mathrm{T}}]}\left[(K_{\mathrm{d}} + L_{\mathrm{T}} + P_{\mathrm{T}}) - \sqrt{(-K_{\mathrm{d}} - L_{\mathrm{T}} - P_{\mathrm{T}})^2 - 4L_{\mathrm{T}}P_{\mathrm{T}}}\right] \tag{2}$$

where $P_T = [P] + [PL]$ is the total protein concentration; $L_T = [L] + [PL]$ is the total ligand/titrant concentration; $\Delta\delta_{obs} = f_b\Delta\delta_{max}$ is the observed chemical shift with f_b the fraction of bound protein, $[PL]/[P_T]$; and $\Delta\delta_{max}$ is the maximum chemical shift change for a specific residue given by the difference $\delta_{free} - \delta_{bound}$ [16, 35].

6. From the above analysis, a K_d is estimated for each of the interacting residues, and the final K_d value is their average with an error estimated of the statistical analysis of these values.
7. Repeat **steps 1–6** for the reverse titration experiment to evaluate the K_d of the interaction.

This analysis can be performed in some cases also in the intermediate exchange regime, if the line broadening of the signals is not significant enough.

3.3 Virtual Screening Using Pharmacophore Modeling

1. Using a protein–ligand structure file for the protein under investigation, load it in the Pharmit main page (http://pharmit.csb.pitt.edu/). A dropdown menu with the available small molecules existent in the structure appears; the one interacting with the binding site should be selected (*see* **Note 3**).
2. After submitting the structure file, the main 3D window appears with the structure, and a defined pharmacophore model based on the protein–ligand interactions is detected. On the left panel, under the Pharmacophore tab, one can switch on and off the available pharmacophore features (hydrogen bond donors, acceptors, hydrophobic, aromatic, etc.). Under the Shape tab, the exclusive shape for the receptor is selected, given that adequate information on the binding site residues is present. Under the Filters tab, and Hit Reduction tab, the maximum values for hits per conformation and molecule can be set to 1. When all parameters of the pharmacophore model are set, from the dropdown menu on the top left, one can select the MolPort database to be screened and click on Search MolPort.
3. Results immediately start to appear on the right panel, next to the 3D panel. Once the search has finished, a message below the hit list appears stating "Showing *i* to *j* of *j* hits." Each hit has an RMSD value of fitting (lowest value means better fitting) to the pharmacophore model, and they can be clicked on one by one, to evaluate the fitting. Alternatively, the hit list can be downloaded as an sdf file and visualized in another molecule visualization software, such as PyMOL (https://pymol.org/) or Chimera (https://www.cgl.ucsf.edu/chimera/) (*see* **Note 4**).
4. After evaluating the top-ranked compounds, the user should select a number of as much diverse hits, based on their chemical features and general preference. The list of selected molecules' IDs can be pasted to the MolPort website, where a list of available ones, along with their physicochemical properties and price per mg, can be seen and consecutively purchased for testing.

3.4 Protein–Ligand Interaction Evaluation

3.4.1 Saturation Transfer Difference (STD)

1. Prepare a solution containing the protein of interest at a concentration circa 50 μM. Acquire a ^{1}H spectrum (reference spectrum protein), using pulse sequence zgesgp.
2. Acquire a ^{1}H spectrum of each ligand (reference spectrum ligands), using stock solutions and pulse sequence zgesgp.
3. Prepare mixtures of protein–ligands, where ligands have to be at least at 20 excess (these are going to be used for the initial screening). If there are different chemical ligand structures, try to divide the molecules at different batches so as to be easier to identify the characteristic signals of each one. Acquire a ^{1}H

spectrum as described previously (**steps 1** and **2**), and run the STD experiment on each sample using the pulse program stddiffgp19.3. Finally, after processing, three different spectra are obtained. The spectrum representing the STD results from the subtraction of the "on" from the "off" resonance experiment. Presence of signals means binding. Identify the bound molecules by comparing the signals of this spectrum to the reference one.

4. To compare the "binding strength" regarding the ligands whose binding was confirmed through **step 3**, prepare the protein–ligand mixtures. In this case the protein–ligand molar excess has to be equal to 100. These samples are going to be used in order to discriminate which chemical group of each ligand binds tighter to the target protein. Prepare one sample for each of the desirable ligands for study according to the results of the screening experiment. Run a series of STD experiments, using the pulse program stddiffgp19.3 on each sample choosing different saturation times from 0.25 to 5 s (a number of ten different saturation times is appropriate in order to have the appropriate number of points for a reliable curve) (*see* **Note 5**).
5. Phase, correct the baseline, and calibrate (if it is necessary) all spectra. Keep in mind that you have to keep the parameters same for all the spectra of each ligand.
6. Integrate the first spectrum reference.
7. Integrate the following spectra using the previous (**step 6**) integration file.
8. The amplification factor should be calculated for the bound protons of each ligand using the STD amplification factor in Eq. 3:

$$\text{STDamp} = \frac{\text{STD}_{\text{diff}}\ \text{intensity of resonance}\ x}{\text{STD}_{\text{off}}\ \text{intensity of intensity}\ x} \times \text{ligand excess} \quad (3)$$

9. Create a diagram for each ligand, and plot the *STDamp* factor for each proton as a function of saturation time.
10. To compare the "binding strength" of the protons, in order to conclude at their contribution proximity to the protein, select the proton STDamp values at one saturation time. Set the highest as 100% and calculate the STD% for the remaining protons.
11. Prepare mixtures of the protein in different protein–ligand molar ratios, e.g., 5, 10, 20, 30, 40, 50, 70, 80, 90, and 100 molar excess for each ligand. This will be used for the K_d analysis. To compare the "binding strength" of the protons, in order to conclude at their contribution proximity to the

protein, select the proton *STDamp* values at one saturation time. Set the highest to 100% and calculate the STD % for the remaining protons.

12. Based on Eq. 4

$$\mathrm{Astd} = \frac{a_{\mathrm{std}} * [L]}{K_{\mathrm{d}}[L]} \times \text{ligand excess} \tag{4}$$

where a_{std} = maximum amplification factor.

Plot Astd as a function of ligand concentration [L]. Calculate the K_{d} for each proton using fitting according to the hyperbolic Michaelis–Menten equation.

3.4.2 Chemical Shift Mapping

1. The general procedure in order to achieve the determination of the binding site is the same as Subheading 3.2 (*see* **Note 6**).
2. The CSD diagrams (as many as the ligands of interest) indicate the residues that are implicated in binding. Moreover, the binding mode (fast or slow exchange regime) can provide information about the binding strength.

3.4.3 Determination of Intermolecular NOEs

1. Prepare a sample containing the protein and the ligand at the selected molar ratio.
2. Acquire a ^{15}N-HSQC spectrum in order to ensure that the complex of interest is fully formed.
3. Apply edited-edited TOCSY and NOESY experiments to acquire the information about the ligand assignment (*see* **Note 7**).
4. Perform the ligand assignment at its complex form.
5. Apply filtered-edited NOESY experiments to acquire the intermolecular NOEs.
6. Analyze and compare these results using the information obtained by **steps 3** and **4** to discriminate the bound ligand protons.

4 Notes

1. Phosphate buffers are preferred as they introduce no extra signals. However, HEPES, Tris, etc. may be used, if this is necessary for protein stability. The pH should be neutral or slightly acidic, and salt concentration should not exceed 100 mM.
2. The filtered-edited experiments are applied in protein complexes, where one partner is labeled and the other is not, with the aim to identify intermolecular NOE between partners that differ in "NMR active" nuclei (^{13}C/^{15}N; usually is one of the

protein partners) or in naturally abundant nuclei ($^{12}C/^{14}N$; is the other protein, a small organic molecule, or a RNA/DNA molecule). The term "filtered" is used to indicate the suppression of the proton resonances attached to a certain nucleus (usually the "NMR active" $^{13}C/^{15}N$), and it takes place through the *J*-coupling between the bonded ^{1}H to the atoms with the heteronuclear spins ^{13}C or ^{15}N. The term "editing" is used to indicate the observation of a particular ^{1}H according to the presence or absence of coupling to the heteronuclei ^{13}C and ^{15}N. Therefore, these isotope filtered edited techniques (and the appropriate pulse sequences) provide the possibility of the discrimination between protons belonging to isotope-labeled or unlabeled molecules allowing the intermolecular NOEs between them [36].

3. In case no protein–ligand structure is available, the protein interface data can be used to manually build a pharmacophore query with software such as MOE, LigBuilder, LigandScout, PharmaGist, or Pharmer.
4. Since results are obtained relatively fast, it is recommended that following inspection, the parameters for the screening are modified, and the process is repeated until the user obtains as much diverse molecule hits.
5. For the calculation of *Astd*, change the parameters so as the relaxation delay is 1 s more than the saturation time.
6. If a different solvent than the protein buffer is used, a titration of this buffer has to be conducted using the same steps. Titrate the protein only with the ligand buffer using the same quantity, and follow the same steps (e.g., the same % of solvent as in the ligand titration) in order to check whether the solvent causes CSD to the protein signals by itself. In addition, this provides the opportunity to create CSD diagram derived from the solvent titration, which can be subtracted from the CSD induced by the tested ligand. This results to the valid actual calculation of the CSD.
7. The spectra have to be recorded at the complex-containing sample. A ligand-only-containing sample is not useful because of the chemical shift changes induced at the ligand's proton upon the binding.

References

1. Pellecchia M, Sem DS, Wüthrich K (2002) NMR in drug discovery. Nat Rev Drug Discov 1(3):211–219. https://doi.org/10.1038/nrd748
2. Cosconati S, Marinelli L, Trotta R et al (2009) Tandem application of virtual screening and NMR experiments in the discovery of brand new DNA quadruplex groove binders. J Am Chem Soc 131(45):16336–16337. https://doi.org/10.1021/ja9063662
3. Shuker SB, Hajduk PJ, Meadows RP et al (1996) Discovering high-affinity ligands for

proteins: SAR by NMR. Science 274 (5292):1531–1534. https://doi.org/10.1126/science.274.5292.1531
4. O'Connell MR, Gamsjaeger R, Mackay JP (2009) The structural analysis of protein–protein interactions by NMR spectroscopy. Proteomics 9(23):5224–5232. https://doi.org/10.1002/pmic.200900303
5. Cala O, Guillière F, Krimm I (2014) NMR-based analysis of protein–ligand interactions. Anal Bioanal Chem 406(4):943–956. https://doi.org/10.1007/s00216-013-6931-0
6. Davis B (2013) Screening protein–small molecule interactions by NMR. In: Protein–ligand interactions: methods and applications. Humana Press, Totowa, NJ, pp 389–413
7. Fielding L (2003) NMR methods for the determination of protein–ligand dissociation constants. Curr Top Med Chem 3(1):39–53. https://doi.org/10.2174/1568026033392705
8. Heller M, Kessler H (2001) NMR spectroscopy in drug design. Pure Appl Chem 73 (9):1429–1436. https://doi.org/10.1351/pac200173091429
9. Dias DM, Ciulli A (2014) NMR approaches in structure-based lead discovery: recent developments and new frontiers for targeting multiprotein complexes. Prog Biophys Mol Biol 116(2):101–112. https://doi.org/10.1016/j.pbiomolbio.2014.08.012
10. Palmer AG (2014) Chemical exchange in biomacromolecules: past, present, and future. J Magn Reson 241:3–17. https://doi.org/10.1016/j.jmr.2014.01.008
11. Wrabl JO, Gu J, Liu T et al (2011) The role of protein conformational fluctuations in allostery, function, and evolution. Biophys Chem 159(1):129–141. https://doi.org/10.1016/j.bpc.2011.05.020
12. Motlagh HN, Li J, Thompson EB et al (2012) Interplay between allostery and intrinsic disorder in an ensemble. Biochem Soc Trans 40 (5):975–980. https://doi.org/10.1042/BST20120163
13. Boehr DD, Nussinov R, Wright PE (2009) The role of dynamic conformational ensembles in biomolecular recognition. Nat Chem Biol 5 (11):789–796. https://doi.org/10.1038/nchembio.232
14. Baldwin AJ, Kay LE (2009) NMR spectroscopy brings invisible protein states into focus. Nat Chem Biol 5(11):808–814. https://doi.org/10.1038/nchembio.238
15. Birkou M, Chasapis CT, Marousis KD et al (2017) A residue specific insight into the Arkadia E3 ubiquitin ligase activity and conformational plasticity. J Mol Biol 429 (15):2373–2386. https://doi.org/10.1016/j.jmb.2017.06.012
16. Williamson MP (2013) Using chemical shift perturbation to characterise ligand binding. Prog Nucl Magn Reson Spectrosc 73:1–16. https://doi.org/10.1016/j.pnmrs.2013.02.001
17. Roberts G, Lian L-Y (2011) Protein NMR spectroscopy: practical techniques and applications. John Wiley & Sons, Chichester
18. Katsila T, Spyroulias GA, Patrinos GP et al (2016) Computational approaches in target identification and drug discovery. Comput Struct Biotechnol J 14:177–184. https://doi.org/10.1016/j.csbj.2016.04.004
19. Matsoukas M-T, Aranguren-Ibáñez Á, Lozano T et al (2015) Identification of small-molecule inhibitors of calcineurin-NFATc signaling that mimic the PxIxIT motif of calcineurin binding partners. Sci Signal 8(382):ra63. https://doi.org/10.1126/scisignal.2005918
20. Kritsi E, Matsoukas M-T, Potamitis C et al (2016) Exploring new scaffolds for angiotensin II receptor antagonism. Biorg Med Chem 24 (18):4444–4451. https://doi.org/10.1016/j.bmc.2016.07.047
21. Villoutreix BO, Lagorce D, Labbé CM et al (2013) One hundred thousand mouse clicks down the road: selected online resources supporting drug discovery collected over a decade. Drug Discov Today 18(21):1081–1089. https://doi.org/10.1016/j.drudis.2013.06.013
22. Sunseri J, Koes DR (2016) Pharmit: interactive exploration of chemical space. Nucleic Acids Res (W1):W442–W448. https://doi.org/10.1093/nar/gkw287
23. Angulo J, Nieto PM (2011) STD-NMR: application to transient interactions between biomolecules—a quantitative approach. Eur Biophys J 40(12):1357–1369. https://doi.org/10.1007/s00249-011-0749-5
24. Cala O, Krimm I (2015) Ligand-orientation based fragment selection in STD NMR screening. J Med Chem 58(21):8739–8742. https://doi.org/10.1021/acs.jmedchem.5b01114
25. Meyer B, Peters T (2003) NMR spectroscopy techniques for screening and identifying ligand binding to protein receptors. Angew Chem Int Ed 42(8):864–890. https://doi.org/10.1002/anie.200390233
26. Japelj B, Ilc G, Marušič J et al (2016) Biosimilar structural comparability assessment by NMR: from small proteins to monoclonal antibodies. Sci Rep 6:32201. https://doi.org/10.1038/srep32201

27. Cui Y, Wen J, Sze KH et al (2003) Interaction between calcium-free calmodulin and IQ motif of neurogranin studied by nuclear magnetic resonance spectroscopy. Anal Biochem 315 (2):175–182. https://doi.org/10.1016/S0003-2697(03)00007-1
28. Otting G, Wüthrich K (1989) Extended heteronuclear editing of 2D ^{1}H NMR spectra of isotope-labeled proteins, using the X (ω1, ω2) double half filter. J Magn Reson 85 (3):586–594. https://doi.org/10.1016/0022-2364(89)90249-7
29. Folmer RH, Hilbers CW, Konings RN et al (1995) A ^{13}C double-filtered NOESY with strongly reduced artefacts and improved sensitivity. J Biomol NMR 5(4):427–432. https://doi.org/10.1007/BF00182287
30. Vaynberg J, Fukuda T, Chen K et al (2005) Structure of an ultraweak protein–protein complex and its crucial role in regulation of cell morphology and motility. Mol Cell 17 (4):513–523. https://doi.org/10.1016/j.molcel.2004.12.031
31. Breeze AL (2000) Isotope-filtered NMR methods for the study of biomolecular structure and interactions. Prog Nucl Magn Reson Spectrosc 36(4):323–372. https://doi.org/10.1016/S0079-6565(00)00020-0
32. Keller R (2004) The computer aided resonance assignment tutorial. Cantina Verlag, Goldau, Switzerland
33. Delaglio F, Grzesiek S, Vuister GW et al (1995) NMRPipe: a multidimensional spectral processing system based on UNIX pipes. J Biomol NMR 6(3):277–293. https://doi.org/10.1007/BF00197809
34. Baker KA, Hilty C, Peti W et al (2006) NMR-derived dynamic aspects of N-type inactivation of a Kv channel suggest a transient interaction with the T1 domain. Biochemistry 45(6):1663–1672. https://doi.org/10.1021/bi0516430
35. Markin CJ, Spyracopoulos L (2012) Increased precision for analysis of protein–ligand dissociation constants determined from chemical shift titrations. J Biomol NMR 53(2):125–138. https://doi.org/10.1007/s10858-012-9630-9
36. Bertini I, McGreevy KS, Parigi G (2012) NMR of biomolecules: towards mechanistic systems biology. John Wiley & Sons, Chichester. https://doi.org/10.1002/9783527644506

Chapter 19

The Use of Dynamic Pharmacophore in Computer-Aided Hit Discovery: A Case Study

Ugo Perricone, Marcus Wieder, Thomas Seidel, Thierry Langer, and Alessandro Padova

Abstract

In recent years pharmacophore modeling has become increasingly popular due to the development of software solutions and improvement in algorithms that allowed researchers to focus on interactions between protein and ligands instead of technical details of the software. At the same time, progress in computer hardware made molecular dynamics (MD) simulations on regular PC hardware possible. MD simulations are usually used, within the virtual screening process, to take into account the flexibility of the target and studying it in more realistic way. In order to do so, it is customary to use simulations before the virtual screening process and then use them for collecting some specific conformation of the target used. Furthermore, some researchers have demonstrated that the use of multiple crystal structures of the same protein can be valuable to better explore the role of the ligand within the binding pocket and then evaluate the most important interactions that are created during the host-guest recognition process. Findings derived from the MD analysis, especially focused on interactions, can be in fact exploited as features for pharmacophore generation or constraints to be used in the molecular docking as integrated steps of the whole virtual screening process. In this chapter, we will present the recent advances in the field pharmacophore modeling combined with the use of MD, a field well explored by our research group in the last 2 years.

Key words Pharmacophore modeling, Molecular dynamics, Dynamic pharmacophore, Structure-based drug design, Virtual screening

1 Introduction

Computer-aided molecular modeling (CAMM) emerged in the 1970s as a tool for the hit and lead identification phase of the modern drug discovery process. The rapid progress in protein crystallography made it possible to use the structure of the binding site in order to design ligands. Over the years there have been several successful applications of computer-aided molecular modeling for the hit discovery and hit to lead development of subsequently approved drugs (e.g., captopril and haloperidol) [1, 2]. The importance of in silico methods for the modern hit

Thomas Mavromoustakos and Tahsin F. Kellici (eds.), *Rational Drug Design: Methods and Protocols*, Methods in Molecular Biology, vol. 1824, https://doi.org/10.1007/978-1-4939-8630-9_19,

discovery process is increasing due to the high costs of experimental testing and the relatively cheap methods computer-aided molecular design can offer to reduce the number of compounds that have to be experimentally validated. This development is backed by the increasing number of crystallized protein and ligand structures that have been made available in public databases in recent years. The two main techniques used in structure-based CAMM are molecular docking and pharmacophore modeling [3–15]. Both methods aim to reduce the amount of molecules that have to be tested experimentally by filtering huge virtual screening libraries—a process called virtual screening (VS). The aim of VS is the retrieval of a small subset of calculated active compounds of the virtual screening database. The two methods use different approaches to achieve this goal—but both exploit properties of the protein and ligand structure in order to evaluate possible protein-ligand interactions and use the interaction patterns for subsequent virtual screening [4, 5, 11, 16, 17]. Both techniques—in their basic form—consider the protein structure as rigid and use only a single possible conformation of the protein-ligand complex as basis for generating the interactions information. But proteins are inherently dynamic entities—ignoring their dynamic nature and using only a single snapshot of the protein-ligand complex may heavily affect the virtual screening process. This issue is aggregated by the fact that the detection of interactions between the ligand and the protein is sensitive to the position of the involved atoms [18, 19]. Receptor and ligand flexibility along with possible-induced conformational changes have to be considered to correctly estimate the binding mode and thermodynamic properties in the binding process [20]. In order to overcome the limitations of regarding only a static protein-binding site for VS, several approaches have been introduced to consider protein flexibility [5, 21].

For molecular docking the most typically used modifications are side-chain flexibility [22], soft docking, induced fit [23, 24], and conformational ensemble-based docking [25, 26]. The mentioned approaches modify the docking algorithm—but there are also approaches that use the basic molecular docking protocol and include protein flexibility by using multiple protein crystal structures. The assumption is that they represent a conformational ensemble of the protein conformation and therefore represent the protein flexibility [27–30]. The quality of this approach is heavily influenced by the number of protein structures used and only useful for proteins that have multiple crystal structures available [31–34].

But there are other possibilities to generate conformational ensembles besides crystallography—one would be molecular dynamics (MD) simulations [35–38]. MD simulations have been demonstrated to be helpful in order to study the dynamic behavior of biomolecules [39]; furthermore, they constitute the basis for more advanced techniques such as the calculation of protein-ligand binding free energy [40]. The use of MD simulations—to be included in the experimental design of virtual screening campaigns—has been demonstrated to be very helpful to retrieve information about protein conformations or ligand-protein interaction dynamics [41, 42]. The correct incorporation of protein dynamics for molecular modeling still remains a nontrivial task. And also not necessarily one that will be rewarded: it has been demonstrated that incorporating protein flexibility could rise the false-positive rate since a greater number of molecules can be adapted to different conformations of the binding pocket [43, 44].

A recently developed method based on MD simulations prior to virtual screening is the relaxed complex scheme (RCS) approach [45]. Other approaches use the conformational ensemble of the receptor generated by MD simulations—the so-called receptor conformation ensemble (RCE). Martiny et al. combined docking with the hierarchical conformational cluster generated from the RCE [46]. Another remarkable approach to overcome protein rigidity has been adopted by Rueda et al. In this method, the conformational changes are gathered as collective movements generated by MD simulation and represent the starting point for cross-docking [47].

In the last years, receptor flexibility has been also assessed using a potential grid representing the receptor deformed through the use of selected collective movements and global structural changes caused by ligand binding [48]. However, considering a large number of modeled conformations may sometimes lead to less predictive VS results compared to those obtained by using the best performing crystal or NMR structures. Often, this is attributed to the possibility of generating non-native protein-ligand conformations [49, 50].

Structure-based pharmacophore models are very sensitive to small coordinate changes of the protein-ligand complex. The starting point of structure-based pharmacophore modeling is usually the coordinate set retrieved from the Protein Data Bank (PDB) [51] which just represent a single conformation of the protein-ligand complex. Moreover, the protein structures solved by X-ray crystallography may be affected by errors such as crystal contacts and solvent effects; for this reason, the reliability of protein-ligand coordinates has been frequently questioned [52, 53]. It is extremely important to consider proteins and small molecules as inherently dynamic and take into consideration a wide range of motions, reflecting the vibrations of individual bonds to collective, large structural movements. The use of a single snapshot of a dynamic system provides neither information about the conformational flexibility of the ligand nor about motions of the residues in and near the binding pocket [54, 55], and therefore a pharmacophore model generated from such a single structure might include features that are artifacts, caused either by crystal packing effects or by the single set of coordinates of the structure.

Recently, several approaches have been suggested to incorporate the dynamic behavior of protein-ligand complexes for pharmacophore modeling [40, 56–62]. The multi-complex pharmacophore model approach derives pharmacophore models from multiple PDB crystal structures of the same protein co-crystallized with different small molecules. Protein-ligand interaction patterns were extracted from the available structures and merged in pharmacophore maps [9, 14]. This approach, however, remains limited to those proteins presenting a high number of crystal structures available with co-crystallized ligands presenting the same binding mode. Using MD simulations to generate conformational ensembles is also a standard method for structure-based pharmacophore modeling. Choudhury et al. presented an approach to build multiple pharmacophore models from MD simulation ranking them based on docking and screening results [59].

Another issue that has to be carefully regarded is the chemical structure of the ligand within the binding pocket. Especially for pharmacophore modeling, the initial ligand can strongly influence the pharmacophore hypothesis. But proteins are promiscuous in their interactions, and a variety of ligands with diverse shape, size, and composition can bind. Therefore it can be reasonable to use multiple active ligand as starting point for further molecular modeling [40, 58–61].

The authors of this chapter have been actively publishing in the field of structure-based pharmacophore modeling combined with MD simulations. The field of structure-based pharmacophore modeling with flexible protein-ligand conformation is young and has been without systematic investigations in the dynamic of pharmacophore features during MD simulations. A first systematic publication exploring the behavior and stability of pharmacophore features during MD simulations was published in 2016 [63]. We were able to show that different pharmacophore feature types behave differently during the dynamic and that new feature appear during the MD simulation that were—using only the coordinate set obtained from the MD simulation—otherwise inaccessible. The frequency information obtained for every pharmacophore feature was subsequently used to construct complementary pharmacophore features in a follow-up publication.

Recently, we presented a new method called "common hits approach" that performs consensus pharmacophore-based VS on the conformational ensemble of the protein-ligand structure obtained by using MD simulations [64]. Using this technique we were able to increase our virtual screening results significantly in a test set of 40 protein-ligand systems compared to the pharmacophore model that was generated using the coordinate set obtained from the PDB database.

Additionally, we have presented a workflow that can potentially help reducing the bias of pharmacophore models introduced by the usage of a single initial ligand. This approach also uses MD simulations to sample the dynamic of the protein-ligand system. A case study was performed using the PPAR-α receptor as test system. Three different ligands and multiple MD runs allowed us to explore possible interactions in the binding pocket. Subsequently, the method used for this approach called MYSHAPE (Molecular dYnamics SHAred PharmacophorE) [65] will be presented and analyzed. The starting point of this method were three crystal structures of the same receptor with different ligands co-crystallized in the same binding site [51]. For each chosen structure, three MD simulations were performed, and ligand-protein interactions were analyzed and collected. A pharmacophore model was subsequently created using the common feature pattern of the three ligands during the MD simulations.

We have found that the MYSHAPE approach improved the virtual screening performance for the PPAR-α receptors [65]. In order to validate the approach, a comparison between the virtual screening results using MYSHAPE and the pharmacophore model obtained using the PDB coordinate set was performed. The MYSHAPE approach was able to increase the screening capability. The use of the shared interaction pattern retrieved from the multiple MD simulations improved the early recognition of active compounds. Comparing the MYSHAPE method to the reference pharmacophore model, the robust initial enrichment (RIE) passed from 3.45 to 6.1. The early recognition in the virtual screening process is raised from 2% to 5% of the screened library.

The strength of the MYSHAPE protocol is its ease of use compared to the improvement of virtual screening results. The success of the method is due to the use of multiple frames to generate pharmacophore models and its combination with molecular docking. The MD simulations on multiple crystal structures of the same protein but with different ligands is an interesting approach to retrieve additional pharmacophore features that could be missed by the use of a single ligand and could represent a guide to improve the pharmacophore hypothesis. In the following page, the general workflow of the protocol is described (Fig. 1).

2 Materials

2.1 Choice, Preparation, and Preliminary Study of Systems

The starting point for the MYSHAPE model generation is to have multiple PDB crystal structures of the same protein and different ligands collected from the PDB database http://www.rcsb.org/pdb/home/home.do. It is a database containing three-dimensional structural data of large biological molecules, such as proteins and nucleic acids. The data are typically acquired by X-ray crystallography, NMR spectroscopy, or cryo-electron microscopy.

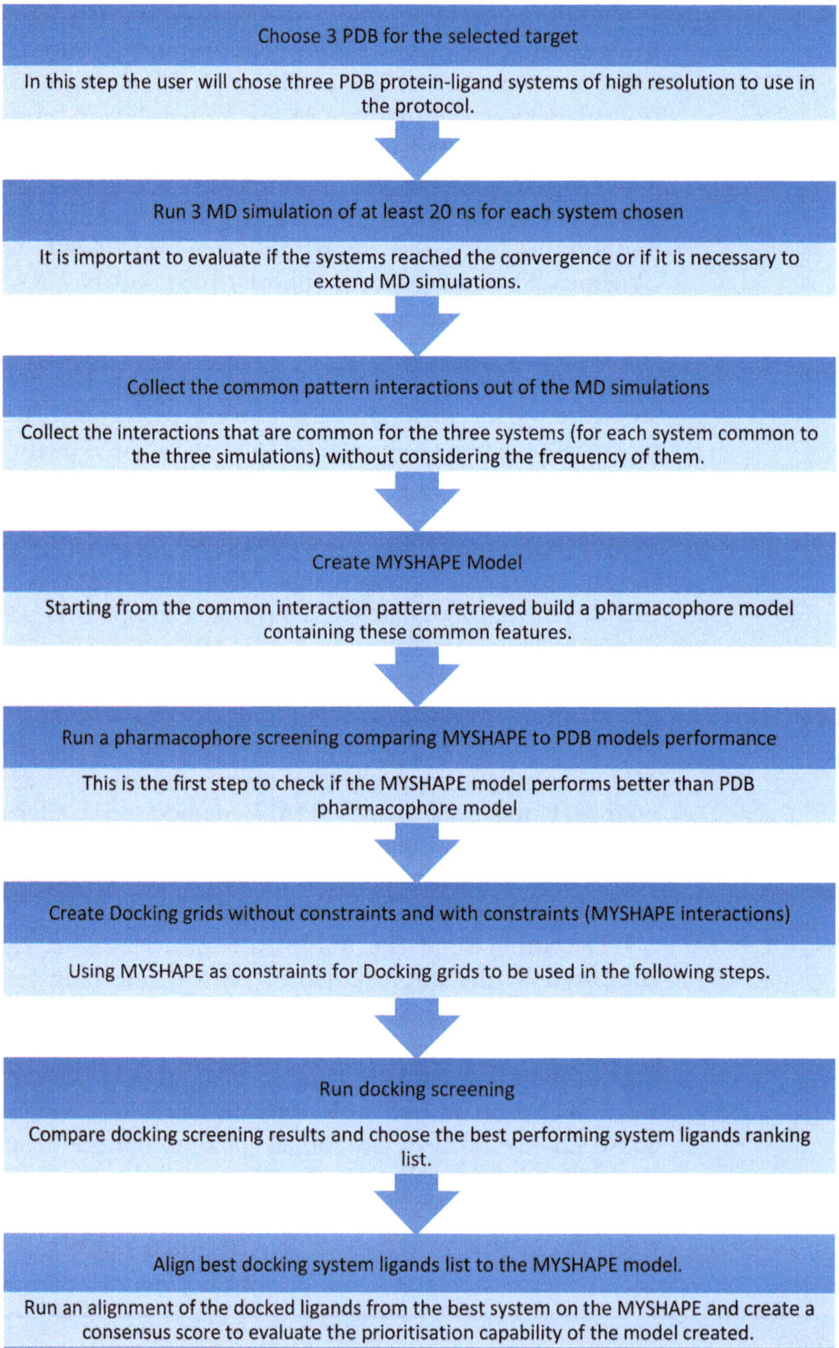

Fig. 1 General workflow for MYSHAPE creation and use

2.2 System Quality Assessment

In order to evaluate the electron density map fitting of the PDB structure, several tools are available but not always easy to understand for non-crystallographer. The most useful and easy to use tools for this issue are VHELIBS [66] and PDBe from EMBL-EBI (http://www.ebi.ac.uk/pdbe/). These software packages exploit the electron density information collected in the PDB file and, thanks to a graphical interface, give users the possibility to see the correctness of the ligand and protein-binding site electron density adherence. In our works we used VHELIBS software to analyze the electron density map quality.

2.3 PDB Preparation

It is good practice for the PDB structure preparation to have a fixed workflow in order to gradually remove all the threads that could be present within the structure used. The most frequent preparation steps for a PDB crystal structure are missing hydrogen atoms, atoms and loops, uncertain protonation states of both protein and ligand, and reversed side-chain residue positions. In order to prepare the crystal structure, many software can be used. In our works, we adopted the protein preparation wizard [67] provided by Schrödinger LTD. This tool is partially an open source. The part relative to missing loops and chains is not free, but the user can use MODELLER [68], a free tool for homology modeling and missing atom and loop fixing.

2.4 Molecular Dynamics

MD simulations can be run with several software available—open source or commercial. What is crucial for such an approach is the use of a tool that allows to collect different frames from the trajectory produced, in order to analyze the protein-ligand structures in every frame collected. In our works we performed MD runs using DESMOND 4.2 and the OPLS2005 force field [69, 70].

2.5 Pharmacophore Generation

In order to construct the MYSHAPE pharmacophore model, we used LigandScout 4.1 [71, 72]. The software allows users to import PDB structures and create structure-based pharmacophore maps. The software also allows modifying pharmacophore features by adding, removing, or customizing them.

2.6 Docking

GLIDE [73, 74] software from Schrödinger was used to build the docking grid to use for successive virtual screening. This software lets the user to create docking grids based on interaction constraints observed, for example, on previous analysis. Standard precision (SP) and extra precision (XP) molecular dockings with and without constraints were performed using GLIDE [73, 74].

2.7 Ligand Selection and Preparation

In order to validate the virtual screening performance of the pharmacophore models and the docking grids, databases with known active and inactive compounds are generated. Using compounds with known activity makes it possible to test the capability of pharmacophore models and docking approaches to differentiate between active compounds and inactive molecules—which is the ultimate goal of both methods. Both the active and decoy molecules must be optimized prior to be used for the retrospective virtual screening. The correct protonation state can be assessed using different tools; in our case, we adopted the LigPrep plugin provided by the MAESTRO software.

2.8 Virtual Screening

Once the pharmacophore maps and docking grids are created, retrospective virtual screening campaigns are run in order to evaluate if the model created thus worked well on the prioritization of actives toward decoys. In order to make this evaluation, ROC curve and enrichment parameters are used.

3 Methods

3.1 Choice, Preparation, and Preliminary Study of Systems

3.1.1 System Quality Assessment

The starting point of the MYSHAPE workflow is the selection of a system for which multiple crystal structures of the same protein co-crystallized with different ligands are present.

The selections of such a system should be governed by the following criteria: high resolution of the crystal structure (below 2.0 Å, if possible), no metal ions in the binding pocket (unless the used force field has established parameters for the metal), and only one ligand co-crystallized. One of the first parameters to be evaluated is the electron density (ED) map quality of the crystal (Fig. 2).

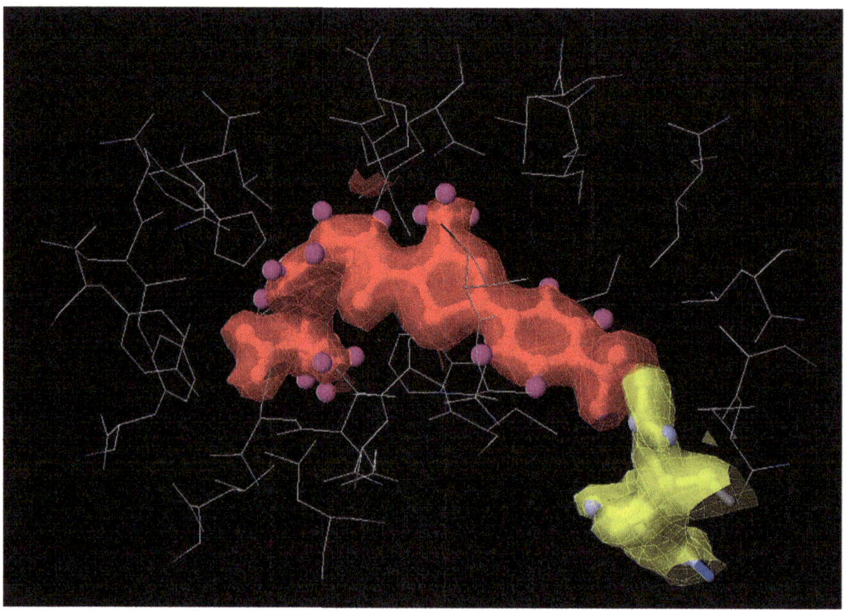

Fig. 2 VHELIBS analysis of the electron density (ED). In red the ED of the ligand is shown; in yellow the ED of the binding site side chains is shown

A useful additional quality check is the validation of the electron density of the binding site and the ligand using VHELIBS [66]. This software visualizes the electron density and checks the quality of the geometry.

3.1.2 PDB Preparation

The quality of the protein-ligand structure is of highest importance for structure-based pharmacophore modeling. The preparation of the crystal structure coordinate set in order to generate a complete, digital representation of the protein-ligand complex is of highest priority. Common issues that arise at this stage are missing hydrogen atoms, missing heavy atoms or amino acids, and undefined protonation state of amino acids or ligand.

There are multiple software solutions that can aid at this phase—we used the protein preparation wizard [67] provided by Schrödinger.

Subsequently, the individual steps of the workflow are described:

1. Analysis of the bond order and hydrogen atoms is added according to the structure.
2. Missing atoms or amino acids are inserted. Co-crystallized water is removed, unless it has been previously demonstrated that these water molecules are crucial for ligand recognition.
3. Ligand protonation state is calculated for the used pH and the ligand. This is done using Hammett and Taft methods in combination with tools for tautomer and isomerization calculation. For each ligand selected, all the possible states will be presented with the relative energy state penalty. We usually use the lowest energy state penalty protonation state of the ligand.
4. Optimize the protonation state of the protein and the ligand considering the H-bond network using PropKa 3.1 [75, 76] at the desired pH.

3.1.3 Molecular Dynamics

The minimum requirements for the workflow are three 20 ns MD simulations for every protein-ligand system (*see* **Note 1**). In order to better explore all the possible molecular conformations, we suggest to use different initial velocities for each simulation. The root-mean-square deviation of the protein during the MD simulations should be monitored in order to avoid using simulations with large protein movement. RMSD values of the aligned protein (on the first frame) should range between 2 and 3 Angströms; the ligand RMSD values (also aligned on the first frame) should be similar.

The MD simulations were performed using DESMOND 4.2 and the OPLS2005 force field [69, 70].

System Preparation

The system should be solvated using an orthorhombic boxes filled with TIP3P [77] water molecules. Ions can be added to neutralize charges in the protein and ligand system. Usually it is recommended to add ions to mimic a physiological osmolarity with 0.15 M NaCl.

System Minimization

An energy minimization is recommended ahead of every MD simulation. Usually, 2000 iterations are performed until a convergence of the total energy is reached at about 1 Kcal/mol/Å. Steepest descent [78] (SD) can be used for the minimization protocol. In the *advanced option* panel, the user can customize the associated parameters for the steepest descendent method associated with optimization algorithm. Also, combining SD with the limited-memory Broyden-Fletcher-Goldfarb-Shanno (LBFGS) is a popular choice for the energy minimization [79, 80].

MD Production Run

The first step of the MD simulation, after the minimization, is the equilibration. Usually the equilibration takes place at 300 K and 1.013 bar pressure.

The production simulation should be performed using the NPT ensemble. The simulations must be performed using a thermostat (like Nose-Hoover) and a barostat (like Martyna-Tobias-Klein).

In order to keep the hydrogen-heavy atom bonds rigid, the SHAKE algorithm is utilized. The usual integration time step is 2 fs. The long-range interaction cutoff radius of 9 Å should be used in combination with smooth particle mesh Ewald summation. We recommend writing coordinate sets every 20 ps—for a 20 ns simulation; this results in 1000 frames.

3.1.4 Shared Feature Evaluation

One of the key steps of the described method is the combination of the common ligand-protein pharmacophore interaction pattern out of the three different systems simulations. Using the MD trajectory, DESMOND is able to show the interaction frequency between ligand atoms and amino acids—but, in this way, not all interactions are shown (frequently, hydrophobic interactions are not shown). For this reason, it is necessary to use raw data files produced by DESMOND during the simulation in which every interaction between the ligand and the protein is reported for each time step.

Using this data, a shared pharmacophore model based on the common interactions of the MD simulations will be created. Only common interactions that were present for the three ligands in all MD simulations are considered. Based on this the term "Molecular dYnamics SHAred PharmacophorE" model (MYSHAPE model) has been created to indicate that the pharmacophore model is based on the shared interactions observed in the different systems during the MD simulations (*see* **Note 2**).

3.1.5 MYSHAPE Model Pharmacophore Generation

In order to construct the MYSHAPE, pharmacophore model LigandScout 4.1 [71, 72] was used. The software allows users to modify pharmacophore models by adding, removing, or customizing features. The following workflow should be followed:

1. Import the different crystal structures of the protein-ligand complex in LigandScout and generate for each complex a structure-based pharmacophore model (PDB pharmacophore model).
2. Copy the PDB pharmacophore models generated together with the different ligands in the alignment view and align them.
3. Generate a shared PDB pharmacophore model. This step generates a model containing only the features that are common for the three PDB pharmacophore models.
4. Add pharmacophore features on the aligned ligand that are found during the MD simulation but are not present in the original shared pharmacophore model. Make sure that these newly added pharmacophore features are present during all MD simulations.
5. The tolerance radius for newly added pharmacophore features should be increased by 0.15 Å in order to compensate for small deviations in the 3D coordinates of the different ligands.

3.1.6 Docking Grid Generation

In the original description of the method, GLIDE [73, 74], from the Schrödinger software package, is used to build the docking grid for the subsequent VS.

Starting from the common ligand-protein interaction pattern observed during the MD simulations, docking grid constraints can be created on the GLIDE grid panel. This step is based on the chemical intuition of the modeler in order to identify regions of the grid that should be restraint using the interaction pattern during the MD simulations.

In order to validate this step, it is useful to generate two grids (one with constraints retrieved from MD simulations and one without constraints) for each protein-ligand system.

3.1.7 Selection and Preparation of the Screening Test Set

In order to validate the virtual screening performance, it is necessary to prepare a screening library with known active and inactive compounds and evaluate the usefulness of the method to discriminate between both categories. A convenient resource for such screening library is the DUD-E database [81] or DecoyFinder [82]. In the initial publication, we used the DUD-E database [81] to retrieve the screening library and subsequently filtered using KNIME [83]. The filtering step is essential to remove duplicate molecules. Both active and decoy molecules must be optimized at the correct pH value, and 3D conformations of the molecules must be created prior to using them for retrospective virtual screening purpose. This can be done using the LigPrep plugin provided by the MAESTRO software suite.

3.2 Virtual Screening Process

3.2.1 Pharmacophore Screening

Once the MYSHAPE model has been created, VS can be performed using LigandScout [71, 72]. After the active and decoy screening libraries are loaded, the screening settings should be further customized. We recommend using the *pharmacophore fit* as scoring function, as well as the "Match all Query Features" as screening mode option. Also, "Stop after first matching conformation" as retrieval mode and zero omitted features should be selected. The last option is the most important one; it ensures that all selected pharmacophore features will be considered for the VS run. After the virtual screening, a receiver operating characteristic (ROC) graphs will be generated, and the area under the curve (AUC) of the ROC as well as the enrichment factor (EF) should be calculated. These results should be used to validate the VS performance of the MYSHAPE model and compare it to the PDB pharmacophore model (*see* **Note 3**).

3.2.2 Molecular Docking Screening

Standard precision (SP) and/or extra precision (XP) molecular docking using constraints and without constraints should be performed using GLIDE on the three crystal structures selected. Using the GLIDE docking panel, ligands should be considered flexible, and Epik state penalties should be added to the docking score. ROC graphs and robust initial enrichment (RIE) [84–86] should be used to evaluate the virtual screening capability of the docking runs. The RIE and the ROC value can be easily generated using the "enrichment calculator" python script provided by Schrodinger. We suggest not to use the EF to evaluate screening performance because each docking run can produce a ranked list with different length, and the EF is influenced by the length of the final list. We recommend that the users should choose the ROC and RIE values to compare results (*see* **Note 4**).

3.2.3 Pharmacophore Alignment and Ranking of Docked Conformations of Ligands

Import into LigandScout [71, 72] the list of docked molecules from the best performing PDB system and calculate pharmacophore alignment scores based on MYSHAPE pharmacophore model. This step is made in order to create the following consensus score to prioritize actives. The different rankings can be evaluated using the EF at different percentages of the screening dataset with particular attention to the early enrichment [84–86].

Furthermore, for the best performing system, a consensus score is calculated that combined the pharmacophore and docking score as shown in Eq. (1).

$$\text{Consensus score} = \left(\frac{\text{docking score}}{\text{maxdocking score}} + \frac{\text{pharmacophore score}}{\text{maxpharmacophore score}}\right) \quad (1)$$

4 Notes

1. *Molecular dynamics:* The choice of three short simulations instead of one, but longer, is explained considering that in this way, it's possible to better explore eventual ligand-protein conformational changes as reported in the literature [87–89].
2. *Shared feature evaluation:* It is noteworthy that the frequency of appearance of each feature during MD simulation is not important in this approach; we have moreover demonstrated that feature frequency is not related to its importance in the pharmacophore generation [63, 90].
3. *Pharmacophore screening:* In case of multiple hydrophobic features very close in space, we suggest to interpolate them increasing the feature of the resultant one of 0.30 Å to better consider the feature volume.
4. *Molecular docking screening:* In contrast to pharmacophore modeling, the AUC is not calculated for different fractions of the screening database, but a numeric representation of the receiver operator characteristic area underneath the curve is obtained. This ROC value can be interpreted as the probability that an active will appear before an inactive compound and is calculated as follows (Eq. 2):

$$\mathrm{ROC} = \left(\frac{\mathrm{AUAC}}{\mathrm{Ri}} - \frac{\mathrm{Ra}}{2\mathrm{Ri}}\right) \quad (2)$$

where AUAC is the area under the accumulation curve, Ri is the ratio of inactive molecules to the total number of compounds in the screening library, and Ra is the ratio of active compounds to the total number of entries in the screening library.

References

1. DesJarlais RL, Seibel GL, Kuntz ID et al (1990) Structure-based design of nonpeptide inhibitors specific for the human immunodeficiency virus 1 protease. Proc Natl Acad Sci U S A 87(17):6644–6648. https://doi.org/10.1073/pnas.87.17.6644
2. Acharya KR, Sturrock ED, Riordan JF et al (2003) Ace revisited: a new target for structure-based drug design. Nat Rev Drug Discov 2(11):891–902. https://doi.org/10.1038/nrd1227
3. Spyrakis F, Benedetti P, Decherchi S et al (2015) A pipeline to enhance ligand virtual screening: integrating molecular dynamics and fingerprints for ligand and proteins. J Chem Inf Model 55(10):2256–2274. https://doi.org/10.1021/acs.jcim.5b00169
4. Kapetanovic IM (2008) Computer aided drug discovery and development: in silico-chemico-biological approach. Chem Biol Interact 171 (2):165–176. https://doi.org/10.1016/j.cbi.2006.12.006
5. Cerqueira NMFSA, Gesto D, Oliveira EF et al (2015) Receptor-based virtual screening protocol for drug discovery. Arch Biochem Biophys 582:56–67. https://doi.org/10.1016/j.abb.2015.05.011
6. Chang CA, Ai R, Gutierrez M et al (2012) Homology modeling of cannabinoid receptors: discovery of cannabinoid analogues for therapeutic use. In: Baron R (ed) Computational drug discovery and design. Methods in molecular biology (methods and protocols).

Springer, New York. https://doi.org/10.1007/978-1-61,779-465-0_35

7. Ou-Yang S-S, Lu J-Y, Kong X-Q et al (2012) Computational drug discovery. Acta Pharmacol Sin 33(9):1131–1140. https://doi.org/10.1038/aps.2012.109
8. Dias R, de Azevedo WF (2008) Molecular docking algorithms. Curr Drug Targets 9(12):1040–1047. https://doi.org/10.2174/138945008786949432
9. Wu F, Xu T, He G et al (2012) Discovery of novel focal adhesion kinase inhibitors using a hybrid protocol of virtual screening approach based on multicomplex-based pharmacophore and molecular docking. Int J Mol Sci 13(12):15668–15678. https://doi.org/10.3390/ijms131215668
10. Agrawal R, Jain P, Dikshit SN et al (2013) Ligand-based pharmacophore detection, screening of potential pharmacophore and docking studies, to get effective glycogen synthase kinase inhibitors. Med Chem Res 22(11):5504–5535. https://doi.org/10.1007/s00044-013-0547-y
11. Dror O, Schneidman-Duhovny D, Inbar Y et al (2009) Novel approach for efficient pharmacophore-based virtual screening: method and applications. J Chem Inf Model 49(10):2333–2343. https://doi.org/10.1021/ci900263d
12. Langer T (2011) Pharmacophores for medicinal chemists: a personal view. Future Med Chem 3(8):901–904. https://doi.org/10.4155/fmc.11.34
13. Wolber G, Sippl W (2015) Pharmacophore identification and pseudo-receptor modeling. In: Wermuth CG et al (eds) The practice of medicinal chemistry, 4th edn. Academic Press, London, pp 489–510. https://doi.org/10.1016/B978-0-12-417,205-0.00021-3
14. Yang S-Y (2010) Pharmacophore modeling and applications in drug discovery: challenges and recent advances. Drug Discov Today 15(11-12):444–450. https://doi.org/10.1016/j.drudis.2010.03.013
15. Langer T, Wolber G (2004) Pharmacophore definition and 3D searches. Drug Discov Today Technol 1(3):203–207. https://doi.org/10.1016/j.ddtec.2004
16. Tutone M, Perricone U, Almerico AM (2017) Conf-VLKA: a structure-based revisitation of the virtual lock-and-key approach. J Mol Graph Model 71:50–57. https://doi.org/10.1016/j.jmgm.2016.11.006
17. Jorgensen WL (2004) The many roles of computation in drug discovery. Science 303(5665):1813–1818. https://doi.org/10.1126/science.1096361
18. Teague SJ (2003) Implications of protein flexibility for drug discovery. Nat Rev Drug Discov 2(7):527–541. https://doi.org/10.1038/nrd1129
19. B-Rao C, Subramanian J, Sharma SD (2009) Managing protein flexibility in docking and its applications. Drug Discov Today 14(7-8):394–400. https://doi.org/10.1016/j.drudis.2009.01.003
20. Gallicchio E, Levy RM (2011) Advances in all atom sampling methods for modeling protein-ligand binding affinities. Curr Opin Struct Biol 21(2):161–166. https://doi.org/10.1016/j.sbi.2011.01.010
21. Chen YC (2015) Beware of docking! Trends Pharmacol Sci 36(2):78–95. https://doi.org/10.1016/j.tips.2014.12.001
22. Shin WH, Kim JK, Kim DS et al (2013) GalaxyDock2: protein-ligand docking using beta-complex and global optimization. J Comput Chem 34(30):2647–2656. https://doi.org/10.1002/jcc.23438
23. Sherman W, Day T, Jacobson MP et al (2006) Novel procedure for modeling ligand/receptor induced fit effects. J Med Chem 49(2):534–553. https://doi.org/10.1021/jm050540c
24. Koska J, Spassov VZ, Maynard AJ et al (2008) Fully automated molecular mechanics based induced fit protein-ligand docking method. J Chem Inf Model 48(10):1965–1973. https://doi.org/10.1021/ci800081s
25. Bolia A, Gerek ZN, Ozkan SB (2014) BP-dock: a flexible docking scheme for exploring protein-ligand interactions based on unbound structures. J Chem Inf Model 54(3):913–925. https://doi.org/10.1021/ci4004927
26. Ivetac A, McCammon JA (2011) Molecular recognition in the case of flexible targets. Curr Pharm Des 17(17):1663–1671. https://doi.org/10.2174/138161211796355056
27. Forman-Kay JD (1999) The "dynamics" in the thermodynamics of binding. Nat Struct Biol 6:1086–1087. https://doi.org/10.1038/70008
28. Nichols SE, Baron R, McCammon JA (2012) On the use of molecular dynamics receptor conformations for virtual screening. In: Baron R (ed) Computational drug discovery and design. Methods in molecular biology (methods and protocols), vol 819. Springer, New York, NY. https://doi.org/10.1007/978-1-61,779-465-0_7
29. Totrov M, Abagyan R (2008) Flexible ligand docking to multiple receptor conformations: a practical alternative. Curr Opin Struct Biol 18

(2):178–184. https://doi.org/10.1016/j.sbi.2008.01.004

30. Verkhivker GM, Bouzida D, Gehlhaar DK et al (2002) Complexity and simplicity of ligand-macromolecule interactions: the energy landscape perspective. Curr Opin Struct Biol 12 (2):197–203. https://doi.org/10.1016/S0959-440X(02)00310-X
31. Abagyan R, Rueda M, Bottegoni G (2010) Recipes for the selection of experimental protein conformations for virtual screening. J Chem Inf Model 50(1):186–193. https://doi.org/10.1021/ci9003943
32. Isvoran A, Badel A, Craescu CT et al (2011) Exploring NMR ensembles of calcium binding proteins: perspectives to design inhibitors of protein-protein interactions. BMC Struct Biol 11:24. https://doi.org/10.1186/1472-6807-11-24
33. Miteva MA, Robert CH, Maréchal JD et al (2011) Receptor Flexibility in ligand docking and virtual screening. In: Miteva MA (ed) In silico lead discovery. Bentham Science Publishers, Emirate of Sharjah
34. Osguthorpe DJ, Sherman W, Hagler AT (2012) Generation of receptor structural ensembles for virtual screening using binding site shape analysis and clustering. Chem Biol Drug Des 80(2):182–193. https://doi.org/10.1111/j.1747-0285.2012.01396.x
35. Asses Y, Venkatraman V, Leroux V et al (2012) Exploring c-Met kinase flexibility by sampling and clustering its conformational space. Proteins 80(4):1227–1238. https://doi.org/10.1002/prot.24021
36. Degliesposti G, Portioli C, Parenti MD et al (2011) BEAR, a novel virtual screening methodology for drug discovery. J Biomol Screen 16 (1):129–133. https://doi.org/10.1177/1087057110388276
37. Hou T, Wang J, Li Y et al (2011) Assessing the performance of the MM/PBSA and MM/GBSA methods: 1. The accuracy of binding free energy calculations based on molecular dynamics simulations. J Chem Inf Comput Sci 51(1):69–82. https://doi.org/10.1021/ci100275a
38. Proctor EA, Yin S, Tropsha A et al (2012) Discrete molecular dynamics distinguishes nativelike binding poses from decoys in difficult targets. Biophys J 102(1):144–151. https://doi.org/10.1016/j.bpj.2011.11.4008
39. Karplus M, McCammon JA (2002) Molecular dynamics simulations of biomolecules. Nat Struct Biol 9:646–652. https://doi.org/10.1038/nsb0902-646
40. Deng J, Lee KW, Sanchez T et al (2005) Dynamic receptor-based pharmacophore model development and its application in designing novel HIV-1 integrase inhibitors. J Med Chem 48(5):1496–1505. https://doi.org/10.1021/jm049410e
41. Ogrizek M, Turk S, Lesnik S et al (2015) Molecular dynamics to enhance structure-based virtual screening on cathepsin B. J Comput Aided Mol Des 29(8):707–712. https://doi.org/10.1007/s10822-015-9847-2
42. Tutone M, Chinnici A, Almerico AM et al (2016) Design, synthesis and preliminary evaluation of dopamine-amino acid conjugates as potential D1 dopaminergic modulators. Eur J Med Chem 124:435–444. https://doi.org/10.1016/j.ejmech.2016.08.051
43. Barril X, Morley SD (2005) Unveiling the full potential of flexible receptor docking using multiple crystallographic structures. J Med Chem 48(13):4432–4443. https://doi.org/10.1021/jm048972v
44. Bolstad ESD, Anderson AC (2009) In pursuit of virtual lead optimization: pruning ensembles of receptor structures for increased efficiency and accuracy during docking. Proteins 75 (1):62–74. https://doi.org/10.1002/prot.22214
45. Amaro RE, Baron R, McCammon JA (2008) An improved relaxed complex scheme for receptor flexibility in computer-aided drug design. J Comput Aided Mol Des 22 (9):693–705. https://doi.org/10.1007/s10822-007-9159-2
46. Martiny VY, Carbonell P, Lagorce D et al (2013) In silico mechanistic profiling to probe small molecule binding to Sulfotransferases. PLoS One 8(9):e73587. https://doi.org/10.1371/journal.pone.0073587
47. Rueda M, Bottegoni G, Abagyan R (2009) Consistent improvement of cross-docking results using binding site ensembles generated with elastic network normal modes. J Chem Inf Model 49(3):716–725. https://doi.org/10.1021/ci8003732
48. Leis S, Zacharias M (2011) Efficient inclusion of receptor flexibility in grid-based protein-ligand docking. J Comput Chem 32:3433–3439. https://doi.org/10.1002/jcc.21923
49. Korb O, Olsson TSG, Bowden SJ et al (2012) Potential and limitations of ensemble docking. J Chem Inf Model 52(5):1262–1274. https://doi.org/10.1021/ci2005934
50. Sgobba M, Caporuscio F, Anighoro A et al (2012) Application of a post-docking procedure based on MM-PBSA and MM-GBSA on single and multiple protein conformations. Eur J Med Chem 58:431–440. https://doi.org/10.1016/j.ejmech.2012.10.024

51. Berman HM, Westbrook J, Feng Z et al (2000) The protein data bank. Nucleic Acids Res 28 (1):235–242. https://doi.org/10.1093/nar/28.1.235
52. Liebeschuetz J, Hennemann J, Olsson T et al (2012) The good, the bad and the twisted: a survey of ligand geometry in protein crystal structures. J Comput Aided Mol Des 26 (2):169–183. https://doi.org/10.1007/s10822-011-9538-6
53. Reynolds CH (2014) Protein-ligand cocrystal structures: we can do better. ACS Med Chem Lett 5(7):727–729. https://doi.org/10.1021/ml500220a
54. Mirjalili V, Feig M (2013) Protein structure refinement through structure selection and averaging from molecular dynamics ensembles. J Chem Theory Comput 9(2):1294–1303. https://doi.org/10.1021/ct300962x
55. Whitesides GM, Krishnamurthy VM (2005) Designing ligands to bind proteins. Q Rev Biophys 38(4):385–395. https://doi.org/10.1017/S0033583506004240
56. Deng J, Sanchez T, Neamati N et al (2006) Dynamic pharmacophore model optimization: identification of novel HIV-1 integrase inhibitors. J Med Chem 49(5):1684–1692. https://doi.org/10.1021/jm0510629
57. Bowman AL, Makriyannis A (2011) Approximating protein flexibility through dynamic pharmacophore models: application to fatty acid amide hydrolase (FAAH). J Chem Inf Model 51(12):3247–3253. https://doi.org/10.1021/ci200371z
58. Carlson HA, Masukawa KM, Rubins K et al (2000) Developing a dynamic pharmacophore model for HIV-1 integrase. J Med Chem 43 (11):2100–2114. https://doi.org/10.1021/jm990322h
59. Choudhury C, Priyakumar UD, Sastry GN (2015) Dynamics based pharmacophore models for screening potential inhibitors of mycobacterial cyclopropane synthase. J Chem Inf Model 55(4):848–860. https://doi.org/10.1021/ci500737b
60. Mallik B, Morikis D (2005) Development of a quasi-dynamic pharmacophore model for anti-complement peptide analogues. J Am Chem Soc 127(31):10967–10976. https://doi.org/10.1021/ja051004c
61. Saez NJ, Mobli M, Bieri M et al (2011) A dynamic pharmacophore drives the interaction between Psalmotoxin-1 and the putative drug target acid-sensing ion channel 1a. Mol Pharmacol 80(5):796–808. https://doi.org/10.1124/mol.111.072207
62. Thangapandian S, John S, Lee Y et al (2011) Dynamic structure-based pharmacophore model development: a new and effective addition in the histone deacetylase 8 (HDAC8) inhibitor discovery. Int J Mol Sci 12 (12):9440–9462. https://doi.org/10.3390/ijms12129440
63. Wieder M, Perricone U, Boresch S et al (2016) Evaluating the stability of pharmacophore features using molecular dynamics simulations. Biochem Biophys Res Commun 470 (3):685–689. https://doi.org/10.1016/j.bbrc.2016.01.081
64. Wieder M, Garon A, Perricone U et al (2017) Common hits approach: combining pharmacophore modeling and molecular dynamics simulations. J Chem Inf Model 57(2):365–385. https://doi.org/10.1021/acs.jcim.6b00674
65. Perricone U, Wieder M, Seidel T et al (2017) A molecular dynamics-shared pharmacophore approach to boost early-enrichment virtual screening: a case study on peroxisome proliferator-activated receptor α. ChemMedChem 12(16):1399–1407. https://doi.org/10.1002/cmdc.201600526
66. Cereto-Massague A, Ojeda MJ, Joosten RP et al (2013) The good, the bad and the dubious: VHELIBS, a validation helper for ligands and binding sites. J Cheminform 5:1–9. https://doi.org/10.1186/1758-2946-5-36
67. Madhavi Sastry G, Adzhigirey M, Day T et al (2013) Protein and ligand preparation: parameters, protocols, and influence on virtual screening enrichments. J Comput Aided Mol Des 27(3):221–234. https://doi.org/10.1007/s10822-013-9644-8
68. Eswar N, Webb B, Marti-Renom MA et al (2007) Comparative protein structure modeling using Modeller. Curr Protoc Bioinformatics 2:Unit 2.9. https://doi.org/10.1002/0471250953.bi0506s15
69. Guo Z, Mohanty U, Noehre J et al (2010) Probing the alpha-helical structural stability of stapled p53 peptides: molecular dynamics simulations and analysis. Chem Biol Drug Des 75(4):348–359. https://doi.org/10.1111/j.1747-0285.2010.00951.x
70. Shivakumar D, Williams J, Wu YJ et al (2010) Prediction of absolute solvation free energies using molecular dynamics free energy perturbation and the OPLS force field. J Chem Theory Comput 6(5):1509–1519. https://doi.org/10.1021/ct900587b
71. Wolber G, Langer T (2005) LigandScout: 3-D pharmacophores derived from protein-bound ligands and their use as virtual screening filters. J Chem Inf Model 45(1):160–169. https://doi.org/10.1021/ci049885e

72. Wolber G, Seidel T, Bendix F et al (2008) Molecule-pharmacophore superpositioning and pattern matching in computational drug design. Drug Discov Today 13(1-2):23–29. https://doi.org/10.1016/j.drudis.2007.09.007
73. Halgren TA, Murphy RB, Friesner RA et al (2004) Glide: a new approach for rapid, accurate docking and scoring. 2. Enrichment factors in database screening. J Med Chem 47 (7):1750–1759. https://doi.org/10.1021/jm030644s
74. Friesner RA, Banks JL, Murphy RB et al (2004) Glide: a new approach for rapid, accurate docking and scoring. 1. Method and assessment of docking accuracy. J Med Chem 47 (7):1739–1749. https://doi.org/10.1021/jm0306430
75. Olsson MHM, Søndergaard CR, Rostkowski M et al (2011) PROPKA3: consistent treatment of internal and surface residues in empirical p K a predictions. J Chem Theory Comput 7(2):525–537. https://doi.org/10.1021/ct100578z
76. Søndergaard CR, Olsson MHM, Rostkowski M et al (2011) Improved treatment of ligands and coupling effects in empirical calculation and rationalization of p K a values. J Chem Theory Comput 7(7):2284–2295. https://doi.org/10.1021/ct200133y
77. Mark P, Nilsson L (2001) Structure and dynamics of the TIP3P, SPC, and SPC/E water models at 298 K. J Phys Chem A 105 (43):9954–9960. https://doi.org/10.1021/jp003020w
78. Meza JC (2010) Steepest descent. Wiley Interdiscip Rev Comput Stat 2(6):719–722. https://doi.org/10.1002/wics.117
79. Andrew G, Gao J (2007) Scalable training of L1 -regularized log-linear models, In: Proceedings of the 24th international conference on Machine learning - ICML '07, pp. 33–40
80. Malouf R (2002) A comparison of algorithms for maximum entropy parameter estimation, In: Proceeding of the 6th conference on Natural language learning - COLING-02, pp. 1–7
81. Mysinger MM, Carchia M, Irwin JJ et al (2012) Directory of useful decoys, enhanced (DUD-E): better ligands and decoys for better benchmarking. J Med Chem 55 (14):6582–6594. https://doi.org/10.1021/jm300687e
82. Cereto-Massagué A, Guasch L, Valls C et al (2012) DecoyFinder: an easy-to-use python GUI application for building target-specific decoy sets. Bioinformatics 28 (12):1661–1662. https://doi.org/10.1093/bioinformatics/bts249
83. Berthold MR, Cebron N, Dill F et al (2009) KNIME - the Konstanz information miner. SIGKDD Explor 11(1):26–31. https://doi.org/10.1145/1656274.1656280
84. Zhao W, Hevener KE, White SW et al (2009) A statistical framework to evaluate virtual screening. BMC Bioinformatics 10:225. https://doi.org/10.1186/1471-2105-10-225
85. Truchon JF, Bayly CI (2007) Evaluating virtual screening methods: good and bad metrics for the "early recognition" problem. J Chem Inf Model 47(2):488–508. https://doi.org/10.1021/ci600426e
86. Fawcett T (2006) An introduction to ROC analysis. Pattern Recognit Lett 27 (8):861–874. https://doi.org/10.1016/j.patrec.2005.10.010
87. Buch I, Giorgino T, De Fabritiis G (2011) Complete reconstruction of an enzyme-inhibitor binding process by molecular dynamics simulations. Proc Natl Acad Sci U S A 108 (25):10184–10110,189. doi:https://doi.org/10.1073/pnas.1103547108
88. Legge FS, Budi A, Treutlein H et al (2006) Protein flexibility: multiple molecular dynamics simulations of insulin chain B. Biophys Chem 119(2):146–157. https://doi.org/10.1016/j.bpc.2005.08.002
89. Perez JJ, Tomas MS, Rubio-Martinez J (2016) Assessment of the sampling performance of multiple-copy dynamics versus a unique trajectory. J Chem Inf Model 56(10):1950–1962. https://doi.org/10.1021/acs.jcim.6b00347
90. Wieder M, Perricone U, Seidel T et al (2016) Comparing pharmacophore models derived from crystal structures and from molecular dynamics simulations. Monatsh Chem 147 (3):553–563. https://doi.org/10.1007/s00706-016-1674-1

Chapter 20

Rational Development of MAGL Inhibitors

Carlotta Granchi, Flavio Rizzolio, Isabella Caligiuri, Marco Macchia, Adriano Martinelli, Filippo Minutolo, and Tiziano Tuccinardi

Abstract

Hit identification and hit-to-lead optimization are key steps of the early drug discovery program. Starting from the X-ray crystal structure of the human monoacylglycerol lipase (*h*MAGL), we herein describe the computational and experimental procedures that we applied for identifying and optimizing a new active inhibitor of this target enzyme. A receptor-based virtual screening method is reported in details, together with enzymatic assays and a first round of hit optimization.

Key words Hit identification, Hit-to-lead optimization, Monoacylglycerol lipase inhibitors, Virtual screening, MAGL

1 Introduction

The endocannabinoid system is mainly constituted by two cannabinoid receptors (CB_1 and CB_2), the endocannabinoids anandamide (AEA) and 2-arachidonylglycerol (2-AG), which are naturally produced in the human body and act as agonists of the cannabinoid receptors. Other components of the endocannabinoid system are the enzymes that regulate the catabolism of the endocannabinoids, such as fatty acid amide hydrolase (FAAH), which hydrolyzes AEA into arachidonic acid (AA) and ethanolamine, and monoacylglycerol lipase (MAGL), which transforms 2-AG into AA and glycerol. MAGL is a cytosolic membrane-associated serine hydrolase located in the presynaptic terminals. Residues Ser122-Asp239-His269 have been identified as the catalytic triad of MAGL, but the three cysteines (Cys201, Cys208, Cys242) that are close to the catalytic triad seem to be necessary for the stabilization of MAGL conformation and for its interaction with substrates. The MAGL active site is mainly composed of (a) an acyl chain-binding pocket, in which the acyl chain of the substrate nicely fits; (b) an alcohol-binding channel, which accommodates the glycerol moiety of the natural substrate; and (c) a glycerol exit channel, from which

Thomas Mavromoustakos and Tahsin F. Kellici (eds.), *Rational Drug Design: Methods and Protocols*, Methods in Molecular Biology, vol. 1824, https://doi.org/10.1007/978-1-4939-8630-9_20,

leaving group glycerol exits the enzyme cavity [1]. A functional proteomic analysis of a panel of aggressive and nonaggressive human cancer cell lines from multiple tumors of origin has been performed, in order to identify enzyme activities that contribute to cancer pathogenesis. MAGL expression was found to be consistently elevated in aggressive cancer cells and in primary tumors relative to their nonaggressive counterparts. Moreover, MAGL regulates many lipid signaling pathways; therefore, its inhibition represents an interesting approach for the treatment of several pathologies [2]. On the one hand, MAGL inhibition in the brain and in peripheral tissues, such as the liver and lung, leads to a decrease in the arachidonic acid level, thus reducing the precursor for the synthesis of pro-inflammatory prostaglandins. At the same time, the increased levels of 2-arachidonylglycerol, which acts as agonist on CB_1 and CB_2 and results from MAGL inhibition, lead to an enhancement of cannabinoid signaling. These two effects are synergistically beneficial mainly for the treatment of neurodegenerative diseases, inflammatory pathologies, and pain. On the other hand, since MAGL is abnormally expressed in several types of cancer, the block of MAGL in cancer cells reduces the formation of free fatty acids, and therefore, the production of protumorigenic lipid modulators is negatively affected, and cancer growth is impaired [3]. Consequently, a great interest for the discovery of MAGL inhibitors has led many research groups from both academy and pharmaceutical industry to the synthesis of various chemical classes of compounds, but unfortunately most of the compounds so far developed are characterized by an irreversible inhibition mechanism [4]. In fact, irreversible MAGL inhibitors have showed several drawbacks in animal models, thus hampering the possibility of in vivo MAGL inhibition studies: after repeated in vivo administration of irreversible inhibitors, the positive effects of MAGL inhibition were lost, producing a general cannabinoid desensitization and, in some cases, also a physical dependence [5]. In order to overcome these problems, the use of inhibitors characterized by a reversible behavior is preferred, since they should leave the endocannabinoid system substantially intact. To the best of our knowledge, only few examples of reversible MAGL inhibitors have been reported in literature [6, 7]. Therefore, our goal is the identification of reversible MAGL inhibitors that are able to temporarily inhibit the enzyme.

Herein, we report the process of design and development we have followed for the production of this new series of MAGL inhibitors.

2 Virtual Screening Studies

Different MAGL crystal structures are deposited in the RCSB Protein Data Bank; [8] however, only one of them describes the interaction of a reversible ligand with the enzyme (compound ZYH, 3PE6 PDB code) [9]. The graphical analysis of the interactions of this compound highlighted an elevated number of lipophilic interactions and two critical H-bonds between the carbonylic function of the inhibitor and the nitrogen backbone of A51 and M123.

2.1 Database Generation

The Asinex Gold and Asinex Platinum commercial databases (corresponding to a total of 319,911 compounds) were downloaded from the website (http://www.asinex.com/libraries-html/) and subjected to conformational analysis by using Omega 2.4.6 [10, 11]. Starting from the default parameters, only the maxconfs command (which sets the maximum number of conformations to be generated) was changed to 10,000.

2.2 Shape Similarity-Based Filter

Using as a template structure the ZYH ligand extracted from the complex with MAGL, the entire Asinex dataset was filtered using the ROCS software [12] by applying the default procedure and selecting the compounds possessing a Tanimoto Combo score higher than 0.70. From this analysis, 319,207 molecules were rejected and only 704 were further taken into account.

2.3 Consensus Docking Filter

The consensus docking technique consists in the comparison of the binding poses obtained for one compound by using different docking methods. This approach was found to predict ligand binding poses better than the single docking procedures [13] and showed to be a promising strategy for improving performance and hit rates of VS campaigns [14]. Furthermore, this technique was successfully employed for the identification of new non-covalent fatty acid amide hydrolase and lactate dehydrogenase inhibitors [15, 16]. The filtered 704 compounds were docked into the MAGL binding site (3PE6 PDB code) by using DOCK [17], GOLD [18], FRED [19], and AutoDock [20] software. For all the four docking calculations, the binding site region was defined by considering the reference ligand as the central group of a box of 10 Å in the *x*, *y*, and *z* directions. For each ligand, the four resulting docking poses were clusterized by applying a threshold of 2.0 Å. Only the ligands that showed a single cluster (i.e., the ligands that showed a common disposition for all the four docking procedures) were analyzed. Then, due to the important role of the H-bond between the carbonyl oxygen of the reference ligand and the nitrogen backbone of A51 and M123, only the 37 compounds that formed H-bonds with these two residues were taken into account (*see* **Note 1**).

2.4 Molecular Dynamic (MD) Simulations and Visual Clustering

The 37 compounds obtained by the previous VS steps were subjected to MD simulations by using AMBER 11 [21]. The complexes were solvated with a 10 Å water cap. Sodium ions were added as counterions to neutralize the system. After two preliminary minimization steps, 5 nanoseconds of MD simulation were then carried out with a time step of 2.0 fs and a cutoff of 10 Å. Constant-volume periodic boundary MD was carried out for 300 ps, during which the temperature was raised from 0 to 300 K, followed by 4.7 ns of constant pressure periodic boundary MD. For the ligands, general AMBER force field (GAFF) parameters were assigned, and partial charges were calculated using the AM1-BCC method as implemented in the Antechamber software from AMBER 11. The MD trajectories produced by the 37 ligand-protein complexes were analyzed, and all the ligands that maintained at least one of the two H-bonds with the backbone of A51 and M123 for at least the 75% of MD simulation were further considered. By applying this filter, 22 compounds were rejected, and the remaining 15 compounds were visually checked and clustered on the basis of their similarity. Eight different clusters were identified, and thus eight representative compounds were chosen.

3 MAGL Inhibition Assay

The eight selected compounds were purchased and subjected to a MAGL inhibition assay (IC_{50} evaluation).

3.1 Material

1. 96-well microtiter plates.
2. Tris buffer 10 mM, pH 7.2 containing EDTA 1 mM and 0.1 mg/mL of bovine serum albumin.
3. 4-Nitrophenylacetate substrate (4-NPA) at a final concentration of 100 μM.
4. Compounds with a final concentration ranging from 200 to 0.0128 μM (seven double points with a 1:5 dilution).
5. MAGL enzyme (11 ng/well).

For each well, the final volume of 200 μL was reached by the sum of 150 μL of 4-NPA 133.3 μM (dissolved in Tris buffer 10 mM pH 7.2 containing EDTA 1 mM), 10 μL of DMSO containing the appropriate amount of compound, and 40 μL of MAGL (dissolved in Tris buffer 10 mM pH 7.2 containing EDTA 1 mM). After the reaction had proceeded for 30 min, absorbance values were then measured by using a Victor X3 PerkinElmer instrument at 405 nm. IC_{50} values were obtained using the sigmoidal dose-response fitting of GraphPad Prism software. To remove possible false-positive results, for each compound concentration, a blank analysis was carried out, and the final absorbance results were obtained by

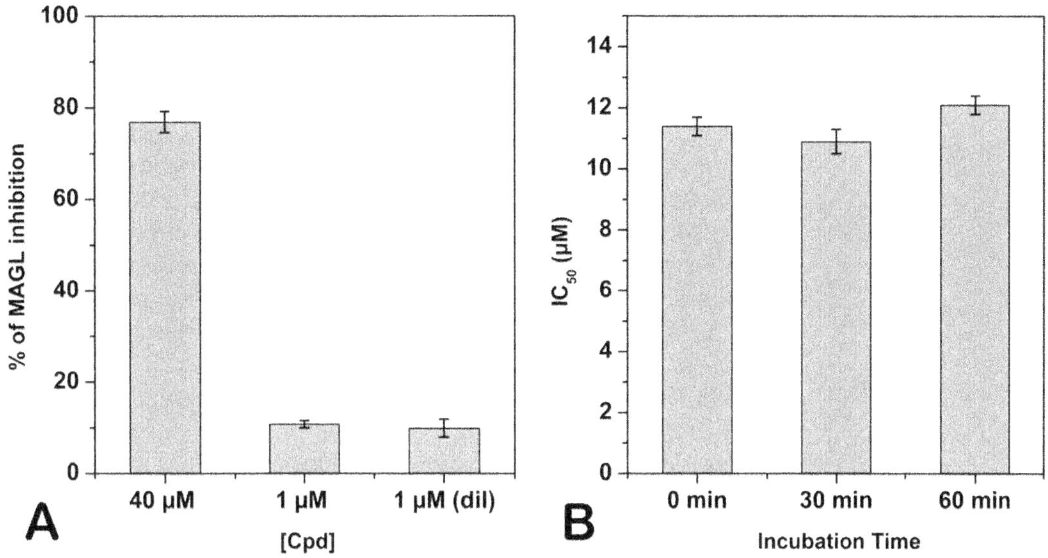

Fig. 1 Compound **1**-*h*MAGL inhibition analysis. (**a**) Dilution assay: the first two columns indicate the inhibition percentage of compound **1** at a concentration of 40 μM and 1 μM. The third column indicates the inhibition percentage of compound **1** after dilution (final concentration = 1 μM). (**b**) IC_{50} (μM) values of **1** at different preincubation times with *h*MAGL (0 min, 30 min, and 60 min)

detracting the absorbance produced by the presence of all the components except MAGL in the same conditions.

Among the eight tested compounds, one compound (**1**) showed an appreciable MAGL inhibitory activity with an IC_{50} value of 11.7 μM [22].

3.2 Reversible Inhibition Analysis

In order to analyze the inhibition mechanism of compound **1**, the effects of dilution and preincubation on its inhibitory ability were evaluated. In the dilution experiments, if **1** is an irreversible inhibitor, then its inhibition potency should not drop upon dilution, whereas inhibition levels should be substantially reduced upon dilution in the presence of a reversible compound [23]. As shown in Fig. 1a, **1** produced a reversible inhibition of MAGL, since the inhibition produced by 40 μM of this compound was significantly higher than that observed with a 40× dilution, which instead appears to be similar to that produced by a 1 μM concentration of the same compound. In the preincubation test, the activity of **1** was tested at different preincubation times of the inhibitor with the enzyme. In principle, an irreversible inhibitor will increase its capacity to block the enzyme with increasingly longer incubation times in the presence of the enzyme prior to addition of the substrate; a constant IC_{50} value, conversely, supports a reversible mechanism. As expected, compound **1** did not show any significant increase in its ability to block MAGL activity after 30 and 60 min (Fig. 1b), thus suggesting that its effect on MAGL activity is reversible.

4 Hit-to-Lead Phase

Figure 2 shows the binding mode of compound **1**. The amidic C=O group of the compound forms two H-bonds with the nitrogen backbone of A51 and M123, and the 4-chlorobenzoyl moiety is directed toward an open cavity of the protein showing lipophilic interactions with L148, L213, and L241. The 4-methoxyphenyl fragment interacts into a small pocket of the protein showing lipophilic interactions with the side chains of Y194 and V270.

As a first step in the optimization of this compound, we explored its interactions inside the pocket delimited by E53, R57, Y58, Y194, V270, and H272. On this basis, the *p*-methoxyphenyl ring present in the amidic portion of the initial compound was replaced by differently substituted aryl groups. Hence, we explored the *ortho/meta/para* effects generated by the presence in the amidic phenyl ring of halogen atoms (F, Cl, Br, I), methyl, trifluoromethyl, methoxy, trifluoromethoxy, hydroxy, amino, and nitro substituents [24]. This fragment analysis was limited to small substituents because as reported below the modeling studies suggested the presence of a small pocket. The in vitro enzymatic assays for these derivatives highlighted that one compound, the *m*-hydroxy-substituted derivative **2**, showed a high inhibition activity (IC_{50} = 0.84 μM), which is about 14-fold more potent than that displayed by the starting lead compound **1**. In order to characterize the binding disposition of this new inhibitor, compound **2** was subjected to docking calculations. As expected, the overall disposition of this molecule is very similar to that observed for compound **1**; however, the *m*-hydroxyphenyl fragment is inserted into a small

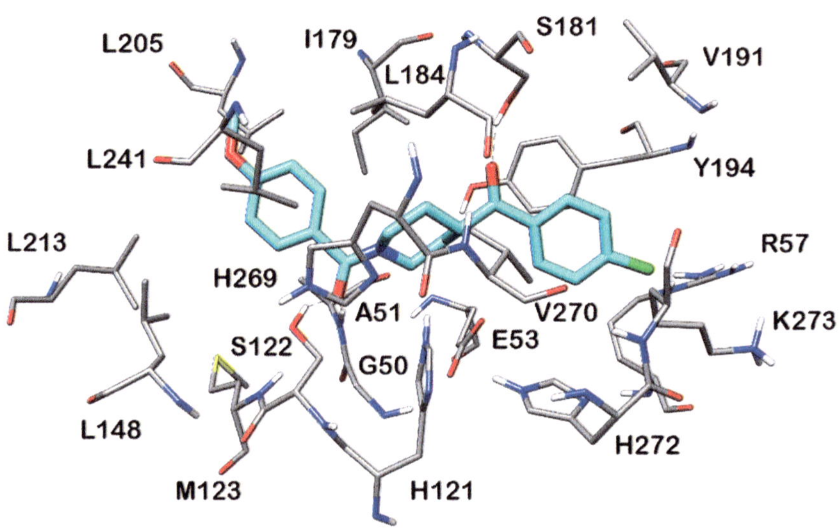

Fig. 2 Minimized average structures of compound **1** docked into *h*MAGL

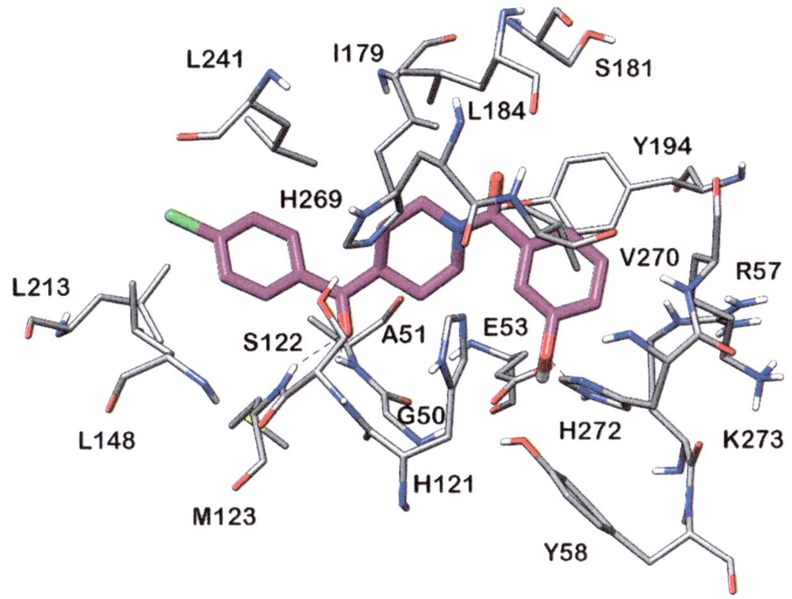

Fig. 3 Minimized average structures of compound **2** docked into *h*MAGL

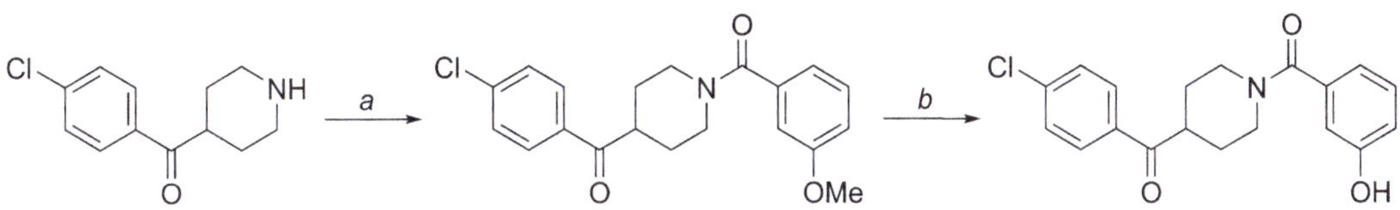

Fig. 4 Synthesis of compound **2**. Reagents and conditions: (**a**) 3-methoxybenzoic acid (1 eq), HATU (1.05 eq), DIPEA (4 eq), dry DMF, RT, 6–8 h; (**b**) 1 M BBr_3, dry CH_2Cl_2, −78 to 0 °C, then RT, 1 h

pocket of the protein and shows lipophilic interactions between its aryl ring and residues Y194 and V270. Very importantly, the *m*-hydroxyl participates to a highly energetic H-bond network with residues E53 and H272, where it behaves as an H-bond acceptor with H272 and as a H-bond donor with E53 (Fig. 3). It was interesting to note that, by analyzing the main crystal structures of *h*MAGL [1, 9, 25, 26] and superimposing them with the *h*MAGL-**2** complex, the hydroxyl group of the ligand replaces a structural water molecule that normally acts as a H-bond bridge between E53 and H272, thus supporting the high activity of this compound.

Compound **2** was obtained following the synthetic pathway reported in Fig. 4, consisting in an amide coupling between commercially available 3-methoxybenzoic acid and 4-(4-chlorobenzoyl)piperidine **3** in the presence of HATU as the condensing agent and DIPEA as the base in dry *N*,*N*-dimethylformamide as the solvent. Methoxylated intermediate **4** was subjected to a BBr_3-promoted deprotection to obtain the hydroxy-substituted derivative **2** with very good yield.

5 Cell Viability Assays

5.1 Materials

5.1.1 Western Blot Analysis

Instruments: (1) WB apparatus, Mini-Protean system, PowerPac™ universal power supply (Bio-Rad Laboratories, CA, US). (2) Imaging instrument: ChemiDoc Imager instrument (Bio-Rad Laboratories, CA, US).

Consumables:

(1) Radioimmunoprecipitation assay (RIPA) buffer (25 mM Tris pH 8, 150 mM NaCl, 0.1% SDS, 0.5% sodium deoxycholate, 1% NP-40)
(2) Complete-EDTA protease inhibitors (Roche, Switzerland)
(3) Nitrocellulose membrane (Whatman International Ltd., UK)
(4) Running (25 mM Tris, 192 mM glycine, 0.1% SDS) and transfer buffers (25 mM Tris, 192 mM glycine, 20% methanol)
(5) Laemmli buffer (2×: 65.8 mM Tris–HCl, pH 6.8, 26.3% (w/v) glycerol, 2.1% SDS, 0.01% bromophenol blue)
(6) Eight % polyacrylamide gels (Sigma-Aldrich, MO, US)
(7) Skim milk (Euroclone, Italy)
(8) Tris-buffered saline Tween 20 solution (TBS-T, 20 mM Tris, pH 7.5, 150 mM NaCl, 0.1% Tween 20)
(9) Primary antibodies: vinculin (sc-7649, Santa Cruz, CA, US); MAGL (Ab24701, Abcam, UK)
(10) Secondary antibodies: goat anti-rabbit IgG (H + L) Cross-Adsorbed, HRP (31462); Donkey anti-Goat IgG Cross-Adsorbed, HRP (PA1-86326)
(11) LiteAblot extend chemiluminescent developer (Euroclone, Italy)

5.1.2 Cell Viability Analysis

Instruments: (1) biosafety cabinet BioAir class II (Euroclone, Italy). (2) CO_2 IncuSafe incubator (Panasonic Biomedical, UK). (3) Microplate reader F200 (Tecan, Switzerland).

Consumables:

(1) OVSAHO, OVCAR3, COV318, and CAOV3 ovarian cancer cell lines
(2) Cell culture media (Euroclone, Italy)
(3) PBS (137 mM NaCl, 12 mM phosphate, 2.7 mM KCl, pH 7.4)
(4) Trypsin-EDTA (Sigma-Aldrich, MO, US)
(5) 96-well microplates (Becton Dickinson, NJ, US)
(6) CellTiter-Glo luminescent cell viability assay (Promega, WI, US)

To select which ovarian cancer cells overexpress the MAGL protein, a Western blot analysis was done on OVSAHO, OVCAR3, COV318, and CAOV3 cell lines. Cancer cells (1x10 [6]) were pelleted at 200 g for 5 min, washed three times with 1 mL of PBS, and resuspended into RIPA buffer supplemented with a protease inhibitor mixture (concentration 20×) for protein extraction.

Fifty microgram of proteins were diluted in loading buffer (Laemmli buffer) in a total volume of 20 μL and run in a precast 8% denaturating polyacrylamide gel (100 V, 2 h). After electrophoresis, the proteins were transferred on nitrocellulose membrane at 100 V for 1 h. To prevent nonspecific binding of antibodies, the membranes were blocked with 20 mL of 5% (w/v) skim milk in TBS-T for 20 min and incubated overnight at 4 °C with 2 mL of primary antibodies in agitation (vinculin and MAGL, dilution 1:1000). The membranes were washed three times with 10 mL of TBS-T for 10 min, in agitation. After washing, membranes were incubated for 1 h with 10 mL of secondary antibodies (dilution 1:10000) in 5% milk TBS-T at room temperature, developed with 1 mL of chemiluminescence solution, and visualized with ChemiDoc Imager instrument. This analysis highlighted an overexpression of MAGL in OVCAR3 and CAOV3 compared to OVSAHO and COV318 cell lines. Following, compound **2** was tested in in vitro experiments to evaluate its cytotoxicity potency against these cells. Cells were maintained in cell culture media at 37 °C in a humidified atmosphere containing 5% CO_2. Normal (1.5 × 10 [4]) and tumor (5 × 10 [2]) cells were plated in 96-well culture plates in a volume of 100 μL. The day after seeding, 100 μL of vehicle or compounds were added to the cell culture at a final concentration ranging from 200 to 0.02 μM (serial dilution of 1:10). After 96 h, the cell media was eliminated, and the cells were incubated with 20 μL of CellTiter-Glo luminescent cell viability assay for 10 min. Luminescence was measured with a Tecan F200 instrument. IC_{50} values were calculated from logistical dose-response curves. Samples were run in triplicate and error bars represent standard deviations. Interestingly, compound **2** caused a considerable inhibition of cell viability, with IC_{50} values ranging from about 30 to 45 μM in the OVCAR3 and CAOV3 cell lines, whereas it proved to be remarkably less potent against the two ovarian cancer cells that do not overexpress MAGL (OVSAHO and COV318). Furthermore, **2** proved to be completely inactive also against noncancerous human fibroblast lung cells (MRC5, $IC_{50} > 200$ μM).

6 Notes

1. Once a virtual screening study is concluded, in case of success (i.e., identification of active compounds), a crucial step is the identification and removal of false-positive or promiscuous compounds. Identification of these molecules at this level will avoid waste of time and resources at the lead optimization level. Therefore, a pan-assay interference compounds (PAINS) analysis is always suggested [27].
   (a) Following the analysis reported by Baell and Holloway [27], the presence of certain substructural features could support the presence of PAINS. The corresponding filters have been included in the Filter-it™ software and can be used for removing or further analyze compounds that possess the substructural features shared by the most common PAINS.
   (b) Another important aspect that should be considered out is the evaluation of interference problems: some compounds can be recognized as active only because they possess a coloration or another property that might interfere with the assay. For this reason, a deep analysis of the characteristics of the compounds should always be carried out, as well as the experimental evaluation of their activities by using a different readout method.
   (c) Some compounds show aggregation properties, and therefore, they result to be active in experimental assays, although they do not inhibit the target at its binding site. In order to prevent this possibility, the use of detergents such as Triton or bovine serum albumin in experimental assays is recommended.
   (d) As reported by Walters and co-workers [28], promiscuous enzymatic inhibition could be due in some cases to covalent reaction with cysteines in multiple proteins. In order to analyze this possible behavior, the inhibition activity should also be tested in the presence of the thiol-containing agent 1,4-dithio-DL-threitol (DTT). If the presence of DTT determines a decrease of the ligand inhibition activity, then the ligand likely binds cysteines.

References

1. Labar G, Bauvois C, Borel F et al (2010) Crystal structure of the human monoacylglycerol lipase, a key actor in endocannabinoid signaling. Chembiochem 11(2):218–227. https://doi.org/10.1002/cbic.200900621
2. Nomura DK, Long JZ, Niessen S et al (2010) Monoacylglycerol lipase regulates a fatty acid network that promotes cancer pathogenesis. Cell 140(1):49–61. https://doi.org/10.1016/j.cell.2009.11.027

3. Mulvihill MM, Nomura DK (2013) Therapeutic potential of monoacylglycerol lipase inhibitors. Life Sci 92(8-9):492–497. https://doi.org/10.1016/j.lfs.2012.10.025
4. Scalvini L, Piomelli D, Mor M (2016) Monoglyceride lipase: structure and inhibitors. Chem Phys Lipids 197:13–24. https://doi.org/10.1016/j.chemphyslip.2015.07.011
5. Schlosburg JE, Blankman JL, Long JZ et al (2010) Chronic monoacylglycerol lipase blockade causes functional antagonism of the endocannabinoid system. Nat Neurosci 13 (9):1113–1119. https://doi.org/10.1038/nn.2616
6. King AR, Dotsey EY, Lodola A et al (2009) Discovery of potent and reversible monoacylglycerol lipase inhibitors. Chem Biol 16 (10):1045–1052. https://doi.org/10.1016/j.chembiol.2009.09.012
7. Hernandez-Torres G, Cipriano M et al (2014) A reversible and selective inhibitor of monoacylglycerol lipase ameliorates multiple sclerosis. Angew Chem Int Ed Engl 53:13765–13770. https://doi.org/10.1002/anie.201407807
8. Berman HM, Westbrook J, Feng Z et al (2000) The Protein Data Bank. Nucleic Acids Res 28:235–242. https://doi.org/10.1093/nar/28.1.235
9. Schalk-Hihi C, Schubert C, Alexander R et al (2011) Crystal structure of a soluble form of human monoglyceride lipase in complex with an inhibitor at 1.35 A resolution. Protein Sci 20(4):670–683. https://doi.org/10.1002/pro.596
10. OMEGA, version 2.4.6 (2013) Santa Fe, NM: OpenEye Scientific Software. www.eyesopen.com
11. Hawkins PC, Nicholls A (2012) Conformer generation with OMEGA: learning from the data set and the analysis of failures. J Chem Inf Model 52(11):2919–2936. https://doi.org/10.1021/ci300314k
12. ROCS, version 3.2.1 (2013) Santa Fe, NM: OpenEye Scientific Software. www.eyesopen.com
13. Tuccinardi T, Poli G, Romboli V et al (2014) Extensive consensus docking evaluation for ligand pose prediction and virtual screening studies. J Chem Inf Model 54 (10):2980–2986. https://doi.org/10.1021/ci500424n
14. Poli G, Martinelli A, Tuccinardi T (2016) Reliability analysis and optimization of the consensus docking approach for the development of virtual screening studies. J Enzyme Inhib Med Chem 31:167–173. https://doi.org/10.1080/14756366.2016.1193736
15. Poli G, Giuntini N, Martinelli A, Tuccinardi T (2015) Application of a FLAP-consensus docking mixed strategy for the identification of new fatty acid amide hydrolase inhibitors. J Chem Inf Model 55(3):667–675. https://doi.org/10.1021/ci5006806
16. Granchi C, Capecchi A, Del Frate G et al (2015) Development and validation of a docking-based virtual screening platform for the identification of new lactate dehydrogenase inhibitors. Molecules 20(5):8772–8790. https://doi.org/10.3390/molecules20058772
17. DOCK, version 6.0 (1998) Molecular design institute. University of California, San Francisco, CA
18. Verdonk ML, Mortenson PN, Hall RJ et al (2008) Protein-ligand docking against non-native protein conformers. J Chem Inf Model 48(11):2214–2225. https://doi.org/10.1021/ci8002254
19. FRED, version 2.2 (2010) Santa Fe, NM, USA: OpenEye Scientific Software. www.eyesopen.com
20. Morris GM, Huey R, Lindstrom W et al (2009) AutoDock4 and AutoDockTools4: automated docking with selective receptor flexibility. J Comput Chem 30(16):2785–2791. https://doi.org/10.1002/jcc.21256
21. Case DA, Darden TA, III TEC, Simmerling CL, Wang J, Duke RE et al (2010) AMBER 11. University of California, San Francisco, CA
22. Tuccinardi T, Granchi C, Rizzolio F et al (2014) Identification and characterization of a new reversible MAGL inhibitor. Bioorg Med Chem 22(13):3285–3291. https://doi.org/10.1016/j.bmc.2014.04.057
23. Granchi C, Rizzolio F, Bordoni V et al (2016) 4-Aryliden-2-methyloxazol-5(4H)-one as a new scaffold for selective reversible MAGL inhibitors. J Enzyme Inhib Med Chem 31 (1):137–146. https://doi.org/10.3109/14756366.2015.1010530
24. Granchi C, Rizzolio F, Palazzolo S et al (2016) Structural optimization of 4-chlorobenzoylpiperidine derivatives for the development of potent, reversible, and selective monoacylglycerol lipase (MAGL) inhibitors. J Med Chem 59(22):10299–10314. https://doi.org/10.1021/acs.jmedchem.6b01459
25. Bertrand T, Auge F, Houtmann J et al (2010) Structural basis for human monoglyceride lipase inhibition. J Mol Biol 396(3):663–673. https://doi.org/10.1016/j.jmb.2009.11.060
26. Griebel G, Pichat P, Beeske S et al (2015) Selective blockade of the hydrolysis of the

endocannabinoid 2-arachidonoylglycerol impairs learning and memory performance while producing antinociceptive activity in rodents. Sci Rep 5:7642. https://doi.org/10.1038/srep07642

27. Baell JB, Holloway GA (2010) New substructure filters for removal of pan assay interference compounds (PAINS) from screening libraries and for their exclusion in bioassays. J Med Chem 53(7):2719–2740. https://doi.org/10.1021/jm901137j

28. Dahlin JL, Nissink JW, Strasser JM et al (2015) PAINS in the assay: chemical mechanisms of assay interference and promiscuous enzymatic inhibition observed during a sulfhydryl-scavenging HTS. J Med Chem 58(5):2091–2113. https://doi.org/10.1021/jm5019093

Chapter 21

Application of Virtual Screening Approaches for the Identification of Small Molecule Inhibitors of the Methyllysine Reader Protein Spindlin1

Chiara Luise and Dina Robaa

Abstract

Computer-based approaches represent a powerful tool which helps to identify and optimize lead structures in the process of drug discovery. Computer-aided drug design techniques (CADD) encompass a large variety of methods which are subdivided into structure-based (SBDD) and ligand-based drug design (LBDD) methods. Several approaches have been successfully used over the last three decades in different fields. Indeed also in the field of epigenetics, virtual screening (VS) studies and structure-based approaches have been applied to identify novel chemical modulators of epigenetic targets as well as to predict the binding mode of active ligands and to study the protein dynamics.

In this chapter, an iterative VS approach using both SBDD and LBDD methods, which was successful in identifying Spindlin1 inhibitors, will be described. All protocol steps, starting from structure-based pharmacophore modeling, protein and database preparation along with docking and similarity search, will be explained in details.

Key words Computer-aided drug design, Virtual screening, Structure-based pharmacophore, Docking, Database preparation, Similarity search, Spindlin1, Methyllysine reader proteins, Epigenetics

1 Introduction

The term epigenetics is defined as "the study of mitotically and/or meiotically heritable changes in gene function that cannot be explained by changes in the DNA sequence" [1]. Although each cell in the organism holds the same DNA sequence, the gene expression pattern differs between the various cell types, resulting, for instance, in different phenotypes. This is attributed to epigenetic mechanisms, which play a pivotal role in the control of gene expression by determining which sets of genes are actively transcribed and which are silenced. The epigenetic machinery is highly complex and dynamic in nature; it comprises diverse molecular mechanisms which mainly include DNA methylation, histone modification/remodeling, and noncoding RNAs [2, 3]. Aberrant

Thomas Mavromoustakos and Tahsin F. Kellici (eds.), *Rational Drug Design: Methods and Protocols*, Methods in Molecular Biology, vol. 1824, https://doi.org/10.1007/978-1-4939-8630-9_21, © Springer Science+Business Media, LLC, part of Springer Nature 2018

epigenetic regulation can contribute to the development of various diseases ranging from cancer [4, 5] to neurological [6], autoimmune, and inflammatory disorders [7, 8] as well as cardiovascular diseases [9]. As a consequence, proteins regulating the epigenome have become major targets for drug discovery and development. Indeed, recent years have seen the emergence of several new drugs, already approved by the FDA or currently in clinical trials [10].

In eukaryotic cells, the ca. 2-m-long, negatively charged DNA is packed by small, basic proteins, called histones, into chromatin to fit into the cell nucleus. The basic repeating unit of chromatin is the nucleosome, which consists of approximately 147 base pairs of DNA wrapped around an octamer of histone proteins [11]. Chromatin exits in two forms: euchromatin, the less condensed form associated with transcriptionally active genomic regions, and heterochromatin, the highly condensed and transcriptionally inactive form [11, 12]. Histone modifications, also referred to as posttranslational modifications (PTMs), are one of the major mechanisms by which the DNA-histone and histone-histone interactions are modified, allowing the chromatin to switch between transcriptionally active and inactive forms. PTMs are highly dynamic processes which majorly occur at the protruding histone tail regions, but also at the core of histone proteins, resulting in the so-called "histone code" [13, 14]. This is controlled by the interplay of various proteins, which have been classified as writers (enzymes which introduce specific histone marks), erasers (enzymes which remove specific histone modifications), and readers (proteins recognizing specific PTMs). Numerous types of histone PTMs have been reported to date including acetylation, methylation, phosphorylation, sumoylation, succinylation, and ubiquitinylation [15].

PTMs are believed to regulate the chromatin structure and function by either directly altering the packaging of chromatin (e.g., by modifying the charge state of histone residues and, hence, the association with the negatively charged DNA) or by recruiting specific binding domains ("reader domains"), the latter mechanism affects further downstream signaling cascades [16, 17]. So far, readers of methyllysine, acetyllysine, methylarginine, as well as phosphorylated serine and threonine histone marks have been discovered [16, 18]. The recent discovery of small molecule inhibitors that disrupt the binding of acetyllysine motifs to the BET bromodomains (acetyllysine reader domains) was a major breakthrough which demonstrated the druggability of these reader domains. More promising is the fact that several of these newly discovered inhibitors are currently undergoing clinical trials [19].

Another important and large group of reader proteins comprise the methyllysine reader domains which are subdivided in three major families: the plant homeodomain (PHD) zinc finger proteins, the WD40 repeat domain-containing proteins, and the so-called Royal family of reader proteins. The latter encompasses four subfamilies: Tudor-, chromo-, Pro-Trp-Trp-Pro (PWWP), and malignant brain tumor (MBT) repeat domain-containing proteins. Characteristic for all the methyllysine reader domains is a cage-like substructure made up of two to four aromatic acid residues ("aromatic cage"), which promotes the binding to the positively charged methylated lysine residues majorly through cation-π interactions [16]. Culminating evidence has clearly indicated that various methyllysine reader proteins are implicated in the pathogenesis of human diseases, most importantly cancer. As is the case with many epigenetic regulators, the validity of the discovered methyllysine reader proteins as novel therapeutic targets has still to be proven. Hence, small molecule inhibitors, which can selectively prevent the binding of these reader proteins to their histone substrates, are highly needed both as chemical probes and as potential therapeutics for the treatment of various diseases. To date, several inhibitors of methyllysine reader domains have been reported, including small molecule inhibitors of the MBT domains [20–22], the Tudor domains 53BP1 [23] and Spindlin1 [24–26], and the chromodomain CBX7 [27, 28]. For more detailed information, the readers are referred to the following reviews [29–31].

Computer-based approaches represent a powerful tool which helps to identity and optimize lead structures in the process of drug discovery. Computer-aided drug design techniques (CADD) encompass a large variety of methods which are subdivided into structure-based (SBDD) and ligand-based drug design (LBDD) methods. While SBDD exploits information about the 3D structure of the protein target (from crystal structures or generation of homology models), LBDD requires sufficient knowledge about active ligands. In many cases, a combined structure-based and ligand-based approach can also be used. In the field of epigenetics, in silico studies have been utilized to identify novel chemical modulators of epigenetic targets as well as to predict the binding mode of active ligands and to study the protein dynamics [32, 33]. Indeed, several virtual screening (VS) studies and structure-based approaches have been successfully used to identify new epigenetic modulators, like inhibitors of *Schistosoma mansoni* HDAC8 (SmHDAC8) [34], the histone acetyltransferase p300 [35], the NAD^+-dependent histone deacetylases Sirt1/Sirt2 and Sirt6 [36–40], the protein arginine methyltransferase PRMT1 [41, 42], and JumonjiC domain-containing histone demethylases [43].

In the context of methyllysine readers, Kireev et al. reported the finding of L3MBTL1 inhibitors by means of VS of a collection of commercially available databases (ChemNavigator iResearch Library, ca. 50,000,000 compounds, of which around 6,000,000 are purchasable) followed by in vitro screening of the identified hits. Prior the VS, they filtered the database by two different procedures: first, a 2D substructure search was performed to retrieve compounds bearing a lysine mimicking substructure, and, second, a pharmacophore-based VS was employed using the crystal structure of L3MBTL1 with the histone peptide substrate. The pharmacophore hits were subsequently docked into the crystal structure of L3MBL1 in complex with the histone substrate. The hits were finally tested using an AlphaScreen assay, which resulted in the identification of a set of L3MBTL1 inhibitors with IC_{50} values in the low micromolar range [44]. We have also recently reported on the identification of small molecule inhibitors of the methyllysine reader Spindlin1 by employing an iterative VS campaign using both structure-based and ligand-based methods while validating the hits using an established AlphaLISA assay [25].

In this chapter, we will describe an example of a CADD workflow, which can be used to identify novel inhibitors of methyllysine readers, here exemplified with the methyllysine reader Spindlin1.

The Tudor-like domain-containing protein Spindlin1 recognizes the H3K4me3 (H3 trimethylated at lysine 4) mark [45, 46], and its affinity toward the histone substrate is increased when the arginine residue in position 8 is asymmetrically dimethylated (H3R8me2a) [47]. Very recently, the recognition of H4K20me3 (H4 trimethylated at lysine 20) by Spindlin1 has been described [48]. Spindlin1 was found to be overexpressed in several types of malignant tumors including ovarian cancer, certain types of liver tumors, non-small cell lung cancers, liposarcoma, metastatic breast cancer, and triple-negative breast cancer [49–53]. Additionally, several studies have demonstrated a role of *Spindlin1* in the progression of tumor [50, 51, 54, 55]. Several crystal structures of Spindlin1 have been reported, both in apo form [56] and in complex with histone peptides [46, 47]; the latter was used as a basis for the herein described VS approach. Only very recently, a co-crystal structure of Spindlin1 in complex with a small molecule inhibitor was reported [24].

Spindlin1 is composed of three structurally homologous Tudor-like domains, where H3K4me3 is mainly bound to domain II. Importantly, the trimethylated lysine is embedded in an aromatic cage, which is composed of the aromatic amino acid residues Phe141, Trp151, Tyr170, and Tyr177. The trimethylated lysine is stabilized in this aromatic cage mainly by cation-π interactions and to a lesser extent by hydrophobic van der Waals contacts. Crystal structures of Spindlin1 in complex with the histone substrate clearly show that the peptide residues flanking the trimethylated lysine exhibit extensive interactions with the outer groove of Spindlin1. Ala1 and Arg2 of the histone peptide are inserted in electronegative regions, where salt bridges are formed between Ala1 and the protein residues Glu142 and Asp189 and between Arg2 and Asp184. Moreover, the backbone of Thr3 of the peptide undergoes two H-bond interactions with the backbone of Glu142. Several water-mediated H-bond interactions can also be observed [46, 47].

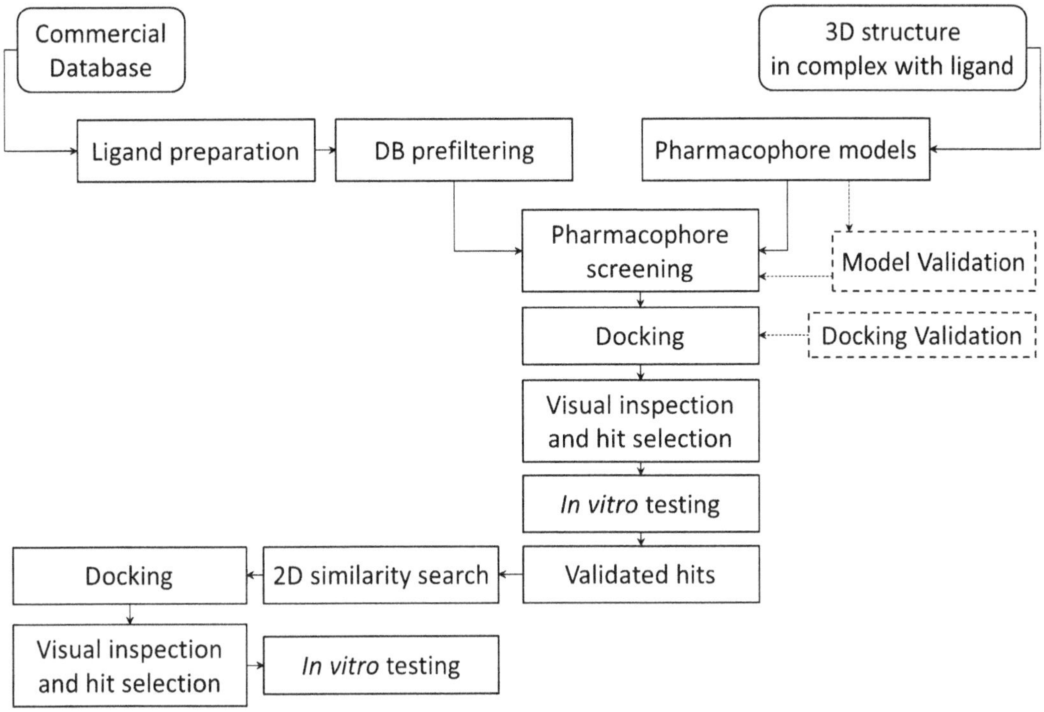

Fig. 1 Iterative VS workflow used for the identification of the methyllysine reader protein Spindlin1. Validation studies, here outlined by dashed lines, were not performed in the described study; however, they can be implemented if enough information is available on active and inactive ligands

Figure 1 illustrates the VS workflow which can be used to identify novel modulators of different biological targets and was successfully applied to identify Spindlin1 inhibitors. The first steps encompass a pharmacophore-based VS approach using databases of commercially available compounds. The commercial databases could be filtered according to several criteria, including substructure searches to only retain compounds which contain some essential features (here, e.g., a positively charge N-atom to occupy the aromatic cage of the methyllysine reader). Structure-based pharmacophore models are generated based on the crystal structure of the target protein with active ligands. Several pharmacophore models can generally be used to screen the databases. Notably, pharmacophore-based screening serves as filter to select the compounds which could possibly mimic the interactions of the active ligands with the protein binding site. To better evaluate the pharmacophore hits, docking into the crystal structure of the protein is usually performed; this gives a more realistic binding mode and helps ranking the compounds according to their docking score. Consequently, the top-ranked compounds are visually inspected, and the most promising compounds are selected ("cherry picking") to be submitted to in vitro screening using an established assay. If active compounds are retrieved from the biological assay, LDBB methods, like 2D similarity searches, can be applied to search for further active derivatives. Again here, docking of the obtained hits is commonly performed.

2 Materials

VS has emerged as a powerful tool for the identification of novel and diverse structures in the CADD scenario since it represents a rational, fast, and cost-effective pre-filtering method, which serves to reduce the number of compounds prior to biological testing [57]. VS allows the discovery of novel bioactive molecules (hits) from very large compound collections (databases) by screening them using different techniques. VS approaches are generally classified based on the information they rely on (*see* **Note 1**, for some general remarks on VS).

2.1 Pharmacophore-Based VS

A pharmacophore is defined as "the ensemble of steric and electronic features that is necessary to ensure the optimal molecular interactions with a specific biological target structure and to trigger (or to block) its biological response" [58]. Pharmacophore models can be generated by two different approaches: ligand-based pharmacophore model, where a common model(s) is generated based on the alignment of the 3D structures of active molecules [59], and structure-based pharmacophore model, which is only applicable when the 3D structure of the target protein is available, preferably in complex with an active ligand. Structure-based models reflect both the information about the binding interactions between the active ligand and the protein (chemical features such as H-bond donors/acceptors, ionizable groups, and hydrophobic moieties are included) as well as size and shape restrictions of the binding pocket (e.g., exclusion volumes are generated) [59].

In this chapter, we describe the use of LigandScout [60] for structure-based pharmacophore generation. Other available pharmacophore modeling software include MOE [61], PHASE (Schrödinger) [62, 63], Discovery Studio [64, 65], and Pharmer (freeware program) [66] (*see* **Note 2a**).

2.2 Structure-Based VS

Structure-based VS (SBVS) methods rely on the availability of the 3D structure of the target protein, preferably in complex with a ligand [67, 68]. Available 3D structures of the protein can be obtained from the Protein Data Bank (PDB) [69, 70], which to this day holds over 120,000 3D structures of protein solved by X-ray crystallography, NMR, and to a lesser extent electron microscopy. In case no crystal structures are available, building a homology model using programs like MODELLER [71, 72] or webservers like SWISS-MODEL [24, 73] can be a useful alternative.

- Molecular docking is the most commonly used SBVS method and can be defined as conformational and orientational sampling of the ligand in the binding site of the receptor. The binding affinity is then predicted by means of a scoring function. Protein-ligand docking is the most commonly applied structure-based method in drug discovery. The compounds are docked, scored, and ranked according to the used docking algorithm and scoring function [74, 75]. Often only the top-ranked compounds are considered for further biological screening.

In the methods part, docking procedure using GLIDE is described [76–78]. Other commonly used docking software include GOLD [79] and the freeware programs DOCK [80] and AutoDock [81, 82] (*see* **Note 1f**).

2.3 Ligand-Based VS

Ligand-based VS (LBVS) relies on the concept that similar compounds usually show similar biological effects. For this purpose, large compound databases can be screened for compounds which show similarity to known active compounds to identify further potentially active compounds. LBVS encompass a large variety of methods, including substructure searches, 2D similarity, 3D similarity, machine learning methods, etc. [83]. Molecular fingerprints are one of most commonly used techniques for similarity searching. These are bit strings, which mark the presence or absence of a chemical fragment or feature by "1" and "0," respectively. Here again, there is a large variety of fingerprints, using different techniques for encoding chemical structures, which would yield a different set of hits [84]. Similarity indices, like the Tanimoto coefficient, are computed to compare the bits for the query ligand and the ligands in the screening library. Here we will describe a chemical similarity search using BIT_MACCS fingerprints [85] which is implemented in the MOE software package [61].

2.4 VS Databases

Virtual chemical databases are essential for all VS approaches. Currently, there are a large number of public databases which are freely available and can be downloaded in different formats like ZINC [86, 87], ChemSpider [88], and NCI Database [89]. Databases of different chemical vendors such as ChemBridge [90], ChemDiv [91], Princeton [92], Maybridge [93], etc. can also be downloaded from the ZINC website or directly from the vendor's website. In the described approach, the two commercial databases ChemBridge [90] and ChemDiv [91] were used for VS, which were downloaded from the ZINC website.

When dealing with huge databases, pre-filtering methods are often applied prior to VS in order to reduce the number of compounds. These filters are based on the physicochemical properties of the compounds like the Lipinski's rule of five for drug-likeness [94], Oprea's criteria for lead-likeness [95], etc. Moreover, substructure searches can be performed to ensure that that screened compounds include fragments which are known to be essential for the activity, e.g., only compounds bearing a N^+ were kept in the described study. Another filter, which is now increasingly used, is the PAINS filter. Pan-assay interference (PAINS) compounds are chemical compounds which tend to show promiscuous activity against numerous proteins and are hence often identified as false positives. These compounds contain substructures (e.g., possess intrinsic redox reactivity, are unstable or reactive, induce protein aggregation, etc.) which tend to bind non-specifically to many biological targets and are often detected as false positives [96–98] (*see* **Note 3a**).

3 Methods

CADD encompass a variety of powerful tools which can be used in the hit identification as well as the hit optimization steps in the process of drug discovery. In this part, we will present in details the methods used in an iterative VS approach, which was successful in identifying Spindlin1 inhibitors. When used in the appropriate context, this workflow (or a modified one thereof) can be applied to other biological targets as well.

3.1 Pharmacophore-Based VS

3.1.1 Structure-Based Pharmacophore Generation Using LigandScout

The following protocol shows the structure-based pharmacophore model generation of Spindlin1 [PDB 4H75 used as example [46]] by LigandScout 3.1 [60]. The program, after searching for interactions between the ligand (here, the co-crystalized peptide substrate) and the protein, automatically suggests pharmacophoric features. The selection of the right chemical features is an important step for the development of a high-quality pharmacophore model; therefore, the suggested features might need to be manually curated. Moreover, some pharmacophoric features can be deleted or disabled, and others can be added. In some cases, like for the peptide, too many features might be assigned; in this case, only the important peptide residues can be used for the pharmacophore generation (*see* **Note 2b**, on pharmacophore validation). A structure-based pharmacophore also allows the generation of excluded volumes that correspond to regions of space where the protein residues reside and, hence, are restricted from being occupied by the ligand.

1. Download the crystal structure of Spindlin1 with H3K4me3 residues 1–8 (PDB ID: 4H75) from the PDB in the *Structure-Based Perspective* of LigandScout's graphical user interface (GUI).

2. Delete peptide residues 6–8.
3. Identify the peptide residues of interest (residues 1–5); if they are recognized as macromolecule, mark them as core molecule by using the *Move to Core* icon in the toolbar. Then check the hybridization states and the bond orders, as they might need to be adjusted properly.
4. Analyze the water molecules in the binding site, and delete the unnecessary ones (*see* **Note 1c**); in this case, keep only water molecule numbers 415 and 416.
5. Select the core molecule, and generate a preliminary pharmacophore model by using the *Create Pharmacophore* icon in the toolbar. Visually inspect the pharmacophore model, and check if the essential features, like the cationic feature denoting the positively charged ammonium group of K4me3, are present. If required, edit the pharmacophore features. As an example:
   - Remove the hydrophobic feature generated for the lysine aliphatic chain.
   - Remove the H-bond donor features assigned for Ala1 backbone NH_3^+ and Arg2 side chain.
6. Generate the excluded volume by using the *Add Exclusion Volume Coat* option via Menu > Pharmacophore > Add Exclusion Volumes Coat.
7. Based on the generated model (Fig. 2), create different pharmacophore models by alternatively enabling and disabling some features; here the cationic feature denoting the positively charged ammonium group of K4me3 was always kept, since it was considered as an essential feature.
8. Save the constructed pharmacophore models in the required format, PMZ.

3.1.2 Database Preparations

Here, we describe the preparation of the databases of commercially available compounds by means of MOE followed by the generation of a multiconformational database using LigandScout [60, 61].

1. The first step is to download the database of commercially available compounds from vendor websites, for example, as SD file.
2. Convert the downloaded database into MDB file format by simply opening it in a new MOE Database Viewer (DBV).
3. In MOE, generate the 3D structures (if necessary) and clean up the database. The 2D structures can be converted into 3D structures simultaneously during the cleaning procedure. The cleaning procedure consists mainly of a wash step, which includes salt stripping, protonation states generation at pH 7,

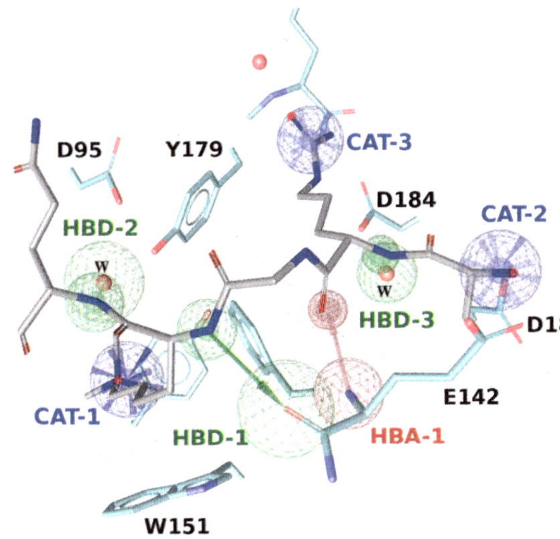

Fig. 2 Structure-based pharmacophore model generated using LigandScout. Blue spheres indicate a cationic feature (CAT), two green spheres and an arrow denote an H-bond donor feature (HBD, vector type), and two red spheres and an arrow denote an H-bond acceptor feature (HBA, vector type). The N-terminal residues of H3K4me3 are shown as gray sticks, the binding pocket residues as cyan sticks, and water molecules as red spheres

and rebuilding of 3D molecules if needed. The *Wash* panel is reached through DBV > Compute > Molecule > Wash.

4. Once the structures are "washed," energy minimization should be carried out. This step is needed for optimizing bond lengths, bond angles, and torsional angles. Several force fields, such as MMFF94(s/x), Amber12:EHT, or OPLS-AA, are available in MOE; here MMFF94x was used. The *Energy Minimization* panel is reached through DBV > Compute > Molecule > Energy Minimize.
5. Calculate the desired molecular descriptors. Different 2D and 3D molecular descriptors, like molecular weight (MW), topological surface area (TPSA), LogP, number of H-bond donors/acceptors, and so on, can be generated. This can be done through the *Calculate Descriptors* panel in MOE; it is reached via DBV > Compute > Descriptors > Calculate. Furthermore, physicochemical descriptor-based profiles, such as Lipinski's rule of five for drug-likeness [94], Oprea's criteria for lead-likeness [95], and the relative number of violations, can be computed. By calculating such properties, the compounds can be tagged and easily filtered.
6. At this point, filters can be applied to reduce the number of compounds for the subsequent pharmacophore screening

procedure by eliminating structures with undesirable properties. For example, by filtering the compounds based on specific molecular properties like MW or based on their drug-likeness/lead-likeness. Other kinds of filters that can be applied are structure filters depending on criteria defined by the user. This can be done by retrieving only the structures that contain a specific feature necessary for the binding of the molecule to the target, like a lysine mimetic moiety for methyllysine reader proteins. For instance, in the Spindlin1 case, all compounds with a molecular weight > 500 Da as well as compounds containing no positively charged N atoms (N^+) (*see* **Note 3b**) or H-bond donors can be filtered out. This can be performed in the DBV of MOE by right-clicking on the column of the desired property and then *selecting* and specifying the desired value, e.g., weight < 500, etc. (*see* **Note 3** for remarks on the filtering steps).

7. Export the prepared and filtered database in SD format. If the database is too big, it can be divided into smaller databases.
8. Multiconformational datasets of the prepared database(s) can be generated through LigandScout, and at the same time, the output can be saved in LDB format. Two different algorithms for conformer ensemble generation are implemented in LigandScout, Omega and iCon. Here, Omega-fast was used as a setting for conformational generation. For using Omega, an OpenEye license is required [99]. Generally, the conformers can be generated either through CLI or via the *Create Screening Database* icon of the *Screening Perspective* in the GUI. In both cases the user can choose among two different conformer generation types, which differ in the number of generated conformers:
   - Icon-fast, iCon high-throughput settings with 25 conformers per structure
   - Icon-best, iCon high-quality settings with 200 conformers per structure
   - Omega-fast, Omega high-throughput settings with 25 conformers per structure
   - Omega-best, Omega high-quality settings with 500 conformers per structure

In the case of large databases, as is the case here, it is highly recommended to use the CLI (idbgen module) to generate the multiconformational database.

Command line example: *idbgen -i [input file] -o [output file] -t omega-fast*

Supported input file formats are *.sdf, *.smi, *.mol2, and *.ldb, and output files, *.ldb.

Other arguments which can be specified in the idbgen module can be found by typing in CLI: *idbgen -h all.*

Alternatively, the conformers can be generated by using other programs. In this case, it is necessary to convert the database into LDB format before using it for pharmacophore screening in LigandScout.

9. Once the database is fully prepared and saved as LDB format, it can be used for pharmacophore-based VS in LigandScout.

3.1.3 Pharmacophore Screening

After generating the pharmacophore models (Subheading 3.1.1) and preparing the databases (Subheading 3.1.2), the next step is to run the pharmacophore screening using LigandScout.

The pharmacophore-based VS can be run both from CLI and GUI.

- Procedures of the screening using GUI:

  1. The constructed pharmacophore models have to be copied into the *Screening Perspective.*
  2. Load the prepared databases in the *Screening Perspective* through the *Load Database* icon; more than one database can be picked and screened against the selected pharmacophore. The uploaded databases have to be marked; thus, mark in green the screening databases.
  3. Choose the pharmacophore model(s) to be used. Different pharmacophore models can be screened at the same time during the VS; nevertheless, the performance will be related to the number of available processors.
  4. The screening settings can be customized in the *Screening* panel by toggling on the *Show Advanced Options.* The user can choose the scoring function, the screening mode, the retrieval mode of the conformers, the number of features to omit or required depending on the selected screening mode, and whether to check or not the exclusion volume.
  5. After choosing the settings, start the screening process by pressing the *Perform Screening* icon.
  6. When the screening process is finished, the hits that match the pharmacophore will be shown in the *Library view.* Go through the results and analyze how the molecules are aligned to the pharmacophore in the 3D view. Save the retrieved pharmacophore hits in SD format for further docking studies.

- Procedures of the screening using CLI:
  As aforementioned, when screening a large database, it is highly recommended to use the CLI and multiple cores for one screening job. One has to bear in mind that the pharmacophore

screening uses a lot of the computer resources, so it is usually not advisable to run several screening jobs simultaneously. The command line script is run by using the iscreen module implemented in LigandScout. Default settings were used.

Command line: *iscreen -q [query-pharmacophore].pmz or pml -d [database to screen].ldb -o [hit list].sdf or ldb -x multi*

For more arguments in the iscreen command, type *iscreen -h all* in the CLI.

3.2 Docking of Pharmacophore Hits

There are diverse ways to prioritize and select the hits retrieved from the pharmacophore-based VS for in vitro testing; one of these is by docking the obtained pharmacophore hits into the crystal structure used for the structure-based pharmacophore generation.

Several software packages, such as Glide [76, 77], GOLD [79], ParaDocks [100], AutoDock Vina [81], MOE [101], and many others, are available for performing protein-ligand docking. In this subsection, we describe the docking procedures by means of Glide [78]. However, before performing docking studies, other preparation steps, like protein preparation, grid generation, and ligand preparations, are required. In the following section, the general procedures of these steps utilizing Maestro GUI, Release 2014-2, are described.

3.2.1 Protein Preparation

This step is necessary for preparing the protein in a format that is suitable for modeling calculations. Indeed, hydrogens need to be added, bond orders and formal charges need to be assigned, and the structure needs to be minimized and optimized. The whole process is done through the *Protein Preparation Wizard* panel [102, 103] reachable from the toolbar and which consists of three tabs.

1. *Import and Process* tab. Download the desired PDB structure [PDB ID 4H75 used as example [46]] or directly import it by specifying the PDB code. Click *Preprocess* to add hydrogens and assign bond orders. Water molecules far away from the co-crystalized peptide can be removed. In some cases, it is recommended to only keep the water molecules which should be considered for docking and delete all others from the very beginning.
2. *Review and Modify* tab. Here analyze the non-protein residues (het), like peptide and co-crystallized buffer molecules, and delete the latter since they are not needed as well as the undesired water molecules near them. Run Epik by pressing *Generate States* to generate probable ionization and tautomeric states of the peptide at the specified pH range [104–106]. The pH range should be chosen according to the target; in this case, we used pH 7.0 ± 1.0.

3. *Refine* tab. First, optimize the hydrogen bonding network and the orientation of asparagine (Asn), glutamine (Gln), and histidine (His) residues, and predict the protonation state of the side chains, as well as the tautomeric state of histidine, at pH 7.0 by means of PROPKA. When the optimization has finished, the different protonation states and tautomers can be analyzed and changed if necessary by pressing the *Interactive Optimizer* button and then *Analyze Network* (*see* **Note 1b**). Then, the selection of the water molecules can be refined by choosing them according to the number of hydrogen bonds they form. For example, remove water molecules with less than 3 H-bond with non-water molecule. Hence, only one water molecule (HOH416), located between Met140 and Asp184, was kept and considered in the docking procedure. Notably, this is the same water molecule which was used during the pharmacophore models generation. Finally, subject the structure to a restrained energy minimization step using the default setting, OPLS_2005 force field [107] and 0.3 Å as RMSD of the atom displacement for terminating the minimization.

3.2.2 Grid Generation for Docking

Include the prepared protein in the Workspace. Then use the *Receptor Grid Generation* panel for setting up and calculating the grid. Open the panel through Tasks > Docking > Grid Generation. Define the K4me3 and Thr3 residues of H3K4me3 as the centroid of the grid box.

3.2.3 Ligand Preparation

Since in this section docking of hits retrieved from pharmacophore VS are taken as an example, the ligands have already been prepared before submitting the database to the VS. Thus, LigPrep [104] is skipped, and the pharmacophore hits were only energy minimized in MOE and saved as SD file.

3.2.4 Docking

Before performing docking of the obtained pharmacophore hits compounds, it is a good practice to verify and validate the docking parameters by re-docking and enrichment studies. Nevertheless, since no information on active ligands was available at that point, these studies could not be performed (*see* **Note 1** for information regarding docking and their limits).

When the grid and the ligands are ready, ligand docking can be executed using Glide [78].

1. Open the *Ligand Docking* panel; it is reachable through Tasks > Docking > Glide Docking.
2. In the *Setting* tab, choose the receptor grid. Then set the docking method to be used, and choose standard precision (SP) for docking.

3. Define the ligand sampling method. This option allows choosing among flexible docking and rigid docking; docking should be performed using the default option flexible docking.
4. In the *Ligand* tab, select the file containing the ligands to be docked.
5. In the *Output* tab, diverse settings can be set. Choose the output file type and format, the number of poses per ligand to include in the post-docking minimization step, and the number of poses per ligand to be written in the output file. Moreover, pre-residue interaction scores can be calculated and reported in the output file; and a separate report file can be generated if the option is marked. In the process of VS, only the top-scored pose is output; this is set by—Write out at most: 1 poses per ligand.
6. In the job settings, define whether to incorporate the output automatically in the project and the number of processors and subjobs to be used. So, run the job.
7. Analyze the output file, which contains only the ligand poses that successfully passed through the several Glide's docking steps. The visual inspection of the top-ranked docking poses that show significant interactions with the residues of the binding should guide the selection of the compounds for the in vitro testing. For Spindlin1, for example, the compounds showing a protonated aliphatic nitrogen rightly positioned in the aromatic cage can be considered for further analysis (*see* **Note 1e**).

3.3 Similarity Search

In the described study, some of the most promising hits were purchased and submitted to in vitro testing using an AlphaLISA assay. Some of these hits were found to inhibit Spindlin1 with IC_{50} values in the micromolar range, which allowed us to run a ligand-based VS using a similarity search [108, 109] in order to search for further derivatives and/or structural analogues of these active hits. This should help not only finding new hit compounds but also developing a SAR. Here, we describe a 2D fingerprint similarity search approach using MACCS fingerprint implemented in MOE [61, 85].

1. Open in MOE the previously prepared (but not filtered) commercial databases to be screened (database preparation as described before in Subheading 3.1.2; required steps before running the similarity search are from 1 to 5).
2. Calculate the type of fingerprint to be applied for screening the database via DBV > Compute > Fingerprint > Calculate. In this panel, the user can select the key fingerprint method, for example, BIT_MACCS (MACCS structural keys bit packed).

3. Load the active hit compounds in the MOE window to use as query molecules.
4. Open the *Search* panel through DBV > Compute > Fingerprint > Search. Here set the Tanimoto coefficient (Tc) cutoff value to be used as similarity index. Then in the MOE window, choose the active hit and select it; thus, allowing the option *Form query from selected atoms only.* Manage the *Visibility and Selection Action* options according to your needs.

   BIT_MACCS and Tanimoto coefficient are the default settings for the key fingerprints and the similarity metric, but they can be changed via *Set Fingerprint* in the *Search* panel. Clearly, before choosing another key fingerprint method, the respective fingerprint type needs to be calculated in the screening database.
5. Run the screening by the *Search* button.
6. After performing the screening, save the results as SD format, and use the saved database(s) for subsequent docking studies (as described in Subheading 3.2.4).

3.4 Evaluation of the Pan-Assay Interference (PAINS) Behavior

In the Database Preparation Subheading 3.1.2, we have already discussed the possibility to study the drug-likeness and lead-likeness behavior by calculating the Lipinski's rule of five and the Oprea's lead-likeness criteria in MOE [61, 94, 95]. In this subsection, we assess the pan-assay interference (PAINS) behavior [96–98] (*see* **Note 3a**).

PAINS filter can be applied during the database preparation; nevertheless, it is time-consuming for huge databases. Hence, it can be applied later only to the retrieved VS hits for identifying the "hitters" compounds (promiscuous compounds which are known to be active in multiple assays) prior the in vitro testing. Following are the details for performing the PAINS filter in Canvas (Schrödinger suite) [110].

1. Import the compounds into the Canvas project.
2. Open the *Structure Filter* panel by Structure > Structure Filter. Here use PAINS1, PAINS2, and PAINS3 which contain the three different PAINS subsets described in the publication [97].

4 Notes

1. VS is a powerful tool for the identification of novel and diverse hits; these hits are usually only active in the μM range. The weak activity of the obtained hits is not necessarily a drawback of VS. With the help of VS, promising lead scaffold can be obtained which can be subsequently optimized during the lead

optimization studies. Here, mostly more accurate and computationally expensive methods are applied. There are diverse limitations of structure-based drug design, which need to be considered and addressed, if possible.

(a) The main docking programs do not take protein flexibility into account; on the other hand, docking programs which consider protein flexibility to some extent have been recently developed (e.g., GOLD [79], Induced Fit (Schrödinger) [111], AutoDock4 [112]). Alternatively, ensemble docking can be performed for overcoming the protein flexibility issue using either an ensemble of X-ray structures or snapshots retrieved from molecular dynamics (MD) simulations. However, both flexible docking and ensemble docking demand more computation time as to be infeasible for VS campaigns.

(b) The protonation states of the amino acids in the binding site should be carefully analyzed when protein preparation is performed. Particular attention has to be given to the protonation state and tautomeric form of histidine, if present in the binding site.

(c) The correct placement of water molecules within the binding site is still challenging. Analysis of the water molecules should always be done before starting any VS study.

(d) Docking score (scoring function) represents a prediction of the binding affinity of a determined docking pose. However, it does not account for (de)solvation and entropic contributions; as a consequence, docking scores usually fail in accuracy.

(e) Docking methods are usually able to provide good enrichment of active compounds; however, docking scores often show unsatisfactory/poor correlation with the experimentally determined binding affinity. More accurate methods such as binding free energy (BFE) calculations, instead, show better correlation. Even so, they are highly computationally expensive and time-consuming, hence not feasible for VS of huge databases. BFE calculation methods (e.g., MMPB(GB)SA and QM/MM-GBSA) [113] from different software, such as AMBER [114] and Schrödinger [115], can be employed for rescoring the top-ranked compounds.

(f) When active and inactive compounds are known, validation studies of the different software, different settings, and docking scores are highly recommended.

2. Pharmacophore-based VS:
   (a) Comparative VS studies using different pharmacophore modeling software have shown that they often result in highly variable hit lists; i.e., there is a small overlap between the pharmacophore hits obtained using different software. This is due to the difference in feature definition and search algorithm implemented in the diverse software. Therefore, it is recommended to employ different software or at least to screen different pharmacophore models [116].
   (b) If there are any known active and inactive ligands, it is highly recommended to evaluate and validate the ability of the generated pharmacophore models to discriminate between active and inactive ligands by screening them before running the pharmacophore screening. In case of absence of known inactive ligands, decoys represent a valuable alternative for benchmarking studies [117–120]. This could not be performed in the herein described example, since there were no reported active ligands. If the results of the validation tests are not satisfying, refine and improve the pharmacophore model(s) that fails, and test it again. Only the pharmacophore models that pass the validation screenings should be used for the subsequent VS campaigns. For validation, usually ROC curves and other useful statistics like area under the curve (AUC) and enrichment factors (EF) are calculated [121, 122].
3. Be careful when applying filters. Do not over-filter. It is important to remember that VS hits are only starting points for further optimization steps. Some physicochemical properties can also be later optimized.
   (a) In recent years, there is a growing tendency to remove promiscuous compounds from screening databases or from the obtained VS hits prior in vitro screening by using PAINS filter. However, it has to be noted that some concerns have been raised about the use of PAINS filters, since it can lead to discard high-quality chemical probes and drug candidates [123–125]. Indeed, PAINS were found among 6–7% of approved drugs [124, 125].
   (b) In the hereby described VS campaign, the compounds were filtered for positively charged N atoms (N^+) in order to fit in the aromatic cage. The right position of this group and the relative interaction formed in the binding site were also an important discriminator when analyzing the docking poses for selecting the compounds for in vitro testing. It should, however, be mentioned that

some reported inhibitors of methyllysine readers do not bear a lysine mimetic group, i.e., no protonated NH group. Co-crystal structures of these inhibitors in complex with the respective target protein show that an aromatic moiety of the inhibitor is responsible for the binding to the aromatic cage by undergoing π-π stacking.

References

1. Russo VEA, Martienssen RA, Riggs AD (1996) Epigenetic mechanisms of gene regulation. Cold Spring Harbor Laboratory Press, Plainview, NY, p 692
2. Egger G, Liang G, Aparicio A, Jones PA (2004) Epigenetics in human disease and prospects for epigenetic therapy. Nature 429 (6990):457–463. https://doi.org/10.1038/nature02625
3. Handy DE, Castro R, Loscalzo J (2011) Epigenetic modifications: basic mechanisms and role in cardiovascular disease. Circulation 123 (19):2145–2156. https://doi.org/10.1161/CIRCULATIONAHA.110.956839
4. Dawson MA, Kouzarides T (2012) Cancer epigenetics: from mechanism to therapy. Cell 150(1):12–27. https://doi.org/10.1016/j.cell.2012.06.013
5. Sharma S, Kelly TK, Jones PA (2010) Epigenetics in cancer. Carcinogenesis 31(1):27–36. https://doi.org/10.1093/carcin/bgp220
6. Lardenoije R, Iatrou A, Kenis G et al (2015) The epigenetics of aging and neurodegeneration. Prog Neurobiol 131:21–64. https://doi.org/10.1016/j.pneurobio.2015.05.002
7. Fogel O, Richard-Miceli C, Tost J (2017) Epigenetic changes in chronic inflammatory diseases. Adv Protein Chem Struct Biol 106:139–189. https://doi.org/10.1016/bs.apcsb.2016.09.003
8. Zhang Z, Zhang R (2015) Epigenetics in autoimmune diseases: pathogenesis and prospects for therapy. Autoimmun Rev 14 (10):854–863. https://doi.org/10.1016/j.autrev.2015.05.008
9. Nuhrenberg T, Gilsbach R, Preissl S et al (2014) Epigenetics in cardiac development, function, and disease. Cell Tissue Res 356 (3):585–600. https://doi.org/10.1007/s00441-014-1887-8
10. Jones PA, Issa JP, Baylin S (2016) Targeting the cancer epigenome for therapy. Nat Rev Genet 17(10):630–641. https://doi.org/10.1038/nrg.2016.93
11. Luger K, Mader AW, Richmond RK et al (1997) Crystal structure of the nucleosome core particle at 2.8 A resolution. Nature 389 (6648):251–260. https://doi.org/10.1038/38444
12. Kornberg RD, Lorch Y (1999) Twenty-five years of the nucleosome, fundamental particle of the eukaryote chromosome. Cell 98 (3):285–294. https://doi.org/10.1016/S0092-8674(00)81958-3
13. Cosgrove MS, Boeke JD, Wolberger C (2004) Regulated nucleosome mobility and the histone code. Nat Struct Mol Biol 11 (11):1037–1043. https://doi.org/10.1038/nsmb851
14. Rothbart SB, Strahl BD (2014) Interpreting the language of histone and DNA modifications. Biochim Biophys Acta 1839 (8):627–643. https://doi.org/10.1016/j.bbagrm.2014.03.001
15. Huang H, Sabari BR, Garcia BA et al (2014) SnapShot: histone modifications. Cell 159 (2):458–458.e1. https://doi.org/10.1016/j.cell.2014.09.037
16. Musselman CA, Lalonde ME, Cote J et al (2012) Perceiving the epigenetic landscape through histone readers. Nat Struct Mol Biol 19(12):1218–1227. https://doi.org/10.1038/nsmb.2436
17. Taverna SD, Li H, Ruthenburg AJ et al (2007) How chromatin-binding modules interpret histone modifications: lessons from professional pocket pickers. Nat Struct Mol Biol 14(11):1025–1040. https://doi.org/10.1038/nsmb1338
18. Patel DJ, Wang Z (2013) Readout of epigenetic modifications. Annu Rev Biochem 82:81–118. https://doi.org/10.1146/annurev-biochem-072711-165700
19. Brand M et al (2015) Small molecule inhibitors of bromodomain-acetyl-lysine interactions. ACS Chem Biol 10(1):22–39. https://doi.org/10.1021/cb500996u
20. James LI, Barsyte-Lovejoy D, Zhong N, Krichevsky L et al (2013) Discovery of a chemical probe for the L3MBTL3 methyllysine reader domain. Nat Chem Biol 9(3):184–191. https://doi.org/10.1038/nchembio.1157

21. James LI, Korboukh VK, Krichevsky L et al (2013) Small-molecule ligands of methyllysine binding proteins: optimization of selectivity for L3MBTL3. J Med Chem 56 (18):7358–7371. https://doi.org/10.1021/jm400919p
22. Herold JM, Wigle TJ, Norris JL et al (2011) Small-molecule ligands of methyl-lysine binding proteins. J Med Chem 54(7):2504–2511. https://doi.org/10.1021/jm200045v
23. Perfetti MT, Baughman BM, Dickson BM et al (2015) Identification of a fragment-like small molecule ligand for the methyl-lysine binding protein, 53BP1. ACS Chem Biol 10 (4):1072–1081. https://doi.org/10.1021/cb500956g
24. Bae N, Viviano M, Su X et al (2017) Developing Spindlin1 small-molecule inhibitors by using protein microarrays. Nat Chem Biol 13 (7):750–756. https://doi.org/10.1038/nchembio.2377
25. Robaa D, Wagner T, Luise C et al (2016) Identification and structure-activity relationship studies of small-molecule inhibitors of the methyllysine reader protein Spindlin1. ChemMedChem 11(20):2327–2338. https://doi.org/10.1002/cmdc.201600362
26. Wagner T, Greschik H, Burgahn T et al (2016) Identification of a small-molecule ligand of the epigenetic reader protein Spindlin1 via a versatile screening platform. Nucleic Acids Res 44(9):e88. https://doi.org/10.1093/nar/gkw089
27. Ren C, Morohashi K, Plotnikov AN et al (2015) Small-molecule modulators of methyl-lysine binding for the CBX7 chromodomain. Chem Biol 22(2):161–168. https://doi.org/10.1016/j.chembiol.2014
28. Ren C, Smith SG, Kyoko Y et al (2016) Structure-guided discovery of selective antagonists for the chromodomain of polycomb repressive protein CBX7. ACS Med Chem Lett 7(6):601–605. https://doi.org/10.1021/acsmedchemlett.6b00042
29. Wagner T, Robaa D, Sippl W et al (2014) Mind the methyl: methyllysine binding proteins in epigenetic regulation. ChemMedChem 9(3):466–483. https://doi.org/10.1002/cmdc.201300422
30. Milosevich N, Hof F (2016) Chemical inhibitors of epigenetic methyllysine reader proteins. Biochemistry 55(11):1570–1583. https://doi.org/10.1021/acs.biochem.5b01073
31. Teske KA, Hadden MK (2017) Methyllysine binding domains: structural insight and small molecule probe development. Eur J Med Chem 136:14–35. https://doi.org/10.1016/j.ejmech.2017.04.047
32. Andreoli F, Del Rio A (2015) Computer-aided molecular design of compounds targeting histone modifying enzymes. Comput Struct Biotechnol J 13:358–365. https://doi.org/10.1016/j.csbj.2015.04.007
33. Medina-Franco JL (2016) Epi-informatics: discovery and development of small molecule epigenetic drugs and probes. Elsevier, Amsterdam, p 424
34. Kannan S, Melesina J, Hauser AT et al (2014) Discovery of inhibitors of Schistosoma mansoni HDAC8 by combining homology modeling, virtual screening, and in vitro validation. J Chem Inf Model 54 (10):3005–3019. https://doi.org/10.1021/ci5004653
35. Bowers EM, Yan G, Mukherjee C et al (2010) Virtual ligand screening of the p300/CBP histone acetyltransferase: identification of a selective small molecule inhibitor. Chem Biol 17(5):471–482. https://doi.org/10.1016/j.chembiol.2010.03.006
36. Pulla VK, Alvala M, Sriram DS et al (2014) Structure-based drug design of small molecule SIRT1 modulators to treat cancer and metabolic disorders. J Mol Graph Model 52:46–56. https://doi.org/10.1016/j.jmgm.2014.06.005
37. Pulla VK, Sriram DS, Viswanadha S et al (2016) Energy-based pharmacophore and three-dimensional quantitative structure-activity relationship (3D-QSAR) modeling combined with virtual screening to identify novel small-molecule inhibitors of silent mating-type information regulation 2 homologue 1 (SIRT1). J Chem Inf Model 56 (1):173–187. https://doi.org/10.1021/acs.jcim.5b00220
38. Schiedel M, Rumpf T, Karaman B et al (2016) Structure-based development of an affinity probe for Sirtuin 2. Angew Chem Int Ed Engl 55(6):2252–2256. https://doi.org/10.1002/anie.201509843
39. Uciechowska U, Schemies J, Neugebauer RC et al (2008) Thiobarbiturates as sirtuin inhibitors: virtual screening, free-energy calculations, and biological testing. ChemMedChem 3(12):1965–1976. https://doi.org/10.1002/cmdc.200800104
40. Parenti MD, Grozio A, Bauer I et al (2014) Discovery of novel and selective SIRT6 inhibitors. J Med Chem 57(11):4796–4804. https://doi.org/10.1021/jm500487d
41. Heinke R, Spannhoff A, Meier R et al (2009) Virtual screening and biological

characterization of novel histone arginine methyltransferase PRMT1 inhibitors. ChemMedChem 4(1):69–77. https://doi.org/10.1002/cmdc.200800301
42. Spannhoff A, Heinke R, Bauer I et al (2007) Target-based approach to inhibitors of histone arginine methyltransferases. J Med Chem 50(10):2319–2325. https://doi.org/10.1021/jm061250e
43. Roatsch M, Robaa D, Pippel M et al (2016) Substituted 2-(2-aminopyrimidin-4-yl)pyridine-4-carboxylates as potent inhibitors of JumonjiC domain-containing histone demethylases. Future Med Chem 8 (13):1553–1571. https://doi.org/10.4155/fmc.15.188
44. Kireev D, Wigle TJ, Norris-Drouin J et al (2010) Identification of non-peptide malignant brain tumor (MBT) repeat antagonists by virtual screening of commercially available compounds. J Med Chem 53 (21):7625–7631. https://doi.org/10.1021/jm1007374
45. Wang W, Chen Z, Mao Z et al (2011) Nucleolar protein Spindlin1 recognizes H3K4 methylation and stimulates the expression of rRNA genes. EMBO Rep 12 (11):1160–1166. https://doi.org/10.1038/embor.2011.184
46. Yang N, Wang W, Wang Y et al (2012) Distinct mode of methylated lysine-4 of histone H3 recognition by tandem tudor-like domains of Spindlin1. Proc Natl Acad Sci U S A 109(44):17954–17959. https://doi.org/10.1073/pnas.1208517109
47. Su X, Zhu G, Ding X et al (2014) Molecular basis underlying histone H3 lysine-arginine methylation pattern readout by Spin/Ssty repeats of Spindlin1. Genes Dev 28 (6):622–636. https://doi.org/10.1101/gad.233239.113
48. Shanle EK, Shinsky SA, Bridgers JB et al (2017) Histone peptide microarray screen of chromo and Tudor domains defines new histone lysine methylation interactions. Epigenetics Chromatin 10:12. https://doi.org/10.1186/s13072-017-0117-5
49. Jiang F, Zhao Q, Qin L et al (2006) Expression, purification, crystallization and preliminary X-ray analysis of human spindlin1, an ovarian cancer-related protein. Protein Pept Lett 13(2):203–205. https://doi.org/10.2174/092986606775101661
50. Wang JX, Zeng Q, Chen L et al (2012) SPINDLIN1 promotes cancer cell proliferation through activation of WNT/TCF-4 signaling. Mol Cancer Res 10(3):326–335. https://doi.org/10.1158/1541-7786.MCR-11-0440
51. Franz H, Greschik H, Willmann D et al (2015) The histone code reader SPIN1 controls RET signaling in liposarcoma. Oncotarget 6(7):4773–4789. https://doi.org/10.18632/oncotarget.3000
52. Drago-Ferrante R, Pentimalli F, Carlisi D et al (2017) Suppressive role exerted by microRNA-29b-1-5p in triple negative breast cancer through SPIN1 regulation. Oncotarget 8 (17):28939–28958. https://doi.org/10.18632/oncotarget.15960
53. Chen X, Wang YW, Xing AY et al (2016) Suppression of SPIN1-mediated PI3K-Akt pathway by miR-489 increases chemosensitivity in breast cancer. J Pathol 239(4):459–472. https://doi.org/10.1002/path.4743
54. Yuan H, Zhang P, Qin L et al (2008) Overexpression of SPINDLIN1 induces cellular senescence, multinucleation and apoptosis. Gene 410(1):67–74. https://doi.org/10.1016/j.gene.2007.11.019
55. Zhang P, Cong B, Yuan H et al (2008) Overexpression of spindlin1 induces metaphase arrest and chromosomal instability. J Cell Physiol 217(2):400–408. https://doi.org/10.1002/jcp.21515
56. Zhao Q, Qin L, Jiang F et al (2007) Structure of human spindlin1. Tandem tudor-like domains for cell cycle regulation. J Biol Chem 282(1):647–656. https://doi.org/10.1074/jbc.M604029200
57. Shoichet BK (2004) Virtual screening of chemical libraries. Nature 432 (7019):862–865. https://doi.org/10.1038/nature03197
58. Wermuth CG, Ganellin CR, Lindberg P et al (1998) Glossary of terms used in Medicinal Chemistry (IUPAC Recommendations 1998). Pure Appl Chem 70(5):1129–1143. https://doi.org/10.1351/pac199870051129
59. Vuorinen A, Schuster D (2015) Methods for generating and applying pharmacophore models as virtual screening filters and for bioactivity profiling. Methods 71:113–134. https://doi.org/10.1016/j.ymeth.2014.10.013
60. Wolber G, Langer T (2005) LigandScout: 3-D pharmacophores derived from protein-bound Ligands and their use as virtual screening filters. J Chem Inf Model 45(1):160–169. https://doi.org/10.1021/ci049885e
61. Molecular Operating Environment (MOE), 2013.08; Chemical Computing Group

ULC, 1010 Sherbooke St. West, Suite #910, Montreal, QC, Canada, H3A 2R7 2017
62. Dixon SL, Smondyrev AM, Knoll EH et al (2006) PHASE: a new engine for pharmacophore perception, 3D QSAR model development, and 3D database screening: 1. Methodology and preliminary results. J Comput Aided Mol Des 20 (10–11):647–671. https://doi.org/10.1007/s10822-006-9087-6
63. Dixon SL, Smondyrev AM, Rao SN (2006) PHASE: a novel approach to pharmacophore modeling and 3D database searching. Chem Biol Drug Des 67(5):370–372. https://doi.org/10.1111/j.1747-0285.2006.00384.x
64. Godden JW, Furr JR, Xue L et al (2004) Molecular similarity analysis and virtual screening by mapping of consensus positions in binary-transformed chemical descriptor spaces with variable dimensionality. J Chem Inf Comput Sci 44(1):21–29. https://doi.org/10.1021/ci0302963
65. Barnum D, Greene J, Smellie A, Sprague P (1996) Identification of common functional configurations among molecules. J Chem Inf Comput Sci 36(3):563–571. https://doi.org/10.1021/ci950273r
66. Koes DR, Camacho CJ (2011) Pharmer: efficient and exact pharmacophore search. J Chem Inf Model 51(6):1307–1314. https://doi.org/10.1021/ci200097m
67. Cheng T, Li Q, Zhou Z et al (2012) Structure-based virtual screening for drug discovery: a problem-centric review. AAPS J 14 (1):133–141. https://doi.org/10.1208/s12248-012-9322-0
68. Cole JC et al (2011) The basis for target-based virtual screening: protein structures, in Virtual Screening Wiley-VCH Verlag GmbH p 87–114
69. Berman HM, Westbrook J, Feng Z et al (2000) The protein data bank. Nucleic Acids Res 28(1):235–242
70. www.rcsb.org
71. Wilks ES (1995) Polymer Nomenclature and Structure - a Comparison of Systems Used by Chemical Abstracts Service, the International Union of Pure and Applied Chemistry, Mdl-Information-Systems-Inc, and Dupont. Abstracts of Papers of the American Chemical Society, 210:27-Cinf
72. Sali A, Blundell TL (1993) Comparative protein modelling by satisfaction of spatial restraints. J Mol Biol 234(3):779–815. https://doi.org/10.1006/jmbi.1993.1626
73. Biasini M, Bienert S, Waterhouse A et al (2014) SWISS-MODEL: modelling protein tertiary and quaternary structure using evolutionary information. Nucleic Acids Res 42 (Web Server issue):W252–W258. https://doi.org/10.1093/nar/gku340
74. Verdonk ML, Berdini V, Hartshorn MJ et al (2004) Virtual screening using protein-ligand docking: avoiding artificial enrichment. J Chem Inf Comput Sci 44(3):793–806. https://doi.org/10.1021/ci034289q
75. Chen YC (2015) Beware of docking! Trends Pharmacol Sci 36(2):78–95. https://doi.org/10.1016/j.tips.2014
76. Friesner RA, Banks JL, Murphy RB et al (2004) Glide: a new approach for rapid, accurate docking and scoring. 1. Method and assessment of docking accuracy. J Med Chem 47(7):1739–1749. https://doi.org/10.1021/jm0306430
77. Halgren TA, Murphy RB, Friesner RA et al (2004) Glide: a new approach for rapid, accurate docking and scoring. 2. Enrichment factors in database screening. J Med Chem 47 (7):1750–1759. https://doi.org/10.1021/jm030644s
78. Small-Molecule Drug Discovery Suite 2014–1 (2014) Glide, version 6.2, Schrödinger, LLC, New York, NY
79. Jones G, Willett P, Glen RC et al (1997) Development and validation of a genetic algorithm for flexible docking. J Mol Biol 267 (3):727–748. https://doi.org/10.1006/jmbi.1996.0897
80. Irwin JJ, Shoichet BK, Mysinger MM et al (2009) Automated docking screens: a feasibility study. J Med Chem 52(18):5712–5720. https://doi.org/10.1021/jm9006966
81. Trott O, Olson AJ (2010) AutoDock Vina: improving the speed and accuracy of docking with a new scoring function, efficient optimization, and multithreading. J Comput Chem 31(2):455–461. https://doi.org/10.1002/jcc.21334
82. Morris GM, Huey R, Lindstrom W et al (2009) AutoDock4 and AutoDockTools4: automated docking with selective receptor flexibility. J Comput Chem 30 (16):2785–2791. https://doi.org/10.1002/jcc.21256
83. Lill M (2013) Virtual screening in drug design. In: Kortagere S (ed) In silico models for drug discovery. Humana Press, Totowa, NJ, pp 1–12
84. Eckert H, Bajorath J (2007) Molecular similarity analysis in virtual screening: foundations, limitations and novel approaches. Drug Discov Today 12(5–6):225–233.

https://doi.org/10.1016/j.drudis.2007.01.011

85. Durant JL, Leland BA, Henry DR et al (2002) Reoptimization of MDL keys for use in drug discovery. J Chem Inf Comput Sci 42 (6):1273–1280. https://doi.org/10.1021/ci010132r
86. Irwin JJ, Sterling T, Mysinger MM et al (2012) ZINC: a free tool to discover chemistry for biology. J Chem Inf Model 52 (7):1757–1768. https://doi.org/10.1021/ci3001277
87. Sterling T, Irwin JJ (2015) ZINC 15-ligand discovery for everyone. J Chem Inf Model 55 (11):2324–2337. https://doi.org/10.1021/acs.jcim.5b00559
88. http://www.chemspider.com/
89. https://cactus.nci.nih.gov/download/nci/
90. Groom CR, Bruno IJ, Lightfoot MP, Ward SC (2016) The Cambridge structural database. Acta Crystallogr B 72(2):171–179. https://doi.org/10.1107/S2052520616003954
91. http://www.chemdiv.com/screening-libraries/
92. http://www.princetonbio.com/
93. http://www.maybridge.com/
94. Lipinski CA, Lombardo F, Dominy BW, Feeney PJ (2001) Experimental and computational approaches to estimate solubility and permeability in drug discovery and development settings. Adv Drug Deliv Rev 46 (1–3):3–26. https://doi.org/10.1016/S0169-409X(00)00129-0
95. Oprea TI (2000) Property distribution of drug-related chemical databases. J Comput Aided Mol Des 14(3):251–264. https://doi.org/10.1023/A:1008130001697
96. Baell J, Walters MA (2014) Chemistry: chemical con artists foil drug discovery. Nature 513 (7519):481–483. https://doi.org/10.1038/513481a
97. Baell JB, Holloway GA (2010) New substructure filters for removal of pan assay interference compounds (PAINS) from screening libraries and for their exclusion in bioassays. J Med Chem 53(7):2719–2740. https://doi.org/10.1021/jm901137j
98. Dahlin JL, Inglese J, Walters MA (2015) Mitigating risk in academic preclinical drug discovery. Nat Rev Drug Discov 14(4):279–294. https://doi.org/10.1038/nrd4578
99. Hawkins PCD, Skillman AG, Warren GL et al (2010) Conformer generation with OMEGA: algorithm and validation using high quality structures from the protein databank and Cambridge structural database. J Chem Inf Model 50(4):572–584. https://doi.org/10.1021/ci100031x
100. Meier R, Pippel M, Brandt F et al (2010) ParaDockS: a framework for molecular docking with population-based metaheuristics. J Chem Inf Model 50(5):879–889. https://doi.org/10.1021/ci900467x
101. Corbeil CR, Williams CI, Labute P (2012) Variability in docking success rates due to dataset preparation. J Comput Aided Mol Des 26(6):775–786. https://doi.org/10.1007/s10822-012-9570-1
102. Schrödinger Release 2014–2 (2014) Protein Preparation Wizard, Epik version 2.8, Impact version 6.3, Prime version 3.6; Schrödinger, LLC, New York, NY
103. Sastry GM, Adzhigirey M, Day T et al (2013) Protein and ligand preparation: parameters, protocols, and influence on virtual screening enrichments. J Comput Aided Mol Des 27 (3):221–234. https://doi.org/10.1007/s10822-013-9644-8
104. Schrödinger Release 2014–1 (2014) Epik, version 2.8, Schrödinger, LLC, New York, NY
105. Greenwood JR, Calkins D, Sullivan AP, Shelley JC (2010) Towards the comprehensive, rapid, and accurate prediction of the favorable tautomeric states of drug-like molecules in aqueous solution. J Comput Aided Mol Des 24(6–7):591–604. https://doi.org/10.1007/s10822-010-9349-1
106. Shelley JC, Cholleti A, Frye LL et al (2007) Epik: a software program for pK a prediction and protonation state generation for drug-like molecules. J Comput Aided Mol Des 21 (12):681–691. https://doi.org/10.1007/s10822-007-9133-z
107. Banks JL, Beard HS, Cao Y et al (2005) Integrated modeling program, applied chemical theory (IMPACT). J Comput Chem 26 (16):1752–1780. https://doi.org/10.1002/jcc.20292
108. Cereto-Massague A, Ojeda MJ, Valls C et al (2015) Molecular fingerprint similarity search in virtual screening. Methods 71:58–63. https://doi.org/10.1016/j.ymeth.2014.08.005
109. Muegge I, Mukherjee P (2016) An overview of molecular fingerprint similarity search in virtual screening. Expert Opin Drug Discov 11(2):137–148. https://doi.org/10.1517/17460441.2016.1117070
110. Schrödinger Release 2014–1 (2014) Canvas, version 1.9, Schrödinger, LLC, New York, NY

111. Sherman W, Day T, Jacobson MP et al (2006) Novel procedure for modeling ligand/receptor induced fit effects. J Med Chem 49 (2):534–553. https://doi.org/10.1021/jm050540c
112. Osterberg F, Morris GM, Sanner MF et al (2002) Automated docking to multiple target structures: incorporation of protein mobility and structural water heterogeneity in AutoDock. Proteins 46(1):34–40. https://doi.org/10.1002/prot.10028
113. Genheden S, Ryde U (2015) The MM/PBSA and MM/GBSA methods to estimate ligand-binding affinities. Exp Opin Drug Discov 10 (5):449–461. https://doi.org/10.1517/17460441.2015.1032936
114. Case DA, Cheatham TE III, Darden TA, Duke RE, Giese TJ, Gohlke H et al (2017) AMBER 2017. University of California, San Francisco, CA
115. Schrödinger Release 2017-1 (2017) Prime, Schrödinger, LLC, New York, NY
116. Spitzer GM, Heiss M, Mangold M et al (2010) One concept, three implementations of 3D pharmacophore-based virtual screening: distinct coverage of chemical search space. J Chem Inf Model 50(7):1241–1247. https://doi.org/10.1021/ci100136b
117. Mysinger MM, Carchia M, Irwin JJ et al (2012) Directory of useful decoys, enhanced (DUD-E): better ligands and decoys for better benchmarking. J Med Chem 55 (14):6582–6594. https://doi.org/10.1021/jm300687e
118. Cereto-Massague A, Guasch L, Valls C et al (2012) DecoyFinder: an easy-to-use python GUI application for building target-specific decoy sets. Bioinformatics 28 (12):1661–1662. https://doi.org/10.1093/bioinformatics/bts249
119. Graves AP, Brenk R, Shoichet BK (2005) Decoys for docking. J Med Chem 48 (11):3714–3728. https://doi.org/10.1021/jm0491187
120. Wallach I, Lilien R (2011) Virtual decoy sets for molecular docking benchmarks. J Chem Inf Model 51(2):196–202. https://doi.org/10.1021/ci100374f
121. Truchon JF, Bayly CI (2007) Evaluating virtual screening methods: good and bad metrics for the "early recognition" problem. J Chem Inf Model 47(2):488–508. https://doi.org/10.1021/ci600426e
122. Clark RD, Webster-Clark DJ (2008) Managing bias in ROC curves. J Comput Aided Mol Des 22(3–4):141–146. https://doi.org/10.1007/s10822-008-9181-z
123. Lagorce D, Oliveira N, Miteva MA, Villoutreix BO (2017) Pan-assay interference compounds (PAINS) that may not be too painful for chemical biology projects. Drug Discov Today 22(8):1131–1133. https://doi.org/10.1016/j.drudis.2017.05.017
124. Capuzzi SJ, Muratov EN, Tropsha A (2017) Phantom PAINS: problems with the utility of alerts for pan-assay INterference CompoundS. J Chem Inf Model 57(3):417–427. https://doi.org/10.1021/acs.jcim.6b00465
125. Senger MR et al (2016) Filtering promiscuous compounds in early drug discovery: is it a good idea? Drug Discov Today 21 (6):868–872. https://doi.org/10.1016/j.drudis.2016.02.004

Chapter 22

Designing Natural Product Hybrids Bearing Triple Antiplatelet Profile and Evaluating Their Human Plasma Stability

Antonis Tsiailanis, Maria Tsoumani, Evgenios K. Stylos, Maria V. Chatziathanasiadou, Tahsin F. Kellici, Thomas Mavromoustakos, Alexandros D. Tselepis, and Andreas G. Tzakos

Abstract

Cardiovascular diseases (CVDs) are becoming major contributors to the burden of disease due to genetic and environmental factors. Despite current standard oral care, cardiovascular risk remains relatively high. A triple antiplatelet therapy with a cyclooxygenase-1 (COX-1) inhibitor, a $P2Y_{12}$ receptor antagonist, and a protease-activated receptor-1 (PAR-1) antagonist has been established in the secondary prevention of atherothrombosis in patients with acute myocardial infraction and in those with peripheral artery disease. However, due to the combinatorial use of three different drugs, patients receiving this triple therapy are exposed to enhanced risk of bleeding. Conforming to polypharmacology principles, the discovery of a single compound that can simultaneously block the three platelet activation pathways (PAR-1, $P2Y_{12}$, and COX-1) is of importance. Natural products have served as an inexhaustible source of bioactive compounds presenting a diverse pharmaceutical profile, including anti-inflammatory, antioxidant, anticancer, and antithrombotic activity. Indeed, principal component analysis indicated that natural products have the potential to inhibit the three aforementioned pathways, though existed reports refer to single inhibition mechanism on specific receptor(s) implicated in platelet activation. We thus set out to explore possibilities that take advantage of this potential of natural products and shape the basis to produce novel compounds that could simultaneously target PAR-1, $P2Y_{12}$, and COX-1 platelet activation pathways. Polyunsaturated fatty acids (PUFAs) have multiple effects leading to improvements in blood pressure and cardiac function and arterial compliance. A promising approach to achieve the desirable goal is the bioconjugation of natural products with PUFAs. Herein, we describe the principles that should be followed to develop molecular hybrids bearing triple antiplatelet activity profile.

Key words Triple antiplatelet activity, Flavonoids, Liquid chromatography, Plasma stability, LC-MS, Polyunsaturated fatty acids

1 Introduction

Antiplatelet therapy possesses a significant role in the current drug-oriented treatment of cardiovascular diseases (CVD) [1]. The

Thomas Mavromoustakos and Tahsin F. Kellici (eds.), *Rational Drug Design: Methods and Protocols*, Methods in Molecular Biology, vol. 1824, https://doi.org/10.1007/978-1-4939-8630-9_22,

recent guidelines of the European Society of Cardiology and the American Heart Association recommend that patients with an acute coronary syndrome (ACS) should be treated with dual antiplatelet therapy receiving an ADP receptor antagonist (ticagrelor, prasugrel, or clopidogrel) and aspirin [2]. Also, very recently the FDA approved the use of vorapaxar, a PAR-1 antagonist, on top of the dual antiplatelet therapy with clopidogrel and aspirin in the secondary prevention of atherothrombosis and acute myocardial infarction [3]. Despite the use of dual antiplatelet therapy (consisting of aspirin and a $P2Y_{12}$ receptor antagonist), residual CVD still remains [4]. Recently, trials have tested the hypothesis whether the simultaneous use of three antiplatelet agents, i.e., a cyclooxygenase (COX)-2 inhibitor (aspirin), a $P2Y_{12}$ receptor antagonist (clopidogrel), and a protease-activated receptor-1 (PAR-1) antagonist (vorapaxar), could represent a more efficient approach for the secondary prevention of atherothrombotic events. Nonetheless, this triple antiplatelet regimen is associated with an increased risk of moderate or severe bleeding [5, 6]. Therefore, it is of utmost importance the development of novel antiplatelet agents with increased efficacy and safety profile that can inhibit simultaneously the three pathways but also reduce bleeding complications.

Recently, our group [7] demonstrated the capacity of an olive leaf extract to efficiently inhibit platelet aggregation and also determined the plant extract components responsible for this platelet inhibition profile mediated through the $P2Y_{12}$ and PAR-1 receptors. This suggested that natural products, derived from plants, could serve as potent compounds with inhibitory platelet activity. Flavonoids, a diverse class of natural products, not only are correlated with lower risk of CVD when they are present in high levels in dietary sources [8, 9], but they also bear important platelet antiaggregatory activities. Despite the therapeutic potential of natural products, their application in medicine is limited due to their low bioavailability, as the numerous phenol groups impede their transportation through the lipophilic cell membrane [10]. In our recent study [11], we established a novel hybrid that inhibited platelet aggregation by conjugating the flavonoid naringenin to the omega-3 fatty acid 4′-docosahexaenoic (DHA). Here, we summarize the criteria for the effective design, development, and, in particular, the principles that influence the selection of a flavonoid hybrid for multiple antiplatelet activity. In order to assess which natural product bears a potential triple antiplatelet activity, in silico studies were performed. In silico calculations have been increasingly deployed in unraveling the mechanism of action of natural compounds. To explore the chemical space sampled by the hybrids and to allow a visual representation of their location in the chemical space defined by different approved antithrombotic drugs and the parent compound, principal component analysis (PCA) was conducted. After the chemical synthesis of the hybrid, human plasma stability studies were conducted, in order to evaluate its stability. Finally, the antiplatelet profile of the hybrid was tested through an in vitro platelet aggregation assay using established agonists of $P2Y_{12}$ receptor, PAR-1 and cyclooxygenase-1.

2 Materials

2.1 In Silico Studies of Natural Compounds

1. All compounds along with conjugates are sketched using Schrödinger Release 2015-2, Maestro Version 10.5 [12] and minimized using Schrödinger Release 2015-2, LigPrep 3.4 [13], and the OPLS3 [14] force field.
2. The topological, physicochemical descriptors as also the descriptors that predict the absorption, distribution, metabolism, and excretion of the compounds are calculated using the Small-Molecule Drug Discovery Suite 2015-2, QikProp 4.4 [15].
3. The PCA is performed using the cheminformatics package Schrödinger Release 2015-2, Canvas 2.4 [16].

2.2 Synthesis, Purification, and Characterization of Polyphenolic Conjugate

1. Naringenin, *cis*-4,7,10,13,16,19-docosahexaenoic acid (DHA).
2. Trifluoroacetic acid (peptide synthesis grade).
3. N,N′-Dicyclohexylcarbodiimide (DCC).
4. Dimethylaminopyridine (DMAP).
5. HPLC Dionex UltiMate 3000.
6. EVOQ Elite ER triple quadrupole mass spectrometer.

2.3 Liquid Chromatography and Mass Spectrometry

1. Rosmarinic acid (internal standard).
2. Regenerated cellulose membrane syringe filters 0.2 μm.
3. Cellulose nitrate filters, 0.2 μm pore size, for mobile phase filtering.
4. Methanol, water, and formic acid (LC-MS grade).
5. Mobile phase A: water containing 0.1% (v/v) formic acid.
6. Mobile phase B: methanol containing 0.1% (v/v) formic acid
7. Drug-free human plasma for the stability studies.
8. C18 column 100 mm × 2.1 mm, 2.6 μm, with proguard column 2.1 mm.
9. Triple quadrupole mass spectrometer coupled to ultra-high performance liquid chromatography (UHPLC) system is utilized for the detection and quantification of the compounds.

2.4 Platelet Preparation and Activation

2.4.1 Buffers

1. Use as anticoagulant acid citrate dextrose (ACD) solution, which consists of 75 mM trisodium citrate dihydrate, 42 mM citric acid monohydrate, and 139 mM anhydrous D(+)glucose. To prepare this anticoagulant, dissolve 2.2 g of trisodium citrate dihydrate, 0.8 g of citric acid monohydrate, and 2.5 g of anhydrous D(+)glucose in distilled H_2O in a final volume of 100 mL.
2. Prepare 10 mM PBS (pH 7.4) by dissolving 8.1816 g NaCl, 1.3800 g $NaH_2PO4\ H_2O$, and 1.7795 g $Na_2HPO4\ 2H_2O$ in 1 L of distilled H_2O, and adjust pH to 7.4.
3. Prepare 1% (w/v) ammonium oxalate solution by dissolving 0.5 g of ammonium oxalate in 50 mL of distilled H_2O and used for platelet count.

2.4.2 Platelet Agonists

1. **Adenosine diphosphate (ADP)**: Prepare a stock solution of 10 mM of ADP by dissolving 2.5 mg ADP in 5 mL of normal saline. Store this solution in aliquots at −80 °C. Aliquots of this solution are diluted 1:10 (v/v) with normal saline to prepare working solutions of 1 mM ADP which are also stored in aliquots at −80 °C. For the platelet aggregation assays, add 5 μL from the working solution to 495 μL sample in order to obtain 10 μM ADP, final concentration.
2. **Arachidonic acid (AA)**: This reagent is supplied as 10 mg in ampule with a purity of higher than 98.5%. Prepare a stock solution of 50 mM of AA solution by reconstitution with 655 μL absolute ethanol. Store the reconstituted AA reagent frozen in aliquots in the dark at −80 °C. For platelet aggregation assay, add 5 μL of the stock solution to 495 μL sample in order to obtain 500 μM AA, final concentration.
3. **Thrombin receptor-activating peptide-6 (TRAP-6)**: This reagent is supplied as 5 mg in a vial. Prepare a stock solution of 5 mM of TRAP-6 by reconstitution with 1335 μL of normal saline. Store this solution in aliquots at −80 °C. Aliquots of this solution are diluted 1:5 (v/v) with normal saline to prepare working solutions of 1 mM TRAP-6, which are also stored in aliquots at −80 °C. For the platelet aggregation assays, add 5 μL from the working solution to 495 μL of sample in order to obtain 10 μM TRAP-6, final concentration.

2.4.3 Antibodies

Fluorescently labeled monoclonal antibodies are PAC-1-FITC, anti-CD62P-PE, and anti-CD61-PerCP.

3 Methods

3.1 Principal Component Analysis (PCA)

1. Select representative antithrombotic drugs (Fig. 1) that act as $P2Y_{12}$ receptor antagonists (ticlopidine, prasugrel, clopidogrel, and their active metabolites ticagrelor and cangrelor), glycoprotein IIb/IIIa inhibitors (eptifibatide, tirofiban), phosphodiesterase inhibitors (dipyridamole, cilostazol), PAR-1 antagonists (vorapaxar, atopaxar), and cyclooxygenase-1 inhibitors (triflusal, acetyl salicylic acid), for the PCA.
2. Explore the chemical property space of 13 approved antithrombotic drugs bearing different mode of action: COX-1 inhibitors, ADP receptor $P2Y_{12}$ antagonists, and PAR-1 antagonists (*see* **Note 1**).
3. Calculate a set of 8 physicochemical and stereochemical properties for all 13 compounds using QikProp 4.4: molecular weight (MW), hydrogen bond donors (HBD), hydrogen bond acceptors (HBA), predicted octanol/water partition coefficient ($logP_{oct/wat}$), predicted aqueous solubility (logS), polar surface area (PSA), and the total solvent accessible surface divided in its hydrophobic (FOSA) and hydrophilic (FISA) components (Fig. 2).
4. Perform the PCA using the cheminformatics package Canvas 2.4 (Figs. 3 and 4).

3.2 Synthesis of DHA-Polyphenol Hybrids

1. Flavonoids bearing phenol hydroxyl groups able to be conjugated with the carboxylic group of DHA using dicyclohexylcarbodiimide (DCC) as the coupling reagent and 4-dimethylaminopyridine (DMAP) as the catalyst as shown in Fig. 5 (Steglich esterification) (*see* **Note 2**). Thin-layer chromatography (TLC) shows the formation of a new spot and almost consumption of the starting material.
2. Conduct the purification with high-performance liquid chromatography (HPLC) using the Chromeleon program (*see* **Note 3**).
3. Perform the characterization of the analogue with ^{1}H-NMR and ^{13}C-NMR spectroscopy. A Bruker AV-500 spectrometer equipped with a TXI CryoProbe and a Bruker Advance 400 MHz spectrometer equipped with a z-gradient unit (Bruker BioSpin, Rheinstetten, Germany) are used. The NMR system is controlled by the software TopSpin 2.1.

3.3 Liquid Chromatography and Mass Spectrometry Operational Conditions for DHA-Polyphenol Analogue

1. Dissolve the compounds in 80:20 (H_2O:MeOH) solvent at a concentration of 0.1 mg/mL for direct infusion in the MS, in order to determine the fragmentation pattern (transitions) of the parent compounds, for their determination and quantitation, in the multiple reaction monitoring (MRM) mode of the mass spectrometer.

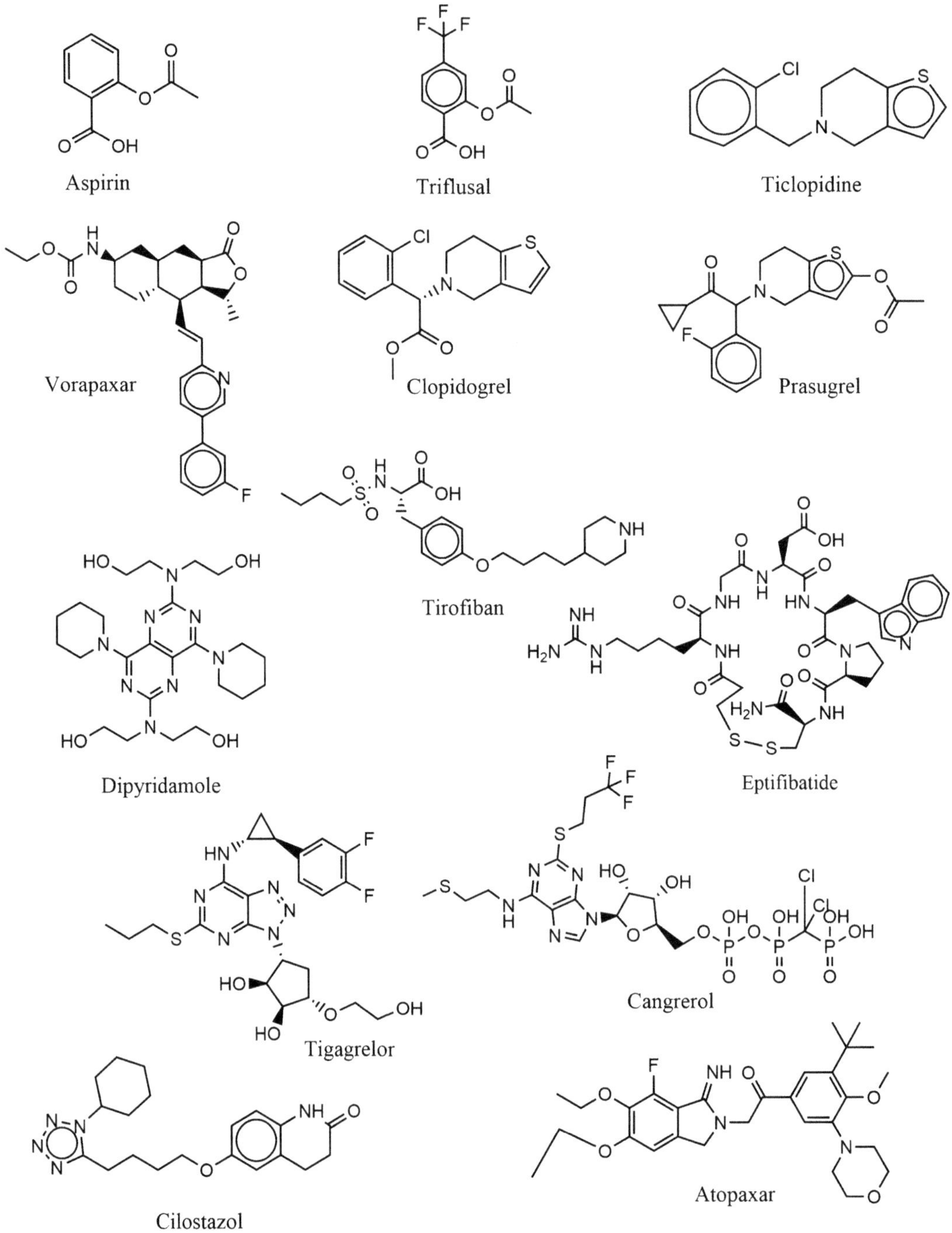

Fig. 1 Structures of antithrombotic drugs used for the PCA

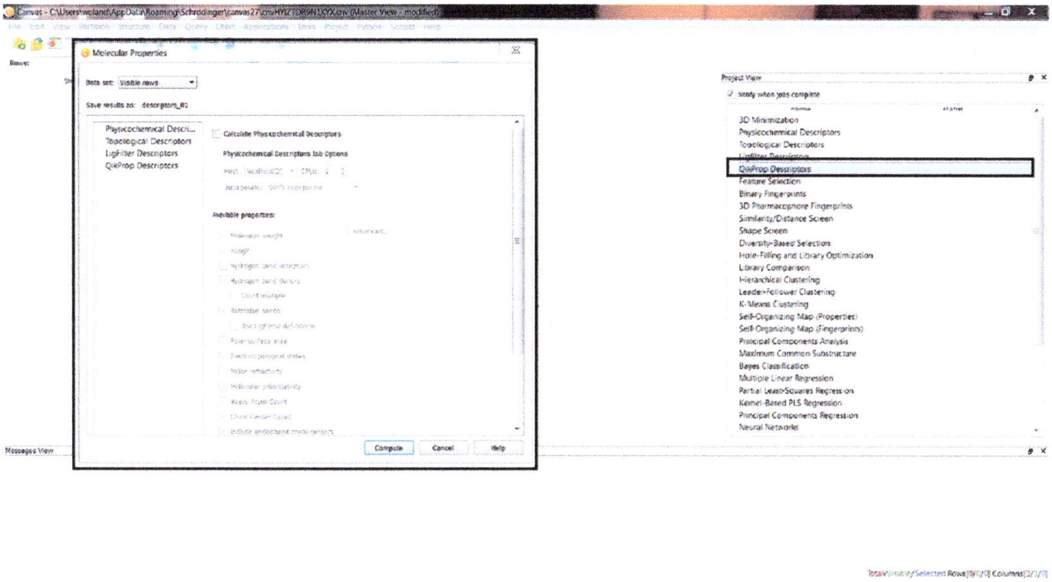

Fig. 2 The Canvas workspace. After importing the sketched structures in Canvas, right-click on the "QikProp Descriptors" button and press "Open". The "Molecular Properties" window will appear. Select the desired descriptors and press "Compute"

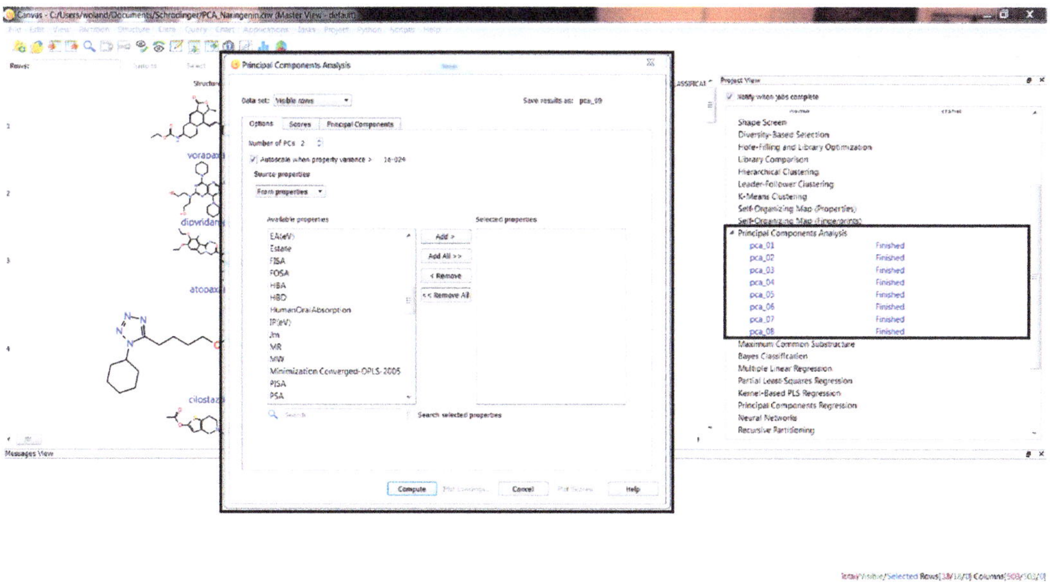

Fig. 3 After computing the chosen descriptors, right-click on the "Principal Components Analysis" button and press "Open". In the window that appears, you can select the number of principal components you want to use as well as the source of these properties that can be fingerprints or properties. After we have computed the properties, we will select this option. After selecting the desired properties that will be used in the PCA, we press "Add" and then "Compute." The PCA is then visualized by pressing "Plot Scores"

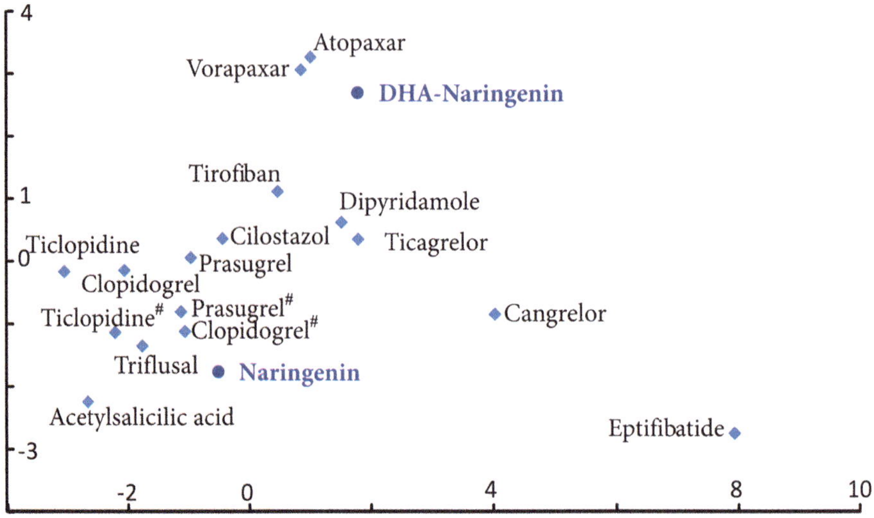

Fig. 4 PCA of the antithrombotic drugs (blue diamond). (#) pinpoints the metabolites of the relevant drugs. The DHA-naringenin and naringenin are illustrated as purple bullets (This figure is modified from the corresponding work of *Stylos* et al.) [11]

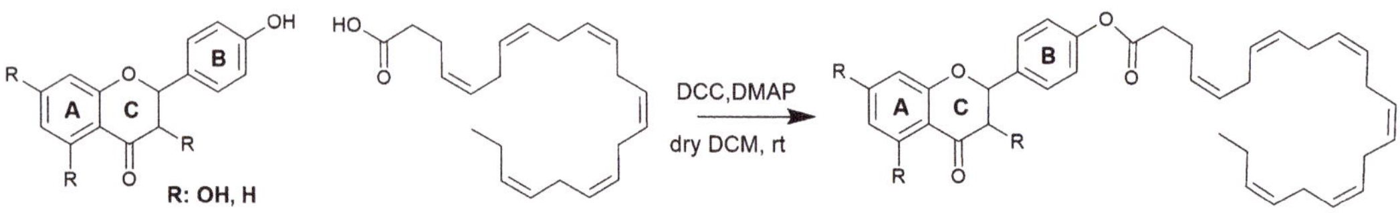

Fig. 5 Synthesis of the polyphenol-PUFA molecular hybrid

2. Using the multiple reaction monitoring (MRM) method, calculate the most prevalent product ions for the determination and quantification of the tested compounds.
3. Prepare fresh samples at a concentration of 1 μM by dissolving the compounds in 50:50 (H_2O/MeOH) in order to determine the optimal chromatographic conditions for the separation of the compounds. The optimum mobile phase is determined to be of 0.1% formic acid in phases A and B since it demonstrated improved peak shapes and increased signal (*see* **Note 4**).
4. The optimal gradient profile for DHA-polyphenol at a constant flow rate of 300 μL/min is initial phase (B) concentration 5%, increased to 95% within 2.5 min, then kept constant for 2 min, and reduced to 5% till the end of the run.
5. The optimal gradient profile for polyphenol at flow rate of 250 μL is initial phase (B) concentration 15%, increased to 95% within 2.5 min, then kept constant for 2 min, and reduced to 15% till the end of the run.
6. Set the analysis run time at 6 min.

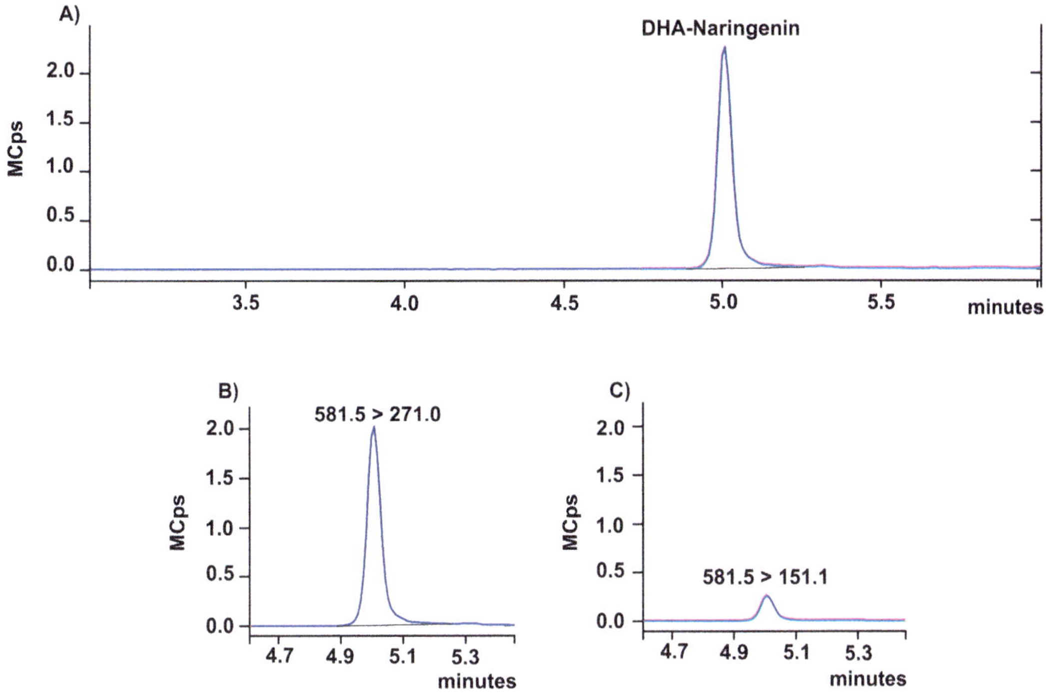

Fig. 6 Representative chromatograms of (**a**) naringenin and (**b**, **c**) of the two main transitions of naringenin, where the retention time and their peaks are illustrated

7. Maintain the column stable at 40 °C and autosampler at 25 °C (*see* **Note 5**).
8. On the same chromatographic runs, optimize the various parameters of mass spectrometer like nebulizer, spray voltage, and heated probe temperature using the MRM mode, in order to obtain a consistent and reliable response for all compounds.
9. The optimal conditions for all compounds are found to be: spray voltage (−) set to 4000 V, heated probe gas flow to 50 units, heated probe temperature at 350 °C, cone gas flow to 20 units, cone temperature at 200 °C, and nebulizer gas flow to 40 units.
10. Set the injection volume 5 μL (Figs. 6 and 7).
11. Bruker's EVOQ Elite ER triple quadrupole is used for the determination and quantification of all compounds.

3.4 Plasma Preparation

1. Leave the free-drug human plasma, stored in aliquots in −20 °C, to thaw in room temperature prior to plasma stability assays (*see* **Note 6**).
2. Check all plasma samples for transparency. In the case of cloudy or precipitated samples, use a new batch of plasma.

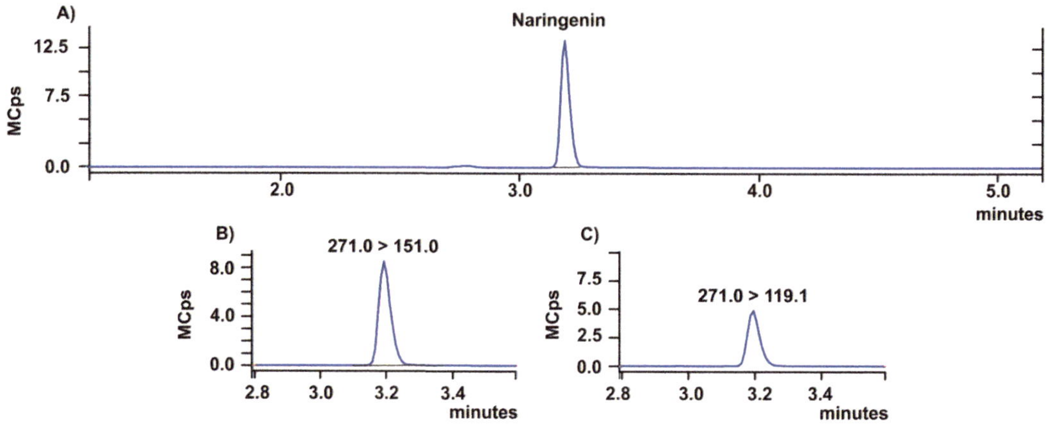

Fig. 7 Representative chromatograms of (**a**) DHA-naringenin and (**b**, **c**) of the two main transitions of DHA-naringenin, where the retention time and their peaks are illustrated

3.5 Human Plasma Stability of Polyphenolic Conjugate

1. Dissolve DHA-polyphenol analogue in DMSO to a final concentration of 40 μM (*see* **Note 7**).
2. Use rosmarinic acid as internal standard (IS), and dilute in MeOH to a final concentration of 40 μM.
3. Add 5 μL of the analogue in eppendorf tubes containing 195 μL of human plasma (adjust pH to 7.4), and place it in a water bath incubator set at 37 °C for 0, 7.5, 15, 30, 45, 60, 90, and 120 min.
4. Add 395 μL of MeOH to each sample in order to quench the reactions, along with 5 μL of rosmarinic acid (IS).
5. Vortex-mix and centrifuge at 10,000 × *g* for 10 min.
6. Then, take the supernatant, filter, and transfer it to vials for LC-MS analysis.
7. Study each sample at triplicates, and design the plot of the mean concentration against time for all compounds (*see* **Note 8**).
8. Analyze immediately the same samples for the determination of the released naringenin after the hydrolysis of the 4′-DHA-naringenin hybrid from the plasma esterases.
9. In order to evaluate the chemical hydrolysis of DHA-polyphenol analogue, conduct the same assay using human plasma first incubated at 52 °C for 24 h (*see* **Note 9**). Design the plot of the percentage of the remaining compound in each time point in comparison to the 0 time point, against time.

3.6 Determination of the Antiplatelet Activity of Various Compounds

In order to determine the antiplatelet activity of various compounds, we use platelet aggregometry and flow cytometry techniques.

3.6.1 Platelet Aggregation Assays

Blood withdrawal: Venous blood samples are withdrawn from an antecubital vein of apparently healthy volunteers (aged 22 to 45 years, not taking antiplatelet drugs or other drugs likely to interfere with platelet function for at least 2 weeks prior to blood sampling), using a 21 gauge butterfly needle. The first 2 mL of blood drawn is discarded. Blood is gently mixed with the ACD anticoagulant into plastic (polypropylene) tubes at a ratio of 9:1 (v/v).

3.6.2 Preparation of Platelet-Rich Plasma (PRP) and Platelet-Poor Plasma (PPP)

1. Centrifuge anticoagulated blood samples at 120 × *g* for 15 min at room temperature without using a brake.
2. Carefully collect the 1/3 of the supernatant (PRP) with a pipette, and transfer it to a polypropylene tube. Centrifuge the remaining plasma with blood cells at 1500 × *g* for 15 min at room temperature without using a brake. Carefully collect the ¾ of the supernatant plasma (PPP) with a pipette, and transfer it to a new polypropylene tube.

3.6.3 Platelet Count

1. Dilute PRP 1:20 (v/v) with 1% ammonium oxalate solution, and 10 μL of the diluted PRP is placed to the Neubauer plate and allowed in a moist petri dish for 20 min to settle down the platelets.
2. Count platelets in the large center square of the Neubauer plate using a light microscope with a 40× objective lens. Calculate the platelet count in the PRP using the following equation: number of platelets/μL PRP = (total number of platelets in the central square/number of small squares) × 1000.
3. For the aggregometry assay, adjust the platelet count in PRP to 250,000 platelets/μL by using autologous PPP.

3.6.4 Test Procedure

1. Measure the platelet aggregation in a four-channel platelet aggregometer (CHRONO-LOG Lumi-Aggregometer, Model 700), equipped with the AGGRO/LINK software package (Fig. 8) (*see* **Notes 10–12**).
2. Before measurement, warm the aggregometer channels to 37 °C.
3. Set all channels to reference channel #1 PPP.
4. Prepare a blank sample by pipetting 0.5 mL PPP into a siliconized glass P/N 312 cuvette (CHRONO-LOG), without a stir bar, which is placed into the reference channel.
5. Place aliquots of 0.5 mL PRP in siliconized glass P/N 312 cuvettes, containing Teflon-coated stir bars. Perform platelet

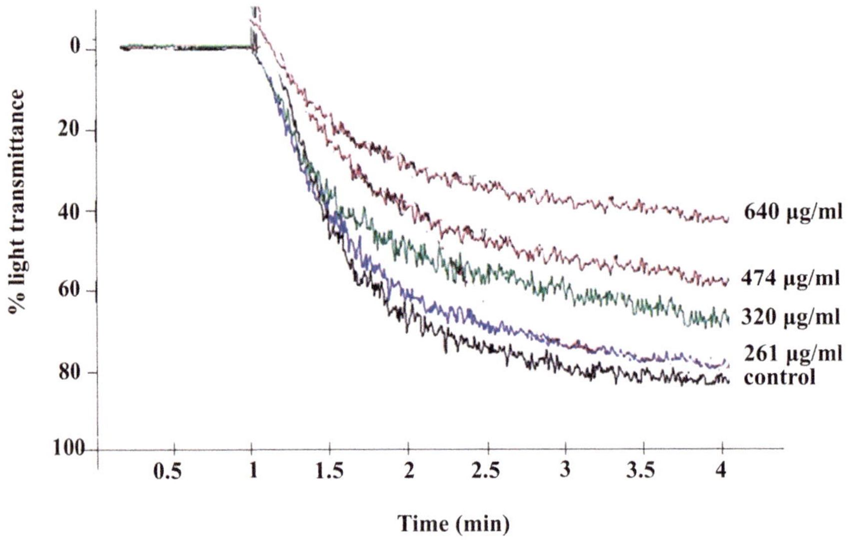

Fig. 8 DHA-naringenin dose-response aggregation curves demonstrating the inhibition of platelet aggregation induced by TRAP (10 μM)

aggregation at 37 °C under continuous stirring at 1200 rpm using magnetic teflon coated stir bars. In control experiments, PRP is preincubated in the cuvette in the presence or absence of <0.5% (v/v) DMSO for 1 min, and then platelets are activated with ADP (10 μM), AA (500 μM), and TRAP-6 (10 μM).

6. The light transmittance of the PRP relative to the PPP blank is recorded automatically. A decrease in optical density reflects an increase in platelet aggregation.
7. Dissolve an appropriate mass (in mg) of each tested compound in DMSO in order to get solutions of 1 mM concentration. Further dilute each one of these solutions with DMSO in order to prepare solutions with various concentrations to enable the study of the dose-dependent inhibitory effect of each compound.
8. In each aggregation assay, use a standard volume of 5 μL from each solution, which is preincubated with 495 μL of PRP in the aggregation cuvette under stirring at 37 °C for 1 min before the initiation of aggregation with ADP, AA, or TRAP-6, at the above concentrations.
9. The maximal aggregation, achieved within 4 min after the addition of each agonist, is determined and expressed as a percentage of 100% light transmission calibrated for each specimen (maximal percentage of aggregation (MPA)).
10. The MPA in the presence of each inhibitory compound, in relation to MPA in the absence of the compound, is used to

calculate the values of platelet aggregation inhibition (IPA) induced by each compound using the following formula:

IPA (%) = (MPA in activated platelets in the presence of DMSO—MPA in the presence of each compound)/(MPA in activated platelets in the presence of DMSO) × 100.

11. The inhibitory potency of each compound is also expressed as IC_{50} values (concentration that induces 50% inhibition of platelet aggregation), which are determined from inhibition profiles in semilogarithmic graphs.

3.7 Flow Cytometry Assays: Membrane Expression of the Integrin Receptor $\alpha_{IIb}\beta_3$ (PAC-1 Binding) and P-Selectin

1. *Blood withdrawal:* As it is described above
2. *Preparation of PRP:* As it is described above
3. *Test procedure:*
   (a) In eppendorf tubes, prepare the following samples: (a) 90 μL of PRP (250,000 platelets/μL) + 5 μL of DMSO+ 5 μL of PBS, (b) 90 μL of PRP (250,000 platelets/μL) + 5 μL of DMSO+ 5 μL of ADP or TRAP (50 mM final concentration for ADP and TRAP), (c) 90 μL of PRP (250,000 platelets/μL) + 5 μL of tested compound +5 μL of PBS, (d) 90 μL of PRP (250,000 platelets/μL) + 5 μL of tested compound +5 μL of ADP or TRAP.
   (b) Incubate the samples for 5 min at 37 °C without stirring but under gentle mixing (low rpm).
   (c) Transfer 5 μL of inactivated or activated platelets to round-bottom BD Falcon tubes where they are incubated with 5 μL of anti-CD61-PerCP, 5 μL of anti-CD62P-PE, and 5 μL of PAC-1-FITC. Add 30 μL of 10 mM PBS at pH 7.4.
   (d) Mix the tubes and incubate the samples for 20 min in the dark at room temperature.
   (e) Add 450 μL of 10 mM PBS at pH 7.4 to each tube and mix in vortex (high rpm).
   (f) Perform flow cytometric analysis using a FACSCalibur flow cytometer (Becton-Dickinson, San Jose, CA, USA). First, platelets are identified with anti-CD61, which labels all platelets. Then they are gated according to staining for the platelet-specific antigen, CD61-PerCP. The gated events are further analyzed in histograms (FL-1 for PAC-1 and FL-2 for P-selectin membrane expression) using the mean fluorescence intensity (MFI). Flow cytometry results are presented as the MFI of the activated sample minus the MFI of the inactivated sample.
   (g) Process numeric data using CellQuest software (Becton-Dickinson).

4 Notes

1. Before implementation of the PCA, it is necessary to standardize the original data by subtracting the mean from each feature and dividing by its respective standard deviation. This step is necessary, because the features present different scales, which yields heterogeneous variances.
2. The reaction should performed with dry conditions (nitrogen gas, dry solvents), and also in dark, due to the sensitivity of the DHA, and also in order to increase the yield of the reaction.
3. Since all polyunsaturated fatty acids are very hydrophobic molecules, during purification with HPLC, we expect the product in the organic phase.
4. Different mobile phases have to be evaluated through different runs to determine the optimum peak shapes and chromatographic conditions.
5. This is important in order to avoid sensitivity and repeatability issues caused by temperature fluctuations.
6. Human plasma samples spiked with the compounds should be freshly prepared on the day of the analysis or prepared as frozen stocks and thawed immediately prior to analysis. Blood and blood-related products may contain harmful pathogens so strict adherence to biosafety rules is mandatory.
7. Since DMSO is used for the preparation of the plasma samples, the percentage of DMSO in the final volume should be kept at low levels since low enzyme activity could be attributed to high percentage of DMSO in plasma.
8. Variability on plasma stability results could be attributed to differences in the expression levels of hydrolytic enzymes between each batch of plasma that will be used for the assay. An up to 20-fold difference could occur that alters the position of a drug in a project that performs plasma stability assays utilizing different plasma batches [17, 18].
9. This step is conducted to eliminate esterase activity.
10. All aggregation assays must be completed within 3 h of blood collection.
11. For the assessment of PRP quality, it is highly recommended for the hemolyzed samples to be discarded.
12. The platelet aggregation tracing should be evaluated based on the following: (a) presence of shape change, (b) length of the lag phase, (c) slope of aggregation, (d) maximal amplitude or % aggregation, (e) amplitude or % aggregation at the end of the monitoring period, (f) deaggregation, (g) visual examination of the aggregation tracings, and (h) presence of a "secondary wave" [19].

References

1. Tsoumani ME, Tselepis AD (2017) Antiplatelet agents and anticoagulants: from pharmacology to clinical practice. Curr Pharm Des 23 (9):1279–1293. https://doi.org/10.2174/1381612823666170124141806
2. Hamm CW, Bassand JP, Agewall S et al (2011) ESC Guidelines for the management of acute coronary syndromes in patients presenting without persistent ST-segment elevation: The Task Force for the management of acute coronary syndromes (ACS) in patients presenting without persistent ST-segment elevation of the European Society of Cardiology (ESC). Eur Heart J 32(23):2999–3054. https://doi.org/10.1093/eurheartj/ehr236
3. Diehl P, Bode C, Duerschmied D (2015) Clinical potential of vorapaxar in cardiovascular risk reduction in patients with atherosclerosis. Ther Clin Risk Manag 11:1133–1138. https://doi.org/10.2147/TCRM.S55469
4. Costa F, Windecker S, Valgimigli M (2017) Dual antiplatelet therapy duration: reconciling the inconsistencies. Drugs 77(16):1733–1754. https://doi.org/10.1007/s40265-017-0806-1
5. Agarwal N, Jain A, Mahmoud AN et al (2017) Safety and efficacy of dual versus triple antithrombotic therapy in patients undergoing percutaneous coronary intervention. Am J Med 130(11):1280–1289. https://doi.org/10.1016/j.amjmed.2017.03.057
6. Moschonas IC, Goudevenos JA, Tselepis AD (2015) Protease-activated receptor-1 antagonists in long-term antiplatelet therapy. Current state of evidence and future perspectives. Int J Cardiol 185:9–18. https://doi.org/10.1016/j.ijcard.2015.03.049
7. Kontogianni VG, Tsoumani ME, Kellici TF et al (2016) Deconvoluting the dual antiplatelet activity of a plant extract. J Agric Food Chem 64(22):4511–4521. https://doi.org/10.1021/acs.jafc.6b00544
8. Hertog MG, Feskens EJ, Hollman PC et al (1993) Dietary antioxidant flavonoids and risk of coronary heart disease: the Zutphen Elderly Study. Lancet 342(8878):1007–1011
9. Palomo I, Toro C, Alarcon M (2008) The role of platelets in the pathophysiology of atherosclerosis (review). Mol Med Rep 1(2):179–184
10. Manach C, Williamson G, Morand C et al (2005) Bioavailability and bioefficacy of polyphenols in humans. I. Review of 97 bioavailability studies. Am J Clin Nutr 81 (1 Suppl):230S–242S
11. Stylos E, Chatziathanasiadou MV, Tsiailanis A et al (2017) Tailoring naringenin conjugates with amplified and triple antiplatelet activity profile: Rational design, synthesis, human plasma stability and in vitro evaluation. Biochim Biophys Acta 1861(11 Pt A):2609–2618. https://doi.org/10.1016/j.bbagen.2017.08.018
12. Schrödinger Release 2015–2 (2015) Maestro, version 10.5, Schrödinger, LLC, New York, NY
13. Schrödinger Release 2015–2 (2015) LigPrep, version 3.4, Schrödinger, LLC, New York, NY
14. Harder E, Damm W, Maple J et al (2016) OPLS3: a force field providing broad coverage of drug-like small molecules and proteins. J Chem Theory Comput 12(1):281–296. https://doi.org/10.1021/acs.jctc.5b00864
15. Small-Molecule Drug Discovery Suite 2015–2 (2015) QikProp, version 4.4, Schrödinger, LLC, New York, NY
16. Schrödinger Release 2015–2 (2015) Canvas, version 2.4, Schrödinger, LLC, New York, NY
17. Di L, Kerns EH, Hong Y et al (2005) Development and application of high throughput plasma stability assay for drug discovery. Int J Pharm 297(1–2):110–119. https://doi.org/10.1016/j.ijpharm.2005.03.022
18. Kerns EH, Di L (2008) Chapter 12 - plasma stability. In: Drug-like properties: concepts, structure design and methods. Academic Press, San Diego, CA, pp 169–177. https://doi.org/10.1016/B978-012369520-8.50013-9
19. Cattaneo M, Cerletti C, Harrison P et al (2013) Recommendations for the standardization of light transmission aggregometry: a consensus of the working party from the platelet physiology subcommittee of SSC/ISTH. J Thromb Haemost. https://doi.org/10.1111/jth.12231

Chapter 23

Pharmacophore Generation and 3D-QSAR Model Development Using PHASE

Eleni Vrontaki and Antonios Kolocouris

Abstract

Nowadays, the prediction of biological activity of novel compounds is one of the major challenges in drug design. Toward this aim a useful procedure is the development and application of predictive computational models using three-dimensional quantitative structure-activity relationship (3D-QSAR) methods, which can decrease the cost and time of biological experiments. In this chapter, the use of application PHASE is analyzed, which is a recent but already widespread method for pharmacophore- or atom-based 3D-QSAR model building. The main steps of procedure provided by PHASE are described, and a general workflow and important practical notes are referred. An attempt in order to design new chemotypes with enhanced cytotoxicity against K562 cells is also provided as an example for the 3D pharmacophore model generation on 33 novel (E)-α-benzylthiochalcones.

Key words 3D-QSAR, Chalcones, Pharmacophore alignment, Pharmacophore model, PHASE

1 Introduction

Hitherto, rational drug design procedures are extensively applied to obtain lead compounds for further development. Studies of quantitative structure-activity relationship (QSAR) aim to decrease the number of potential drugs to be tested for their biological activity. In this way the efficiency of producing new lead compounds is increased, while the human resources, time, consumable, and costs decrease.

Although in drug discovery structure-based computational studies are desirable, in the cases where macromolecular structure is not available or poorly modeled, ligand-based design procedures can be applied to build a 3D pharmacophore. The definition of 3D pharmacophores in modeling has been established by providing several advantages in the early stages of rational drug design since chemical characteristics, which are considered important for ligand binding to the protein and biological activity, can be identified. As in structure-based drug design, screening based on

Thomas Mavromoustakos and Tahsin F. Kellici (eds.), *Rational Drug Design: Methods and Protocols*, Methods in Molecular Biology, vol. 1824, https://doi.org/10.1007/978-1-4939-8630-9_23, © Springer Science+Business Media, LLC, part of Springer Nature 2018

pharmacophores allows the recovery of ligands with structurally diverse bioisosteric scaffolds, which could not be detected by systemic derivatization of already synthesized chemical compounds.

Since three decades, the most used ligand-based methodologies for 3D-QSAR modeling are CoMFA and CoMSIA, developed by Cramer and Klebe [1, 2], respectively, and implemented as tools in commercial programs (like SYBYL [3]). In this chapter, PHASE (**Ph**armacophore **A**lignment and **S**coring **E**ngine), a more recently developed but already widespread friendly-user method for 3D-QSAR model building, will be analyzed. PHASE, an application provided by Schrödinger and supported by a Maestro panel, is a comprehensive, self-contained tool, where 3D models of structurally similar or/and diverse compounds can be developed. These 3D models can be either pharmacophore-based or atom-based models [4–6].

For a set of molecules with high activities, and using a range of scoring techniques, PHASE identifies common pharmacophore hypotheses, which convey characteristics of 3D structures that are supposedly critical of their activity. It performs systematic explorations of rotatable bonds and calculates the associated conformational energies, retaining only the most reasonable energy conformers. PHASE is a versatile product for pharmacophore perception by building a pharmacophore hypothesis, structure alignment, activity prediction, and 3D database searching for matches to a pharmacophore hypothesis [4].

2 Materials

A computational workflow was developed to build a 3D-QSAR model in order to understand the structural characteristics that affect the cytotoxicity of studied molecules in the K562 cell line [7] (*see* **Notes 1–3**).

1. A dataset of 33 (E)-α-benzylthiochalcones (Fig. 1) was taken from the literature [8] that have defined stereochemistry and well defined in vitro cytotoxicity values (*see* **Note 4**). The IC_{50} values of the 33 chemicals are ranging from 0.2 to 75 μM (*see* **Notes 5** and **6**).
2. The development of common pharmacophore hypothesis (CPH) and alignment based on it were carried out using PHASE software, version 4.3 by Schrödinger (2015) [6]. The present procedure runs on a 2.0 GHz Pentium with four processors on a Windows platform.

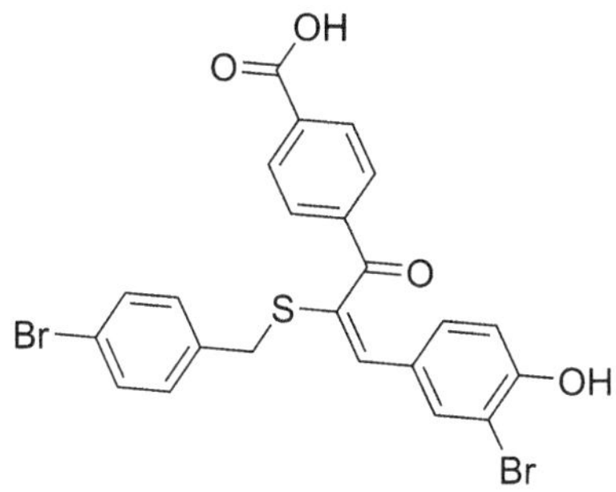

6ab

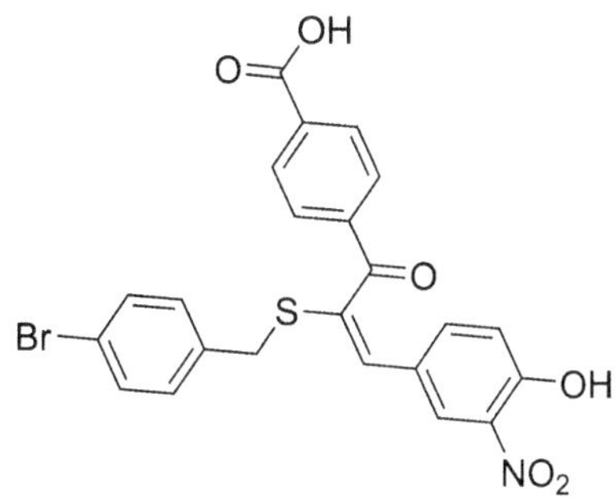

6ac

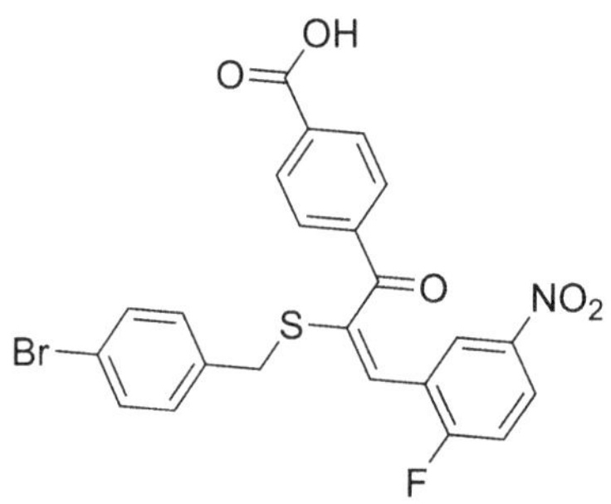

6ad

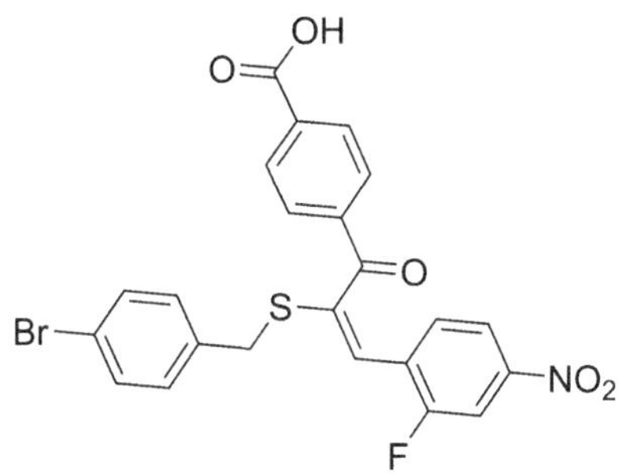

6ag

Fig. 1 Structures of (E)-α-benzylthiochalcones included in the studied dataset

3 Methods

The structures of the molecules were built using ChemBioDraw Ultra 14.0 [9], and their SMILE strings were imported in the project table of Maestro 10.2, the graphical user interface (GUI) by Schrödinger [10]. Then, all the structures were imported from the project table in the **Develop Common Pharmacophore Hypotheses** panel of PHASE workflow, and the cytotoxicity (pIC_{50} values) was selected to be used as the experimental activity variable. Active and inactive thresholds of pIC_{50} were applied to the dataset of compounds; molecules with pIC_{50} values $\geq$6.50 were considered to be active, and molecules with pIC_{50} values $\leq$5.00 were considered to be inactive. The remaining molecules were considered to be moderately active. Therefore, the pharm set comprises six actives and five inactives.

The procedure followed in PHASE 4.3 to build a model consists of five main steps:

1. **Prepare ligands**: The molecules are introduced and prepared utilizing the LigPrep [11], which adds hydrogens, converts 2D

structures to 3D, generates tautomers and stereoisomers, and, optionally, neutralizes charged structures or determines the most probable ionization state at a user-defined pH value. Then, the production of multiple conformations of molecules (conformational analysis) is applied using one of two search methods, ConfGen or Mixed MCMM/LMOD, in which the second one uses a combined Monte Carlo Multiple Minimum and low-mode conformational searching [12]. Both of these approaches employ the MacroModel [13] conformational search engine. Finally, all molecules are minimized by the force field OPLS_2005 [14]. Thereafter, the limits for activity values are defined, separating the compounds into three groups, one including active compounds, one with inactive compounds, and one with compounds having intermediate potencies (*see* **Notes 7** and **8**).

2. **Create sites**: Chemical features are used to define pharmacophore sites. These pharmacophore sites are characterized by type, location, and, if it is applicable, directionality. The pharmacophore features provided by PHASE are hydrogen bond acceptor (A), hydrogen bond donor (D), hydrophobe (H), negative ionizable (N), positive ionizable (P), and aromatic ring (R). In addition, users may define up to three custom feature types (X, Y, Z) to account for characteristics that do not fit clearly into any of the above categories.
3. **Find common pharmacophores**: Using the results of the previous step, pharmacophore hypotheses are searched that are common to all active molecules (*see* **Note 9**). The search spans one or more families of pharmacophores, known as variants. The user can choose the number of site points in the pharmacophore, filter out variants that have too many or too few of a particular kind of feature, and select a set of variants from the filtered list. The user can also set a lower limit on the number of ligands that must match a pharmacophore before it can be considered to be a hypothesis.
4. **Score hypotheses**: In this step the alignment of all molecules in the model is achieved. The models are classified based on a function that depends on:
   - The quality of alignment (RMSD)
   - The definition of a vector that measures the angle deviation between the vector characteristics in the molecules
   - The definition of a score based on the overlap of stereochemical models of heavy atoms in each pair of molecules
5. **Build QSAR model**: The dataset is randomly divided into two groups, the training set and the test set, at a user-defined ratio. The structures are aligned to the optimal pharmacophore, and

a rectangular grid is formed that encircles the aligned molecules. The partial least squares (PLS) analysis is used to calculate the standard deviation. Favorable and unfavorable sites are represented by cubes of different colors.

As aforementioned, in PHASE, there are six built-in pharmacophore features: hydrogen bond acceptor (A), hydrogen bond donor (D), hydrophobic group (H), negatively charged group (N), positively charged group (P), and aromatic ring (R). Each pharmacophore feature is defined by a set of SMARTS patterns, with the exception of the default hydrophobic features (H) and aromatic rings (R). Special algorithms applied to detect these features automatically and more efficiently than would be possible using the SMARTS patterns. All user-defined patterns are specified as SMARTS patterns and assigned one of the three possible geometries, which define the physical characteristics of the site:

- Point: the site is located on a single atom in the SMARTS query.
- Vector: the site is located on a single atom in the SMARTS query, and it is assigned directionality according to one or more vectors originating from the atom.
- Group: the site is located at the center of a group of atoms in the SMARTS query. For aromatic rings, the site is assigned directionality, defined by a vector that is normal to the plane of the ring.

Common pharmacophores were then identified using a tree-based partitioning technique, which groups together similar pharmacophores according to their intersite distances (i.e., the distance between a pair of sites in the pharmacophore). After applying the default pharmacophore features for each molecule, common pharmacophores containing five sites (*see* **Notes 10–12**) were generated using a terminal box size of 1 Å and with the requirement that all actives should match. A total of 3450 five-featured common pharmacophore hypotheses (CPHs) belonging to five variants (AAHRR = 272, HHRRR = 887, AHRRR = 909, AHHRR = 1275, AARRR = 107) were subjected to stringent scoring function analysis with respect to actives using default parameters for site, vector, and volume terms (*see* **Note 13**). The overall maximum root-mean-square deviation (RMSD) value of the intersite distances between an active ligand and the reference ligand of pharmacophore must be 1.2 Å. The hypotheses that emerged from this process were subsequently scored with respect to the five inactive compounds.

All pharmacophore hypotheses that survived the scoring process were subsequently used to build atom-based QSAR models in PHASE. The dataset of molecules was divided randomly into training set and test set in a 75:25 ratio by selecting **sample uniformly**

over activity coordinate. Therefore, the training set consists of 25 molecules and the test set consists of 8 molecules. The training set and test set molecules were aligned on these CPHs and analyzed by PLS analysis described in PHASE [4, 5]. The PHASE descriptors serve as independent variables and the activity values as dependent variables. Four PLS factors were selected, as, and atom-based linear regression models were built containing one, two, three, and four PLS factors using the training set. The predictive activity of each analysis was determined using the test set, i.e., the compounds that are not included in the training set. The statistical parameters shown in the QSAR results table are:

- SD: the standard deviation of regression; the RMS error in the fitted activity values distributed over n-m-1 degrees of freedom (n = training set ligands, m = PLS factors).
- R-squared: the coefficient of determination. A value of 0.90, i.e., means that the model accounts for 90% of the variance in the observed activity data. R-squared is always between 0 and 1, while values greater than 0.80 are considered satisfactory.
- F: the ratio of the model variance to the observed activity variance. Statistically, the larger the value of F, the more important is the regression.
- P: the significance level of F when treated as a ratio of Chi-squared distributions. A P value of 0.05, i.e., means that F is significant at the 95% level.
- Stability: the stability of the model prediction when changing the training set. The maximum value is 1. This factor is important to compare models from different pharmacophore hypotheses.
- RMSE: the RMS error in the test set predictions.
- Q-squared: directly analogous to R-squared but based on the test set predictions. Values greater than 0.65 are considered satisfactory (*see* **Notes 14** and **15**).
- Pearson-R: Pearson coefficient value for the correlation between the predicted and observed activity for the test set.

The best common pharmacophore hypotheses using PHASE based on site, vector, and volume alignment of active compounds were the five-featured CPHs with IDs AHHRR.423 and AAHRR.76. Two regression models were derived with four PLS factors. The results of these models are shown in Table 1. The best-fitted model based on statistical results of QSAR analysis was AHHRR.423, and the pharmacophore hypothesis is displayed in Fig. 2. The pharmacophore contains a red sphere that indicates the hydrogen bond acceptor site (A), two green spheres that indicate the hydrophobic regions (H), and two orange tori that show the

Table 1
Statistical parameters and results of the QSAR models with PHASE

ID	AHHRR.423	AAHRR.76
# PLS factors	4	4
SD	0.0819	0.0779
R-squared	0.9884	0.9895
F	425.6	471.4
P	4.854e−019	1.769e−019
Stability	0.7288	0.7124
RMSE	0.1922	0.3774
Q-squared	0.9418	0.7756
Pearson-R	0.9776	0.9525

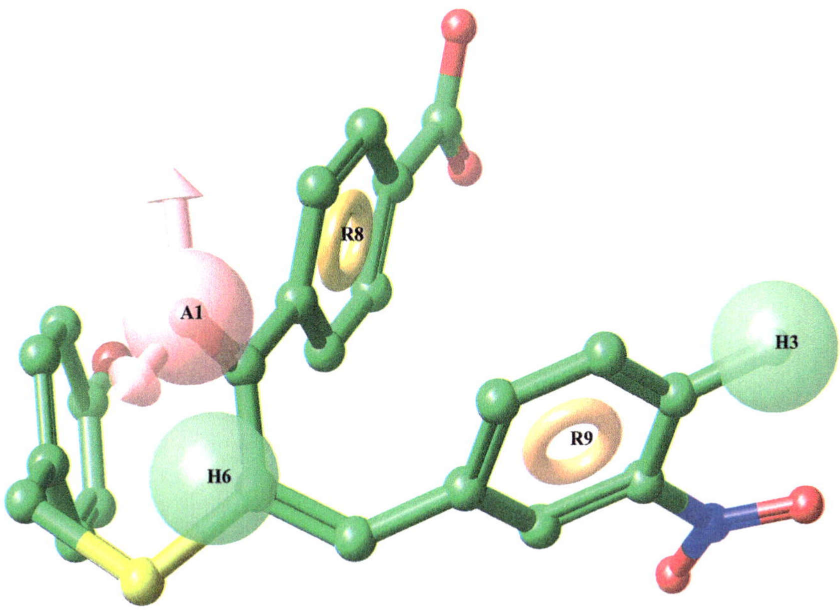

Fig. 2 The best common pharmacophore hypothesis for reference compound (ID AHHRR.423). Pharmacophore features are represented by light red sphere for hydrogen bond acceptor (A) with the arrows pointing in the direction of lone pairs, green sphere for hydrophobic groups (H), and orange torus for aromatic rings (R)

aromatic rings (R). The result of the dataset alignment is depicted in Fig. 3.

As it is observed from the pharmacophore hypothesis (Fig. 2), a hydrophobic group is required at the right side of the scaffold and, more specifically, at the para position of right phenyl ring. Nevertheless, some compounds from the studied dataset bear no group in

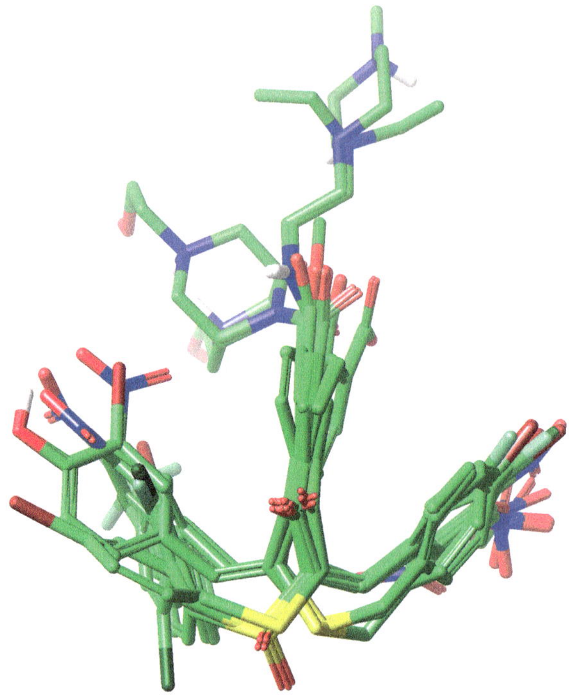

Fig. 3 The common pharmacophore hypothesis-based alignment of all (E)-α-benzylthiochalcones

this position (i.e., **6ad**, Fig. 1) and other bear polar groups, such as –OH and –NO_2 (**6ab**, **6ac**, and **6ag**, Fig. 1). This justifies the low activity of these molecules (*see* **Note 16**).

The statistical results of the 3D-QSAR model summarized in Table 1 were excellent, with R-squared = 0.9884, Q-squared = 0.9418, and Pearson-R = 0.9776. The QSAR results can also be visualized using 3D plots of pharmacophore (Fig. 4). In these plots, the atom-based PHASE 3D-QSAR model is represented by colored regions (blue and red cubes) according to the sign of their coefficient values. The blue cubes refer to positive coefficients in which the feature is crucial for the increase of activity, whereas the red cubes refer to negative coefficients indicating that the feature substitution is responsible for the decrease of activity. In the present PHASE QSAR model, hydrophobic/nonpolar, negatively and positively charged, and electron-withdrawing parameters are contributing to activity and are discussed separately.

In Fig. 4a the effects of the hydrophobic model are visualized. The map shows a big blue region around the left phenyl ring, indicating that hydrophobic groups are favored for increased activity. Similarly, around the right phenyl ring hydrophobic groups are favored, except from the meta-position, where red cubes are visualized. In this map, a big red region above the right phenyl ring is showed, which indicates that polar groups in this area increase the

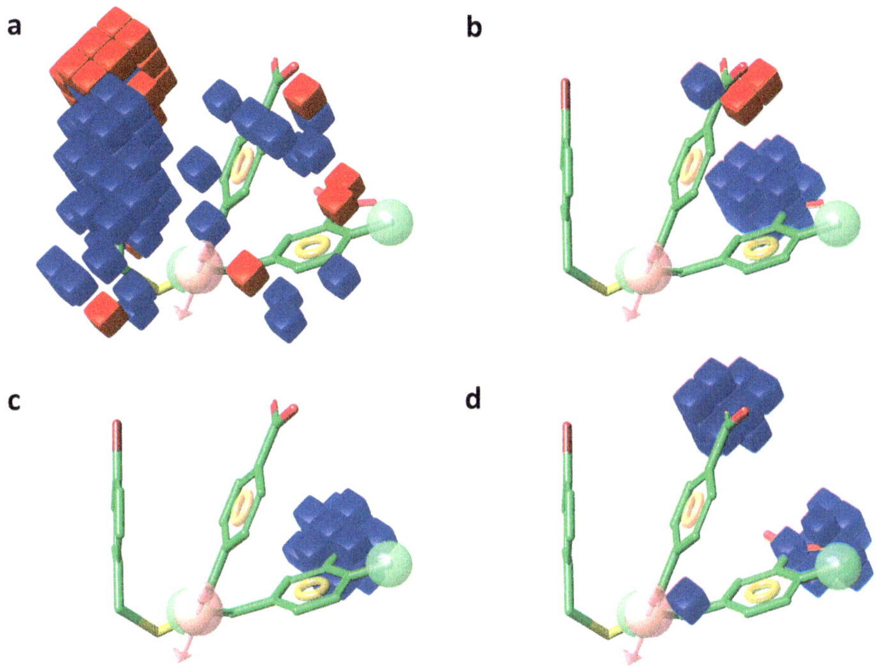

Fig. 4 PHASE 3D-QSAR visual plots displayed for compound **6c**. (**a**) Hydrophobic, (**b**) negative ionic, (**c**) positive ionic, and (**d**) electron-withdrawing model, where blue cubes indicate positive coefficient (increase activity) and red cubes indicate negative coefficients (decrease activity)

activity. In general, the blue cubes around the nitro group in compound **6c** (reference compound) show that in this region a charged (positively and/or negatively) or an electron-withdrawing group increases the activity (Fig. 4b–d). Therefore, the $-NO_2$ group at the p-position of left phenyl ring is the best choice, as well as –CN group. In addition, around the carboxyl group of compound **6c** in Fig. 4b**,** there are both blue and red cubes. This means that negatively charged groups are favored near the blue cubes and are disfavored near the red ones. In this position, an electron-withdrawing group (i.e., a hydrogen bond acceptor) is favored.

The workflow followed in the present study is described below:

1. In the graphical user interface (GUI) of Schrödinger, Maestro, choose one of the following in the main window:
   - Applications → Phase → Develop Common Pharmacophore Hypotheses.
   - Tasks → Pharmacophore Modeling → Develop Common Hypotheses and the Develop Common Pharmacophore Hypotheses panel opens.

2. In the first tab called **Prepare Ligands**, there are no entries in the Ligands table, so now the structures can be added to the PHASE workflow. Click **From File**, **From Run**, or **From Project.**
3. If you click **From File**, select the file and click **Open** (*see* **Notes 17** and **18**).
4. The **Choose Activity Property** dialog box opens. Choose **All properties** from the **Subset** option menu (*see* **Notes 19** and **20**).
5. Select <**none**> property or choose "Activity," if you have already added a column named "Activity" and containing the activity values of the studied compounds as a new property in the imported file, and click **OK**. The Ligands table is now filled with copies of the structures from the file (*see* **Note 21**).
6. Click on **Clean Structures**, which is an interface to LigPrep. The dialog box opens, and you can set options for generation of stereoisomers and ionization states, and click **Start** to run the job to perform the cleanup.
7. Click on **Generate conformers**. Set your options, and click **Start** to run the conformational search job.
8. Click **Activity Thresholds**. Set a threshold for the active ligands and a threshold for the inactive ligands, in order to define the set of ligands (the **Pharm Set**) that will be used for model development (*see* **Notes 22** and **23**).
9. Click **Next** to proceed to the next step, **Create Sites**.
10. Click the **Create Sites** button near the top of the panel.
11. Click **Start** in the Create Sites—Start dialog box (*see* **Note 24**).
12. Click **Next** to proceed to the next step. The **Find Common Pharmacophores** step is displayed.
13. Choose the number of sites from the **Number of sites** option menu (*see* **Note 10**).
14. Specify the number of actives or active groups to match in the **Must match** section.
15. Set limits on the minimum and maximum number of features of each type in the **Feature frequencies** table (*see* **Note 25**).
16. Select variants from the **Variant list** and click **Find**.
17. Click **Start** in the **Find Common Pharmacophores—Options** dialog box (*see* **Note 26**).
18. Click **Next** to enter the **Score Hypotheses** step.
19. Click **Score Actives** (*see* **Note 27**).
20. Click **Start**, and click **Start** again in the Start dialog box.
21. Click **Score Inactives** (*see* **Note 28**).

22. Click **Start**, and click **Start** again in the Start dialog box.
23. Click **Rescore**.
24. Enter 0.3 in the reference ligand activity text box and click **OK**.
25. Click twice on the **Post-hoc** column heading, to sort the hypotheses in descending order by this score.
26. Click **Alignment Options** below the Alignments table. The **Alignment Options** dialog box opens.
27. Select **Align non-model ligands**. You can also require certain features to match by clicking on them and then click **OK** (*see* **Notes 29–32**).
28. Select the best **Post-hoc** and a reference ligand and click **Next** to enter the **Build QSAR Model** step (*see* **Note 33**).
29. The **Build QSAR Model** step is displayed. In the Random training set type 75% and click **Apply** (*see* **Note 34**).
30. Click **Options**.
31. In Training set, select by clicking only the option **Sample uniformly over activity coordinate**.
32. In QSAR model, set Grid spacing to 1.0 and Maximum PLS Factors to 5 (*see* **Note 35**).
33. Under Model type, ensure that atom-based is selected, and click **OK**.
34. Click **Build Models** and then **Start**.
35. When run finishes, place the most active ligand in the Workspace, and click **QSAR Visualization**.
36. Ensure that all items in the **View effects** from list are present and that **Combine effects** is not selected.
37. Ensure that **Workspace ligands** is selected under **View volume** occupied by.
38. Choose (D) H-bond donor in the **View effects** from list and the Effect option menu.
39. Select the number of PLS factors that gave the best statistics.
40. Then, do the same procedure replacing the most active ligand in the workspace with the least active ligand, and notice that the workspace contains many more red cubes than blue cubes, indicating a preponderance of unfavorable interactions (*see* **Note 36**).
41. Continue the same procedure choosing the other effects from list and using the most and least active ligand each time.

4 Notes

1. CoMFA/CoMSIA model based on an atom-based alignment using the lower energy conformer of each compound provided no satisfactory results while with the use of PHASE obtained excellent results.
2. The conformations of all compounds obtained from the alignment of pharmacophoric points can be also used in other 3D-QSAR models.
3. PHASE can also be applied on docked poses skipping the first step of workflow (**Prepare Ligands** step) (*see* ref. [15]).
4. Compound **6t** of the original dataset is excluded from this study as it contains sulfoxide instead of sulfur dioxide group and behaved as an outlier in the generated model.
5. Molecules with activities spanning about three log units of K_i or IC_{50} values are required for the 3D-QSAR studies.
6. The activity values should be in logarithmic unit ($-logIC_{50}$).
7. The preparation of molecules can precede their insertion into the PHASE table. In this case, you can skip the step of **Prepare Ligands**.
8. Separate stereoisomers, if necessary, by selecting the relevant ligands in the table and choosing **Separate stereoisomers** from the shortcut (right-click) menu.
9. The set of actives should contain as much structural diversity as possible, so that the resulting pharmacophore models are applicable across different chemical families.
10. You can choose any number between 3 and 7 for **Maximum number of sites** and **Minimum number of sites** options. The default is 5 for both of the options.
11. In the present study, three- and four-featured pharmacophores were not included in the **Find Common Pharmacophores** step, since the CPHs might not contain all required features and therefore might not discriminate between actives and inactives very well.
12. The compounds of the dataset are similar enough, and therefore six- and seven-featured common pharmacophores are not recommended to be selected.
13. Several of the scores in the survival score formula have zero weights. By default, none of these optional scores contribute to the ranking of the hypotheses. However, all individual components of the score are reported, so you can always consider selectivity, if you so desire, when making choices among hypotheses that have very similar overall scores.

14. The R-squared value always increases as the number of PLS factors increases, but the same is not necessarily true of Q-squared.
15. To increase the Q- and R-squared values, you should start changing the ligands from training to test set and vice versa.
16. The inactive compounds **6ab**, **6ac**, and **6ag** have a hydrophobic group at the p-position of the left phenyl ring. For this reason, these compounds in the present pharmacophore alignment have to "flip" horizontally in order to align the hydrophobic substitution at the para position of ring in the pharmacophore. This conformational change could not be necessarily obtained in a docking-based alignment.
17. To add ligands, select **From File** containing all the structures and stored in *.mae or *.maegz forms.
18. In case you import multiple conformers for each ligand, you can normally see only a single conformation for each ligand in the workspace.
19. In **Choose Activity Property** dialog box, you should select the property to use as the experimental activity variable.
20. In **Choose Activity Property** dialog box, ensure that **Convert property values** is not selected.
21. The pIC50-Exp data which are contained in the **Activity column** should be typed by hand, if there is no data in the imported file with the structures.
22. The **Pharm set** column is blank for ligands whose activity falls between activity thresholds.
23. Clear the **Pharm Set** column for any test set ligands that are assigned to the active or the inactive set by selecting the assigned ligands and control-clicking in the column for one of ligands until the selected rows are blank in this column. The values cycle through active, inactive, and blank when you click. The test set ligands should not be part of the pharm set because the pharm set is used to develop the pharmacophore model, and the test set is used to validate the model.
24. The **Create Sites** job requires less than a minute on a 2 GHz Pentium 4 processor. Incorporation of results does not add any new information to the Ligands table.
25. The possible common pharmacophores that PHASE can identify depend on the number of features of each type that are available in the ligand set (listed in the **Available** column of the **Feature frequencies** table).
26. In the **Find Common Pharmacophores—Options** dialog box, the parameters are kept as default, i.e., minimum intersite

distance, 2.0 Å; maximum tree depth, 5; initial box size, 32.0 Å; and final box size, 1.0 Å.

27. In **Score Actives** panel, the parameters of the survival score formula are kept as default, except for weights of the selectivity score and the number of matches that defined 0.0 and 1.0, respectively.
28. In **Score Inactives** panel, leave the inactives weight at its default value of 1.0.
29. In the **Score Hypotheses** step, the **Alignments** table is filled with a record for each ligand, when you select a hypothesis from the above table. The rows for the ligands not used for the model are dark gray, indicating that no alignment is done for these ligands. There is also a blue row in the **Alignments** table, indicating that it is the reference ligand, i.e., the ligand from which the hypothesis came.
30. **Fitness** measures the quality of each alignment using a weighted sum of alignment and volume scores, just as in the total scoring function. For the reference ligand, the fitness score is the 3.0, the maximum possible score.
31. For the generation of the QSAR model, modeled (actives) and non-modeled molecules in the dataset are aligned based on the matching with at least all the pharmacophoric features.
32. The "non-model" ligands are those that are not in the pharm set (inactives and moderately actives) or do not match all sites in the selected hypothesis.
33. It is not necessary that there is a connection between the score and the quality of the QSAR model with the top-scoring hypotheses. Therefore, when you build QSAR models, you should try several hypotheses to ensure that you have a good model.
34. In the **Alignments** table, all ligands are placed in the training set by default, so you should separate them into the training and test sets that you want, by clicking in the proper cell of the **QSAR Set** column, to change the value from training to test.
35. In **Build QSAR Model** step, the maximum number of PLS factors that can be taken is N/5, where N is the number of ligands present in the training set.
36. Move the positive and negative coefficient threshold sliders to an intermediate value, such as 0.015 and −0.015. You are viewing only those cubes whose regression coefficients exceed the intermediate thresholds you set.

Acknowledgments

The corresponding author Eleni Vrontaki (E.V.) acknowledges funding by State Scholarships Foundation (IKY postdoctoral fellowship, MIS 5001552, NSRF 2014–2020).

References

1. Cramer RD III, Bunce JD, Patterson DE, Frank IE (1988) Cross validation, bootstrapping, and partial least squares compared with multiple regression in conventional QSAR studies. Quant Struct Act Relat 7(1):18–25. https://doi.org/10.1002/qsar.19880070105
2. Klebe G, Abraham U, Mietzner T (1994) Molecular similarity indexes in a comparative-analysis (Comsia) of drug molecules to correlate and predict their biological activity. J Chem 37(24):4130–4146. https://doi.org/10.1021/jm00050a010
3. SYBYL/QSAR and COMFA, version 8.0 (2007) Tripos Inc., St Louis, MO
4. Dixon SL, Smondyrev AM, Knoll EH et al (2006) PHASE: a new engine for pharmacophore perception, 3D QSAR model development, and 3D database screening: 1. Methodology and preliminary results. J Comput Aided Mol Des 20(10–11):647–671. https://doi.org/10.1007/s10822-006-9087-6
5. Dixon SL, Smondyrev AM, Rao SN (2006) PHASE: a novel approach to pharmacophore modeling and 3D database searching. Chem Biol Drug Des 67(5):370–372. https://doi.org/10.1111/j.1747-0285.2006.00384.x
6. PHASE, version 4.3 (2015) Schrödinger, LLC, New York, NY
7. Vrontaki E, Melagraki G, Voskou S et al (2017) Development of a predictive pharmacophore model and a 3D-QSAR study for an in silico screening of new potent Bcr-Abl kinase inhibitors. Mini Rev Med Chem 17(3):188–204. https://doi.org/10.2174/1389557516999160629101709
8. Reddy MV, Pallela VR, Cosenza SC et al (2010) Design, synthesis and evaluation of (E)-alphabenzylthiochalcones as novel inhibitors of BCR-ABL kinase. Bioorg Med Chem 18(6):2317–2326. https://doi.org/10.1016/j.bmc.2010.01.051
9. ChemBioDraw Ultra 14.0, ChemBioOffice (2014) PerkinElmer
10. Maestro 10.2 (2015) Graphical User Interface, Schrödinger, LLC, New York, NY
11. LigPrep, version 3.4 (2015) Schrödinger, LLC, New York, NY
12. Kolossvary I, Guida WC (1996) Low mode search. An efficient, automated computational method for conformational analysis: application to cyclic and acyclic alkanes and cyclic peptides. J Am Chem Soc 118 (21):5011–5019. https://doi.org/10.1021/ja952478m
13. MacroModel, version 10.8 (2015) Schrödinger, LLC, New York, NY
14. Kaminski GA, Friesner RA, Tirado-Rives J, Jorgensen WL (2001) Evaluation and reparameterization of the OPLS-AA force field for proteins via comparison with accurate quantum chemical calculations on peptides. J Phys Chem B 105(28):6474–6487. https://doi.org/10.1021/jp003919d
15. Vrontaki E, Melagraki G, Afantitis A et al (2017) Searching for novel Janus kinase-2-inhibitors using a combination of pharmacophore modeling, 3D-QSAR studies and virtual screening. Mini Rev Med Chem 17 (3):268–294. https://doi.org/10.2174/1389557516666160919163930

Chapter 24

Design of Drugs by Filtering Through ADMET, Physicochemical and Ligand-Target Flexibility Properties

Marlet Martínez-Archundia, Martiniano Bello, and Jose Correa-Basurto

Abstract

There is a synergistic interaction between medicinal chemistry, chemoinformatics, and bioinformatics. The last one includes analyses of sequences as well as structural analysis which employ computational techniques such as docking studies and molecular dynamics (MD) simulations. Over the last years these techniques have allowed the development of new accurate computational tools for drug design. As a result, there have been an increased number of publications where computational methods such as pharmacophore modeling, de novo drug design, evaluation of physicochemical properties, and analysis of ADMET (absorption, distribution, metabolism, excretion, and toxicity) properties have been quite useful for eliminating the compounds with poor physicochemical or toxicological properties. Furthermore, using MD simulations and docking analysis, it is possible to estimate the binding energy of the protein-ligand complexes by using scoring functions, as well as to structurally depict the binding pose of the compounds on proteins, in order to select the best evaluated compounds for subsequent synthetizing and evaluation through biological assays. In this work, we describe some computational tools that have been used for structure-based drug design of new compounds that target histone deacetylases (HDACs), which are known to be potential targets in cancer and parasitic diseases.

Key words Histone deacetylases, Rational drug design, *ADMET* properties, Pharmacophore modeling, Docking analysis, Molecular dynamics simulations

1 Introduction

The use of computational methods for drug design of new compounds for a specific target is commonly known as computer-assisted molecular design. Genomics, proteomics, and bioinformatics have helped to discover new therapeutic targets. Many three-dimensional (3D) structures of therapeutic targets have been solved through some specialized experimental techniques such as X-ray crystallography, nuclear magnetic resonance (NMR), and super-resolved fluorescence microscopy (SRFM), which shows a 3D image of a single molecule [1, 2]. Knowledge of the 3D target structure is crucial as input information for computational methodologies employed in drug design because in many cases, the

Thomas Mavromoustakos and Tahsin F. Kellici (eds.), *Rational Drug Design: Methods and Protocols*, Methods in Molecular Biology, vol. 1824, https://doi.org/10.1007/978-1-4939-8630-9_24,

initial structure determines the success or failure of the theoretical study. Nevertheless, despite the knowledge of the 3D structure of a protein, rational drug design of a new compound that can interact with a therapeutic target is still a challenge [3]. On the other side, virtual screening technique has been used to screen large libraries of compounds that could complement targets of known 3D structures and even to test the ligands that are predicted to bind with high affinity to the proteins of interest [4].

Two approaches are used in virtual screening.

1. The structure-based drug design (SBDD) methodology is applied when the 3-D structure of the therapeutic target is available through experimental methods (X-ray, NMR, or SRFM). This approach currently represents a core component of modern drug discovery (*see* **Note 1**) [5]. With regards to this issue, Molecular dynamics (MD) simulations help to obtain refined structures of the protein of study and to get energetic information about the receptor-ligand interactions whereas docking studies investigate the binding between two molecules, namely a receptor and a ligand, which are included in the SBDD approach.
2. In the case when there is no 3D structure available, virtual screening of compound libraries can be performed through ligand-based searches. This approach is based on the analysis and comparison of molecular properties and receptor affinity data for known ligands, without accounting for the 3D structure of the receptor. Thus, in this case, ligand-based drug design (LBDD) methodology is highly recommended. Some of the ligand-based drug design methods are the similarity search techniques through 2D/3D descriptors, QSAR (quantitative structure-activity relationship or quantitative relation of the structural changes of a set of compounds with the changes in activity), development of pharmacophore models (identification of the set of structural characteristics of a ligand directly related to the key interaction sites of a receptor), and shape matching techniques (overlapping the form of two ligands) [7–10].

Thus, virtual screening tools inevitably require the knowledge of the activity of some compounds or the structure of the biological target.

A typical virtual screening cascade contains different filtering steps that reduce the number of candidate compounds to be examined experimentally, such as the minimum in nine orders of magnitude, finishing with the most promising compounds for clinical testing. These filters are applied sequentially according to the level of required computational effort used by each of the techniques (from lowest to highest calculation cost) and complexity of the information needed. For the identification of hits, it is necessary to start from the conformational analysis of the structures of the generated library of compounds. Starting from this library of compounds, a prescreening is performed in which the selected molecules show structures and properties of drugs (***drug-likeness***), as well as good *ADMET* (absorption, distribution, metabolism, elimination, and toxicity) properties [11], in order to simultaneously optimize the potency and pharmacokinetics. Then, 2D/3D filters are applied to select compounds focused on a type of physical structure required for the interaction with the therapeutic target. The next step is usually the search for pharmacophoric models enabling an even more focused selection of the compounds according to some structural and 3D characteristics. Once the library has been sufficiently focused, the method proceeds with the lead discovery and optimization phase. Here, techniques such as docking analysis focus on sampling ligand-receptor poses by employing a scoring function for the evaluation of the ligand-macromolecule interactions [12]. Moreover, the best conformations obtained by docking all of the molecules from a database can be refined through MD simulation approaches combined with more sophisticated methods of binding free energy estimation. Finally, based on these structured-based drug design techniques, a new library of compounds can be proposed.

In this chapter is described a protocol which includes the basic techniques present in a typical virtual screening workflow. First, a library of compounds is compiled containing the known active compound (reference compounds) and drug-like compounds (based on structure-based pharmacophore models) to be screened (*see* **Note 2**). As a first step in the virtual screening, filters are used on the library of compounds to eliminate the structures that have non-drug properties in terms of their functional groups and physical properties (drug-likeness). The filters used to consider a drug-like compound are the following: Lipinski's "rule of five" filters the molecules according to their molecular weight ($\leq$500 g/mol), lipophilicity, as measured by the octanol-water partition coefficient (LogP) ($\leq$5), and the number of hydrogen bond donors ($\leq$5) and acceptors ($\leq$10). In the second step, ligand-based filters (ADME properties) are applied for the compounds. Finally, docking-based and MD simulation filters are applied to select only the compounds with the best affinity properties to the target of interest.

2 Materials

1. 2D structures of the small organic molecules were drawn with ACD/ChemSketch 14.01 software (http://www.acdlabs.com/resources/freeware/chemsketch/). The matrix Z of each molecule was created using the GaussView 5.0.9 package.

This program was installed on an Intel Core i3 CPU with 4 GB of RAM and a Windows 64-bit operating system. The molecules were submitted to a geometric and energetic optimization by the semiempirical molecular orbitals AM1 (Austin Model 1) method using the GAUSSIAN 09 W 9.5 program [13].

2. The physicochemical and *ADMET* properties were determined by two online servers, Molinspiration (http://www.molinspiration.com), Osiris explorer (http://www.organic-chemistry.org/prog/peo), and Data Warrior V 4.5.2.
3. AutoDock 4.2 [14] and AutoDock tools were installed on a workstation with Intel Core 2 Quad CPU with 8 GB of RAM in a Linux 64-bit operating system.
4. NAMD, GROMACS, and AMBER 12 programs were executed on a GeForce GTX 680 GPU on an Intel Core 2 Quad CPU with 16 GB of RAM and a Linux 64-bit operating system.

3 Methods

Previously, there have been some reports that describe strategies that have followed the structure-based design approach [15]. In this section is described the methodology that this group has followed for the design of a set of molecules that show a pharmacophore core and target HDACs. These molecules were evaluated through *ADMET* properties. A schematic representation of the used workflow is given in Fig. 1. Additionally, different protein conformations were taken from MD simulations and were used for further docking analysis [16] (*see* **Note 3**).

3.1 Identification of Pharmacological Target

Histone deacetylases (HDACs) have been described to be involved in gene regulation expression that control various cell biochemical properties, for example, cell proliferation, cell cycle regulation, and apoptosis [17]. Although there are 18 isoforms of HDACs, we have focused on those related to cancer, such as HDAC6, which is a metalloprotein that plays an important role in the biological action triggered by GPER, a membrane protein [18], and HDAC8, which is highly expressed in childhood neuroblastoma [19]. Moreover, HDAC8 has also been implicated in other cancers such as lung, colon, and cervical cancers [20].

Once the pharmacological target related to a particular disease has been identified, an exhaustive search for the crystallographic structure needs to be performed, and if it is available, it can be downloaded from the Protein Data Bank (PDB) (*see* **Note 4**); then, structural preparation of the file is needed, e.g., removal of water molecules, ligands, antibodies, or enzymes that were necessary to crystallize the biological system. Moreover, one has to check if

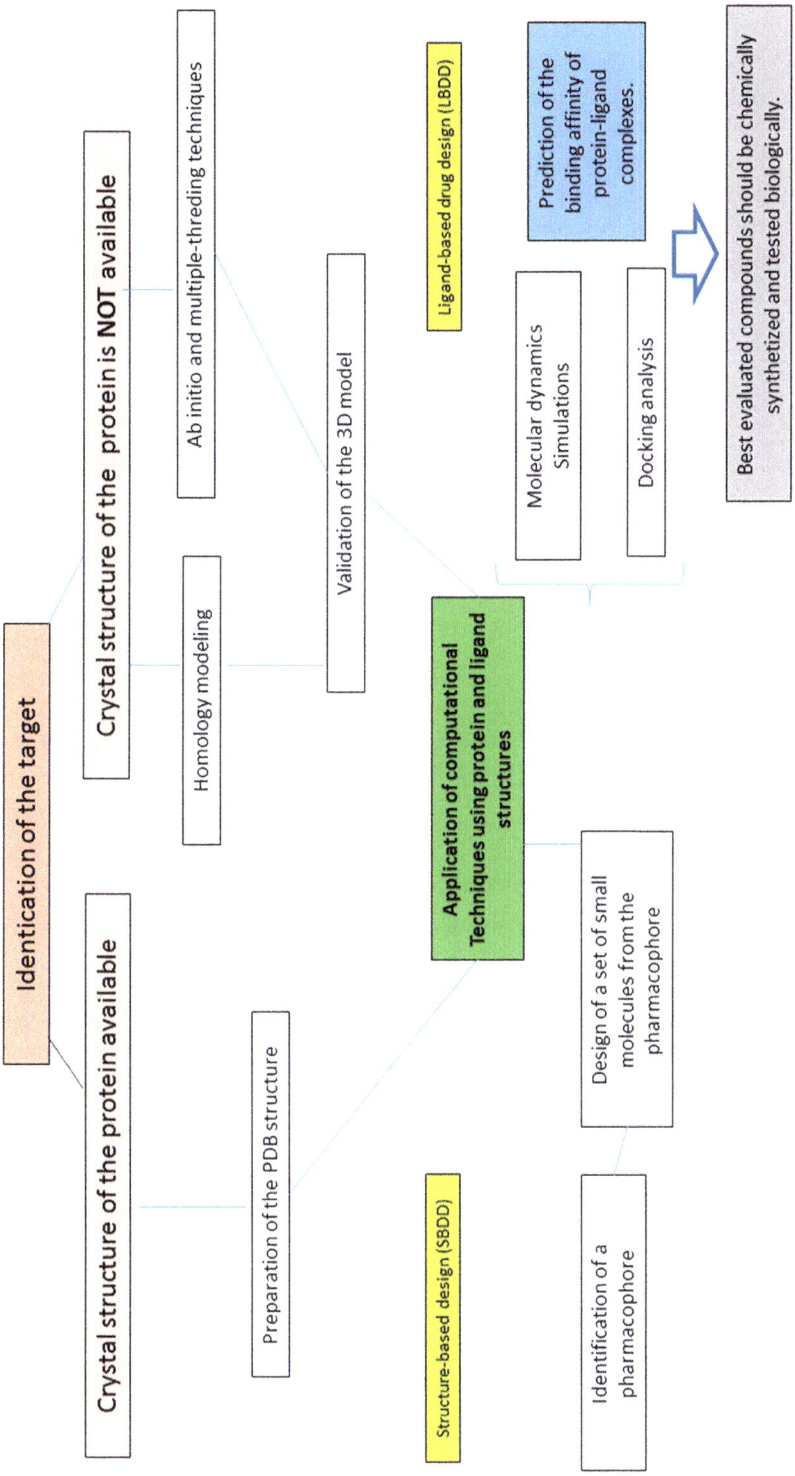

Fig. 1 Schematic representation of rational drug design procedures

there are any deletions or mutations in the crystallographic structure, as well as for the pKa calculation for protein residues, which will allow the establishment of their protonation states. For the cases where there is no crystallographic structure available, homology modeling procedures such as ab initio or a multiple threading technique can be used to build a 3D model of a protein (*see* **Note 5**) however validation of this 3D model is needed before performing other studies [21] (*see* **Note 6**). Additionally, one has to verify that the model shows important structural characteristics such as disulfide bonds, cofactors, and transcriptional modifications.

3.2 Homology Modeling of Histone Deacetylases (HDACs) and Validation of the 3D Models

3.2.1 HDCA6

1. To obtain the 3D model of HDAC6, the protein sequence with NCBI accession number NP_006035.2 was employed after performing multiple sequence alignment studies using BLAST of the HDAC6 protein sequences [22].
2. The I-TASSER server was used to generate the three-dimensional model of the human HDAC6, considering some of the crystal structures available for this protein, which maintained some structural identities (2VCG (37%), 1ZZ0 (37%), 1C3P (29%), 3MEN (36%), 3COY (47%), 3MAX (29%), and 2VQJ (48%), and by combining multiple threading techniques [23].
3. The protein complex, the second catalytic domain of HDAC6 (DD2-HDAC6, G482-G801), was modeled due to the structural complexity of HDAC6 [24].
4. Subsequently, diverse crystal structures of the protein (1 W22, 1 T69, 2V5W, and 3F0R) were checked in order to find the correct location of Zn2+ atoms in the catalytic site [22].
5. Validation of the 3D model was performed using the PROCHECK server [25].

3.2.2 HDCA8

1. To obtain the 3D model of HDAC8, approximately 20 3D models were considered from the PDB (PDB ID: 3SFH, 3SFF, 1 T64, 3MZ3, 3F07, 3EZP, 3EZT, 2V5W, 2V5X, 3F06, 3EW8, 3EWF, 3MZ4, 1 T67, 1 T69, 1VKG, 3MZ6, 3MZ7, 3F0R, and 1 W22) to perform a BLAST analysis.
2. These 3D structures were subjected to sequence alignment using the STRAP program [26].
3. In this structural alignment, the HDAC8 primary sequence (NP_060956.1) was used as reference and was compared with each of the 3D models of HDAC8.
4. Finally, the crystal structure of PDB: 3F07 was chosen for further docking studies because this structure shared the highest percentage of sequence identities [27], and only a few missing residues were added using the MODELLER program.

5. Validation of the 3D model was carried out by redocking the co-crystallized ligand (APHA: 3-(1-methyl-4-phenylacetyl-1H-2pyrrolyl)-N-hydroxy-2-propenamide) of the PDB: 3F07. The binding mode of APHA was reproduced in this constructed 3D model.

3.3 Proposal of a Set of Ligands that Target the Proteins of Pharmacological Interest

Prior to the design of new ligands, it is highly recommended to identify the necessary features that an active ligand should possess, for example, feature chemistry type, three-dimensional conformational positions, and binding poses (*see* **Note 7**), which can be encoded into a pharmacophore model [28]. Indeed, the pharmacophore model can be generated from a set of known ligand complexes [29]. Moreover, information regarding the active sites of the ligands can be applied to create a pharmacophore model [30].

3.3.1 HDCA6

Regarding the HDAC6, a set of phenyl butyric acid derivatives with possible HDAC6 inhibitory activity were designed through in silico methods, considering tubacin (HDAC-selective inhibitor) as a reference [16]. The designed compounds were submitted to theoretical *ADMET* analyses, and their binding properties on different HDAC6 conformers were evaluated through docking calculations. Finally, these in silico studies allowed us to identify a compound named B-R2B [16].

3.3.2 HDC8

With regard to HDAC8, some known HDAC inhibitors (HDACi), suberoylanilide hydroxamic acid (SAHA), valproic acid (VPA), aroyl-pyrrole-hydroxy-amide (APHA-8), and tubacin, were employed to explore their binding properties [27]. Additionally, in another study from our group, some VPA derivatives were designed to target HDAC8. These compounds were evaluated using computational procedures in order to select the best compounds (Gln-VPA) and to synthesize and test them experimentally [31]. Additionally, some other VPA-aryl derivatives have been designed and virtually studied in order to improve the solubility of the former compounds [32, 33].

3.4 Drawing and Parameterization of the Ligands

In all cases, ligands were drawn using ACD/ChemSketch (http://www.acdlabs.com/resources/freeware/chemsketch/) to be built according to their chemical structures considering pKa, chiral center, and other features according to their natural environment. Furthermore, some specialized software products such as *Gaussian View 5.0 package* (used to convert ligands into 3D format (Z-Matrix) and *Gaussian 03 software* were used to perform energetic and geometric optimization of the ligands at different semi-empirical levels [13].

For particular cases, some quantum chemical descriptors were used to select the best compounds using QSAR analyses to obtain reliable data for statistical analyses that yield robust data to select the most promising compounds for the synthesis [33].

3.5 ADMET Analysis

ADMET (absorption, distribution, metabolism, excretion, and toxicity) analysis and the use of the Lipinski rule have revolutionized the drug development pipeline since their exploitation has achieved savings in research costs [34] (*see* **Note 8**). Moreover, it has been observed that ignoring these properties can cause a major cause of failure of drug candidates during late phases of drug development [35].

The servers OSIRIS Property Explorer (http://www.organic-chemistry.org/prog/peo/) and Molinspiration (http://www.molinspiration. com/) have been widely used in order to determine the *ADMET* properties and physicochemical properties of the compounds. After this in silico evaluation, it was possible to select only the ligands that show null or very low predicted toxicity and proper physicochemical properties (non-violations of Lipinski rules) [16]. Thus, a higher probability for the proposed compounds to be successful in the pharmaceutical market is suggested.

3.6 Docking Simulations of the Designed Compounds on Target Structures

Molecular docking studies have been considered one of the most useful methods in SBDD [36] (*see* **Note 9**). In general, the docking process consists first of predicting the ligand conformation (poses) and second of the assessment of the binding affinity of all poses by a score obtained either from a physical or knowledge-based potential. Docking analyses are very useful for the prediction of the binding site of the proteins as well as for the determination of the binding affinities of the compounds on the protein systems (*see* **Note 10**) [8]. Depending on the characteristics (environment and nonprotein components) of the proteins, one should establish a particular docking protocol initializing with the docking validation procedure (*see* **Note 11**).

3.6.1 HDCA6

In the docking analysis on HDAC6, only one monomer (DD2-HDAC6, G482-G801) of the dimeric protein was considered as previously reported [22]. The set of phenyl butyric acid derivatives were docked on different DD2-HDAC6 conformations using the AutoDock 4.2 program [14]. For all cases, blind docking calculations were carried out using a box with the dimensions of 126 Å × 126 Å × 126 Å and a point grid with the spacing of 0.375 Å centered on the protein and applying default settings. Free energy values of docking were calculated using a scoring function inspired by X-Score [37]. After performing *ADMET* and docking analysis, we could identify the compound named B-R2B [16].

3.6.2 HDCA8

For docking studies on HDAC8 [27, 38], some known HDAC inhibitors (HDACi) were employed: suberoylanilide hydroxamic acid (SAHA), valproic acid (VPA), aroyl-pyrrole-hydroxy-amide (APHA-8), and tubacin. These were docked into different conformations of the protein obtained though MD simulations (10, 20, 30, 40, and 50 ns). Docking analyses for HDAC8 inhibitors were performed using AutoDock Vina [37] and considering zinc metal as a cofactor because all ligands show hydroxamic acid that can couple to the metal ion [27]. All docking simulations employed a 126 Å × 126 Å × 126 Å point grid with the 0.375 Å spacing, centered on the protein. The free energy values of docking were calculated using a scoring function inspired by X-Score [37].

3.7 Molecular Dynamics Simulations as a Valuable Tool for Binding Prediction

In parallel with docking simulations, MD simulations provide a better approximation of the binding affinities and modes of the potential compounds on the proteins of pharmacological interest because they permit the consideration of the dynamic aspects of the protein (which are ignored in common docking analysis) by obtaining different conformational states of the protein, better known as snapshots.

3.7.1 HDAC6

After identifying the compound B-R2B from theoretical *ADMET* analysis, the B-R2B-HDAC6 complex was submitted to 100-ns-long MD simulations in order to obtain detailed structural information as well as to obtain different HDAC6 conformers for further docking analysis; the simulations revealed that the B-R2B binding site is located at the entrance of HDAC6 active pocket [16]. In this work, MD simulations were performed with the AMBER 12 package [39]. Technical information about these MD simulations is described in detail in ref. 16.

3.7.2 HDAC8

Through docking analysis and MD simulations, it was possible to elucidate the HDAC8 structural features in order to obtain insights for drug development of new HDAC inhibitors. For HDAC8, classical MD simulations were conducted using the NAMD 2.6 program [40] and the CHARMM22 force field [41] in order to elucidate the HDAC8 structural features to obtain insights for future drug development of new HDAC inhibitors, as well as to obtain different conformations of the protein for further docking studies. Technical information about these MD simulations is described in detail in Ref. [27].

3.8 Selection of the Best Evaluated Ligands

One of the main objectives of the in silico studies is to select the most promising compounds for further studies including their chemical synthesis and testing through biological evaluation assays (*see* **Note 12**).

3.8.1 HDAC6

1. From the in silico studies of this protein, it was possible to estimate the binding free energy of the compounds, thus enabling the selection of the compounds (first generation) that show the highest affinities on HDAC6 from the docking studies.
2. These ligands were structurally modified by including an aromatic group to increase their affinity on DD2-HDAC. Additionally, a second generation of compounds, which preserve better structural similarity to the tubacin structure (named biphenylamides), was generated [16].

3.8.2 HDAC8

In the published work by Sixto Lopez and collaborators, the main objective was to explore the affinity and binding modes of known HDACi (APHA, VPA, SAHA, and tubacin) and then to identify important characteristics that will assist in the future design of new HDAC8-selective inhibitors [27]. In this work, MD simulations and docking studies were employed to depict the binding interactions of the HDACi on the different conformers of HDAC8. Finally, the results suggest that the inhibitors that showed the highest binding free energy were those that established π-π and hydrophobic interactions with the residues of the catalytic pocket, such as tubacin, which was able to interact with the ACSP residues (F152 and Y306), the CS (H180 and H143), and the CS pocket (F207 and F208) through π-π interactions [27].

In another work by Martinez-Pacheco, docking and QSAR studies were performed for 500 aryl-VPA derivatives as possible HDAC8 inhibitors to detect the potential antiproliferative compounds [33].

In order to obtain HDAC inhibitors through chemical synthesis, amide formation was performed to form mono-aryl ligands [16], VPA-aryl derivatives [32, 33], or VPA-amino acid derivatives [31].

4 Notes

1. Target-based drug design requires a 3D structure obtained from PDB or under molecular modeling.
2. Drug design could consider being either target- or ligand-based for building pharmacophore groups.
3. If 3D data is available, the structure is retrieved from PDB and can be subjected to structural refinement (minimization) or MD simulation studies to obtain several conformations, and thus, they can be used for further docking studies.

4. Most of the crystal structures retrieved from PDB (https://www.rcsb.org/pdb/home/home.do) are obtained from X-ray or NMR experimental techniques.
5. In the case when no crystal structure of the protein is available at the Protein Data Bank (PDB), the sequence needs to be downloaded from NCBI or EBI. Then, multiple alignment sequences are performed to select the consensus sequence (which in most of the cases belongs to wild-type sequence). Then, this sequence can be submitted to BLAST analysis in order to identify if there are any crystal structures that belong to these homologous proteins. In some cases, programs such as I-TASSER, Rosetta protein structure prediction, SWISS-MODEL, and many others can be used to build three-dimensional models of the proteins.
6. Once the 3D model is built by molecular modeling techniques, it needs to be evaluated under structural criteria, such as 3D-verify, Errat, or Ramachandran maps.
7. Drug design could be guided by employing a set of small ligands that contain pharmacophores. A pharmacophore model can be used to identify novel ligands through de novo design or virtual screening techniques.
8. After designing hundreds of possible compounds, these compounds have to be subjected to *ADMET* analysis by using several *online* servers (e.g., Molinspiration, Data Warrior), which will help to select the most promising compounds, for example, the compounds that could reach the target efficiently after crossing all biological barriers without any or with minimal side effects, and to discard the compounds that show any toxicity problem.
9. Following the filtering of the compounds through *ADMET* analysis which discard those compounds that showed toxicity properties whereas the best evaluated compounds are subjected to docking analysis by employing a crystal structure of the protein or a 3D built 3D model obtained through molecular modeling methods.
10. From the docking analysis, it is possible to select the compounds that show the highest free binding energy values by applying scoring functions implemented by programs such as AutoDock, and thus, some of the compounds are predicted to be bound with higher affinity on the protein of interest.
11. A validation process is needed before performing docking analysis with the designed ligands. This can be performed by coupling a co-crystallized ligand on the protein of interest and evaluating whether the binding mode is reproducible.

12. Only the best evaluated ligands from the *ADMET* and docking analyses will be synthesized and biologically assayed since they are predicted to show better drug-like properties.

Acknowledgments

This work was supported by CONACYT Mexico (CB-254600 and PDCPN-782), SIP20160204, COFAA-SIP/IPN COFAASIP/IPN and Centro de Nanociencias y Micro y Nanotecnologías del IPN, México, and CYTED: 214RT0482.

References

1. Blundell TL, Abell C, Cleasby A et al (2002) High-throughput X-ray crystallography for drug discovery. In: Flower DR (ed) Drug design: special publication. Royal Society of Chemistry, Cambridge
2. Müntener T, Häussinger D, Selenko P, Theillet FX (2016) In-cell protein structures from 2D NMR experiments. J Phys Chem Lett 7 (14):2821–2825. https://doi.org/10.1021/acs.jpclett.6b01074
3. Mandal S, Moudgil M, Mandal SK (2009) Rational drug design. Eur J Pharmacol 625 (1-3):90–100. https://doi.org/10.1016/j.ejphar.2009.06.065
4. Shoichet BK (2004) Virtual screening of chemical libraries. Nature 432(7019):862–865. https://doi.org/10.1038/nature03197
5. Charifson PS, Kuntz ID (1997) Recent successes and continuing limitations in computer aided drug design. In: Charifson PS (ed) Practical application of computer aided drug design. Dekker, New York
6. Leelananda SP, Lindert S (2016) Computational methods in drug discovery. Beilstein J Org Chem 12:2694–2718. https://doi.org/10.3762/bjoc.12.267
7. Aparoy P, Reddy KK, Reddanna P (2012) Structure and ligand based drug design strategies in the development of novel 5-LOX inhibitors. Curr Med Chem 19(22):3763–3778. https://doi.org/10.2174/092986712801661112
8. Meng XY, Zhang HX, Mezei M, Cui M (2011) Molecular docking: a powerful approach for structure-based drug discovery. Curr Comput Aided Drug Des 7(2):146–157. https://doi.org/10.2174/157340911795677602
9. Acharya C, Coop A, Polli JE, Mackerell AD Jr (2011) Recent advances in ligand-based drug design: relevance and utility of the conformationally sampled pharmacophore approach. Curr Comput Aided Drug Des 7 (1):10–22. https://doi.org/10.2174/157340911793743547
10. Ishikawa T, Hirano H, Saito H et al (2012) Quantitative structure-activity relationship (QSAR) analysis to predict drug-drug interactions of ABC transporter ABCG2. Mini Rev Med Chem 12(6):505–514. https://doi.org/10.2174/138955712800493825
11. Wang Y, Xing J, Xu Y et al (2015) In silico ADME/T modelling for rational drug design. Q Rev Biophys 48(4):488–515. https://doi.org/10.1017/S0033583515000190
12. Bello M, Martínez-Archundia M, Correa-Basurto J (2013) Automated docking for novel drug discovery. Expert Opin Drug Discovery 8(7):821–834. https://doi.org/10.1517/17460441.2013.794780
13. Frisch MJ, Trucks GW, Schlegel HB et al (1998) Gaussian 98, revision A.9. Gaussian, Pittsburgh, PA
14. Morris GM, Huey R, Lindstrom W et al (2009) AutoDock4 and AutoDockTools 4: automated docking with selective receptor flexibility. J Comput Chem 30(16):2785–2791. https://doi.org/10.1002/jcc.21256
15. Anderson AC (2003) The process of structure-based drug design. Chem Biol 10(9):787–797. https://doi.org/10.1016/j.chembiol.2003.09.002
16. Rodríguez-Fonseca RA, Sixto-López Y, Fragoso-Vázquez MJ et al (2017) Design, synthesis and biological evaluation of a phenyl butyric acid derivative, N-(4-chlorophenyl)-4-phenylbutanamide: a HDAC6 inhibitor with anti-proliferative activity on cervix cancer and leukemia cell. Anticancer Agents Med Chem 17 (10):1441–1454. https://doi.org/10.2174/1871520617666170103092851

17. Roper S, Esteller M (2007) The role of histone deacetylases (HDACs) in human cancer. Mol Oncol 1(1):19–25. https://doi.org/10.1016/j.molonc.2007.01.001
18. Lappano R, Pisano A, Maggiolini M (2014) GPER function in breast cancer: an overview. Front Endocrinol 5:66. https://doi.org/10.3389/fendo.2014.00066
19. Oehme I, Deubzer HE, Wegener D et al (2009) Histone deacetylase 8 in neuroblastoma. Clin Cancer Res 15(1):91–99. https://doi.org/10.1158/1078-0432.CCR-08-0684
20. Vannini A, Volpari C, Filocamo G et al (2004) Crystal structure of a eukaryotic zinc-dependent histone deacetylase, human HDAC8, complexed with a hydroxamic acid inhibitor. Proc Natl Acad Sci USA 101 (42):15064–15069. https://doi.org/10.1073/pnas.0404603101
21. Zhou H, Skolnick J (2010) Improving threading algorithms for remote homology modeling by combining fragment and template comparisons. Proteins 78(9):2041–2048. https://doi.org/10.1002/prot.22717
22. Sixto-López Y, Bello M, Rodríguez-Fonseca RA et al (2016) Searching the conformational complexity and binding properties of HDAC6 through docking and molecular dynamic simulations. J Biomol Struct Dyn 35 (13):2794–2814. https://doi.org/10.1080/07391102.2016.1231084
23. Zhang Y (2008) I-TASSER server for protein 3D structure prediction. BMC Bioinformatics 9:40. https://doi.org/10.1186/1471-2105-9-40
24. Haggarty SJ, Koeller KM, Wong JC et al (2003) Domain-selective small-molecule inhibitor of histone deacetylase 6 (HDAC6)-mediated tubulin deacetylation. Proc Natl Acad Sci U S A 100(8):4389–4394. https://doi.org/10.1073/pnas.0430973100
25. Laskowski R, Rullmann JA, MacArthur M et al (1996) AQUA and PROCHECK-NMR: programs for checking the quality of protein structures solved by NMR. J Biomol NMR 8 (4):477–486. https://doi.org/10.1007/BF00228148
26. Gille C, Frommel C (2001) STRAP: editor for STRuctural alignments of proteins. Bioinformatics 17(4):377–378. https://doi.org/10.1093/bioinformatics/17.4.377
27. Sixto-López Y, Gómez-Vidal JA, Correa-Basurto J (2014) Exploring the potential binding sites of some known HDAC inhibitors on some HDAC8 conformers by docking studies. Appl Biochem Biotechnol 173(7):1907–1926. https://doi.org/10.1007/s12010-014-0976-1
28. Van Drie JH (2003) Pharmacophore discovery-lessons learned. Curr Pharm Des 9 (20):1649–1664. https://doi.org/10.2174/1381612033454568
29. Yang SY (2010) Pharmacophore modeling and applications in drug discovery: challenges and recent advances. Drug Discov Today 15 (11-12):444–450. https://doi.org/10.1016/j.drudis.2010.03.013
30. Chia-Hsien L, Hsuan-Cheng H, Hsueh-Fen J (2011) Reviewing ligand-based rational drug design: the search for an ATP synthase. Int J Mol Sci 12(8):5304–5318. https://doi.org/10.3390/ijms12085304
31. Martínez-Ramos F, Luna-Palencia GR, Vásquez-Moctezuma I et al (2016) Docking studies of glutamine valproic acid derivative (S)-5-amino-2-(heptan-4-ylamino)-5-oxopentanoic acid (Gln-VPA) on HDAC8 with biological evaluation in HeLa cells. Anticancer Agents Med Chem 16(11):1485–1490. https://doi.org/10.2174/1871520616666160204111158
32. Prestegui-Martel B, Bermúdez-Lugo JA, Chávez-Blanco A et al (2016) N-(2-hydroxyphenyl)-2-propylpentanamide, a valproic acid aryl derivative designed in silico with improved anti-proliferative activity in HeLa, rhabdomyosarcoma and breast cancer cells. J Enzyme Inhib Med Chem 31(sup3):140–149. https://doi.org/10.1080/14756366.2016.1210138
33. Martínez-Pacheco H, Ramírez-Galicia G, Vergara-Arias M et al (2017) Docking and QSAR studies of aryl-valproic acid derivatives to identify antiproliferative agents targeting the HDAC8. Anticancer Agents Med Chem 17 (7):927–940. https://doi.org/10.2174/1871520616666161019143219
34. Lawless MS, Waldman M, Fraczkiewicz R, Clark RD (2016) Using cheminformatics in drug discovery. Handb Exp Pharmacol 232:139–168. https://doi.org/10.1007/164_2015_23
35. Butina D, Segall K, Frankcombe K (2002) Predicting ADME properties *In silico*: methods and models. Drug Discov Today 7(11): S83–S88. https://doi.org/10.1016/S1359-6446(02)02288-2
36. Ruyck J, Brysbaert G, Blossey R, Lensink M (2016) Molecular docking as a popular tool in drug design, an in silico travel. Adv Appl Bioinform Chem 9:1–11. https://doi.org/10.2147/AABC.S105289

37. Trott O, Olson AJ (2010) AutoDock Vina: improving the speed and accuracy of docking with a new scoring function, efficient optimization and multithreading. J Comput Chem 31 (2):455–461. https://doi.org/10.1002/jcc.21334
38. Bermúdez-Lugo JA, Perez-Gonzalez O, Rosales-Hernández MC et al (2012) Exploration of the valproic acid binding site on histone deacetylase 8 using docking and molecular dynamic simulations. J Mol Model 18 (6):2301–2310. https://doi.org/10.1007/s00894-011-1240-z
39. Case DA, Cheatham TE 3rd, Darden T et al (2005) The Amber biomolecular simulation programs. J Comput Chem 26(16):1668–1688. https://doi.org/10.1002/jcc.20290
40. Phillips JC, Braun R, Wang W et al (2005) Scalable molecular dynamics with NAMD. J Comput Chem 26(16):1781–1802. https://doi.org/10.1002/jcc.20289
41. Brooks BR, Bruccoleri RE, Olafson BD et al (1983) CHARMM: a program for macromolecular energy, minimization, and dynamics calculations. J Comput Chem 4(2):187–217. https://doi.org/10.1002/jcc.540040211

Chapter 25

Reactions in NMR Tubes as Key Weapon in Rational Drug Design

Dimitrios Ntountaniotis

Abstract

NMR spectroscopy is a powerful technique suitable for obtaining detailed structural and dynamic data at atomic resolution. Progress in NMR instrumentation has led the scientific community to produce novel techniques which provide valuable information to resolve demanding and crucial questions of molecular biology and rational drug design. This chapter outlines the progress of NMR spectroscopy in the rational drug design. In addition, it offers an example of a reaction in NMR tube for achieving rational drug design.

Key words NMR spectroscopy for liquids, Structural properties, Drug design and discovery

1 Introduction

The physical phenomenon of nuclear magnetic resonance (NMR) has led scientists to develop many techniques in order to acquire significant structural information. In this context, NMR is a powerful tool used in molecular biology and rational drug design. Nowadays, NMR and X-ray diffraction complement one another, so that researchers are able to resolve important issues of molecular biology and rational drug design [1, 2]. Biological systems resemble like intricate puzzles and NMR has been proven to be the most influential contributor to put "pieces of knowledge" together. Molecular structures' elucidation is a challenging and demanding procedure. Each case of a biological system is characterized by unique features and leads also to distinct problems (in order to obtain all the necessary information). Therefore, it is evident that different NMR techniques are applied with the aim to resolve a variety of biological issues.

There is a basic separation of the broad range of spectroscopic experiments into two kinds: (1) NMR spectroscopy for liquids and (2) NMR spectroscopy for solids (ssNMR). Historically, NMR for

Thomas Mavromoustakos and Tahsin F. Kellici (eds.), *Rational Drug Design: Methods and Protocols*, Methods in Molecular Biology, vol. 1824, https://doi.org/10.1007/978-1-4939-8630-9_25,

liquids is the most common, but during the last decades, ssNMR is developed rapidly.

High-resolution NMR for liquids: A functional advantage of NMR spectroscopy is its ability to attribute data for protein complexes under physiological environment at atomic detail. The saturation transfer difference spectroscopy (STD) is developed in order to identify small ligands which bind a receptor protein [3, 4]. The sensitivity of STD procedure is so high that the binding of the ligand can be detected even if the receptor is at 30-fold lower concentration [3, 4]. The key point is that selective irradiation saturates the spectrum of the receptor in a range that does not include ligand resonances. In case the ligand dissociates sufficiently fast, it is possible to detect saturation as signal reductions in the spectrum of the free ligand.

Isotope labeling method (^{15}N, ^{13}C, ^{2}H) is another common experiment for studying protein-ligand interactions. Recording intermolecular NOEs is an extremely demanding task, because there is the necessity to distinguish weak NOEs among a plethora of strong intramolecular NOEs. In this frame at the past, isotope-filtered NMR experiments have been applied, targeting to comprehend protein interactions [5, 6]. In case of homodimers which have C2 symmetry, a more efficient approach has been applied [7, 8]. The idea is to mix a deuterated ^{15}N-labeled protein and an unlabeled binding protein. As a result, the ^{15}N-dispersed 3D NOESY-HSQC spectrum of the complex is appropriate to record intermolecular NOEs between aliphatic protons of non-labeled protein and amide protons of the ^{15}N-labeled protein. One major difference (from the pulse sequences applied in filtering experiments) is that the pulse sequence is shorter and this fact leads to higher sensitivity [3].

In general integral membrane proteins (IMPs) are very significant in cell communication with the environment. Solution NMR spectroscopy has been used to shed light on these molecular mechanisms and reveal detailed information [9]. Fluorine labeling of IMPs is being developed rapidly during the last decade. For example, conformational changes in β2-adrenergic receptor were studied when a covalent modification of cysteines with a ^{19}F-labeled compound was applied [10].

The chemical shift index (CSI) is a widely used tool in protein NMR. It is recommended as it can provide information related to the secondary structure (e.g., helices, beta strands, or random coil regions). If the aforementioned data is combined with distance constraints of the protein, then it is possible to determine protein's 3D fold [9, 11].

Historically, significant progress in the scientific effort to develop target-detected NMR methods was made by S. Fesik and colleagues in 1997, when the structure-activity relationship (SAR) for NMR was introduced [12, 13]. In this context, libraries of thousands drug-like fragments are screened by heteronuclear NMR. The idea is to choose ligands with low to medium affinity and establish primary binding sites. Subsequently, a new NMR screening is carried out in order to identify weak ligands which bind to another location near to the first site [13]. In some ideal cases, the described procedure can result to appropriate compounds with paramount importance for several therapeutic targets [13].

Researchers have achieved also to develop a membrane-mimicking environment in order to solubilize IMPs for NMR experiments. The membrane mimetic media are called nanodiscs. They don't contain detergents. As a consequence it is expected that problems related to detergents (e.g., they may alter the interactions with a ligand) [9, 14] are avoided.

Flow NMR spectroscopy is characterized by the fact that the solution sample enters the NMR probe as a flowing stream [15]. Two different approaches are applied. Firstly, the sample is submitted in a separation method (e.g., electrophoresis) prior to NMR experiment. Secondly, the liquid flow is applied only in order to lead the sample into the NMR probe. LC-NMR-MS is an example of this approach, whereas direct-injection NMR (DI-NMR) and flow-injection analysis NMR (FIA-NMR) are the main representatives for the second approach. FIA-NMR is a technique where the sample is injected as a plug in the flow stream and then is introduced to the NMR coil [15–17]. In case of DI-NMR, the sample is injected directly into the coil. The absence of additional solvents makes it feasible to retrieve the sample [15]. For this reason this technique is important for analysis of novel drugs (which are often very expensive). DI-NMR is recommended also, if maximum sensitivity is necessary.

It is evident also that a lot of the aforementioned methods are applied to collect significant data for drug discovery. A variety of questions can be answered. For example, "does a drug bind to the target," "is the target folded," or "what is the stoichiometry of binding" [18]? Furthermore, apart from novel methods, the effort to design innovative NMR equipment is also crucial. For example, the significance to accelerate the drug discovery process by developing high-throughput NMR spectrometers using complementary metal-oxide semiconductor (CMOS) has been already described [19].

NMR is also a powerful tool in specific drug-related issues. After structure-activity optimization has been fulfilled, other problems may still exist. Poor bioavailability is a major concern for medicinal chemists. The synthesis of inclusion complexes has been a widespread idea to ameliorate the bioavailability of drugs. Subsequently, it is necessary to obtain detailed information concerning structural properties of inclusion complexes. NMR spectrometry has been applied in order to understand the complex formation (e.g., ROESY spectroscopy provides data for spatial proximity between the guest and the host molecules) [20].

A variety of examples for exceptional structural information can be found in literature. It is known that the HMBC experiment leads to the assignment of structural fragments through correlations between protons and carbons separated by two or three bonds (2JC,H and 3JC,H). A very interesting paper by Araya-Maturana et al. was published in 2008 [21]. In this report the authors explained several cases with correlations across five bonds.

A different issue resolved often by NMR is to detect different kinds of isomerism (e.g., regioisomerism, stereoisomerism, rotamer formation, etc.) [22]. For example, the determination of enantiomeric excess in chiral compounds is challenging. Organic chemists have used chiral derivatization agents (CDAs) in order to produce diastereoisomers [23]. A lot of effort to achieve the objective of determining the absolute configuration in similar cases via NMR spectroscopy exists for decades [24]. A review with recent advances in multinuclear NMR spectroscopy for chiral recognition has been published in 2017 [25]. Moreover, another demanding and interesting task is to find out the energy barrier between two rotamers. An example was described by Sulima et al., who used the temperature dependence of ^{1}H and ^{13}C coalescence experiments [26]. Conformational and tautomeric eccentricities have been studied using NMR as reported by Hansen et al. [27].

A significant tautomerism study is achieved by ^{15}N NMR. The widespread interest is due to two groups of molecules, pyridine derivatives and Schiff bases, which constitute a variety of biologically active compounds [28].

An additional issue studied also by NMR spectroscopy is to monitor a reaction into a NMR tube. This method has the following advantages: (1) the necessary quantity of a reactant in order to monitor the reaction may be small (consequently it is a cost-effective process); (2) the yield of the reaction may be (often) calculated easily; (3) it is possible to calculate the reaction rate coefficient, k, for simple reactions; (4) it is possible to understand the overall reaction mechanism without disturbing the conditions of the reaction; and (5) a rapid screening of different conditions (of the reaction) may be applicable. The key experimental information is often derived by ^{1}H NMR spectroscopy. The appropriate proton peak (or peaks) of the reactant is selected. The respective proton peak (or peaks) of the product is also monitored. The integration of the aforementioned peaks (both, those of the reactant and those of the product) in successive ^{1}H NMR experiments provides all the necessary data. The percentage of the conversion of the reactant is calculated easily via these spectra. Very useful reactions in NMR tubes have been described in recent years [29–33]. In fact, a lot of technological and experimental setups have been developed in order to apply NMR spectroscopy to more complex reaction systems [33].

^{1}H NMR spectra are appropriate for continuous analysis of the progress of a reaction. An ideal case of a reaction in an NMR tube consists of two reactants. The first reactant is a substance, and the second reactant is its solvent. In this case the spectra may be simpler. ç representative example is described in Subheading 3.1 of this chapter. The methylation reaction discussed at room temperature can be applied to other drug molecules whose the pharmacological properties can be important. In general, the methylation of hydroxyl or phenolic groups leads to ethers which are more lipophilic, a property that sometimes is beneficial for the drug discovery if the initial compound is highly hydrophilic. In addition, the methylation can optimize the physicochemical properties of the molecules.

2 Materials

2.1 General Practical Aspects

1. All samples for liquid NMR spectroscopy should be sufficiently soluble in the respective deuterated solvent.
2. Usually, liquid NMR samples are prepared in 5 mm tubes. For different NMR instruments (e.g., 400, 500, 600 MHz), NMR tubes of different quality are selected as well. In case that the sample dissolves glass, a polytetrafluoroethylene (PTFE) insert or a Kel-F (a fluorochemical product) tube is used.
3. There is a possibility that the tube cap may contaminate the sample. The cap could release materials (e.g., when $CDCl_3$ or DMSO-d6 is used). In this case the researcher could close the tube with Teflon tape and afterward with the cap. It is not recommended to invert the tube, but just to mix with a vortex mixer [34].
4. Rarely the sample is air sensitive; therefore, an inert atmosphere or vacuum is required. If the removal of oxygen is necessary, it is recommended to prepare the sample under argon and run the experiment as soon as possible. Special NMR tubes are commercially available in case it is necessary to prepare samples under vacuum or an inert atmosphere [34].

2.2 Materials for Liquid NMR Experiments

All materials for liquid NMR experiments are stored at 4 °C.

1. CD_3OD (99%+) is purchased from Sigma Aldrich, St. Louis, MO.
2. CD_3CN 99.80% and DMSO-d6 99.96% are purchased from Euriso-Top, Gif-sur-Yvette, Essone, France.
3. Olmesartan is kindly donated by Daiichi Sankyo Pro Pharma Japan.

3 Methods

3.1 Monitoring via ^1H NMR Spectroscopy of the Progress of Transformation of Drug Olmesartan to Its Methyl Ether Analogue: A Pharmacologically Active Compound

1. The in situ formation of a new product is observed when olmesartan (Fig. 1) is dissolved in an NMR tube with CD_3OD.

The new peaks are enhanced with time. For example, the new peak at 5.59 ppm appears (Fig. 2) due to the formation of a new molecule. At a higher temperature (45 °C), the reaction is completed at 90%. The experiment which ensures that the integration of peaks can result in quantitative measurements (in order to compare respective peaks of the reactant and the product) is explained in **Note 1**.

The rationale to exclude three possible reactions (dynamic process, formation of dimer, or lactonization) is explained in **Notes 2–4**. After the completion of the structure elucidation (for further details, please read [35]), it is revealed that the new product is olmesartan methyl ether (Fig. 3).

The resonated peak at 5.59 ppm is attributed to the protons 7 (Fig. 1). Information about the pharmacological characterization of olmesartan methyl ether (in order to understand if this analogue is bound to the AT1 receptor with similar affinity to drugs olmesartan and losartan) is provided in **Note 5**. In the described work, simple NMR experiments (^{1}H) of olmesartan proved to be valuable for many future studies. Impurities (whose structure elucidation is achieved mainly with NMR experiments) of a drug are very significant, because valuable stability issues of the initial drug are comprehensible. Furthermore, the formation of a byproduct may result to

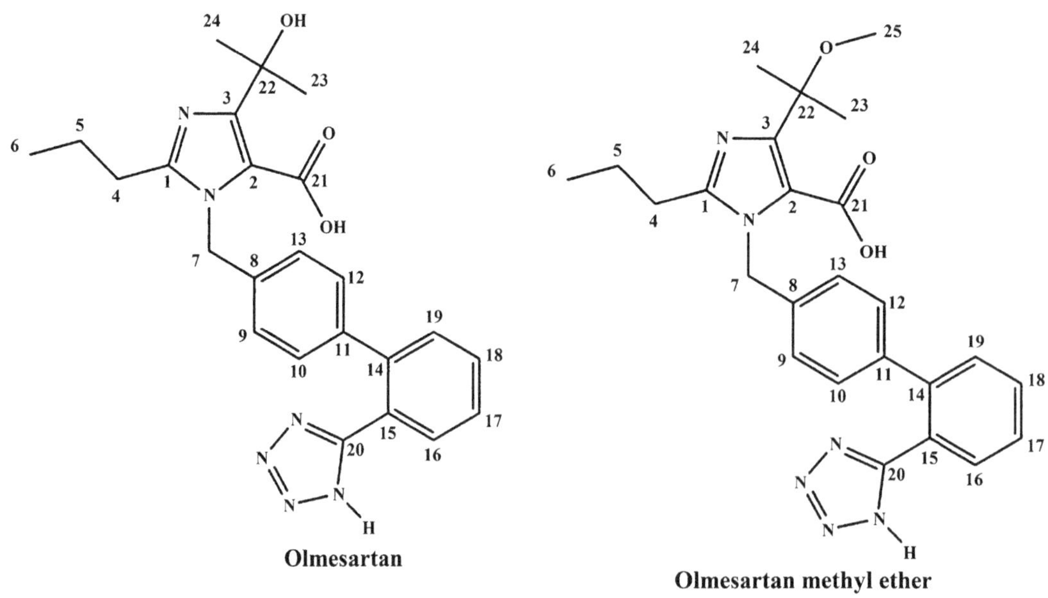

Fig. 1 Olmesartan and olmesartan methyl ether

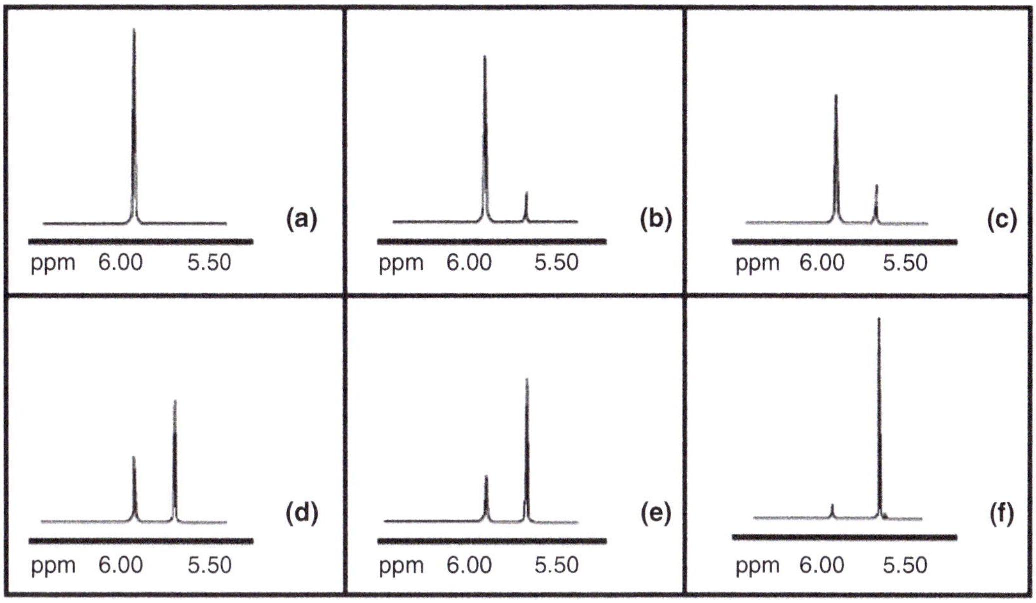

Fig. 2 The peak at 5.59 ppm is enhanced with time. Experimental run after (**a**) dissolution, (**b**) 4 h, (**c**) 16 h, (**d**) 29 h, (**e**) 37 h, (**f**) 70 h

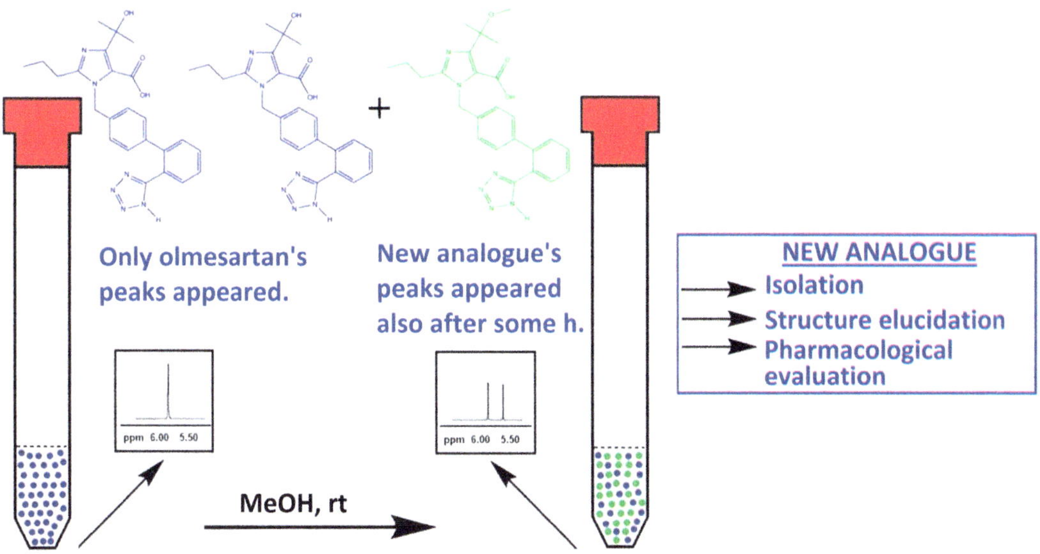

Fig. 3 The formation of olmesartan methyl ether

a synthetic idea which may be applicable in similar cases. Of course all the new impurities could be checked for pharmacological characterization.

In case of olmesartan, the reaction which takes place is the following:

$$C_{24}H_{26}N_6O_3 + CD_3OD \rightarrow C_{25}H_{25}D_3N_6O_3 + HDO \quad (1)$$

2. 3.3 mg of olmesartan is dissolved in CD_3OD and its methyl analogue is dissolved in either CD_3OD or CD_3CN (for further details, please read [35]), in order to obtain NMR spectra. The experiments are performed on a Bruker Avance III spectrometer operating at 600.11 MHz for 1H and at 150.11 MHz for 13C, with a 5 mm inverse detection probe and on a direct-drive Varian 800 MHz NMR spectrometer equipped with a 5 mm cryoprobe. The residual ^{1}H (3.33 ppm) and ^{13}C (49.50 ppm) signals of CD_3OD are used as an internal standard. The pulse sequences included in the libraries of pulse programs are used in order to acquire 1D and 2D (COSY, HSQC, HMBC) NMR spectra.
3. In general the rate v of a reaction $\alpha\varsigma + \beta B \rightarrow \gamma C + \delta D$ is given by the equations

$$v = k\,[A]^x[B]^y \quad (2)$$

$$\text{or } v = -1/\alpha\ \Delta[A]/\Delta t = -1/\beta\Delta[B]/\Delta t = 1/\gamma\ \Delta[\Gamma]/\Delta t = 1/\delta\ \Delta[\Delta]/\Delta t \quad (3)$$

and x, y are not always equal to α and β (stoichiometric coefficients). [A], [B], [C], and [D] represent the concentrations of the substances A, B, C, and D, and t is the time (after the moment the reaction started). k is the reaction rate constant or reaction rate coefficient which depends on temperature and the nature of the reactants. The exponents x and y represent the partial orders of the reaction. The total order is equal to $x + y$. In case x and y are identical (respectively) to α and β, then the reaction takes place with the simple mechanism described by the chemical equation. Otherwise (in case $x \neq \alpha$ and $y \neq \beta$), the reaction mechanism is more complicated, and it can be determined experimentally. The reaction rate constant is calculated via the Arrhenius equation:

$$k = A\ \mathrm{e} - \mathrm{Ea/RT} \quad (4)$$

- Ea is the activation energy per mole of the reactants.
- ς (different from the reactant A) is the pre-exponential factor which is correlated with the conditions of the reaction and the shape and size of reactants.
- T is the temperature.
- R is the gas constant.

For the aforementioned reaction, the rate v is given by the following equation:

$$v = k_{45^\circ C}[C_{24}H_{26}N_6O_3]^x[CD_3OD]^y \quad (5)$$

Figure 4 and Table 1 show the $[C_{24}H_{26}N_6O_3]$ as function of time. The $[C_{24}H_{26}N_6O_3]_{initial}$ (3.3 mg of olmesartan is dissolved in 0.7 mL CD_3OD) is

$[C_{24}H_{26}N_6O_3]_{initial} = 0.0106$ mole/L

$[CD_3OD]$ is calculated easily knowing that the MW of CD_3OD is 36.0665 g/mole and the density of methanol-d_4 is equal to $d_{meth} = 0.888$ g/cm^3)

$[CD_3OD]_{initial} \approx 24.621$ mole/L

In order to calculate the instantaneous rate v at a certain moment t_1, it is possible to design the tangent line of the curve at the point which represents the moment t_1. The slope of the tangent

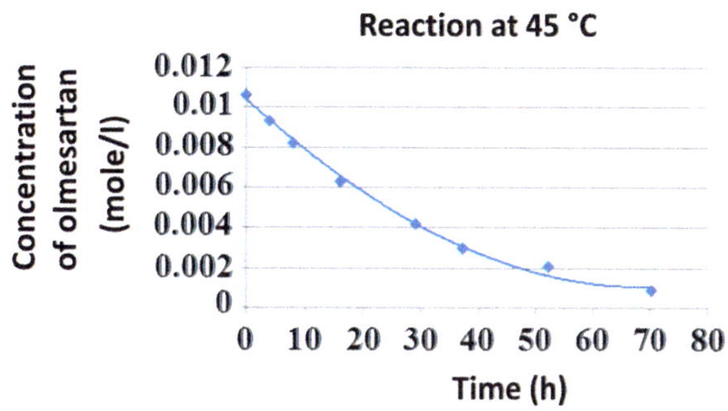

Fig. 4 The concentration of olmesartan as function of time

Table 1
The concentration of olmesartan as function of time

Time (h)	Concentration of olmesartan (mole/l)
0	0.0106
4	0.0093
8	0.0082
16	0.0063
29	0.0042
37	0.0030
52	0.0021
70	0.0009

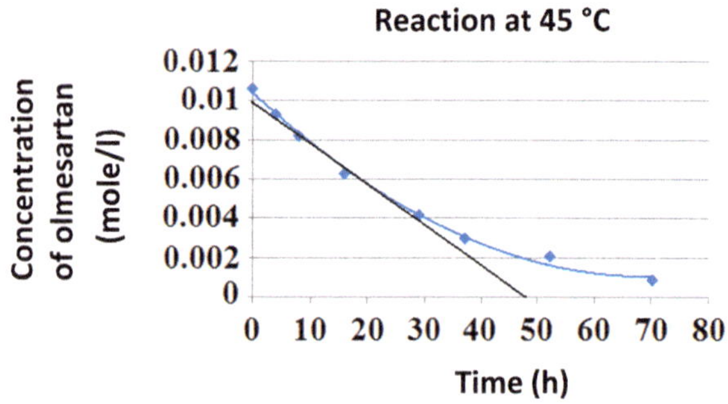

Fig. 5 The slope of the tangent line provides the instantaneous rate v after 16 h of reaction

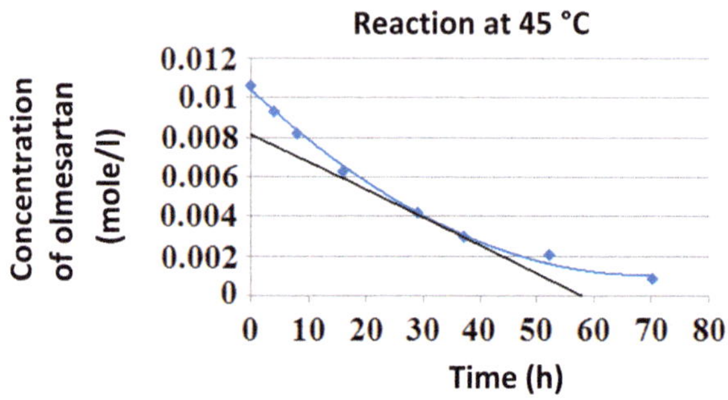

Fig. 6 The instantaneous rate v after 29 h of reaction

line provides the instantaneous rate v at the certain moment t_1. For example, Fig. 5 shows the tangent of the reaction after 16 h and at this moment

$$v = 0.0099/48.3 \text{ mole L}^{-1}\text{ h}^{-1} \approx 0.00020 \text{ mole L}^{-1}\text{ h}^{-1} \quad (6)$$

The application of Eq. (5) after 16 h of reaction gives the following results

$$0.00020 = k_{45^\circ\text{C}}(0.0063)^x(24.621)^y \quad (7)$$

in which it is considered that $[CD_3OD]_{initial}$ has not changed, since CD_3OD is the solvent in the NMR tube.

After 29 h the rate v of a reaction is $v = 0.0081/58.9$ mole $\text{L}^{-1}\text{ h}^{-1} \approx 0.00014$ (Fig. 6). The application of Eq. (5) after 29 h of reaction gives the following results

$$0.00014 = k_{45^\circ\text{C}}(0.0042)^x(24.621)^y \quad (8)$$

If we divide Eqs. (7) and (8), the result is $x \approx 0.88$, and because x is an integer number, $x = 1$.

The stoichiometry of the reaction and Table 1 provide the necessary information in order to calculate that after 29 h the quantity of olmesartan which has reacted is

$[C_{24}H_{26}N_6O_3]_{initial}$-$[C_{24}H_{26}N_6O_3]_{\text{after 29 h}}$ = (0.0106 − 0.0042) mole/L = 0.0064 mole/L

The same concentration of CD_3OD has reacted also. Consequently after 29 h the concentration of CD_3OD in the NMR tube is (24.621 − 0.0064) mole/L = 24.6146 ≈ 24.615 mole/L. Taking into consideration x and y, the new equation is

$$0.00014 = k_{45^\circ C}(0.0042)^1(24.615)^y \quad (9)$$

Similarly, after 16 h of reaction the concentration of CD_3OD which has reacted is equal to (0.0106–0.063) mole/l = 0.0043 mole/L. Consequently, after 16 h the concentration of CD_3OD in the NMR tube is (24.621–0.0043) mole/L = 24.6167 ≈ 24.617 mole/L. Knowing x and y, the new equation is

$$0.00020 = k_{45^\circ C}(0.0063)^1(24.617)^y \quad (10)$$

If we divide Eqs. (9) and (10), the result is $y \approx 0.95$, so the conclusion is that $y = 1$. It is evident that at this point, it is possible to calculate $k_{45^\circ C}$

$0.00020 = k_{45^\circ C}\ (0.0063)^1\ (24.617)^1$ or $k_{45^\circ C} \approx 0.0013\ \text{mole}^{-1}\ \text{l h}$

4 Notes

1. For the kinetic experiments, the relaxation delay of the experiment should be greater compared to 5T1 (relaxation time for the two protons at position 7). Only this way it is ensured that the integration of peaks can result in quantitative measurements. The inversion recovery experiment showed that T1 for the two protons was approximately 0.478. Therefore, for the experiment a relaxation delay of 3 s (> 5 T1) was used. This time is sufficient for quantitative measurements.
2. After the first observation of new peaks in the ^1H spectrum of olmesartan (when the sample is kept in CD_3OD), the case of a dynamic process is examined. In particular, 2D EXSY experiments in CD_3OD (at a temperature range of 25–45 °C and mixing times 0–1200 ms) are performed. The results show an absence of a dynamic process.
3. Subsequently, the possibility that the product could be a dimer is excluded, since the ^1H NMR spectrum of this product in CD_3OD is not identical with those reported in the literature [36].

4. Moreover, the possibility of a lactonization of olmesartan is investigated. This result does not occur, because NMR data are different, when compared to those reported in the literature in DMSO solvent [37].
5. The pharmacological characterization of this molecule shows that this analogue is bound to the AT1 receptor with similar affinity to that of two commercially available drugs (olmesartan and losartan). Furthermore, the proposed mechanism leading to the in situ formation of olmesartan methyl ether led the research team to look for chemical structures of other drugs which may be affected from the same mechanism.

References

1. Carlon A, Ravera E, Andrałojc W et al (2016) How to tackle protein structural data from solution and solid state: an integrated approach. Prog Nucl Magn Reson Spectrosc 92–93:54–70. https://doi.org/10.1016/j.pnmrs.2016.01.001
2. Fello IC, Pierattelli R (eds) (2014) Intrinsically disordered proteins studies by NMR spectroscopy (Advances in Experimental Medicine and Biology). Springer, Switzerland. https://doi.org/10.1007/978-3-319-20164-1
3. Takeuchi K, Wagner G (2006) NMR studies of protein interactions. Curr Opin Struct Biol 16:109–117. https://doi.org/10.1016/j.sbi.2006.01.006
4. Mayer M, Meyer B (1999) Characterization of ligand binding by saturation transfer difference NMR spectroscopy. Angew Chem Int Ed 38 (12):1784–1788. https://doi.org/10.1002/(SICI)1521-3773(19990614)38:12<1784::AID-ANIE1784>3.0.CO;2-Q
5. Carlomagno T, Blommers MJ, Meiler J et al (2003) The high-resolution solution structure of epothilone A bound to tubulin: an understanding of the structure-activity relationships for a powerful class of antitumor agents. Angew Chem Int Ed Engl 42:2511–2515. https://doi.org/10.1002/anie.200351276
6. Otting G, Wuthrich K (1990) Heteronuclear filters in two-dimensional [1H, 1H]-NMR spectroscopy: combined use with isotope labelling for studies of macromolecular conformation and intermolecular interactions. Q Rev Biophys 1990(23):39–96. https://doi.org/10.1017/S0033583500005412
7. Walters KJ, Ferentz AE, Hare BJ et al (2001) Characterizing protein-protein complexes and oligomers by nuclear magnetic resonance spectroscopy. In: James TL, Dötsch V, Schmitz U (eds) Nuclear magnetic resonance of biological macromolecules - Part B (methods in enzymology), vol 339. Elsevier, New York, pp 238–258. https://doi.org/10.1016/S0076-6879(01)39316-3
8. Walters KJ, Matsuo H, Wagner G (1997) A simple method to distinguish intermonomer nuclear Overhauser effects in homodimeric proteins with C2 symmetry. J Am Chem Soc 119(25):5958–5959. https://doi.org/10.1021/ja963309k
9. Maslennikov I, Choe S (2013) Advances in NMR structures of integral membrane proteins. Curr Opin Struct Biol 23(4):555–562. https://doi.org/10.1016/j.sbi.2013.05.002
10. Liu JJ, Horst R, Katritch V et al (2012) Biased signaling pathways in b2-adrenergic receptor characterized by 19F-NMR. Science 335:1106–1110. https://doi.org/10.1126/science.1215802
11. Wishart DS (2011) Interpreting protein chemical shift data. Prog Nucl Magn Reson Spectrosc 58:62–87. https://doi.org/10.1016/j.pnmrs.2010.07.004
12. Shuker SB, Hajduk PJ, Meadows RP, Fesik SW (1996) Discovering high-affinity ligands for proteins: SAR by NMR. Science 274 (5292):1531–1534
13. Middleton DA (2006) NMR methods for characterising ligand-receptor and drug–membrane interactions in pharmaceutical research. In: Webb GA (ed) Annual reports in NMR spectroscopy, vol 60. Elsevier, New York, pp 39–75. https://doi.org/10.1016/S0066-4103(06)60002-1
14. Ritchie TK, Grinkova YV, Bayburt TH et al (2009) Reconstitution of membrane proteins

in phospholipid bilayer nanodiscs. In: Düzgünes N (ed) Liposomes, Part F (methods in enzymology). Elsevier, New York. https://doi.org/10.1016/S0076-6879(09)64011-8

15. Keifer PA (2003) Flow NMR applications in combinatorial chemistry. Curr Opin Chem Biol 7:388–394. https://doi.org/10.1016/S1367-5931(03)00051-6
16. Lenz E, Taylor S, Collins C et al (2002) Flow injection analysis with multiple on-line spectroscopic analysis (UV, IR, 1H-NMR and MS). J Pharm Biomed Anal 27:191–200. https://doi.org/10.1016/S0731-7085(01)00534-9
17. Louden D, Handley A, Taylor S et al (2000) Flow injection spectroscopic analysis of model drugs using on-line UV-diode array, FT-infrared and ^{1}H-nuclear magnetic resonance spectroscopy and time-of-flight mass spectrometry. Analyst 125:927–931. https://doi.org/10.1039/B000696N
18. Renaud J-P, Chung C, Danielson H et al (2016) Biophysics in drug discovery: impact, challenges and opportunities. Nat Rev Drug Discov 15(10):679–698. https://doi.org/10.1038/nrd.2016.123
19. Pourmodheji H, Ghafar-Zadeh E, Magierowski S (2016) A multidisciplinary approach to high throughput nuclear magnetic resonance spectroscopy. Sensors 16(6):E850. https://doi.org/10.3390/s16060850
20. Wei Y, Zhang J, Zhou Y (2017) Characterization of glabridin/hydroxypropyl--cyclodextrin inclusion complex with robust solubility and enhanced bioactivity. Carbohydr Polym 159:152–160. https://doi.org/10.1016/j.carbpol.2016.11.093
21. Araya-Maturana R, Pessoa-Mahana H, Weiss-Lopez B (2008) Very long correlations ($^{n}J_{C,H}$ n>3) in HMBC spectra. Nat Prod Commun 3:445–450
22. Oguadinma P, Bilodeau F, LaPlante R (2017) NMR strategies to support medicinal chemistry workflows for primary structure determination. Bioorg Med Chem Lett 27(2):242–247. https://doi.org/10.1016/j.bmcl.2016.11.066
23. Nardini V, Palaretti V, Jose da Silva GV (2017) Enantiomeric quantification of amines by 1H and 13C NMR: first report of S-citronellal as chiral derivatization agent (CDA). Microchem J 133:208–215. https://doi.org/10.1016/j.microc.2017.03.014
24. Wenzel TJ, Wilcox JD (2003) Chiral reagents for the determination of enantiomeric excess and absolute configuration using NMR spectroscopy. Chirality 15:256–270. https://doi.org/10.1002/chir.10190
25. Silva MS (2017) Recent advances in multinuclear NMR spectroscopy for chiral recognition of organic compounds. Molecules 22:E247. https://doi.org/10.3390/molecules22020247
26. Sulima A, Cheng K, Jacobson AE (2013) Z and E rotamers of N-formyl-1-bromo-4-hydroxy-3-methoxymorphinan-6-one and their interconversion as studied by ^{1}H/^{13}C NMR spectroscopy and quantum chemical calculations. Magn Reson Chem 51:82–88. https://doi.org/10.1002/mrc.3909
27. Hansen PE, Kamounah FS, Hansen BKV et al (2007) Conformational and tautomeric eccentricities of 2-acetyl-1,8-dihydroxynaphthalenes. Magn Reson Chem 45:106–117. https://doi.org/10.1002/mrc.1925
28. Kolehmainen E, Osmialovski B (2012) ^{15}N NMR studies of tautomerism. Int Rev Phys Chem 31:567–629. https://doi.org/10.1080/0144235X.2012.734157
29. Santos R, Fernandes LM, Boto RF et al (2006) NMR spectroscopy study of 2-methylbenzoxazolium salts hydroxylation in DMSO-d_6 solution. Tetrahedron Lett 47:6723–6725. https://doi.org/10.1016/j.tetlet.2006.07.091
30. Rivera A, Núñez ME, Avella E et al (2008) An NMR study of sequential intermediates and collateral products in the conversion of 1,3,6,8-tetraazatricyclo[4.4.1.1^{3,8}]dodecane (TATD) to 1,3,6,8-tetraazatricyclo[4.3.1.1^{3,8}]undecane (TATU). Tetrahedron Lett 49:2154–2158. https://doi.org/10.1016/j.tetlet.2008.01.091
31. Mills A, O'Rourke C (2014) Photocatalytic organic synthesis in an NMR tube: C-C coupling of phenoxyacetic acid and acrylamide. Catal Today 230:256–264. https://doi.org/10.1016/j.cattod.2013.10.083
32. Limtiaco JF, Beni S, Jones CJ (2011) NMR methods to monitor the enzymatic depolymerization of heparin. Anal Bioanal Chem 399:593–603. https://doi.org/10.1007/s00216-010-4132-7
33. Foley DA, Bez E, Codina A et al (2014) NMR flow tube for online nmr reaction monitoring. Anal Chem 86(24):12008–12013. https://doi.org/10.1021/ac502300q
34. http://chem.ch.huji.ac.il/nmr/preparation/preparation.html
35. Ntountaniotis D, Agelis G, Resvani A et al (2014) An efficient synthetic method and theoretical calculations of olmesartan methyl ether: study of biological function of AT1 antagonism. Comb Chem High Throughput

Screen 17:652–662. https://doi.org/10.2174/138620731708140922171503

36. Murakami HT, Konno H, Fukutsu N et al (2008) Identification of a degradation product in stressed tablets of olmesartan medoxomil by the complementary use of HPLC hyphenated techniques. J Pharm Biomed Anal 47:553–559. https://doi.org/10.1016/j.jpba.2008.02.021

37. Zhang, F, Taizhi WU (2004) 4,6-dihydrofuro [3,4-d]imidazole-6-one derivatives and their salts and process for the preparation of the same. WO/2004/083213A1

Chapter 26

Application of Multiscale Simulation Tools on GPCRs. An Example with Angiotensin II Type 1 Receptor

Ismail Erol, Busecan Aksoydan, Isik Kantarcioglu, and Serdar Durdagi

Abstract

G protein-coupled receptors (GPCRs) represent the biggest class of membrane proteins included in signal transduction cascade across the biological lipid bilayers. They are essential target structures for cell signaling and are of great commercial interest to the pharmaceutical industry (~50% of marketed drugs and ~25% of top-selling drugs targeting this receptor family). Recent advances made in molecular biology and computational chemistry open new avenues for the design of new therapeutic compounds. Molecular biology has recently provided the crystal structures of a few ligand-bound GPCRs in active and inactive states, which can be used as accurate templates in modeling studies. Computational chemistry offers a range of simulation, multiscale modeling with ligand- and structure-based approaches, and virtual screening tools for definition and analysis of protein-ligand, protein-protein, and protein-DNA interactions. Development of new approaches and algorithms on statistical methods and free energy simulations help to predict novel optimal compounds. Integrated approach to drug discovery that combines quantum mechanics calculations, molecular docking, molecular dynamics (MD) simulations, quantitative structure-activity relationships (QSAR), and de novo design studies under a single umbrella can be used for decreasing the risk of false-positive results. Each method has its own pros and cons and, when used alone, is not likely to yield very useful results. However, when these methods are combined with positive feedback loops, they may enhance each other and successful drug leads may be obtained. Moreover, investigating the activation mechanisms and atomistic determinants of ligand binding to GPCR targets would allow greater safety in the human life.

Key words GPCRs, AT1, CCR5, CB1, Molecular modeling, Docking, Molecular dynamics (MD) simulations, Homology modeling, Protein engineering, Ligand- and structure-based drug design

1 Introduction

Together with the significant progress made in the understanding of molecular mechanism, structure, dynamics, and function of G protein-coupled receptors (GPCRs), an increasing number of novel findings have associated with genetic mutations in these targets with diverse diseases [1, 2]. Since GPCR targets play important roles in the regulation of membrane excitability, abnormalities in their structure may distort the normal functioning of cells such as

Thomas Mavromoustakos and Tahsin F. Kellici (eds.), *Rational Drug Design: Methods and Protocols*, Methods in Molecular Biology, vol. 1824, https://doi.org/10.1007/978-1-4939-8630-9_26,

cardiac, neurons, and smooth muscle cells [2]. This may lead to neurodegenerative, cardiovascular, or renal diseases. Thus, finding therapeutic small compounds targeting the GPCRs that are involved in such diseases is important [1–14]. Although the classical high-throughput screening methods show limited success in finding new lead compounds, they are costly compared to virtual screening methods. The pharmaceutical industry and related disciplines in academy need more rational approaches in drug design which use and combine recent advances made in molecular biology, molecular biophysics, pharmaceutical chemistry, bioinformatics, structural biology, and computational chemistry.

Computational chemistry provides a range of simulation tools for the description of protein-ligand binding, protein-protein, and protein-DNA interactions. It also utilizes new approaches for molecular modeling tools and statistical methods for analysis of the binding data that help to predict the optimal ligands, drug repositioning for new indications, and rehabilitation of drugs for minimizing the side effects of withdrawn or restricted drugs. One can use all these advances by developing an integrated approach to drug discovery, which will help to rationalize the ligand screening process and facilitate the design of new compounds with optimum binding properties. Thus, defining the activation mechanisms and atomistic determinants of ligand binding to GPCR targets would allow greater safety in the human life.

There are two main hypotheses for the conformational change of GPCRs in response to agonist binding:

1. Conformational selection/change
2. Ligand induction

According to the conformational selection model, there are two states of the GPCRs: active (R*) and inactive (R). Agonists preferentially bind to the receptor in the active state R* and increase the lifetime of active state [14]. The ligand induction hypothesis suggests that transition between the active and inactive states is very rare in the absence of an agonist. Binding of agonist to state R may induce the transition to state R* [1, 14].

Since the most of the crystal structures of both active and inactive forms of proteins from GPCR family (i.e., dopamine-2-receptors (D2R)) are not available, drug/receptor interactions for these targets can be investigated using homology models of target proteins that are derived using available crystal structure from the same family (i.e., dopamine-3-receptors, D3R). Obviously crystallized form (active and inactive state) of the template protein will determine the state of the target protein. If the template protein is crystallized in its inactive form, the derived homology models of protein of interest is in its inactivated form, and according to the activation hypothesis, this state may not be suitable for studying the binding of agonists.

Recently many crystal structures of ligand-bound GPCRs (i.e., β2-adrenergic receptors) have been determined. Currently, there are available proteins that the receptor was stabilized in an active state with a potent agonist or crystallized with agonist bound or inverse agonist bound to GPCRs [1–6]. These have opened a broad avenue of experimental and computational studies that aim to obtain a better understanding of the structure-function relationships and dynamical profiles in GPCRs. On the computational side, rapid developments in high performance computing and computational methodologies have enabled accurate molecular-level simulations of biomolecules and their interactions with ligands. This is particularly important for the design of drugs targeting GPCRs because computational studies can help to relate the functional data on binding of specific drugs to the molecular structure of a GPCR. Binding of a ligand to binding pocket of a GPCR target can stabilize the protein in an active or inactive state. Finding such compounds that bind with high affinity could lead to therapeutic interventions that modulate the function of a receptor as desired.

1.1 GPCRs

GPCRs are located in the plasma membrane and transduce input signals through their interactions with ligands from extracellular (EC) side or from cytoplasmic intracellular (IC) G proteins. All GPCRs share a common α-helical seven transmembrane (TM) domains (Fig. 1).

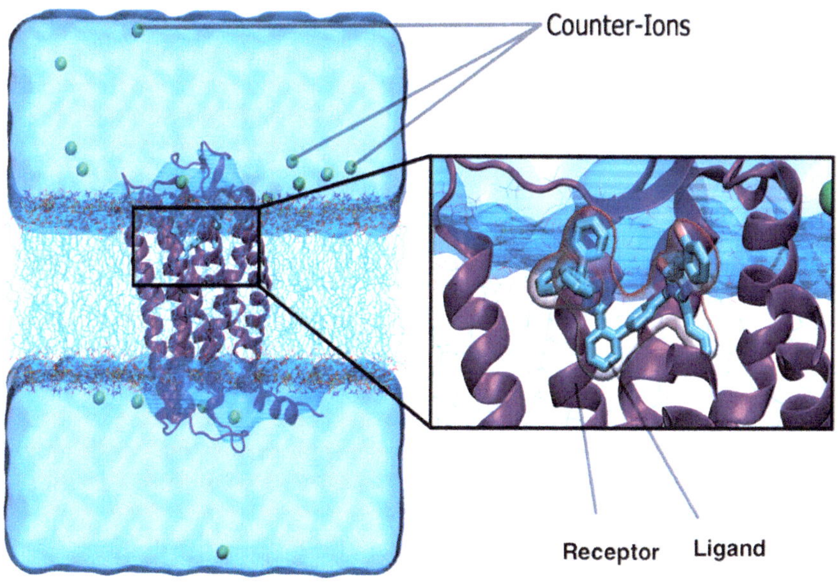

Fig. 1 Side view of a ligand-bound GPCR (shown as ribbon) in the membrane bilayer (shown as sticks; water molecules are shown as surface)

GPCRs bind heterotrimeric G protein complexes that include α, β, and γ subunits. Upon ligand binding, the Gα protein becomes uncoupled from the Gβγ proteins, allowing it to initiate cellular signaling cascades. G protein-mediated signaling starts with binding of a ligand molecule to EC side of GPCR that may lead to activation of target protein. GPCR target is also a guanine nucleotide exchange factor that induces the switch of guanosine diphosphate (GDP)/guanosine triphosphate (GTP) associated with Gα subdomain [3–6]. Because of the conformational changes at activated GPCR, activated GPCR promotes exchange of GTP for GDP on the Gα domain which leads to decomposition of Gα section and Gβγ dimer units. Activated G proteins in this way establish an amplified representation of the activated GPCR. Gα and Gβγ subunits bind to different effectors and thus operate them as either active or inactive in different systems [7, 8]. GPCRs are activated by a diversity of agonists which differ with respect to chemical class, molecular weight, size, and physical properties. It was hypothesized that binding of any agonist induced the active state conformation that activated a single G protein type to initiate an intracellular signal. It is now discovered that GPCR signaling is much more complex than this. Individual GPCRs can activate multiple types of G protein, and signaling can be G protein independent, such as β-arrestin-dependent GPCR activation of MAPK [3–9].

1.2 Structure and Function of GPCRs

GPCRs have a hydrophobic exterior, which makes them insoluble in water and thus hard to crystallize for X-ray diffraction [7]. Although 2D-NMR spectroscopy provides an alternative method and the total number of files deposited to PDB (protein data bank) is increasing in the last years, it has still some limitations related with the size of the proteins. The determination of the crystal structure of the bovine rhodopsin by Palczewski et al. [10] has started a revolution in the field in 2000. The rhodopsin structure provided a great deal of information about how GPCRs looked like and revealed for the first time how a GPCR functions at the atomic level [10]. Rhodopsin is crystallized in the inactive state. Spectroscopic techniques on purified protein preparations helped to understand the structural differences and structural changes during the receptor activation. These observations suggest essential conformational differences between active and inactive states. Information gained from these structures provided structural explanations for the specific domains that are highly conserved among the large class A of GPCRs subgroup (i.e., rhodopsin).

1.3 Impact of GPCRs in Clinical Medicine

Given their large number and diverse distribution and roles in cell physiology and the regulation, GPCRs physiologically have very crucial roles in clinical medicine. A number of diseases linked to GPCRs have been determined. Genetic disorders identified in

GPCRs can influence receptor expression, targeting, and function and also the abilities of receptors to recognize and respond to pharmacological ligands [7–11].

1.4 Protein-Ligand Binding

Accurate prediction of the protein-ligand interactions is one of the major problems in molecular biology. Various experimental techniques are employed for this purpose, e.g., structures of ligand-bound complexes are data mined from X-ray crystallography and NMR, binding energies from rate constants, and specific pairs of residues involved in binding from site-directed mutagenesis studies [2]. While experiments can provide a fairly complete description of a protein-ligand complex, such experiments usually require a great deal of effort and cannot be performed routinely. Similar information on bound complexes may be obtained more easily using molecular modeling techniques such as molecular docking, structure-based pharmacophore modeling (E-pharmacophore), and MD simulations, which have become feasible during the last decade thanks to the rapid growth in computational power. This is a very important consideration in drug discovery process because one has to screen large numbers of ligand candidates to find the most potent one for a given target receptor.

The details of applications of computational tools to different GPCRs will be detailed in this chapter.

1.5 Angiotensin II Type 1 Receptor (AT1R)

The regulation of blood pressure and modulation of salt and fluid balance in body are achieved by a hormone system named renin-angiotensin-aldosterone system (RAAS) [12]. Blood pressure (BP) is the pressure exerted by the circulating blood against the walls of blood vessels. High blood pressure, or hypertension, is one of the cardiovascular risk factors which can also be secondary to several other conditions such as myocardial infarction, stroke, and heart and kidney failure. Hypertension, in the long term, leads to complications caused by narrowing of blood vessels. Therefore, early diagnosis of hypertension is very difficult due to its rare symptoms and complex pathogenesis [13–16]. Angiotensin II (AngII), which is the major bioactive octapeptide (seq. DRVYIHPF), plays an important role in RAAS and the increased arterial blood pressure [12, 17]. AngII mediates many of its actions through binding to two major GPCRs:

1. Angiotensin II type 1 receptor (AT1R)
2. Angiotensin II type 2 receptor (AT2R)

Although most of the functions and physiological properties of AT2R are not well elucidated and thought to have opposite effects compared to the AT1R, many of the effects of AngII are mediated through the activation of the AT1R [17, 18]. AT1R belongs to the class A of GPCR family and is formed by seven transmembrane (TM) domains connected to each other with IC and EC loops [12].

AT1 antagonists are the most recent drug class of molecules against hypertension. There are various in silico studies available not only focused on investigating the molecular basis of actions and further studies of known AT1R antagonists such as telmisartan and losartan but also the development of potent molecules [19–24]. The effects of AT1 antagonists are not limited to cardiovascular diseases. AT1 receptor blockers may be used as potential anticancer agents – due to the inhibition of cell proliferation stimulated by AngII. It is also reported that they can also be used against Alzheimer's disease [25–27]. Therefore, AT1 receptors and the AngII biosynthesis mechanisms are targets for the development of new synthetic drugs and therapeutic treatment of various cardiovascular and such issues.

Recent advances in the studies of AT1R and AT1R blockers were branched several other fields besides the hypertension and other cardiovascular risk factors associated with it. Crowley et al. [28] highlighted the immunologic effects of global RAS manipulation. They stated the differences of immunologic effects between the activation of RAS in hematopoietic cells and RAS stimulation in the kidney and vasculature. There is another study for Alzheimer's disease by Ho et al. [27] which revealed that AT1R blockers may confer the greatest benefit for cognition and risk for Alzheimer's disease, independent of stroke in older adults having antihypertensive treatment. Trofimiuk et al. [29] investigated the effects of candesartan, a standard antihypertensive AT1R blocker, on age-related memory decline and concluded that it potently abolishes some kinds of aging-induced memory impairments in aged rats, but in some circumstances it may even could increase the damage of memory. Dimerization of the AT1R (homo and heterodimers) also constitutes a new trend in drug design and discovery. AbdAlla et al. [30] revealed that specific targeting of the AT1R-B2R heterodimer could pave the way to a new class of drugs that specifically interfere with pathological AngII-AT1R system activation.

Zhang et al. published the first antagonist-bound crystal structure of AT1 receptor with relatively low resolution (2.9 Å) [31]. Same group revealed also inverse agonist-bound AT1R structure, although the structure does not involve short 8th helix which is important in structural dynamics of GPCRs [32]. These two structures assisted to the better understanding of the crucial amino acids at the binding pocket as well as they provided very useful starting structures for molecular docking and molecular dynamics (MD) simulations.

1.6 CB1

Mammalian tissues have two specific cannabinoid receptors, CB1 and CB2. These two receptors are involved in the endocannabinoid system that is a part of the regulation of appetite, cognition, mood, immunity, memory, and pain sensation [33]. CB1 and CB2 receptors are member of the class A, membrane-bound rhodopsin-like receptors of GPCRs. They have common GPCR features like seven TM α-helices that are connected with three EC and three IC loops, with an EC amino-terminal sequence and an IC carboxy-terminal tail [34]. Related CB1 gene is CNR1 that is located on human chromosome 6. CB1 expression level is the highest in central nervous system (CNS) [35]. The CNR1 gene regulation knowledge is limited in literature. Thus, investigation on CB1 has focused mainly on protein-related topics like ligand-receptor binding and protein-protein interactions.

Cannabinoids (CBs) are group of compounds that have effect on cannabinoid receptors CB1 and CB2. They can be divided into three main categories: natural (herbal) or classical CBs, endogenous CBs, and synthetic CBs. Tetrahydrocannabinol (THC), cannabidiol (CBD), and cannabinol are some examples of natural CBs. According to recent pharmacological studies, CBs may have therapeutic potential against various diseases like cancer, depression, chronic pain, AIDS, obesity, diabetes, anorexia, Huntington's disease, and Parkinson's disease. CB1 participates in the regulation of homeostasis [36]. Improving the medicinal properties of known CBs and reducing their side effects are few of the efficient approaches [37–45].

Hua et al. revealed the crystal structure of CB1 with a known three-armed antagonist. This promising article revealed binding pocket networks and sub-pockets of the receptor [46]. Three-armed antagonist is critical for flexibility of receptor in non-signaling conformation. The article clearly explains roles of these arms in binding.

Understanding features of CB1 activation and binding is critical for potential novel therapeutics. Thus, Hua et al. revealed another crystal structure, an agonist-bound CB1 [47]. The most remarkable finding in this article is the fact that agonist binding causes decreased binding pocket volume. This finding may shed light into the elasticity of GPCR's binding cavity. Therefore, in case of targeting a GPCR in structure-based strategies, various receptor models would be a better choice.

Since the allosteric modulators of endocannabinoid system have become a hot topic, various negative (lipoxin A4, hemopressin, pepcan-12, pregnenolone) and positive allosteric modulators (NAM PSNCBAM-1 and RTI-371) are proposed [48].

1.7 CCR5

Acquired immune deficiency syndrome (AIDS) is a fatal and contagious disease that induces serious infections by a virus called human immunodeficiency virus (HIV) which causes to collapse the human immune system by penetrating the immune cells. Although the previous studies about how HIV interacts with human cells provide important advances for the treatment of this disease, there is still a necessity for continuing research since the interaction mechanisms are not resolved yet at molecular level.

HIV replication includes multistate processes, and each step is crucial for a successful replication. Thus, it is important to focus on molecular mechanisms of these steps in atomic scale for the development of potent antiretroviral drugs. The first step is the infection of CD4+ T lymphocytes. The entry of HIV to cell needs cell surface receptors such as CD4 or C-C chemokine receptor type 5 (CCR5) and C-X-C chemokine receptor type 4 (CXCR4) co-receptors. These receptors interact with protein complexes (extracellular GP120 and transmembrane GP41) at the viral envelope. When HIV approaches to a target cell, GP120 protein binds to CD4 receptor. This enhances the co-receptor binding, and then, GP120 changes its conformation. GP41 then unfolds its terminus toward the cell membrane. Viral nucleocapsid enters the cell, then viral RNA strands and three main replication enzymes (integrase, protease, and reverse transcriptase) are released. CCR5 from GPCR family is a critical co-receptor in HIV infection. HIV protein employs CCR5 as a surface co-receptor to enter human cell. The protein GP120 is a glycoprotein which binds to the surface of the HIV and mediates HIV-CCR5 binding. Inhibition of GP120-CCR5 coupling is an effective way of protecting HIV infection [49–58].

2 Materials

The following modules implemented in the Schrodinger molecular modeling package are used in this protocol. Free softwares and webservers are indicated with a star (*), and all these softwares were executed on Linux-/Unix-like operating system.

1. LigPrep [59]
2. QikProp [60]
3. PrepWiz [61, 62] and Prime [63–65]
4. Glide [66–68]
5. OPM server* [69]
6. CHARMM-GUI* [70–74]
7. Gromacs* [75–78]
8. Prime molecular mechanics-generalized born surface area (MM-GBSA) methods [63, 79].
   (a) LigPrep is a module that converts 2D chemical structures into 3D, assigns hydrogens at defined pH level (protonation states), minimizes energies of ligand structures, and finally prepares ligands for further calculations [59].

(b) QikProp is a module that predicts adsorption, distribution, metabolism, and excretion (ADME) properties and some toxicity predictions of compounds [60].

(c) PrepWiz (protein preparation wizard) is a module that adds missing side chains (if any) and fixes loops, creates disulfide bridges, assigns protons (protonation states), and bond orders to the protein structure [61]. Prime is a module that predicts and builds homology model structures based on homolog proteins and refines structures [63].

(d) Glide is the molecular docking module of Schrodinger and predicts possible conformations and interactions between ligands and receptor structures [66].

(e) OPM server is a web server that provides orientations of transmembrane and some peripheral proteins across the lipid bilayer. It can be found at http://opm.phar.umich.edu/server.php [69].

(f) CHARMM-GUI is a web-based input generator for various molecular simulation packages, and it can be found at http://www.charmm-gui.org/ [70].

(g) Gromacs is free and powerful molecular simulation software to perform primarily MD simulations of biochemical systems. It can be found at http://www.gromacs.org/ [75].

(h) Prime MM-GBSA is an approach to calculate binding free energies (Coulomb, vdW, solvent components, etc.) of protein-ligand complex structures using VSGB 2.0 solvation model [63, 79].

3 Methods

In these following two sections, a case study will be represented. First, we will step by step highlight a virtual screening study of a ligand database on GPCRs. Second, we will describe a validation study of identified ligands using MD simulations and free energy calculations.

3.1 Ligand Preparation

In this section, we will prepare the ligand structures for virtual screening.

1. Download the section with the small drug-like molecules from the ZINC database (~18 million).
2. Go to Applications section of Maestro and then LigPrep.
3. Browse downloaded ligand structures, and import them to the workspace.

4. Define force field as such as *OPLS_2005*.
5. Generate possible protonation states at pH 7.4 using Epik.
6. Generate tautomers, determine chiralities, and finally structurally optimize the ligands. If the molecule does not exist in the literature, use 2D Sketcher in Schrodinger.

3.2 In Silico Predictions of Pharmacokinetic Properties

In this section, we will use prepared ligands from previous section, and then we will apply QikProp module of Maestro.

1. Import all ligands into workspace, or browse the pathway of the ligands.
2. Go to Applications section of Maestro and then QikProp.
3. Run the QikProp application.

This module analyzes volume and surface area, charges, and the atom types of the submitted compounds and rapidly reports predictions of pharmacologically relevant properties.

One can eliminate compounds that have higher penalties in respect to their functional groups and other properties such as volume, H-bond donor, H-bond acceptor, logP, molecular weight, hERG inhibition, logK, and Lipinski's rule of five fitting. After eliminating ligands that have higher penalties, the ligand database will be ready for further molecular modeling calculations.

3.3 Protein Preparation

Crystallized protein structures contain heavy atoms of amino acids, metal ions, water molecules, co-crystallized ligands, cofactors, and some other stabilizator compounds. Thus, for the immediate usage in the molecular modeling studies, protein structures need to be prepared.

In this section, we will prepare our protein structure by fixing missing atoms and residues, removing water molecules (beyond given distance from ligand) and ions which are not structural, and adding formal charges and bond orders.

1. Go to Applications section of Maestro and then PrepWiz.
2. In PrepWiz, there are three types of tools: import and process, review and modify, and refine.
3. Start with import and process.
4. There are two options for importing structures into the workspace. One can directly download the target structure from PDB (Protein Data Bank), or it can be imported from working directory.
5. For this protocol, use X-ray structure of angiotensin II type 1 receptor (PDB ID: 4YAY) at 2.9 Å resolution. In PDB, there are two available structures for this protein. Use 4YAY instead of 4ZUD, since the latter structure lacks 8-TM short helix which is known to be important for the signaling and lipid

bilayer interactions. Although, Kellici et al. suggested that there is no significant differences in the binding sites [80].

It must be noted that, in spite of the fact that extracellular loops (ECLs) may also locate peripheral within the GPCR topology, they are also crucial elements for modulating the receptor function [81].

6. Preprocess section of PrepWiz has several options to make structure ready.
7. The stabilizer part corresponding to residues from Asp1002 to Leu1106 is removed from the protein structure.
8. Nonstandard residues (in this case), ZD7, a selective antagonist, are shown in different color at the workspace.
9. Red-colored representation indicates standard residues but contains missing atoms at the side chain. Cyan-colored residues indicate that the adjacent residue is missing. In this case, the following residues contain missing atoms: Lys20, Lys135, Ser136, Arg137, Ile177, Glu185, Leu191, Ile193, Thr198, Lys199, Ile201, Leu205, Phe206, Phe208, Lys224, Asn235, Leu305, Lys308, Tyr312, Gln315, and Leu317. Residues starting from Glu173 to Asn176, Ser186 to Ser189, and Ala225 to Arg234 are missing in the crystal structure. Also at the C-terminal side, last two residues, Lys318 and Tyr319, are missing.
10. Select *assign bond order*, add hydrogens, create zero-order bonds to metals, and create disulfide bonds between sulfur atoms that are within 3.2 Å. AT1 receptor structure has, we have two disulfide bridges between Cys18 and Cys274 and between Cys101 and Cys180.
11. Fill in missing side chains and missing loops with Prime module, and delete waters beyond 5 Å from ligand.
12. If the module reports about the overlapping atoms, first visualize them, probably they are occurred due to lack of H-bond assignment, and go to next step.
13. Use review and modify button to analyze workspace. In this case, since there are no parts or residues that need to be deleted, we only generate states for the ligand. Epik reports five different protonation states for the ligand, ZD7. Original state has penalty of 3.83 kcal/mol, neutral charge, and 4 H-bonds. S2 state has penalty of 0.05 kcal/mol, −1 charge, and 4 H-bonds. S3 state has penalty of 1.55 kcal/mol, neutral charge, and 3 H-bonds. S4 state has penalty of 3.83 kcal/mol, neutral charge, and 4 H-bonds. S5 state has penalty of 3.90 kcal/mol, neutral charge, and 3 H-bonds. Thus, we selected S2 state and proceeded to the final stage with *refine* tab.

14. In this tab, select *sample water orientations* to correctly define H-bonding network, and use PropKA at pH 7.4. PropKA is used to define protonation states of the residues respect to the working pH. Then, click optimization.
15. Since we do not have any crystal waters, skip *remove waters* tab.
16. The last step of the protein preparation is the restrained minimization, in which heavy atoms are restrained, and use 0.3 Å as threshold value to stop minimization where steric clashes are alleviated and side chains are relaxed. Select force field as OPLS_2005, and then click minimize.
17. When the job is completed, we have a fully prepared and optimized protein structure ready for modeling and further calculations.

3.4 OPM Server

In this section we will use OPM server to insert our protein-ligand complex into lipid bilayer. Since all GPCRs are located in biological membranes, to mimic its natural environment, we place our structure into model membranes. For this aim, OPM server is an excellent option to arrange spatial conformation of proteins at the membrane bilayer.

1. Go to OPM server web site, http://opm.phar.umich.edu/
2. Then click PPM server tab.
3. To find orientation of our receptor, provide pdb file of the complex structure, and then click submit.
4. Web server will process our complex, find its spatial conformation, and provide us output.
5. Remove DUMMY atoms from the output structure, and it will be ready to use in MD simulations.

3.5 CHARMM-GUI

In this section we will use CHARMM-GUI web server to generate protein-ligand-membrane system inputs for the MD simulations.

1. Go to http://www.charmm-gui.org/ web site.
2. Click Input Generator tab.
3. Select Membrane Builder and then Bilayer Builder.
4. To construct protein/membrane system, upload oriented complex structure, and select PDB format as PDB.
5. Select Model/Chain.
6. In Model/Chain Selection stage, select hetero under the type tab to include ligand, and proceed to manipulate PDB step.
7. In this section, we provide our hetero chain (ligand) as a SDF file. In this stage CgenFF is used to generate topology and parameter files using ParamChem by the server. Also, in this section, we define the disulfide bridges (CYS18-CYS274, CYS101-CYS180).

8. Generate PDB and Orient Molecule (*see* **Note 1**).
9. When calculations are done, this page reports our ligand analogy quality. Download and check topology for the ligand, and pay attention to penalty values. Higher penalties mean extensive validation is needed.
10. In orientation options, select Use PDB orientation (*see* **Note 2**).
11. Calculate Cross-Sectional Area.
12. Next stage is about lipid bilayer construction. In this step, choose homogeneous lipid, and then give lipids numbers. For our case, number of lipids on top and on bottom are set to 128 and water thickness is 20 Å. DPPC (dipalmitoylphosphatidylcholine) type of phospholipid will be used in rectangular box.
13. Determine the System Size.
14. System-building option is replacement method in our case. Use 0.15 M of NaCl solution to neutralize the system; it will add 60 positive and 75 negative ions and use Monte-Carlo simulations for the ion-placing method.
15. Assemble Components (*see* **Note 3**).
16. Select input generation options (*see* **Note 4**), from the force field options CHARMM36, and define temperature as 310 K; other settings will be default.

3.6 Gromacs

All simulations will be performed with Gromacs 4.6.5 package.

1. A prior energy minimization is applied to the full system using the steepest-descent (SD) integrator for 5000 steps with the initial step size of 0.01 Å (the energy minimization tolerance was set to 1000 kJ/mol).
2. The systems are then equilibrated for 5 ns MD simulations in a total of six different steps using Berendsen barostat and thermostat algorithms.
3. Bond lengths are constrained using LINCS algorithm and particle mesh Ewald (PME) method is used to calculate long-range electrostatic interactions. Cutoff distances for the calculation of Coulomb and van der Waals interactions are both 12 Å.
4. 100 ns and 0.5 μs production runs are performed for different systems with a time step of 2.0 fs using Nose-Hoover thermostat and Parrinello-Rahman barostat.
5. Simulations are run in the NPT ensemble at 310 K and 1 bar with periodic boundary conditions (PBC).

3.7 Prime MM-GBSA

Free energy of binding of the ligands to the receptor can be calculated using post MD simulations method, MM-GBSA. For this aim, three options are available. First we can use a representative structure from the simulation trajectory, second we can extract several frames from the trajectory, and third all frames can be used to calculate binding affinity of the ligand. Accuracy of the calculation will improve from first to last methodology. Here, we will report free energy of binding of the potent inhibitor using one representative structure.

1. Go to Applications section of Maestro, then Prime, and finally MM-GBSA.
2. In the Structures tab, select take complexes from separated ligand and protein structures, and provide ligand and receptor structures separately.
3. In the Options tab, select solvation model as VSGB and force field as OPLS_2005. Use input ligand partial charges.
4. For the protein flexibility, define residues 5 Å away from the ligand, choose sampling method as Minimize, and click Run.

4 Notes

1. We do not choose a special treatment for our structure, since we already prepared it at the beginning.
2. This is done since we already oriented our structure in OPM server.
3. The server will check protein surface and lipid ring penetrations.
4. In our case we only select GROMACS.

Acknowledgements

This study is supported by The Scientific and Technological Research Council of Turkey (TÜBİTAK); Project No: 214Z122.

References

1. Audet M, Bouvier M (2012) Restructuring G-protein- coupled receptor activation. Cell 151(1):14–23. https://doi.org/10.1016/j.cell.2012.09.003
2. Dror RO, Arlow DH, Maragakis P et al (2011) Activation mechanism of the β2-adrenergic receptor. Proc Natl Acad Sci U S A 108 (46):18684–18689
3. Rasmussen SG, Choi H-J, Fung JJ et al (2011) Structure of a nanobody-stabilized active state of the [bgr] 2 adrenoceptor. Nature 469 (7329):175–180
4. Rosenbaum DM, Zhang C, Lyons JA et al (2011) Structure and function of an irreversible agonist-[bgr] 2 adrenoceptor complex. Nature 469(7329):236–240

5. Tuccinardi T, Ferrarini PL, Manera C et al (2006) Cannabinoid CB2/CB1 selectivity. Receptor modeling and automated docking analysis. J Med Chem 49(3):984–994
6. Xu F, Wu H, Katritch V et al (2011) Structure of an agonist-bound human A2A adenosine receptor. Science 332(6027):322–327
7. Conn PM, Ulloa-Aguirre A, Ito J, Janovick JA (2007) G protein-coupled receptor trafficking in health and disease: lessons learned to prepare for therapeutic mutant rescue in vivo. Pharmacol Rev 59(3):225–250
8. Insel PA, Tang C-M, Hahntow I, Michel MC (2007) Impact of GPCRs in clinical medicine: monogenic diseases, genetic variants and drug targets. Biochim Biophys Acta 1768 (4):994–1005
9. Azzi M, Charest PG, Angers S et al (2003) β-Arrestin-mediated activation of MAPK by inverse agonists reveals distinct active conformations for G protein-coupled receptors. Proc Natl Acad Sci 100(20):11406–11411
10. Palczewski K, Kumasaka T, Hori T et al (2000) Crystal structure of rhodopsin: AG protein-coupled receptor. Science 289(5480):739–745
11. Filmore D (2004) It's a GPCR world. Modern Drug Disc 7:24–28
12. De Gasparo M, Catt K, Inagami T et al (2000) International union of pharmacology. XXIII The angiotensin II receptors. Pharmacol Rev 52(3):415–472
13. Carey RM (2008) Pathophysiology of primary hypertension. Comprehensive Physiology
14. Carey RM (2009) AT1 receptors, angiotensin receptor blockade, and clinical hypertensive disease. In: Renin angiotensin system and cardiovascular disease. Springer, Berlin, pp 59–79
15. Naik P, Murumkar P, Giridhar R, Yadav MR (2010) Angiotensin II receptor type 1 (AT 1) selective nonpeptidic antagonists—a perspective. Bioorg Med Chem 18(24):8418–8456
16. WHO (2013) A global brief on Hypertension: Silent killer, global public health crisis. http://apps.who.int/iris/bitstream/10665/79059/1/WHO_DCO_WHD_2013.2_eng.pdf
17. Sallander J, Wallinder C, Hallberg A et al (2016) Structural determinants of subtype selectivity and functional activity of angiotensin II receptors. Bioorg Med Chem Lett 26 (4):1355–1359
18. Kawai T, Forrester SJ, O'Brien S et al (2017) AT1 receptor signaling pathways in the cardiovascular system. Pharmacol Res 125 (Pt A):4–13
19. Kellici TF, Ntountaniotis D, Kritsi E et al (2016) Leveraging NMR and X-ray data of the free ligands to build better drugs targeting GPCRs: the case of AT1R. Curr Med Chem 23 (1):36–59
20. Zervou M, Cournia Z, Potamitis C et al (2013) Insights into the molecular basis of action of the AT1 antagonist losartan using a combined NMR spectroscopy and computational approach. Biochim Biophys Acta 1838 (3):1031–1046
21. Kritsi E, Potamitis C, Durdagi S et al (2013) Molecular insights into the AT1 antagonism based on biophysical and in silico studies of telmisartan. Med Chem Res 22 (10):4842–4857
22. Mavromoustakos T, Agelis G, Durdagi S (2013) AT1 antagonists: a patent review (2008 - 2012). Expert Opin Ther Pat 23 (11):1483–1494
23. Agelis G, Resvani A, Durdagi S et al (2012) The discovery of new potent non-peptide angiotensin II AT1 receptor blockers: a concise synthesis, molecular docking studies and biological evaluation of N-substituted 5-butylimidazole derivatives. Eur J Med Chem 55:358–374
24. Potamitis C, Zervou M, Katsiaras V et al (2009) Antihypertensive drug valsartan in solution and at the AT1 receptor: conformational analysis, dynamic NMR spectroscopy, in silico docking, and molecular dynamics simulations. J Chem Inf Model 49(3):726–739
25. Dolley-Hitze T, Jouan F, Martin B et al (2010) Angiotensin-2 receptors (AT1-R and AT2-R), new prognostic factors for renal clear-cell carcinoma? Br J Cancer 103(11):1698
26. Ge J, Barnes NM (1996) Alterations in angiotensin AT1 and AT2 receptor subtype levels in brain regions from patients with neurodegenerative disorders. Eur J Pharmacol 297 (3):299–306
27. Ho JK, Nation DA (2017) Memory is preserved in older adults taking AT1 receptor blockers. Alzheimer's Res Ther 9(1):33
28. Crowley SD, Rudemiller NP (2017) Immunologic effects of the renin-angiotensin system. J Am Soc Nephrol 28(5):1350–1361
29. Trofimiuk E, Wielgat P, Braszko JJ (2018) Candesartan, angiotensin II type 1 receptor blocker is able to relieve age-related cognitive impairment. Pharmacol Rep 70(1):87–92
30. AbdAlla UQS (2014) Vasopressor meets vasodepressor: The AT1–B2 receptor. Atherosclerosis 39:40
31. Zhang H, Unal H, Gati C et al (2015) Structure of the angiotensin receptor revealed by serial femtosecond crystallography. Cell 161 (4):833

32. Zhang H, Unal H, Desnoyer R et al (2015) Structural basis for ligand recognition and functional selectivity at angiotensin receptor. J Biol Chem 290(49):29127
33. Durdagi S, Kapou A, Kourouli T et al (2007) The application of 3D-QSAR studies for novel cannabinoid ligands substituted at the C1' position of the alkyl side chain on the structural requirements for binding to cannabinoid receptors CB1 and CB2. J Med Chem 50 (12):2875–2885. https://doi.org/10.1021/jm0610705
34. Tuteja N (2009) Signaling through G protein coupled receptors. Plant Signal Behav 4 (10):942–947
35. Matsuda LA, Lolait SJ, Brownstein MJ et al (1990) Structure of a cannabinoid receptor and functional expression of the cloned cDNA. Nature 346(6284):561–564. https://doi.org/10.1038/346561a0
36. Ruginsk SG, Vechiato FM, Uchoa ET et al (2015) Type 1 cannabinoid receptor modulates water deprivation-induced homeostatic responses. Am J Physiol Regul Integr Comp Physiol 309(11):R1358–R1368. https://doi.org/10.1152/ajpregu.00536.2014
37. Chakravarti B, Ravi J, Ganju RK (2014) Cannabinoids as therapeutic agents in cancer: current status and future implications. Oncotarget 5(15):5852–5872. https://doi.org/10.18632/oncotarget.2233
38. Greenberg I, Kuehnle J, Mendelson JH, Bernstein JG (1976) Effects of marihuana use on body weight and caloric intake in humans. Psychopharmacology (Berl) 49(1):79–84. https://doi.org/10.1007/bf00427475
39. Hao S, Avraham Y, Mechoulam R, Berry EM (2000) Low dose anandamide affects food intake, cognitive function, neurotransmitter and corticosterone levels in diet-restricted mice. Eur J Pharmacol 392(3):147–156
40. Martin BR, Compton DR, Thomas BF et al (1991) Behavioral, biochemical, and molecular modeling evaluations of cannabinoid analogs. Pharmacol Biochem Behav 40(3):471–478
41. Howlett AC, Barth F, Bonner TI et al (2002) International Union of Pharmacology. XXVII. Classification of cannabinoid receptors. Pharmacol Rev 54(2):161–202
42. Kempf K, Hector J, Strate T et al (2007) Immune-mediated activation of the endocannabinoid system in visceral adipose tissue in obesity. Horm Metab Res 39(8):596–600. https://doi.org/10.1055/s-2007-984459
43. Hurley MJ, Mash DC, Jenner P (2003) Expression of cannabinoid CB1 receptor mRNA in basal ganglia of normal and parkinsonian human brain. J Neural Transm (Vienna) 110 (11):1279–1288. https://doi.org/10.1007/s00702-003-0033-7
44. Zeng BY, Dass B, Owen A et al (1999) Chronic L-DOPA treatment increases striatal cannabinoid CB1 receptor mRNA expression in 6-hydroxydopamine-lesioned rats. Neurosci Lett 276(2):71–74
45. Denovan-Wright EM, Robertson HA (2000) Cannabinoid receptor messenger RNA levels decrease in a subset of neurons of the lateral striatum, cortex and hippocampus of transgenic Huntington's disease mice. Neuroscience 98(4):705–713
46. Hua T, Vemuri K, Pu M et al (2016) Crystal structure of the human cannabinoid receptor CB1. Cell 167(3):750–762 e714. https://doi.org/10.1016/j.cell.2016.10.004
47. Hua T, Vemuri K, Nikas SP et al (2017) Crystal structures of agonist-bound human cannabinoid receptor CB1. Nature 547 (7664):468–471. https://doi.org/10.1038/nature23272
48. Busquets Garcia A, Soria-Gomez E, Bellocchio L, Marsicano G (2016) Cannabinoid receptor type-1: breaking the dogmas. F1000Res 5:F1000. https://doi.org/10.12688/f1000research.8245.1
49. Acharya P, Dogo-Isonagie C, LaLonde JM et al (2011) Structure-based identification and neutralization mechanism of tyrosine sulfate mimetics that inhibit HIV-1 entry. ACS Chem Biol 6(10):1069–1077. https://doi.org/10.1021/cb200068b
50. Barmania F, Pepper MS (2013) CC chemokine receptor type five (CCR5): An emerging target for the control of HIV infection. Appl Transl Genom 2:3–16
51. Bobyk KD, Mandadapu SR, Lohith K et al (2017) Design of HIV co-receptor derived peptides that inhibit viral entry at submicromolar concentrations. Mol Pharm 14 (8):2681–2689. https://doi.org/10.1021/acs.molpharmaceut.7b00155
52. Curreli F, Kwon YD, Belov DS et al (2017) Synthesis, antiviral potency, in vitro ADMET, and X-ray structure of potent CD4 mimics as entry inhibitors that target the Phe43 cavity of HIV-1 gp120. J Med Chem 60(7):3124–3153
53. Dogo-Isonagie C, Lee S-L, Lohith K et al (2016) Design and synthesis of small molecule-sulfotyrosine mimetics that inhibit HIV-1 entry. Bioorg Med Chem 24 (8):1718–1728
54. Hütter G, Nowak D, Mossner M et al (2009) Long-term control of HIV by CCR5 Delta32/

Delta32 stem-cell transplantation. N Engl J Med 360(7):692–698

55. Moseri A, Biron Z, Arshava B et al (2015) The C4 region as a target for HIV entry inhibitors–NMR mapping of the interacting segments of T20 and gp120. FEBS J 282 (24):4643–4657
56. Pacheco B, Alsahafi N, Debbeche O et al (2017) Residues in the gp41 ectodomain regulate HIV-1 envelope glycoprotein conformational transitions induced by gp120-directed inhibitors. J Virol 91(5):e02219–e02216
57. Platt EJ, Durnin JP, Kabat D (2015) HIV-1 variants that use mouse CCR5 reveal critical interactions of gp120's V3 crown with CCR5 extracellular loop 1. AIDS Res Hum Retroviruses 31(10):992–998
58. Salmas RE, Yurtsever M, Durdagi S (2015) Investigation of inhibition mechanism of chemokine receptor CCR5 by micro-second molecular dynamics simulations. Sci Rep 5:13180
59. Schrödinger Release 2015–2 (2015) LigPrep S, LLC, New York, NY
60. Schrödinger Release 2015–2 (2015) QikProp, Schrödinger, LLC, New York, NY
61. Schrödinger Release 2015–2 (2015) Schrödinger suite 2015-2 protein preparation wizard; Epik S, LLC, New York, NY, 2015; impact, Schrödinger, LLC, New York, NY, 2015; Prime, Schrödinger, LLC, New York, NY
62. Madhavi Sastry G, Adzhigirey M, Day T et al (2013) Protein and ligand preparation: parameters, protocols, and influence on virtual screening enrichments. J Comput Aided Mol Des 27(3):221–234. https://doi.org/10.1007/s10822-013-9644-8
63. Schrödinger Release 2015–2 (2015) Prime S, LLC, New York, NY
64. Jacobson MP, Pincus DL, Rapp CS et al (2004) A hierarchical approach to all-atom protein loop prediction. Proteins 55(2):351–367. https://doi.org/10.1002/prot.10613
65. Jacobson MP, Friesner RA, Xiang Z, Honig B (2002) On the role of the crystal environment in determining protein side-chain conformations. J Mol Biol 320(3):597–608. https://doi.org/10.1016/S0022-2836(02)00470-9
66. Schrödinger Release 2015–2 (2015) Glide S, LLC, New York, NY
67. Friesner RA, Murphy RB, Repasky MP et al (2006) Extra precision glide: docking and scoring incorporating a model of hydrophobic enclosure for protein–ligand complexes. J Med Chem 49(21):6177–6196. https://doi.org/10.1021/jm051256o
68. Halgren TA, Murphy RB, Friesner RA et al (2004) Glide: a new approach for rapid, accurate docking and scoring. 2. Enrichment factors in database screening. J Med Chem 47 (7):1750–1759. https://doi.org/10.1021/jm030644s
69. Lomize MA, Pogozheva ID, Joo H et al (2012) OPM database and PPM web server: resources for positioning of proteins in membranes. Nucleic Acids Res 40(D1): D370–D376. https://doi.org/10.1093/nar/gkr703
70. Jo S, Kim T, Iyer VG, Im W (2008) CHARMM-GUI: a web-based graphical user interface for CHARMM. J Comput Chem 29 (11):1859–1865. https://doi.org/10.1002/jcc.20945
71. Lee J, Cheng X, Swails JM et al (2016) CHARMM-GUI input generator for NAMD, GROMACS, AMBER, OpenMM, and CHARMM/OpenMM simulations using the CHARMM36 additive force field. J Chem Theory Comput 12 (1):405–413. https://doi.org/10.1021/acs.jctc.5b00935
72. Wu EL, Cheng X, Jo S et al (2014) CHARMM-GUI membrane builder toward realistic biological membrane simulations. J Comput Chem 35(27):1997–2004. https://doi.org/10.1002/jcc.23702
73. Jo S, Lim JB, Klauda JB, Im W (2009) CHARMM-GUI membrane builder for mixed bilayers and its application to yeast membranes. Biophys J 97(1):50–58. https://doi.org/10.1016/j.bpj.2009.04.013
74. Jo S, Kim T, Im W (2007) Automated builder and database of protein/membrane complexes for molecular dynamics simulations. PLoS One 2(9):e880. https://doi.org/10.1371/journal.pone.0000880
75. Berendsen HJC, van der Spoel D, van Drunen R (1995) GROMACS: a message-passing parallel molecular dynamics implementation. Comput Phys Commun 91(1):43–56. https://doi.org/10.1016/0010-4655(95)00042-E
76. Abraham MJ, Murtola T, Schulz R et al (2015) GROMACS: high performance molecular simulations through multi-level parallelism from laptops to supercomputers. SoftwareX 1–2:19–25. https://doi.org/10.1016/j.softx.2015.06.001
77. Páll S, Abraham MJ, Kutzner C, Hess B, Lindahl E (2015) Tackling Exascale software challenges in molecular dynamics simulations with GROMACS. In: Markidis S, Laure E (eds) Solving Software Challenges for Exascale: International Conference on Exascale Applications and Software, EASC 2014, Stockholm,

Sweden, April 2–3, 2014, Revised Selected Papers. Springer, Cham, pp 3–27. https://doi.org/10.1007/978-3-319-15976-8_1

78. Pronk S, Páll S, Schulz R et al (2013) GROMACS 4.5: a high-throughput and highly parallel open source molecular simulation toolkit. Bioinformatics 29(7):845–854. https://doi.org/10.1093/bioinformatics/btt055

79. Li J, Abel R, Zhu K et al (2011) The VSGB 2.0 model: a next generation energy model for high resolution protein structure modeling. Proteins 79(10):2794–2812. https://doi.org/10.1002/prot.23106

80. Kellici, TF, Ntountaniotis D, Liapakis G et al (2016) The dynamic properties of angiotensin II type 1 receptor inverse agonists in solution and in the receptor site. Arab J Chem: In Press. https://doi.org/10.1016/j.arabjc.2016.11.014

81. Wheatley M, Wootten D, Conner MT et al (2012) Lifting the lid on GPCRs: The role of extracellular loops. British J Pharmacol 165:1688–1703.

Chapter 27

Angiotensin II Type 1 Receptor Homology Models: A Comparison Between In Silico and the Crystal Structures

Tahsin F. Kellici

Abstract

For many years structural studies of the angiotensin II type 1 receptor (AT1R) solely relied on mutagenesis experiments combined with homology modeling. The recent publication of the co-crystallized structures of AT1R with the antagonists ZD7155 and olmesartan allows comparative studies. In this chapter the binding modes of olmesartan in the crystal structures and the homology models are compared utilizing mutagenesis data. The obtained results suggest that both homology and crystal structures should be used for future rational drug design. Of paramount importance are these co-crystallized structures or homology models to be simulated in a lipid bilayer environment that mimics the biological.

Key words Angiotensin II type 1 receptor, Homology modeling, Induced fit docking, Quantum-polarized ligand docking, Molecular dynamics

1 Introduction

One of the most important issues in the drug discovery is the use of the most proper conformation of the receptor that explains the biological data (Fig. 1). Based on this valuable information, someone can initiate and apply a rational drug design.

This is the case with GPCRs where most of them are not crystallized and yet the rational drug design approaches continue with homology models. One interesting case is the AT1R, which was recently co-crystallized, and therefore one can argue that the future rational drug design must be based upon this co-crystallized receptor with ZD7155 [1] or olmesartan [2] and not to the hitherto developed homology models.

We must point out that homology modeling is a popular method for predicting protein's three-dimensional structure especially in the absence of X-ray crystallography or NMR data. It is based on experimentally structurally elucidated structures of the target's homologues, using the assumption that similar protein sequences should result in similar native conformations. A three-

Thomas Mavromoustakos and Tahsin F. Kellici (eds.), *Rational Drug Design: Methods and Protocols*, Methods in Molecular Biology, vol. 1824, https://doi.org/10.1007/978-1-4939-8630-9_27, © Springer Science+Business Media, LLC, part of Springer Nature 2018

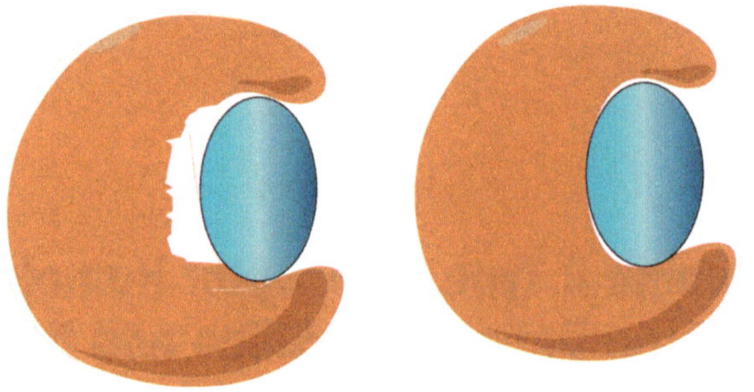

Fig. 1 The best model is the one that ligand induces a perfect fit in the receptor site taking into account the flexibility of both the receptor and ligand. In this case, the model of the receptor shown on the right is more suitable for the ligand

dimensional structure enables the application of computational studies and helps to direct in vitro research in an attempt to reduce the time and funds consumed. The quality of obtained models is mainly governed from the choice of the template. Proteins whose sequence similarity is higher than 50% are considered to provide a reliable model [3].

Reservations must be expressed on considering a priori that crystallographic co-crystallized receptor is the best suitable to be used. These reservations are outlined briefly in the following two reasons:

(a) In order to achieve the co-crystallization of GCPRs, as in the case of AT1R, rigorous conditions are applied, and parts of the receptor might even have to be truncated. In such a case, the deletion of parts of the receptor can dramatically influence the overall conformation of the receptor. Other methods include the usage of fusion proteins such as the T4 lysozyme, mutagenesis for expression and thermostability, and the use of antibodies or nanobodies as crystallization "chaperones" [4].

(b) The environment of the crystallization on GCPRs can differ severely from that of the receptor in the biological system. As it is well known in biological system, GCPRs are surrounded by a lipid bilayer that influences considerably the binding and biological activity of small organic drug molecules. GPCRs are extracted from their native lipid membrane environment and solubilized by detergents before purification. These detergents must efficiently extract the protein from the membrane and be mild enough to maintain the protein stability [4].

These two fundamental reasons should cause a degree of skepticism in terms of the model to use for designing new AT1R antagonists. We thus find legitimate to provide a direct comparison between the most important homology models along the co-crystallized structures. This chapter is devoted to this approach in order for the reader and drug designer to understand the limitations of the co-crystallized GPCRs. More specifically, for our study we will compare the advantages and disadvantages of (a) the co-crystallized structure(s), (b) the homology model based on CXCR4, and (c) the homology model based on rhodopsin.

1.1 Renin-Angiotensin System

Let us give a very brief information on the system that AT1R antagonists act and focus specifically to olmesartan as a case study to show that co-crystallization of a receptor cannot be a panacea in the application of the rational drug design.

Renin-angiotensin system (RAS) is a major system that regulates the blood pressure. It consists of a biocascade of enzymic reactions which results in the production of peptide octapeptide hormone angiotensin II. In pathogenic states, angiotensin II is implicated to cause hypertension through its action on AT1R. A class of molecules called sartans, as the first marketed drug in this series was losartan, acts as antihypertensives by blocking angiotensin II to exert its detrimental effect on AT1R. These Trojan horses are the most recent class of drugs against hypertension that act on the renin-angiotensin system [5, 6] (Fig. 2).

In this chapter, we will provide details of the computational approach used to study the binding of olmesartan and test which conformation between co-crystallized and homology models fits the experimental data. In order to further explore the most suitable receptor, we utilized mutation studies by Miura et al. [7]. These studies are of paramount importance as mutations at different sites of AT1R influence differently the biological activity of AT1 antagonists. Specifically, Miura et al. have reported that mutations in the AT1R such as Y113F, K199Q, H256A, and Q257A lower the binding affinity for olmesartan by 25-, 15-, 16-, and 103-folds, respectively. Moreover the Y113A mutation did not exert any impact on the binding affinity of olmesartan [7–9].

The computational approach consists of induced fit docking (IFD) and molecular dynamics (MD) to describe the binding affinity and stability of olmesartan and olmesartan methyl ether in the receptor using lipid bilayers that simulate the biological environment. IFD and MD were also run in the mutated receptors to examine the consequences of binding and justify the biological results. For completeness of our studies both co-crystallized receptors and homology models have been used. In none of these models, the biological results are justified. The olmesartan molecule showed identical binding affinity scores in the co-crystallized structure or the homology models in non-mutated and mutated structures [10].

The above discussion brings to the point that the crystal structure and homology models of AT1R do not simulate adequately the

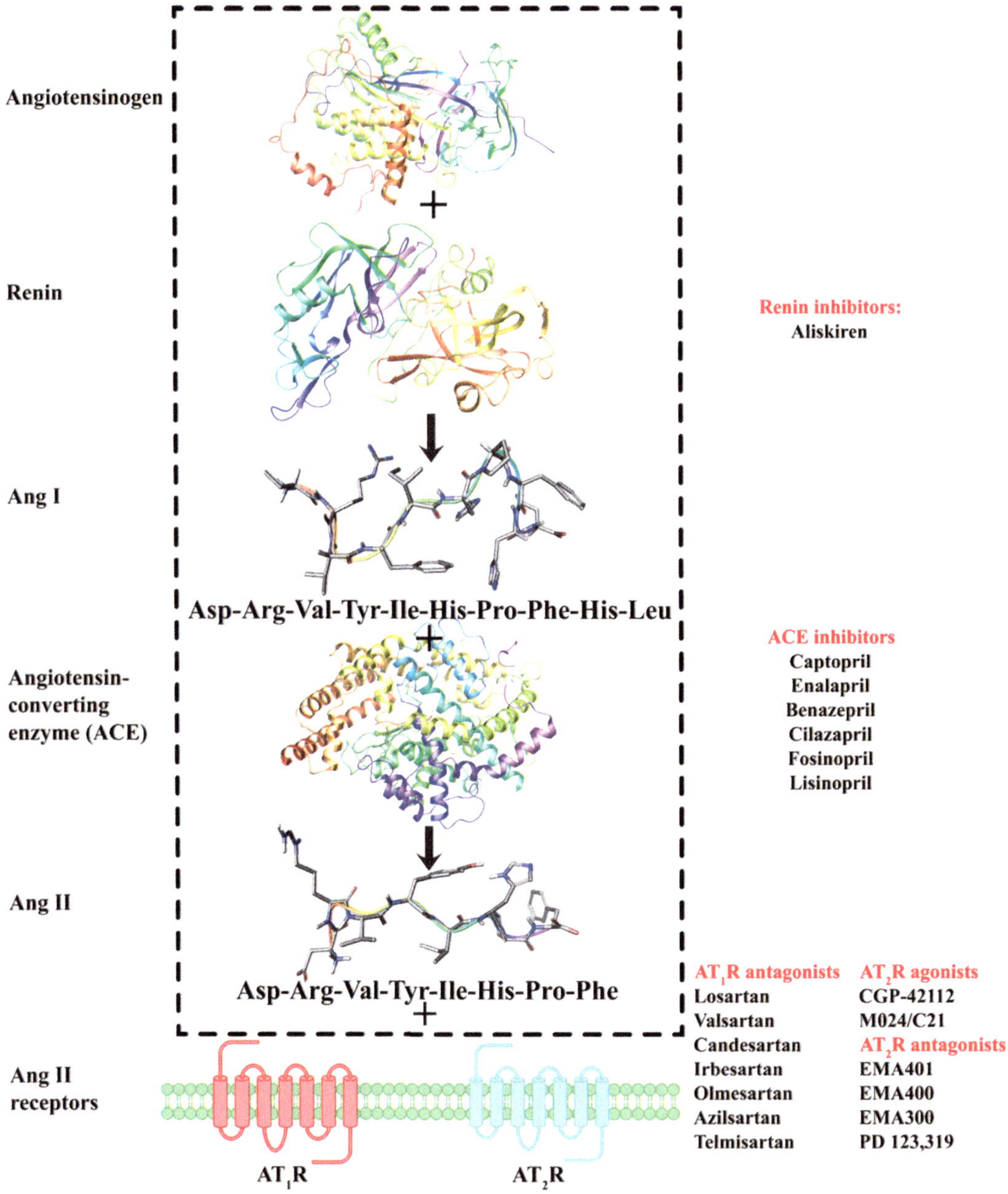

Fig. 2 The RAS and representative drugs that interfere in it [Reproduced from the article by Kellici et al. published in *Molecules* under Creative Commons License 4.0 [6]]

real environment of AT1R. AT1R is incorporated in the lipid bilayer which may interfere in the binding of AT1R antagonists. Mutation of AT1R may break the communication of the lipid bilayer core and AT1R and thus affects significantly the binding of the AT1R. The absence of a real lipid bilayer environment in docking and MD calculations make these inaccurate to simulate the biological results.

An effort is under progress to increase the complexity of the study systems in order to examine whether we can reconcile the discrepancy between the experimental and in silico results.

2 Materials

1. Protein Preparation Wizard [11].
2. QM-polarized ligand docking [12].
3. Induced fit docking [13].
4. Prime [14].
5. Desmond [15].

3 Methods

3.1 Docking Procedure

All the procedures described are applied using the Schrodinger Suite 2015.2. With similar of course manipulations the procedure can be extended to other softwares.

1. The structures of olmesartan and olmesartan methyl ether are designed in Maestro. The crystal structure of olmesartan also can be used (CSD reference code: ZOGSOD [16]).
2. The crystal structures and two homology models of the AT1R are used for the docking procedure. The first model is kindly provided by Prof. T. Tuccinardi and is generated using the bovine rhodopsin crystal structure as template (PDB ID 1U19) [17]. The second model is kindly provided by Dr. M. Matsoukas [18, 19] and is based on the CXCR4 crystal structure with PDB ID 3ODU. Two co-crystallized structures are used [PDB IDs 4YAY (X-ray free-electron laser (XFEL) structure with resolution 2.9 Å) and 4ZUD (resolution 2.8 Å)] [1, 2].
3. The homology models are prepared using the Protein Preparation Wizard. The Protein Preparation Wizard panel has three tabs. In the "Import and Process tab" you can import a protein directly from the RCSB database or the workspace. The Review and Modify tab allows you to delete unwanted chains and waters and fix or delete het groups. In the Refine tab you can optimize orientations of hydrogen-bonded groups and minimize the structure. GPCRs are ionized at a pH of 7.4 using PROPKA [20] and are minimized using the OPLS3 force field [21].
4. Receptor grids for the homology models are generated centroid of the residues Tyr113, Lys199, Tyr253, and His256. The receptor grid for the crystal structure 4YAY is generated

centroid to the co-crystallized ligand ZD7155 while for the crystal structure 4ZUD is generated centroid of olmesartan.

5. The four important mutations according to Miura et al. [7], for each 3D structure of the protein (Y113F, K199Q, H256A, and Q257A) are generated using the "Residue and Loop mutation" panel that can be opened from the Tasks menu in BioLuminate 1.9 [22]. In our case we need to mutate a single residue to a standard amino acid. In order to do so, (a) select "Single mutation" in the Type section, (b) select the residue to be altered either in the Workspace or in the panel's sequence viewer, (c) click Workspace Selection, d) choose the amino acid from the option menu in the Mutated to section, and click Mutate.
6. Refine the mutated structure, by clicking Advanced Refinement Options, and make selections in the Refinement Options dialog box. All residues within 5 Å of the mutation are minimized.
7. Firstly, Schrodinger's docking algorithm Glide is used to predict the binding geometries for the ligand-receptor complexes. The docking calculations are performed with GlideXP (extra precision mode) [23, 24] using standard van der Waals scaling of 0.8.
8. All the resulting poses of olmesartan inside the receptor are used as starting conformations for the QM-polarized ligand docking (QPLD) approach [12]. In this workflow, accurate quantum mechanical charges are generated from the electrostatic potential energy surface of the ligand using the density functional theory (DFT). The level and type chosen of quantum mechanical treatment in the QM charge tab were the B3LYP/6-31G* basis set and the ultrafine SCF accuracy level within the Jaguar module.
9. In the "Redocking" tab ligands are redocked using GlideXP. Afterward the energy parameter by which the final poses are scored in the Final selection tab is selected. The final selection chosen is based on the Emodel score. Since Emodel combines the GlideScore and the internal energy of the ligand conformation, it is a more suitable score to rank the best poses of the same ligand.
10. The five QPLD conformers with best Emodel scores are submitted as starting geometries for the induced fit docking calculations [13, 25]. At the initial stage of docking, side chains of residues within 5 Å of the ligand were trimmed.
11. Three residues that are within 5 Å of the ligand and have the highest B-factors (above 40) are refined using Prime [13].

12. All IFD calculations are run using the implicit membrane option. This is selected in the "Prime refinement" tab. When the user presses the "Set up" button, it sets the membrane to the helices. The implicit membrane is a low-dielectric slab-shaped region, which is treated in the same way as the high-dielectric implicit solvent region. Hydrophobic groups, which normally pay a solvation penalty for creating their hydrophobic pocket in the high-dielectric region, do not pay the same penalty while are in the membrane slab. Conversely, hydrophilic groups lose any short-ranged solvation energy from the high-dielectric region when moving into the low-dielectric region. The implicit membrane model is intended for use with proteins that span the membrane and as such is ideal for GPCRs.
13. The ligands are redocked using the extra precision mode in the "Glide Redocking" tab.
14. The RMSD between the docked structure of olmesartan in the crystal structure 4YAY and the crystallized structure of olmesartan in the AT1R receptor (PDB ID 4ZUD) is found to be 0.3 Å. This pinpoints that the crystal structure 4YAY produces reliable poses and that the selected virtual workflow is suitable.

The results of these computations are given in Fig. 3.

3.2 Molecular Dynamics Simulations

The poses in the two crystal structures with best induced fit score are subjected to molecular dynamics simulations using Desmond 4.2 [15].

1. The receptor is immersed in the DPPC bilayer (*see* **Note 1**). The SPC solvent model is used with an orthorhombic box shape. The OPLS3 force field is used during the building of the system [21].
2. The system is minimized using steepest descent for 2500 maximum iterations until a gradient threshold of 25 kcal mol^{-1} $Å^{-1}$ is reached.
3. The simulation time for the molecular dynamics is set at 300 ns in the NPT ensemble class.
4. The temperature and the pressure are set at 325 K and 1.01325 bar correspondingly. The RESPA integrator is used with a time step of 2.0 fs [26]. The thermostat method used is the Nose-Hoover chain [27], while the Martyna-Tobias-Klein method was used as barostat [28].
5. The cutoff radius is set at 9.0 Å.

The interactions of olmesartan and its methylated analogue during the simulations are shown in Fig. 4.

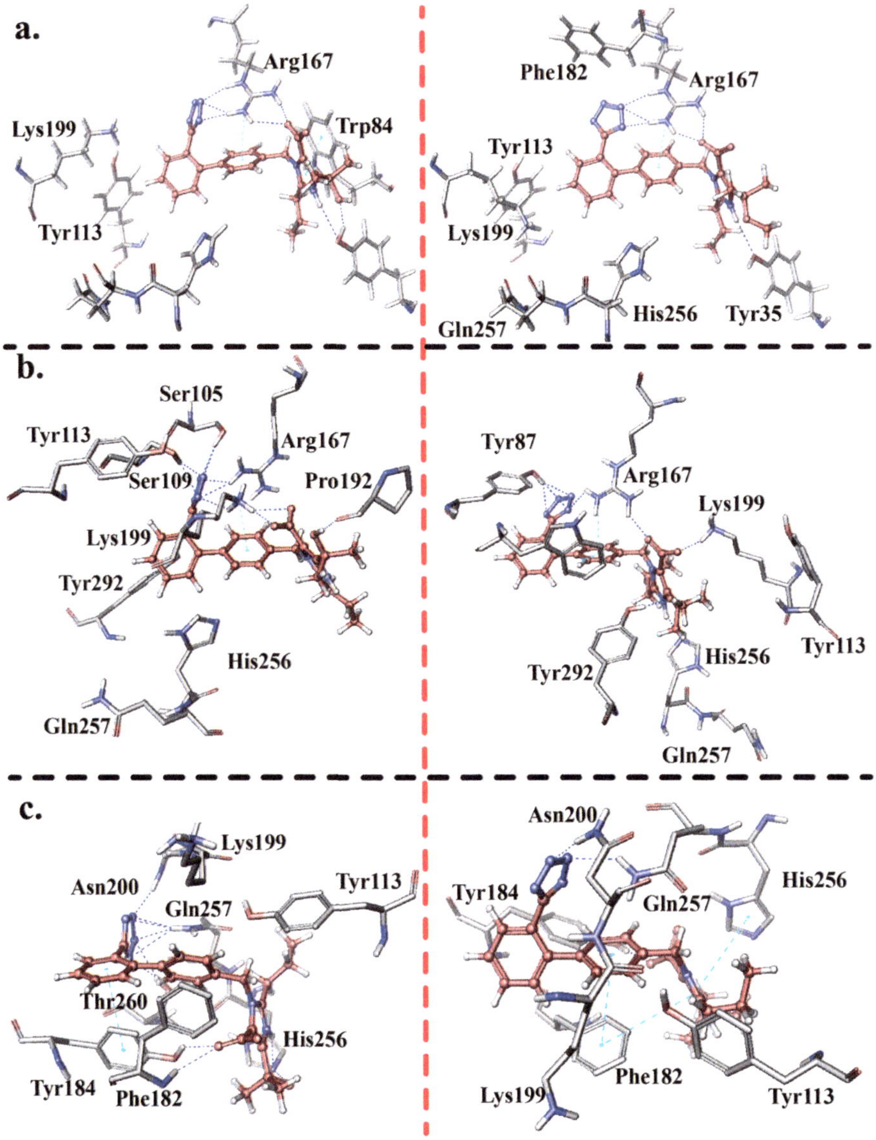

Fig. 3 Most energetically favorable poses of olmesartan (left) and olmesartan methyl ether (right) in the AT1R after applying induced fit docking in the (**a**) crystal structure (PDB ID 4YAY), (**b**) CXCR4 homology model, (**c**) rhodopsin homology. Blue lines represent hydrogen bonds; cyan lines represent π-cation interactions [Reproduced from the article by Kellici et al. published in the *Arabian Journal of Chemistry* under Creative Commons License 4.0 [10]]

3.3 MM-GBSA Calculations

The MM-GBSA calculations were performed using Prime.

1. The DPPC molecules are removed from the trajectories using the delete_atoms.py utility (*see* **Note 2**) and by running the command line

   $SCHRODINGER/run delete_atoms.py -h

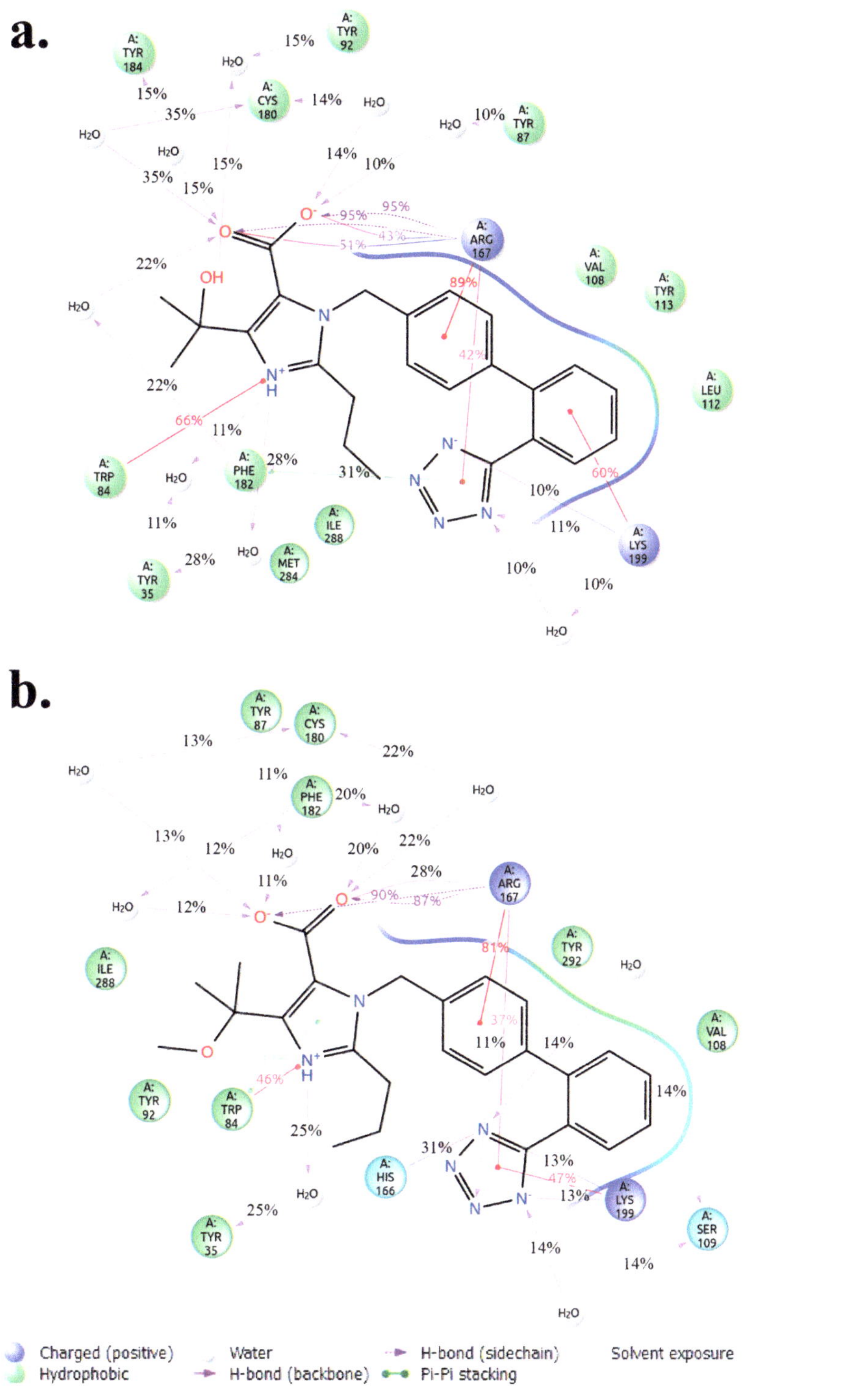

Fig. 4 Protein-ligand interactions during the whole time of simulation for (**a**) olmesartan and (**b**) olmesartan methyl ether [Reproduced from the article by Kellici et al. published in the *Arabian Journal of Chemistry* under Creative Commons License 4.0 [10]]

to see the usage and options for the script. The following command deletes the DPPC molecules from the system:

$SCHRODINGER/run delete_atoms.py -asl "res. DPPC" infile outfile

where infile is your trajectory file and outfile is the name you give the new trajectory file.

2. The binding energy is calculated for a total of 4151 frames of the MD trajectory starting from the 100th ns until the end of the trajectory at the 300th ns using the thermal_mmgbsa.py script. This script takes in a Desmond MD trajectory, splits it into individual frame snapshots, and runs each one through MM-GBSA (after deleting waters and separating the ligand from the receptor).
3. The binding free energy was calculated by the following equation:

$$\Delta G_{\mathrm{Bind}} = \Delta E_{\mathrm{MM}} + \Delta G_{\mathrm{Solv}} + \Delta G_{\mathrm{SA}}$$

where ΔE_{MM} is the difference in the minimized energies between the protein-ligand complexes, ΔG_{Solv} is the difference in the GBSA solvation energy of the protein-ligand complex and sum of the solvation energies for the protein and ligand, and ΔG_{SA} is the difference in the surface area energies for the complex and sum of the surface area energies in the protein and ligand. The contributions to the total energy from different components are also reported in the final output. These components may differ from mutation to mutation (*see* **Notes 3** and **4**).

4 Notes

1. The following reasons favor the use of DPPC bilayers exclusively in this computational study: (a) DPPC's partition coefficient with respect to its aqueous environment, especially in the fluid state, resembles that of natural plasma membranes of the vasculature [29, 30]; (b) Phosphatidylcholines (PCs) are the most abundant lipid species in the plasma membranes of the vascular smooth muscle cells [30] and sarcolemma cardiac membranes [29].
2. The DPPC molecules are not removed automatically from the trajectory by using the thermal_mmgbsa.py script. As a result the delete_atoms.py script must be run first.
3. The Coulomb term especially may differ from mutation to mutation since a mix of charged and neutral residues are added, so fluctuations in this term are not surprising.

4. MD followed by the thermal_mmgbsa,py script is probably not the most exact way of addressing the problem. This approach is missing some reference terms with respect to the unfolded state so it is not scientifically complete. A more exact approach but computationally demanding would be residue scanning or FEP protein mutation.

Acknowledgment

T.K. is extremely grateful to Prof. Thomas Mavromoustakos for his supporting and funding.

References

1. Zhang H, Unal H, Gati C et al (2015) Structure of the angiotensin receptor revealed by serial femtosecond crystallography. Cell 161 (4):833–844. https://doi.org/10.1016/j.cell.2015.04.011
2. Zhang H, Unal H, Desnoyer R et al (2015) Structural basis for ligand recognition and functional selectivity at angiotensin receptor. J Biol Chem 290(49):29127–29139. https://doi.org/10.1074/jbc.M115.689000
3. Rataj K, Witek J, Mordalski S et al (2014) Impact of template choice on homology model efficiency in virtual screening. J Chem Inf Model 54(6):1661–1668. https://doi.org/10.1021/ci500001f
4. Xiang J, Chun E, Liu C et al (2016) Successful strategies to determine high-resolution structures of GPCRs. Trends Pharmacol Sci 37 (12):1055–1069. https://doi.org/10.1016/j.tips.2016.09.009
5. Kellici TF, Ntountaniotis D, Kritsi E et al (2016) Leveraging NMR and X-ray data of the free ligands to build better drugs targeting angiotensin II type 1 G-protein coupled receptor. Curr Med Chem 23(1):36–59. https://doi.org/10.2174/0929867323666151117122116
6. Kellici TF, Tzakos AG, Mavromoustakos T (2015) Rational drug design and synthesis of molecules targeting the angiotensin II type 1 and type 2 receptors. Molecules 20 (3):3868–3897. https://doi.org/10.3390/molecules20033868
7. Miura SI, Fujino M, Hanzawa H et al (2006) Molecular mechanism underlying inverse agonist of angiotensin II type 1 receptor. J Biol Chem 281(28):19288–19295. https://doi.org/10.1074/jbc.M602144200
8. Miura S, Nakao N, Hanzawa H et al (2013) Reassessment of the unique mode of binding between angiotensin II type 1 receptor and their blockers. PLoS One 8(11):e79914. https://doi.org/10.1371/journal.pone.0079914
9. Miura S, Kiya Y, Hanzawa H et al (2012) Small molecules with similar structures exhibit agonist, neutral antagonist or inverse agonist activity toward angiotensin II type 1 receptor. PLoS One 7(6):e37974. https://doi.org/10.1371/journal.pone.0037974
10. Kellici TF, Ntountaniotis D, Liapakis G et al (2016) The dynamic properties of angiotensin II type 1 receptor inverse agonists in solution and in the receptor site. Arab J Chem. https://doi.org/10.1016/j.arabjc.2016.11.014
11. Madhavi Sastry G, Adzhigirey M, Day T et al (2013) Protein and ligand preparation: parameters, protocols, and influence on virtual screening enrichments. J Comput Aided Mol Des 27(3):221–234. https://doi.org/10.1007/s10822-013-9644-8
12. Small-Molecule Drug Discovery Suite 2015–2 (2015) Schrödinger Suite 2015-2-QM-Polarized Ligand Docking protocol; Glide version 6.7, Schrödinger, LLC, New York, NY, 2015; Jaguar version 8.8, Schrödinger, LLC, New York, NY, 2015; QSite version 6.7, Schrödinger, LLC, New York, NY
13. Small-Molecule Drug Discovery Suite 2015–2 (2015) Schrödinger Suite 2015-2 Induced Fit Docking protocol; Glide version 6.7, Schrödinger, LLC, New York, NY, 2015; Prime version 4.0, Schrödinger, LLC, New York, NY
14. Jacobson MP, Pincus DL, Rapp CS et al (2004) A hierarchical approach to all-atom protein

loop prediction. Proteins 55(2):351–367. https://doi.org/10.1002/prot.10613
15. Schrödinger Release 2015–2 (2015) Desmond Molecular Dynamics System, version 4.2, D. E. Shaw Research, New York, NY, 2015. Maestro-Desmond Interoperability Tools, version 4.2, Schrödinger, New York, NY
16. Yanagisawa H, Amemiya Y, Kanazaki T et al (1996) Nonpeptide angiotensin II receptor antagonists: synthesis, biological activities, and structure - activity relationships of imidazole-5-carboxylic acids bearing alkyl, alkenyl, and hydroxyalkyl substituents at the 4-position and their related compounds. J Med Chem 39(1):323–338
17. Tuccinardi T, Calderone V, Rapposelli S et al (2006) Proposal of a new binding orientation for non-peptide AT1 antagonists: homology modeling, docking and three-dimensional quantitative structure-activity relationship analysis. J Med Chem 49(14):4305–4316. https://doi.org/10.1021/jm060338p
18. Matsoukas MT, Cordomi A, Rios S et al (2013) Ligand binding determinants for angiotensin II type 1 receptor from computer simulations. J Chem Inf Model 53(11):2874–2883. https://doi.org/10.1021/ci400400m
19. Matsoukas MT, Potamitis C, Plotas P et al (2013) Insights into AT1 receptor activation through AngII binding studies. J Chem Inf Model 53(11):2798–2811. https://doi.org/10.1021/ci4003014
20. Olsson MHM, Søndergaard CR, Rostkowski M et al (2011) PROPKA3: consistent treatment of internal and surface residues in empirical p K a predictions. J Chem Theory Comput 7(2):525–537. https://doi.org/10.1021/ct100578z
21. Harder E, Damm W, Maple J et al (2016) OPLS3: a force field providing broad coverage of drug-like small molecules and proteins. J Chem Theory Comput 12(1):281–296. https://doi.org/10.1021/acs.jctc.5b00864
22. Zhu K, Day T, Warshaviak D et al (2014) Antibody structure determination using a combination of homology modeling, energy-based refinement, and loop prediction. Proteins 82 (8):1646–1655. https://doi.org/10.1002/prot.24551
23. Small-Molecule Drug Discovery Suite 2015–2 (2015) Glide, version 6.7, Schrödinger, LLC, New York, NY
24. Friesner RA, Murphy RB, Repasky MP et al (2006) Extra precision glide: docking and scoring incorporating a model of hydrophobic enclosure for protein-ligand complexes. J Med Chem 49(21):6177–6196. https://doi.org/10.1021/jm051256o
25. Sherman W, Day T, Jacobson MP et al (2006) Novel procedure for modeling ligand/receptor induced fit effects. J Med Chem 49 (2):534–553. https://doi.org/10.1021/jm050540c
26. Tuckerman M, Berne BJ, Martyna GJ (1992) Reversible multiple time scale molecular dynamics. J Chem Phys 97(3):1990–2001
27. Martyna GJ, Klein ML, Tuckerman M (1992) Nosé-hoover chains: the canonical ensemble via continuous dynamics. J Chem Phys 97 (4):2635–2643
28. Martyna GJ, Tobias DJ, Klein ML (1994) Constant pressure molecular dynamics algorithms. J Chem Phys 101(5):4177–4189
29. Netticadan TJ, Ashavaid TF, Nair KG (1997) Characterisation of the canine cardiac sarcolemma in experimental myocardial ischemia. Indian J Clin Biochem 12(1):49–54. https://doi.org/10.1007/bf02867955
30. Oliveira TR, Lamy MT, De Paula UM et al (2009) Structural properties of lipid reconstructs and lipid composition of normotensive and hypertensive rat vascular smooth muscle cell membranes. Braz J Med Biol Res 42 (9):844–853

INDEX

Thomas Mavromoustakos and Tahsin F. Kellici (eds.), *Rational Drug Design: Methods and Protocosl*, Methods in Molecular Biology, vol. 1824, https://doi.org/10.1007/978-1-4939-8630-9, © Springer Science+Business Media, LLC, part of Springer Nature 2018

P

Q

R

S

T

U

V

W

X

Z

Printed by Printforce, the Netherlands